McGraw-Hill Education Specialty Board Review
Neonatal-Perinatal Medicine

McGraw-Hill Education Specialty Board Review
Neonatal-Perinatal Medicine

Ira Adams-Chapman, MD

Associate Professor of Pediatrics
Director, Developmental Progress Clinic
Emory University School of Medicine
Atlanta, Georgia

David P. Carlton, MD

Emory University
Department of Pediatrics
Atlanta, Georgia

James Moore, MD, PhD

Division Chief for Neonatal-Perinatal Medicine
University of Connecticut School of Medicine
Medical Director, NICU
Connecticut Children's Medical Center
Hartford, Connecticut

New York Chicago San Francisco Athens London Madrid
Mexico City Milan New Delhi Singapore Sydney Toronto

McGraw-Hill Education Specialty Board Review: Neonatal-Perinatal Medicine

1 2 3 4 5 6 7 8 9 0   RMN/RMN   19 18 17 16 15

ISBN 978-0-07-176794-1
MHID 0-07-176794-0

This book was set in Minion Pro by Aptara, Inc.
The editors were Andrew Moyer and Brian Kearns.
The production supervisor was Catherine Saggese.
Project management was provided by Nomeeta Devi, Aptara, Inc.
RR Donnelley was printer and binder.

This book is printed on acid-free paper.

Library of Congress Cataloging-in-Publication Data

Neonatal-perinatal medicine (Moore)
    Neonatal-perinatal medicine / [edited by] James Moore, David P. Carlton,
Ira Adams-Chapman.
        p. ; cm. —   (McGraw-Hill Education specialty board review)
    Includes bibliographical references.
    ISBN 978-0-07-176794-1 (pbk. : alk. paper)
    I. Moore, James (Neonatologist), editor. II. Carlton, David P., editor.
III. Adams-Chapman, Ira, editor. IV. Title. V. Series: McGraw-Hill specialty
board review.
    [DNLM: 1.   Fetal Diseases—Examination Questions. 2.   Infant, Newborn,
Diseases—Examination Questions. 3.   Perinatal Care—Examination Questions.
4.   Pregnancy Complications—Examination Questions. Fetal Diseases / WQ 18.2]
    RG628
    618.3'2075—dc23
                                                              2015033658

McGraw-Hill Education books are available at special quantity discounts to use as premiums
and sales promotions or for use in corporate training programs. To contact a representative,
please visit the Contact Us pages at www.mhprofessional.com.

This book is dedicated to the dedicated healthcare teams and parents who care for medically fragile newborns around the globe. Each of you enhances the care of a child—one patient at a time. We would also like to thank each of the authors who have contributed to this project.

We would like to thank Vicki Williams of Emory University for administrative support to compile this project.

CONTENTS

CONTRIBUTORS

Margaret L.P. Adam, MD
Professor of Pediatrics
Clinical Genetics
University of Washington School of Medicine
Seattle, Washington

Ira Adams-Chapman, MD
Associate Professor of Pediatrics
Director, Developmental Progress Clinic
Emory University School of Medicine
Atlanta, Georgia

Donald L. Batisky, MD
Professor of Pediatrics
Emory University School of Medicine
Director, Pediatric Hypertension Program
Children's Healthcare of Atlanta
Atlanta, Georgia

Christel Biltoft, MD
Instructor
Department of Pediatrics
Emory University School of Medicine
Atlanta, Georgia

Jose Nilo G. Binongo
Associate Research Professor
Department of Biostatistics & Bioinformatics
Rollins School of Public Health
Emory University
Atlanta, Georgia

Michael Briones, DO
Assistant Professor of Pediatrics
Division of Pediatric Hematology and Oncology
Aflac Cancer and Blood Disorders Center
Emory University
Children's Healthcare of Atlanta
Atlanta, Georgia

William A. Carey, MD
Division of Neonatal Medicine
Mayo Clinic
Rochester, Minnesota

David P. Carlton, MD
Professor, Department of Pediatrics
Division Director, Neonatal-Perinatal
 Medicine
Emory University School of Medicine
Atlanta, Georgia

Jodi Chen, MD
Cardiac Intensivist
Fellowship Director - Cardiac Intensive Care
The Children's Hospital of Philadelphia
Assistant Professor of Anesthesia and Critical
 Care Medicine
Assistant Professor of Clinical Pediatrics
University of Pennsylvania School of Medicine
Philadelphia, Pennsylvania

Matthew S. Clifton, MD, FACS, FAAP
Assistant Professor of Surgery and Pediatrics
Emory University School of Medicine
Atlanta, Georgia

Patricia L. Denning, MD
Associate Professor of Pediatrics
NICU Medical Director and Chief of
 Pediatrics
Emory University Hospital Midtown
Emory University School of Medicine
Atlanta, Georgia

Swati V. Elchuri, MD
Assistant Professor of Pediatrics
Division of Pediatric Endocrinology
Emory University School of Medicine
Atlanta, Georgia

Jane E. Ellis, MD, PhD
Assistant Professor
Maternal-Fetal Medicine
Emory University School of Medicine
Medical Director, Emory Regional Perinatal
 Center
Grady Memorial Hospital
Atlanta, Georgia

Eric I. Felner, MD, MSCR
Associate Professor of Pediatrics
Division of Pediatric Endocrinology
Emory University School of Medicine
Atlanta, Georgia

Roshan George, MD
Assistant Professor of Pediatrics
Division of Nephrology
Emory University School of Medicine
Children's Healthcare of Atlanta
Atlanta, Georgia

Shannon E.G. Hamrick, MD
Associate Professor of Pediatrics
Divisions of Neonatology and
    Cardiology
Emory University School of Medicine
Atlanta, Georgia

Joseph A. Hilinski, MD
Associate Professor of Pediatrics
Division of Pediatric Infectious Diseases
Emory University School of Medicine
Atlanta, Georgia

Sarah J. Hill, MD
Fellow Pediatric Surgery
Department of Surgery
Emory University
Atlanta, Georgia

Vijaya Kancherla, PhD
Instructor
Department of Epidemiology
Emory University Rollins
School of Public Health
Atlanta, Georgia

Heidi E.G. Karpen, MD
Assistant Professor of Pediatrics
Neonatal-Perinatal Medicine
Emory University School of Medicine
Atlanta, Georgia

Howard Katzenstein, MD
Professor of Pediatrics
Vanderbilt University School of Medicine
Medical Director
Division of Pediatric Hematology/Oncology
Scott and Tracie Hamilton Chair in Cancer
    Survivorship
Nashville, Tennessee

Sarah Keene, MD
Assistant Professor of Pediatrics and
    Physiology
Neonatal-Perinatal Medicine
Emory University School of Medicine
Atlanta, Georgia

Michael R. Kramer, PhD
Assistant Professor of Epidemiology
Rollins School of Public Health
Emory University
Atlanta, Georgia

Leslie P. Lawley, MD
Assistant Professor of Pediatrics
Division Chief for Pediatric Dermatology
Emory University School of Medicine
Atlanta, Georgia

Nancy A. Louis, MD
Clinical Associate Professor of Pediatrics
Georgia Regents University
Georgia Neonatology, LLC
Athens Regional Medical Center
Atlanta, Georgia

James Moore, MD, PhD
Division Chief for Neonatal-Perinatal Medicine
University of Connecticut School of Medicine
Medical Director, NICU
Connecticut Children's Medical Center
Hartford, Connecticut

Ravi Mangal Patel, MD, MSc
Assistant Professor of Pediatrics
Neonatal-Perinatal Medicine
Emory University School of Medicine
Atlanta, Georgia

Zakiya Pressley Rice, MD
Assistant Professor of Dermatology and
    Pediatrics
Department of Dermatology
Emory University School of Medicine
Atlanta, Georgia

Jessica Roberts, MD
Assistant Professor of Pediatrics
Division of Neonatology
Department of Pediatrics
Emory University School of Medicine
Children's Healthcare of Atlanta
Atlanta, Georgia

Lakshmi Sukumaran, MD
Adjunct Assistant Professor of Pediatrics
Division of Infectious Diseases
Emory University School of Medicine
Atlanta, Georgia

Angela Sun, MD
Assistant Professor of Pediatircs
Division of Genetic Medicine
University of Washington School of Medicine
Seattle, Washington

Christina J. Valentine, MD, MS, RD, FAAP
Associate Professor
Department of Obstetrics and Gynecology
The University of Cincinnati
Medical Director
North American Mead Johnson Nutrition
Glenview, Illinois

Shilpa Vyas-Read, MD
Assistant Professor of Pediatrics
Division of Neonatal-Perinatal Medicine
Emory University School of Medicine
Atlanta, Georgia

Benjamin Watkins, MD
Pediatric Hematology/Oncology
Fellow Aflac Cancer and Blood Disorders
Emory University School of Medicine
Center Children's Healthcare of Atlanta
Atlanta, Georgia

Helen O. Williams, MD
Assistant Professor of Pediatrics
Neonatal-Perinatal Medicine
Emory University School of Medicine
Atlanta, Georgia

Jumi Yi, MD
Assistant Professor of Pediatrics
Division of Infectious Diseases
Emory University School of Medicine
Atlanta, Georgia

PREFACE

This review book represents a comprehensive review of issues related to neonatology, including all of the major subspecialty areas. Clinical scenarios are presented to help the reader develop a differential diagnosis followed by a detailed description of the correct diagnosis including features that define or distinguish it from the other options presented. This interactive feedback approach mirrors the clinical decision making process. This review book is a guide to those interested in learning more about newborn care for the purpose of a clinical neonatology rotations, general knowledge, and review for neonatology board exam preparation. A unique feature about neonatology as a specialty area is that evidence-based practice guidelines are constantly changing. This text reflects contemporary care at the time of publication and specific references are provided for current practice guidelines as applicable. Highlighted throughout the text are clinical pearls and interesting facts for the reader to augment your learning.

The experience and expertise from each of the contributing authors become readily apparent very quickly as you move through the text. Through the efforts of this group of clinician educators and researchers we have compiled a review book which addresses clinical issues in neonatology within a framework that is evidence based and thorough.

Chapter 1
MATERNAL–FETAL MEDICINE

Jane E. Ellis, MD, PhD

CASE 1

Ms. K, a 33-year-old Hispanic female, presents for her new OB visit at 19 weeks. She is obese but reports no other medical problems. Review of her obstetrical history reveals her previous pregnancy resulted in vaginal delivery of a 4,510-g female complicated by a mild shoulder dystocia.

What screening test SHOULD be offered to this patient?
A. Group B streptococcus (GBS) screening
B. Rapid glucose screen (RGS)
C. Amniocentesis
D. Human papillomavirus (HPV) screening

Discussion

The correct answer is **B**. This patient should be offered a RGS for gestational diabetes mellitus (GDM). About 6% to 8% of pregnancies in the United States are affected by diabetes and of this number about 85% have gestational diabetes. GDM is defined as impaired glucose tolerance identified during the pregnant state, and this impairment makes it difficult for a pregnant woman to compensate for insulin resistance caused by hormonal and inflammatory changes occurring during gestation.[1] Risk factors for GDM include ethnicity, obesity, GDM in a prior pregnancy, previous macrosomic baby, any previous laboratory evidence of DM such as an elevated fasting glucose, or previous unexplained stillbirth. GBS is a significant cause of neonatal morbidity and mortality; screening via vaginal/rectal swab is usually offered at 35 to 37 weeks. Amniocentesis is not indicated at this initial visit but could be offered if a maternal serum screen is obtained and is abnormal. Routine screening for HPV is not recommended.

When SHOULD the RGS be offered for this particular patient?
A. At the current visit
B. At a follow-up visit in 2 weeks after an overnight fast
C. At 24 to 28 weeks
D. At 30 to 34 weeks after an overnight fast

Discussion

The correct answer is **A**. Because of her risk factors, this patient should be offered screening at this visit. The RGS consists of a 50-g oral glucose load followed by a venous blood draw 1 hour later to assess maternal blood glucose level. Although the test is most sensitive between 24 and 28 weeks, it can be performed at any gestational age. If Ms. K's test is abnormal (BG >130–140 mg/dL), identification and treatment of the diabetic state early in pregnancy may improve maternal and fetal outcomes. If her 1-hour blood glucose is not elevated, then rescreening should be offered at the standard 24 to 28 weeks. Although fasting may improve the accuracy of the RGS result, fasting is not required and most patients receive their RGS in the nonfasting state.

What is the follow-up recommended for an abnormal RGS?
A. Initiation of oral medication or insulin
B. Initiation of nutritional counseling and glucose monitoring
C. Referral to an endocrinologist for evaluation
D. Follow-up is determined by the value of the RGS

Discussion

The answer is D. If the RGS value is >130 to 140 mg/dL but <200 mg/dL, a 3-hour oral glucose tolerance test (OGTT) is recommended. This test consists of the patient consuming her usual unrestricted diet followed by an overnight fast. A fasting blood glucose level is obtained and a 100-g oral glucose load is then provided. Blood glucose levels are drawn at 1, 2, and 3 hours following the glucose load. If two of the four values obtained from this test are abnormal, the diagnosis of GDM is made and the patient is initially offered nutritional counseling and attempt at management by dietary means and four times per day blood glucose monitoring. If the blood glucose level from the RGS is ≥200 mg/dL, the pregnant woman is considered to have GDM and no 3-hour OGTT is offered. She should receive nutritional counseling, check and record her blood glucose levels each morning upon rising and following each meal, and attempt to control her BG levels via dietary means. If diet alone does not result in blood glucose values <90 mg/dL in the fasting state and <120 mg/dL 2 hours after each meal, then an oral hypoglycemic medication such as glyburide or metformin or subcutaneous insulin may be considered.

Which of the following fetal/neonatal outcomes MAY result from poorly controlled maternal GDM?
A. Large for gestational age fetuses
B. Hyperbilirubinemia
C. Hypoglycemia
D. Structural anomalies of the cardiac or central nervous system
E. All of the above

Discussion

The correct answer is **E**. Adverse pregnancy outcomes often associated with poorly controlled GDM include increased birth weight, increased risk of shoulder dystocia with resulting maternal or neonatal injury, increased likelihood of c-section, neonatal laboratory abnormalities and, if poorly controlled as indicated by a markedly elevated hemoglobin A1C in the first trimester, structural anomalies. Although it is somewhat controversial as to whether treatment of GDM improves pregnancy outcomes, most authorities and professional organizations agree that GDM should be treated. Treatment of GDM may lead to improved pregnancy outcomes and reduce a woman's risk of type II diabetes in later life.

Helpful Hint: The incidence of gestational diabetes appears to be increasing, coincident with and most likely related to the increasing incidence of obesity in pregnancy. Screening should be offered to all pregnant women between 24 and 28 weeks or earlier if risk factors for GDM are present. There are different screening strategies for GDM. The one most often used in the United States is a 1-hour 50-g glucose load followed by a 3-hour OGTT if the 1-hour test is abnormal. An alternative to this two-step method for screening and diagnosis of

gestational diabetes involves a 75-g 2-hour glucose tolerance test. This approach is common in Europe and is used by some providers in the United States. Some obstetricians use the White Classification scale to help counsel pregnant diabetic patients about pregnancy outcome.[2] This scale describes gestational diabetics as having A1 (diet controlled only) or A2 (medication required) diabetes. Classes B, C, D, F, R, H, and T are determined by the age of onset, the duration of diabetes in years, and the vascular disease present or organ system involved. The organ system involved and the degree of impairment in that system may have a significant impact on pregnancy outcomes. Classes B to T are typically managed with diet and insulin therapy. Although this classification system is still used by some providers, the American College of Obstetricians and Gynecologists no longer uses this system. This group places the emphasis on whether diabetes was present prior to pregnancy or is diagnosed during pregnancy.

Objectives

1. Know effects on fetus associated with maternal diabetes
2. Know recommendations for screening and risk factors for gestational diabetes
3. Know classification scale for diabetes associated with pregnancy and how it impacts management
4. Understand delivery-related complications in pregnancy affected by maternal diabetes

CASE 2

Ms. G presents for an initial prenatal care visit for her first pregnancy. She notes significant nausea and vomiting previously but states this has improved. She reports that she has been using an injectable form of birth control and her periods are irregular. She is unsure of her last normal menstrual period (LMP) but thinks it was 19 weeks prior to this visit. Bimanual examination suggests a fundal height (FH) of 15 cm but she is slightly obese so this measurement may not be accurate. Fetal heart tones at 120 bpm were verified by Doppler.

What is the next test or procedure that SHOULD be considered?
A. Maternal serum screening for aneuploidy
B. Obstetric ultrasound for dating
C. 3-hour OGTT
D. Maternal thyroid panel

Discussion

The correct answer is **B**. Ultrasound dating has consistently been shown to be more accurate than LMP or FH in correctly dating a pregnancy.[3] Maternal serum screening should be deferred until the pregnancy is dated since correct dating is essential for accurate interpretation of screening results. She has not had a screening test such as a RGS for diabetes, so the diagnostic 3-hour OGTT is not indicated. Nausea and vomiting are common in early pregnancy and typically resolve by 18 to 20 weeks. Although nausea and vomiting can be associated with maternal thyroid disorders the patient's symptoms have improved making thyroid disease less likely. Maternal thyroid panels are not routinely recommended unless there is a history of thyroid dysfunction. Obstetric ultrasound for dating should be obtained as the next step since optimal management of a pregnancy will depend on the best estimate of gestational age. Accurate estimation of gestational age determines if maternal serum screening is an option and if first- or second-trimester screening should be offered. Three methods to estimate gestational age include the menstrual history, determination of FH, and ultrasonography. Reliance on menstrual history or FH often results in inaccurate dating.[3] Many women are unsure of the first day of their last normal period, and dating based on FH is subject to error due to maternal body habitus, uterine fibroids, multiple gestation, full maternal bladder, and examiner error. The majority of pregnant women will have at least one ultrasound assessment during their pregnancies and dating is often established by this examination.

Helpful Hint: On a first-trimester ultrasound, the most accurate measurement to estimate gestational age is the crown-rump length.[3] The crown-rump length will accurately date a pregnancy to within 3 to 5 days. First-trimester dating by ultrasound is generally considered to provide the best dating for a pregnancy. In the second and third trimesters fetal femur length is the most commonly used single measurement. A combination of biparietal diameter, abdominal circumference, and femur length are typically obtained to provide accurate second- and third-trimester dating.[3] In addition to providing information on gestational age, ultrasound allows assessment of fetal number, fetal viability, and placental location. Fetal anatomy is assessed between 18 and 22 weeks.

The patient has an ultrasound performed and it is determined that she is 16.4 weeks pregnant. Although the fetal anatomy could not be completely evaluated, no obvious abnormalities were noted. A second semester serum screen (quad screen) is obtained and this screen is negative. This patient is not of advanced maternal age and she has no significant medical, surgical, or family history.

What type of ultrasound examination SHOULD be ordered for this patient at her next visit in 4 weeks?
A. No follow-up scan is indicated
B. Limited ultrasound
C. Standard examination
D. Specialized or high-risk scan

Discussion

The answer is C. For this particular patient the standard examination is indicated. During this examination at 20 weeks, fetal number, fetal presentation, fetal heart rate, placental location, and amniotic fluid volume can be assessed. Also during this examination fetal anatomy can be evaluated and described as normal within the limitations of ultrasound or any abnormalities described and follow-up determined. Second- and third-trimester scans can be technically difficult due to fetal position, size or movement, maternal abdominal scars, maternal body habitus, or patient inability to tolerate the examination. If anatomy is not completely visualized follow-up examination should be considered to complete the anatomy and check fetal growth.

A limited ultrasound is an examination that does not entail an attempt to evaluate the fetal anatomy, but is one with a more limited focus. For example, a limited ultrasound might be ordered to check fetal presentation in an early labor patient, assess amniotic fluid volume, or confirm fetal cardiac activity.

A specialized or high-risk scan is usually performed when there is concern for possible fetal anomaly on the basis of patient history (advanced maternal age or previous child with an anomaly), abnormal maternal serum screening, or findings on a standard examination. Other specialized examinations which can be ordered as indicated include evaluation of fetal nuchal translucency in the first trimester, Doppler assessment of fetal or maternal blood vessels, examinations of the cervix, fetal echocardiography, and biophysical profiles. Specialized examinations should be performed by ultrasonographers or physicians with appropriate training and experience.

At 24 weeks' gestation the patient has an abnormal random glucose screen with gestational diabetes confirmed by a 3-hour OGTT. Nutritional counseling and dietary management are attempted and failed. At 30 weeks' gestation the patient is started on an oral hypoglycemic.

What ultrasound assessments, if any, SHOULD be recommended for this patient?
A. A nonstress test every 2 weeks and a fetal growth scan at 36 weeks
B. Biophysical profile twice weekly starting at 32 weeks and a growth scan every 3 to 4 weeks

C. An ultrasound-guided amniocentesis for fetal lung maturity at 39 weeks
D. A weekly nonstress test and a fetal growth scan every week

Discussion

The answer is B. For patients with chronic medical conditions such as hypertensive disorders, autoimmune disorders such as lupus, and pregestational diabetes or gestational diabetes requiring medication antepartum surveillance is recommended.[4] Various strategies for such surveillance exist and the best approach remains controversial. Many perinatal centers use biophysical profiles twice weekly and periodic growth scans for fetal surveillance. A biophysical profile involves assessment of five components: fetal tone, fetal movement, fetal breathing, amniotic fluid pocket of 2 cm or greater, and a reactive nonstress test. Each component is scored as a 0 (absent) or 2 (present). A score of 8/10 or 10/10 is reassuring and significant fetal morbidity or mortality is unlikely within the next 7 days, excluding unpredictable obstetric events such as cord accident. A score of 0, 2, or 4 out of 10 often results in immediate delivery due to concern of fetal well-being. If the score is 6/10, then delivery may be considered if the patient is term or maternal/fetal status is otherwise nonreassuring. If the fetus is preterm or has not yet received antenatal steroids for fetal lung maturity, then continuous fetal heart rate monitoring could be considered while antenatal steroids are being administered, followed by another BPP in 12 to 24 hours.[4] The other testing paradigms above do not have appropriate time intervals for accurate determination of fetal well-being. Amniocentesis for FLM would not typically be recommended for this patient since there is no indication for delivery and her dating should provide confidence of the patient's gestational age.

Helpful Hint: When delivery is considered, effort should be made to ensure that fetal lungs are mature prior to delivery. Amniocentesis is an invasive test that can confirm lung maturity. However, amniocentesis is not required if one of these criteria for confirming a term gestation is met:

• Ultrasound at <20 weeks supports a gestational age of 39 weeks or greater
• Fetal heart tones have been documented by Doppler ultrasound for 30 weeks or more
• It has been 36 weeks since a positive urine or serum pregnancy test was obtained

Objectives

1. Know the general guidelines for use of ultrasonography for the assessment of gestational age and fetal well-being
2. Understand the limitations of ultrasonography for dating
3. Know the various modalities available to assess fetal well-being including ultrasonography, biophysical profile, nonstress test, and contraction stress test
4. Know recommendations for monitoring fetal status in high-risk pregnancies

CASE 3

A 24-year-old nulliparous woman presents for her initial prenatal visit at 20 weeks' gestation. As you review her medical history she tells you she thinks she might have hypothyroidism. She was given an unknown medication which she stopped taking when she found out she was pregnant. In addition to her routine prenatal laboratories you order a thyroid panel, which includes thyroid-stimulating hormone (TSH), free thyroxine (T_4), thyroid-stimulating immunoglobulin, and T_4 index.

Which set of findings WOULD help confirm your suspicion of primary hypothyroidism?
A. Increased TSH and decreased free T_4
B. Decreased TSH and decreased thyroid-stimulating immunoglobulin levels
C. Increased TSH and decreased thyroid-stimulating immunoglobulin levels
D. Decreased TSH and increased free T_4

Discussion

The correct answer is **A**. The most important measurement is the TSH level, which will be increased in primary hypothyroidism.[5] Free T_4 will be decreased in all forms of hypothyroidism. In the management of a pregnant woman with hypothyroidism TSH and a free T_4 level are the most useful for diagnosis and management. The other components of the thyroid panel would not be useful for diagnosing and managing primary hypothyroidism but may useful in assessment of other forms of hypothyroidism.

The results of the patient's thyroid panel suggest that she has primary hypothyroidism.

Which medication SHOULD be prescribed for her?
A. Propylthiouracil (PTU) at a starting dose of 300 to 450 μg daily
B. Levothyroxine at a starting dose of 0.10 to 0.15 mg daily
C. Methimazole at a starting dose of 5 mg daily
D. No treatment is needed during pregnancy but should be deferred until the postpartum period

Discussion

The correct answer is **B**. PTU and methimazole are used in the treatment of hyperthyroidism. Levothyroxine is commonly used for T_4 replacement and the starting dose above is correct. TSH and free T_4 levels should be obtained every 4 weeks after treatment has started and medication adjusted to keep the TSH at the lower end of normal and free T_4 within normal limits. Primary hypothyroidism should be treated promptly and not delayed until the postpartum period.

Helpful Hint: Women with untreated hypothyroidism have a higher incidence of pregnancy complications, including miscarriage, preeclampsia, placental abruption, fetal growth restriction, prematurity, and stillbirth.[6] Early treatment has been demonstrated to improve outcomes. Some studies have suggested that children born to mothers with untreated primary hypothyroidism may have lower IQs.[7] Routine screening for hypothyroidism in pregnant women with no history of thyroid disease is not recommended.[8]

Objectives

1. Understand the management of thyroid abnormalities during pregnancy
2. Understand the relationship between abnormal thyroid function and pregnancy complications

CASE 4

A patient presents for care for her second pregnancy at 24 weeks' gestation having recently arrived from another country. She provided a picture from a dating ultrasound at 18 weeks. A review of prenatal laboratories you ordered reveals that her blood type is A−, antibody positive. She does not remember receiving any injections during the previous pregnancy or in the postpartum period.

What is the NEXT step in her management?
A. Perform ultrasound to confirm gestational age
B. Repeat the laboratory to ensure that the results are correct
C. Ask the laboratory to identify the antibody and provide titers
D. Administer anti-D immune globulin such as Rhogam®

Discussion

The correct answer is **C**. Since dating was by an 18-week ultrasound there is no need to confirm her gestational age.

Maternal type and screen could be repeated but most likely the same result would be obtained. Since antibodies are present, there would be no utility in administering Rhogam®, which is one of several types of anti-D immune globulins available. The laboratory should be contacted and asked to identify as well as provide titers for the antibody. Identity of the antibody and titer are key factors in assessing the possibility of alloimmunization. Maternal alloimmunization significantly affecting a fetus occurs when there is an immune response in the mother to a paternally derived red blood cell antigen inherited by the fetus which is foreign to the mother. Maternal immunoglobulin G antibodies will cross the placenta to bind to these antigens on fetal red blood cells and cause hemolysis.[9] Anti-D immune globulin acts to prevent sensitization although the mechanism by which it acts has not been clearly elucidated. Since it was introduced in 1968 and became widely available, there has been a significant decrease in the number of cases of Rh alloimmunization. It is typically administered at 28 weeks and repeated immediately postpartum in women known to be Rh negative with no antibodies. It may also be indicated in other situations that would potentially result in sensitization, such as following amniocentesis or trauma. Some women are alloimmunized despite prophylaxis. Unfortunately, Rh alloimmunization remains a cause of perinatal morbidity and mortality.[9]

The laboratory identifies the antibody as anti-D with a titer of 1:64.

Which of the following WOULD be a reasonable next step in the evaluation?
A. Ultrasound to evaluate the fetus for signs of compromise
B. Umbilical artery Dopplers
C. Biophysical profile in 2 weeks
D. Immediate delivery of the fetus

Discussion

The answer is **A**. Anti-D antibody is the most common antibody identified and is capable of causing severe fetal anemia. A titer of 1:16 or greater is significant and may result in substantial fetal morbidity. With titers of 1:64 this fetus is a risk for developing anemia. Ultrasound should be performed to determine if signs of hydrops are present, which suggests significant fetal anemia. Umbilical artery velocimetry is useful for fetal evaluation in the setting of intrauterine growth restriction. This fetus needs to be evaluated at least weekly; therefore, performing a biophysical profile in 2 weeks would be inappropriate. Based on the information provided, immediate delivery is not indicated.

Which of the following is NOT a procedure that could be employed to manage this patient during the remainder of her pregnancy?

A. Middle cerebral artery (MCA) Doppler velocimetry
B. Amniocentesis for ΔOD_{450}
C. Fetal blood sampling and intrauterine blood transfusion
D. Uterine artery (UA) Doppler velocimetry

Discussion

The answer is D. There are several procedures available to guide evaluation and treatment of fetal anemia in the setting of alloimmunization. Ultrasonography for the evaluation of fetal hydrops and determination of the peak systolic velocity of blood flow through the MCA are noninvasive means of assessment.[10] Fetal anemia is associated with increased blood flow to the fetal brain as evidenced by increased MCA blood flow and increased peak systolic velocity. Amniocentesis is an invasive test which is employed to withdraw amniotic fluid to allow for assessment of the degree of hemolysis and quantify the severity of fetal anemia by determination of amniotic fluid bilirubin levels. Fluid is analyzed via spectral analysis at a wavelength of 450 nm (ΔOD_{450}) to determine bilirubin levels. Severity of anemia is determined using either the Liley (Fig. 1-1),[11] or Queenan (Fig. 1-2),[12] curves. These curves plot ΔOD_{450} values levels against gestational age in weeks and are divided into zones of fetal risk, ranging from minimal risk to imminent death. If values obtained from amniocentesis fall into a zone on one of these curves suggesting impending fetal death, then fetal blood sampling via the umbilical cord is performed to obtain fetal hematocrit. If blood sampling confirms severe anemia then intrauterine blood transfusion can be considered. Amniocentesis can be performed serially, usually every 10 to 14 days. Delivery rather than transfusion would be considered if the fetus were near term. Doppler assessment of the UA is not usually employed to assess fetal anemia. UA Dopplers are sometimes used to assess uterine blood flow in pregnancies at high risk for the development of preeclampsia.

Helpful Hint: The Liley curve was published in 1961 after demonstration that the bilirubin content of amniotic fluid could be assessed by spectral analysis and provides an assessment of the presence and severity of hemolysis and thus fetal anemia. Analysis provides a value referred to as ΔOD_{450}, which is then plotted on the Liley curve as a function of gestational age (27–42 weeks). There are three zones on the graph which when the ΔOD_{450} value is plotted as a function of gestational

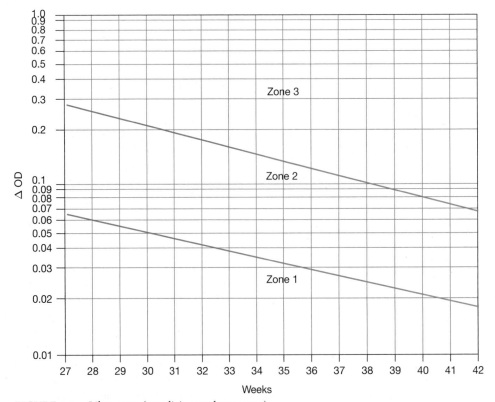

FIGURE 1-1.   Liley curve (emedicine.medscape.com).

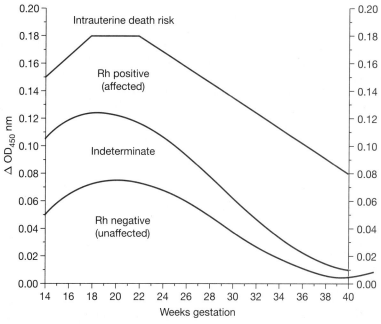

FIGURE 1-2.   Queenan curve (emedicine.medscape.com).

age reveals the fetal risk for anemia. If the value falls in Zone 1 then no anemia or mild anemia is likely. In Zone 2 moderate anemia is likely, while a value in Zone 3 indicates severe anemia and possible impending fetal demise. Use of the Liley curve allows pregnancies affected by alloimmunization to be managed by the degree of anticipated anemia. The Liley curve was later updated by Queenan to allow for the assessment of fetal anemia at earlier gestational ages (14–40 weeks).[12]

To employ the Liley or Queenan curves invasive amniocentesis must be performed. Assessment of the fetal MCA peak systolic velocity has been developed to avoid an invasive procedure and appears to be the most effective noninvasive technique for assessing fetal anemia. It is now widely employed for this purpose and has essentially replaced amniocentesis.[10] Normative tables exist of the peak systolic values at each gestational age. Values greater than 1.5 multiples of the median are predictive of moderate to severe fetal anemia. MCA Dopplers are usually obtained weekly beginning at 16 to 18 weeks' gestation and concluding at 35 weeks.

Objectives

1. Know the effects on the fetus with maternal alloimmunization
2. Know recommendations to assess fetal well-being in pregnancies complicated by alloimmunization
3. Understand management guidelines for pregnancies complicated by alloimmunization

CASE 5

A patient presents for a prenatal visit and growth scan at 30.4 weeks. On examination her fundal height (FH) is 25 cm. Pregnancy dating is by a 13-week ultrasound. Ultrasound is performed to assess fetal growth due to discrepancy between FH and known dates. The estimated gestational weight is 998 g, which is <10th percentile for gestational age. The biophysical profile (BPP) is 8/8.

Which SHOULD be considered next?
A. Dating ultrasound
B. Middle cerebral artery (MCA) Dopplers
C. Umbilical artery (UA) Dopplers
D. Delivery

Discussion

The correct answer is **C**. FH in centimeters should approximate gestational age in weeks.[13] When there is a discrepancy between FH and known gestational age, a growth scan should be considered. This fetus, with an estimated weight of <10th percentile for gestational age, has intrauterine growth restriction (IUGR). Inaccurate dating can lead to the diagnosis of IUGR, but in this case gestational age is accurate due to dating by an early scan. There is no need to perform a dating scan in this scenario. The BPP is reassuring and the amniotic fluid index is appropriate.

The recommended procedure along with today's growth scan and BPP is Doppler assessment of UA blood flow. Normal UA blood flow is characterized by high-velocity diastolic blood flow due to decreased resistance to UA blood flow secondary to the reservoir effect of the placenta. When IUGR exists, diastolic flow in the UA decreases due to increased resistance to blood flow within the placenta. This yields an increased systolic to diastolic (S/D) ratio. If the S/D ratio is elevated, the patient needs to be followed carefully. Absent or reversed end diastolic flow may follow, indicating that severe fetal compromise could be present. MCA Dopplers are typically used in assessment of fetal anemia and not IUGR. Delivery is not yet warranted in the face of reassuring testing.

A review of the measurements of fetal growth parameters reveals that all measurements are less than 10th percentile.

What type of IUGR is present?
A. Symmetric
B. Asymmetric
C. Discordant
D. Nondiscordant

Discussion

The correct answer is **A**. With all measurements of the fetal head, abdomen and extremities measuring <10th percentile symmetric IUGR is assumed to be present and accounts for up to 30% of cases of IUGR. Typical causes of symmetric IUGR include insults that occur early in pregnancy such as infection, exposure to certain medications, chromosomal abnormalities, and congenital malformations. When some fetal measurements are appropriate for gestational age and others are <10th percentile, asymmetric IUGR is present. This growth abnormality often occurs later in pregnancy and is thought to be due in part to placental insufficiency. Attempts should be made to determine the cause of IUGR since this may affect management. Discordant and nondiscordant are typically the terms used to describe patterns of growth based on estimated fetal weights in multiple gestations.

What techniques for antepartum fetal surveillance COULD be employed to follow this patient until delivery occurs?
A. Frequent growth scans
B. Biophysical profiles
C. Umbilical artery Dopplers
D. All of the above

Discussion

The correct answer is **D**. When IUGR is documented by ultrasound, fetal surveillance should be initiated. Close surveillance has been shown to improve fetal outcomes.[14]

A commonly used surveillance paradigm involves performing growth scans every 3 to 4 weeks, twice weekly biophysical profiles, and weekly umbilical artery Dopplers. If testing remains reassuring (normal BPPs and umbilical artery Dopplers) and there are no maternal indications, delivery would be recommended at 39 weeks. If there is evidence of maternal or fetal compromise, delivery may be indicated prior to 39 weeks, following administration of antenatal steroids to enhance fetal lung maturity.

Helpful Hint: Doppler ultrasonography has been shown to reduce the risk of perinatal death when IUGR is present.[14,15] Abnormalities on nonstress testing and biophysical profiles are usually late findings of fetal compromise. Doppler abnormalities such as an elevated S/D ratio, or absent or reversed end diastolic blood flow through the umbilical arteries are typically observed before significant fetal compromise, and early delivery may reduce morbidity and mortality. Doppler assessment of umbilical arteries may help differentiate a normal but small for gestational age fetus from one that is growth restricted. Fetuses with true growth restriction are more likely to have abnormal Doppler studies than are fetuses who are small for gestational age.[15]

Objectives

1. Define IUGR
2. Know recommendations for diagnostic evaluation of pregnancies affected by IUGR
3. Know recommendations for monitoring pregnancies affected by IUGR to ensure fetal well-being

CASE 6

A patient presents for a prenatal visit at 30 weeks. She informs you that she has a history of genital herpes and had multiple outbreaks prior to pregnancy. She states that she had an outbreak at about 16 weeks' gestation but none since that time.

What medication plan SHOULD be considered for this patient?
A. Valacyclovir starting now
B. Acyclovir starting at 36 weeks
C. Valacyclovir at the onset of labor
D. Acyclovir in the postpartum period

Discussion

The correct answer is **B**. Genital herpes simplex virus infection is a common sexually transmitted disease. As many as 50 million adolescent and adults in the United States are considered to have been infected.[16,17] It is estimated that the incidence of new infections during pregnancy is approximately 2% and approximately 75% of women with recurrent genital herpes will have an outbreak during pregnancy.[16,17] Neonatal herpes can occur, although it is more common following a primary maternal infection when antibodies may not be present. The usual route of neonatal infection involves exposure to the virus in the genital tract, although in utero and postnatal infections can occur. Up to 80% of infected infants are born to mothers with no history of HSV infection. Infected neonates may have disease involving only the skin, eyes, or mouth, but disease involving the central nervous system or disseminated disease can occur. Neonatal mortality from CNS disease is thought to be about 4%, while for disseminated disease it may be as high as 30%. The goal of maternal suppressive therapy is to prevent a recurrence of disease at the time of delivery. Several studies supported the practice of offering suppressive therapy at 36 weeks' gestation to prevent neonatal herpes.[18] The antiviral medications acyclovir, valacyclovir, and famciclovir are safe in pregnancy, but acyclovir is the most commonly used. For the patient mentioned above, she is currently asymptomatic at 30 weeks so there is no indication to start medication now. She should be offered suppressive therapy beginning at 36 weeks unless she experiences an outbreak prior to that time, which would require treatment. Treatment at the time of delivery or in the postpartum period would be needed if there is a recurrence during these time periods.

This patient presents to your Labor and Delivery 1 week later with an outbreak of genital herpes and upon presentation experiences preterm premature rupture of membranes.

Once she is admitted, what is the NEXT most appropriate management at this point?
A. Immediate delivery
B. Delivery at 36 weeks
C. Immediate antiviral treatment
D. Antiviral treatment at 36 weeks

Discussion

The correct answer is **C**. Given that she has an outbreak, antiviral treatment is indicated. Treatment at the time of outbreak, especially in the context of ruptured membranes, is indicated to decrease the risk to the fetus. Antiviral treatment should not be delayed until 36 weeks. The question of whether to deliver this patient immediately would be controversial. It would be necessary to weigh the risk of prematurity if delivery occurs against the risk of neonatal herpes. If the patient is remote from term

and has recurrent disease rather than a primary infection there is support for attempting to continue the pregnancy and administer antenatal steroids. Unfortunately, there is no agreement among providers on when the risk of prematurity may outweigh the risk of neonatal herpes. In light of ruptured membranes there is consensus among providers on offering delivery at 34 weeks. If an active herpetic lesion is present when delivery is considered, then cesarean delivery is usually recommended.

Objectives

1. Know guidelines for the management of a pregnancy complicated by genital herpes
2. Know treatment options for pregnant women with active herpes infections
3. Know risks to fetus in a pregnancy complicated by herpes infection

CASE 7

A 42-year-old patient having her first baby presents at 18 weeks for prenatal visit and genetic counseling because of her advanced maternal age status. She is aware that her age may place her at risk for having a fetus with a chromosomal abnormality. She is currently not interested in invasive testing but asks what tests are available to screen for chromosomal abnormalities.

All of the following are considered screening tests EXCEPT
A. Maternal serum screening
B. Free fetal DNA in maternal circulation
C. Amniocentesis
D. High-risk ultrasound

Discussion

The correct answer is **C**. Amniocentesis, which involves the removal of amniotic fluid via maternal transabdominal needle puncture and subsequent analysis of the fluid for fetal karyotype, is an invasive diagnostic procedure.[19] First-trimester maternal serum screening may be offered to patients between 11 and 13.6 weeks' gestation.[20] This testing involves maternal serum analytes of hCG or free hCG and pregnancy-associated protein A (PAPP-A) combined with an ultrasound measurement of fetal nuchal translucency, which is gestational age dependent. A nuchal translucency of >95th percentile for gestational age has been associated with an increased risk for chromosomal abnormalities. The detection rate of first-trimester screening for trisomy 21 and trisomy 18 is about 87% to 90% and 90%, respectively, with a 5% false-positive rate. Risk for open neural tube defects is not calculated since such screening is ideally performed between 16 and 18 weeks; therefore, maternal serum alpha-fetoprotein should be obtained in second trimester to assess this risk. Since this patient is in the second trimester, she can be offered a quad screen, which can be obtained between 14 and 21.6 weeks.[20] A maternal blood sample is required and analyzed for levels of hCG, maternal serum alpha-fetoprotein, estriol, and inhibin A. The detection rate of the quad screen for trisomy 21 is 81%, trisomy 18 is 80%, and open neural tube defect is 80%. There are other forms of screening that combine first- and second-trimester testing. Serum screens do not give a risk for trisomy 13 due to its low rate of occurrence and insufficient normative data. A new screening test has become available and involves the analysis of free fetal DNA in maternal circulation.[21] This test can be performed at any gestational age after 10 weeks and requires only a maternal blood sample. This test reports an accuracy of 99% in detecting cases of T21, T18, and T13. It does not assess the risk for neural tube defects. If this test reveals an increased risk for a chromosomal abnormality, amniocentesis is still recommended for confirmation. A high-risk ultrasound can also be offered as a screening test to look for ultrasound markers associated with chromosomal abnormalities or open neural tube defects. Commonly evaluated markers include an increased nuchal translucency in the first trimester, a thickened nuchal fold in the second trimester, absent nasal bone, echogenic bowel, cardiac abnormalities, and shortened long bones. The patient would need to be counseled that the lack of ultrasound markers may reduce but not eliminate the risk of a fetal chromosomal abnormality.

Helpful Hint: Amniocentesis is a diagnostic test for fetal chromosomal abnormalities. Traditional teaching has been that amniocentesis should be offered to women of advanced maternal age (≥35 years at the time of delivery) and to patients with an abnormal serum screen, abnormal ultrasound findings, previous child with a chromosomal abnormality, or a significant family history amenable to diagnosis with amniocentesis. Recently, the recommendation has been changed and providers are encouraged to make all pregnant women aware of the availability of amniocentesis for prenatal diagnosis.[19]

Objectives

1. Know recommendations for screening of pregnant women with advanced maternal age
2. Know limitations of screening modalities to evaluate for anomalies commonly associated with advanced maternal age

CASE 8

A 24-year-old woman at 39.4 weeks presents to Labor and Delivery with the complaint of regular uterine contractions. Cervical examination shows that she is dilated 1 cm. Her previous child was born vaginally 2 years ago. During her current pregnancy she tested positive for human immunodeficiency virus (HIV). She has been compliant with her highly active antiretroviral therapy (HAART) which was started at 15 weeks. Her viral load is undetectable.

What is the MOST appropriate management for this patient?
A. Initiate oral zidovudine and recommend c-section
B. Initiate oral zidovudine and recommend vaginal delivery
C. Initiate IV zidovudine and recommend c-section
D. Initiate IV zidovudine and recommend vaginal delivery

Discussion

The correct answer is **D**. Great strides have been made in reducing the risk of perinatal transmission of HIV. The risk of transmission with no maternal therapy can be as high as 25%.[22] The combined use of antenatal HAART, IV zidovudine prior to delivery and delivery by c-section when maternal viral loads are >1,000 copies/mL, have reduced this risk to <2%.[22] This patient has an undetectable viral load and without any other indications for cesarean delivery (such as breech presentation) she is a candidate for vaginal delivery. Intrapartum therapy with IV zidovudine is recommended regardless of the route of delivery or viral load. For patients undergoing vaginal delivery, IV zidovudine is started at the time of admission and continues until delivery. If delivery is by c-section, then zidovudine is administered for 3 hours prior to the surgery. Use of oral zidovudine is not recommended. C-section delivery in a patient who is HIV+ is indicated if her viral load is greater than 1,000 copies/mL or for usual obstetric indications such as placenta previa or fetal malpresentation. In resource-poor countries where HAART is not readily available, single dose nevirapine given to a pregnant woman during the intrapartum period and to her newborn has been shown in one study to reduce maternal-to-child transmission by almost 50% among a population of breastfeeding women in Uganda.[23] More recently, the World Health Organization made the recommendation for resource-poor areas that a combination of tenofovir, emtricitabine, and efavirenz be initiated in all HIV-infected pregnant women as soon as their pregnancies are confirmed or if HIV is diagnosed in a pregnant or breastfeeding woman.[24] Data on the use of this regimen is somewhat limited.

Helpful Hint: All pregnant women should be offered HIV testing at their initial prenatal visit. For patients who present for delivery with unknown **HIV** status, rapid HIV testing is available. Administration of IV zidovudine to a laboring patient whose rapid test is positive can still reduce the risk of perinatal transmission to approximately 10%.

Objective

1. Know recommendations for care and management for women known to be HIV positive during pregnancy

CASE 9

A 35-year-old woman at 18 weeks presents for her initial prenatal visit. She reports that she has a seizure disorder which is well controlled on lamotrigine. When she told her neurologist that she was pregnant he added 4 mg of folic acid per day.

Which of the following would NOT be appropriate in the management of this patient?
A. Obtaining a second-trimester serum screen and ordering a high-risk ultrasound
B. Recommending that she should discontinue her lamotrigine and start valproic acid
C. Ordering a RGS at 24 weeks
D. Ordering genetic counseling for AMA and seizure disorder

Discussion

The correct answer is **B**. Up to 0.6% of pregnant women have a seizure disorder.[25] This patient has been well controlled on her current medication so there is no indication for a change in her medications. Although all antiepileptic medications have an associated risk of fetal effects such as craniofacial abnormalities, neural tube defects, and developmental delay, some of the newer medications such as lamotrigine may have a lower risk. Valproic acid has been associated with risk for neural tube defects as high as four- to eightfold and is rarely used in pregnancy. Seizure medications, the seizure disorder or the two acting in combination may produce these undesired effects in 2% to 3% of exposed fetuses. It is important, however, that maternal seizures be well controlled throughout pregnancy and medications should not be withheld or abruptly stopped due to pregnancy. The lowest effective dose of a single medication should be used since fetal effects are most likely to be seen when high doses or multiple medications are used. Folic acid is recommended for patients

on antiepileptic medications since it may help reduce the risk of major malformations. Serum screening in the second trimester is indicated due to the increased risk for open neural tube defect. High-risk ultrasound should be considered in patients who use antiepileptic medications. Neural tube defects can usually be detected by ultrasound unless they are small or skin covered. Screening for diabetes by random glucose screen is typically considered between 24 and 28 weeks. Genetic counseling is recommended for patients of advanced maternal age. Many genetic counselors are also very knowledgeable about the impact of medications on a developing fetus. Genetic counseling may help her better understand the impact of maternal age, seizure disorder, and medications on a fetus. Genetic counseling can also help her interpret her serum screen results and understand options for additional testing such as amniocentesis.

Objectives

1. Know recommendations for care and treatment of mothers with seizure disorder during pregnancy
2. Understand the risk associated with antiseizure medications during pregnancy

CASE 10

A patient is brought to Labor and Delivery at 28 weeks' gestation complaining of severe abdominal pain and heavy vaginal bleeding. This is her first pregnancy and she reports no significant medical history with the exception of occasional substance abuse, primarily crack cocaine, which she reports using several hours prior to presentation. Her blood pressure is 220/114 mm Hg. On examination brisk vaginal bleeding of bright red blood is noted and her abdomen is very hard and tender to palpation. She is placed on the fetal heart rate monitor and late decelerations followed by a prolonged fetal bradycardia are noted.

What is the MOST LIKELY diagnosis?
A. Early preterm labor
B. Maternal pulmonary embolism
C. Placental abruption
D. Uterine rupture

Discussion

The correct answer is **C**. Classic complaints suggesting placental abruption include significant abdominal pain, tetanic contractions, and vaginal bleeding. Placental abruption complicates 1% of pregnancies.[26] Risk factors for abruption include previous history of abruption, hypertensive disorders, multiple gestations, substance abuse, and premature rupture of membranes. Maternal complications may depend on the severity of the abruption and can include obstetric hemorrhage, coagulopathy, renal failure, need for blood transfusion, hysterectomy, and even maternal death. Fetal complications include prematurity, anemia, and fetal death. Patients in early labor may have painful regular contractions with uterine relaxation between contractions but usually do not experience heavy vaginal bleeding. Presenting symptoms of maternal pulmonary embolism may include tachypnea, tachycardia, and various chest complaints. Uterine rupture can present with the same symptoms as described above, but would be unusual in a patient who has not had a previous c-section.

Objectives

1. Identify the classic clinical signs and symptoms associated with a placental abruption
2. Know maternal risk factors that increase the risk for a placental abruption
3. Know potential maternal and fetal complications of pregnancies complicated by placental abruption

CASE 11

A patient presents for ultrasound for fetal growth at 24 weeks. Twin gestation with male fetuses was diagnosed on her first ultrasound at 18 weeks. Fetal anatomy appeared normal. A very thin separating membrane was visualized with one placenta. At that time fetal weights were equivalent with both fetuses measuring about 17 weeks. On today's scan Twin A's weight is 28% greater than Twin B's. Twin A has polyhydramnios while B has oligohydramnios.

What is the MOST LIKELY diagnosis?
A. Twin-to-twin transfusion syndrome
B. Normal twin gestation
C. Chromosomal abnormality in Twin B
D. Ruptured membranes in Twin B

Discussion

The correct answer is **A**. Based on the description these twins appear to be monochorionic diamniotic twins, which means that they share a placenta (monochorionic) but are in separate amniotic sacs (diamniotic). Twin-to-twin transfusion syndrome is a disorder that complicates up to 15% of monochorionic gestations and is a significant cause of mortality.[27] It occurs because of abnormal vasculature of the shared placenta or, specifically, the

presence of ≥1 arteriovenous anastomoses (shunts) within the monochorionic placenta. It should be suspected in monochorionic twins when ultrasound shows gender concordance, thin separating membrane (<2 mm thickness) with asymmetric fluid distribution and discordant fetal growth. The severity of the process may be described by the Quintero Stages I to V.[28] This disorder is progressive and if left untreated fetal mortality of one or both twins may be as high as 90%. Forms of treatment include serial amnioreductions, septostomy, selective feticide, or fetoscopic laser coagulation of abnormal placental vessels. The latter two should be performed only at centers with extensive experience in these procedures.

Helpful Hint: Twins are the most common type of multiple births occurring in up to 33 per 1,000 live births in the United States. Triplet and higher-order multiple births occur at a much less frequent rate of 124 per 100,000 live births. There has been a general increase in the number of multiple gestation births in many countries due to the increasing use of reproductive technology. Classification in terms of type of twinning is based on the organization of the fetal membranes and placenta. Dizygotic twins are the most common type of twin gestation. Dizygotic twins occur when two oocytes are fertilized by two different sperms. Although fertilization occurs during the same cycle, these twins are genetically different. Dizygotic twins implant separately and develop separate membranes and each has its own placenta (see Fig. 1-3). Monozygotic twins occur when a single oocyte is fertilized by a single sperm and the twinning occurs due to division of the blastomere at various stages of development (Fig. 1-4A–C). If the

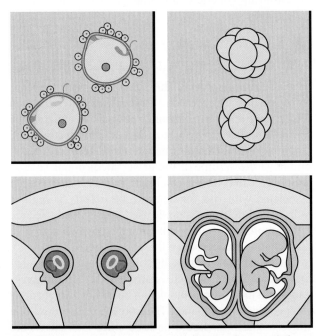

FIGURE 1-3. Dizygotic twins: Fertilization by two different spermatozoa.

division of the blastomere occurs during cleavage, the monozygotic twins implant separately, have separate placentas and do not share fetal membranes. More commonly, the cleavage in the blastocyst stage and both embryos have the same placenta and chorion but each has its own

amnion. The rarest type of monozygotic twin occurs when cleavage occurs in the stage of the double-layer embryo resulting in a shared placenta, chorion, and amniotic cavity.

Multiple gestation pregnancies are at risk for various complications including discordant growth,

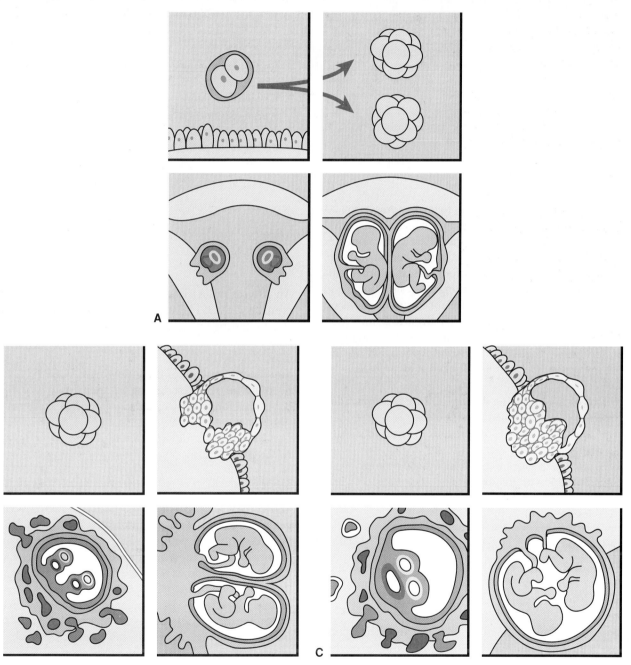

FIGURE 1-4.   Monozygotic twins. (**A**) Fertilization by a single spermatozoon and separation in the cleavage stage. If the division takes place during the cleavage in the 2-cell-blastomere stage, the monozygotic twins implant themselves separately (after the zona pellucida has disappeared), similar to dizygotic twins. They do not share their membranes: each twin has its own placenta, its own chorion and amnion. (**B**) Fertilization by a single spermatozoon and separation occurs in the blastocyst stage. In the majority of the cases, the cleavage occurs in the blastocyst stage. The embryonic bud divides itself in the interior of the same blastocyst cavity into two masses of cells. Both embryos possess the same chorion and the same placenta, but each has its own amnion. (**C**) Fertilization by a single spermatozoon and separation occurs in the double-layer embryo. In rare cases, the cleavage can also take place in the stage of the double-layer embryo, directly before the appearance of the primitive streak. For both twins, this kind of separation leads to a common placenta, a common chorion, and a common amniotic cavity.

malplacentation, cord entanglement (for those with a shared amniotic cavity), and preterm labor. Heightened monitoring is recommended to ensure fetal well-being.

Objectives

1. Recognize the various types of twin pregnancies
2. Know complications associated with twin-to-twin transfusion syndrome
3. Know recommendations for management and care of twin pregnancies associated with discordant growth

CASE 12

A patient whom you have been following presents at 33 weeks' gestation. She was recently evaluated for intense itching assumed to be due to an allergic reaction. Her complete blood cell count and basic chemistries were normal. She reports no relief from topical or oral medications and states that the itching makes her unable to perform her usual activities. Except for excoriations on her abdomen, soles, and palms her physical examination is normal. You repeat her laboratories with the addition of serum bile acids. Her laboratories are again normal but the serum bile acids are elevated at 80 μmol/L.

Which of the following would NOT be recommended for this patient?
A. Administration of betamethasone for fetal lung maturity
B. Initiation of twice weekly biophysical profiles
C. Prescription of ursodiol
D. Planned induction at 40 weeks if spontaneous labor does not occur

Discussion

The correct answer is **D**. This patient most likely has intrahepatic cholestasis of pregnancy, a disorder that affects about 1% of pregnant patients. It is characterized by intense itching, usually of the soles and palms. There may be a transaminitis and elevated serum bile acids.[29] The itching and laboratory abnormalities usually resolve in the mother after delivery. Cholestyramine and ursodiol may be prescribed to relieve itching. Cholestasis of pregnancy is associated with adverse pregnancy outcomes, including preterm delivery, meconium-stained fluid, nonreassuring fetal heart rate tracings, and intrauterine fetal demise. Fetal complications may be increased when maternal bile acid levels exceed 40 μmol/L. Delivery is recommended at 37 to 38 weeks to decrease fetal/neonatal morbidity and mortality.

For this patient, steroids could be administered in preparation for early delivery. Antenatal surveillance via twice weekly biophysical profiles should be considered to ensure fetal well-being or to initiate delivery if there is evidence of compromise. Delaying induction to 40 weeks would not be recommended due to increased fetal morbidity and mortality which may occur after 37 to 38 weeks.[29]

Objectives

1. Recognize the the clinical presentation of cholestasis of pregnancy
2. Know associated pregnancy outcomes for patients with a diagnosis of cholestasis of pregnancy
3. Know recommended surveillance and delivery management for patients with a diagnosis of cholestasis of pregnancy

CASE 13

An 18-year-old African American patient presents for a prenatal visit at 19 weeks. She has been reading about genetic testing and wants to know what screening tests she should consider.

You recommend all of the following EXCEPT
A. Maternal serum screening for aneuploidy
B. Hemoglobin electrophoresis for sickle cell trait or disease
C. Cystic fibrosis mutation testing
D. Fragile X testing

Discussion

The correct answer is **D**. Determining which available genetic tests to offer a patient can be difficult and may need consultation with a genetic counselor. Important factors in the decision may include the patient's age and ethnic background as well as obstetric and family history. All patients who present between 11 and 21.6 weeks should be offered first- or second-trimester serum screening for aneuploidy. As an African American this patient could have sickle cell trait or disease, which can be determined by hemoglobin electrophoresis. If she has sickle cell trait or disease, testing of her partner should be offered to allow for appropriate counseling on the risk to the fetus. Cystic fibrosis is an autosomal recessive disorder with a carrier frequency of 1/24 in patients of Ashkenazi Jewish descent to 1/94 in Asian Americans. It is more common in patients of Northern European descent but with the mixing of racial and ethnic backgrounds that has occurred in many populations the frequency of this disorder has increased among African Americans. The American College of Obstetricians and Gynecologists and the American College of Medical Genetics now recommend that cystic fibrosis testing be offered to women of reproductive age, regardless of ethnic background or other risk factors, along with genetic counseling to explain the complexity of carrier testing.[30] Fragile X, an X-linked dominant disorder, is the most common inherited cause of mental retardation and occurs due to a trinucleotide (CGG) expansion which causes abnormal methylation of the fragile X mental retardation-1 (FMR-1) gene.[31] Normal repeat number is 5 to 40 repeats; with repeats >200 full fragile X syndrome phenotype occurs in males. In males fragile X usually results in moderate mental retardation and characteristic phenotype; females are more mildly affected. Unless there is a family history of fragile X–related disorders, unexplained mental retardation or developmental delay, or premature ovarian failure, fragile X testing is probably not indicated.[31] Genetic testing recommendations change frequently as more testing options become available and providers should keep abreast of these changes.

Objectives

1. Know ACOG recommendations for genetic testing during pregnancy
2. Recognize commonly available genetic tests during pregnancy

CASE 14

A 23-year-old patient presents for her initial prenatal visit at 15 weeks' gestation by early ultrasound. This is her first pregnancy and she reports no significant medical history. Her blood pressure at this visit is 148/97 mm Hg with repeat of 145/92 mm Hg. She is asymptomatic with normal laboratories with the exception of 1+ protein on urinalysis. Fundal height is appropriate and normal fetal heart tones are auscultated with Doppler. She returns at 19 weeks for follow-up and to have her maternal serum screen drawn.

Her blood pressure is 152/97 mm Hg. The most LIKELY diagnosis is

A. Gestational hypertension
B. Chronic hypertension
C. Preeclampsia
D. Chronic hypertension with superimposed pre-eclampsia
E. Eclampsia

Discussion

The correct answer is **B**. Hypertensive disorders complicate up to 22% of pregnancies and are a leading cause of maternal death.[32] Chronic hypertension is hypertension that occurs prior to 20 weeks' gestation, is present prior to the pregnant state, or persists beyond the usual 6-week postpartum period. Gestational hypertension is diagnosed when elevated blood pressure occurs for the first time during the pregnancy with no proteinuria. Preeclampsia is defined as the onset of hypertension (BP >140/90 mm Hg) and proteinuria after 20 weeks' gestation. Preeclampsia superimposed on chronic hypertension is defined as the development of proteinuria of 300 mg or more in a 24-hour urine collection in a woman with documented hypertension prior to 20 weeks or, also, worsening proteinuria or blood pressures, or evidence of end-organ involvement in patients with hypertension and proteinuria documented before 20 weeks. Eclampsia is the occurrence of a seizure in a patient previously diagnosed with preeclampsia. Chronic hypertension occurs in about 5% of pregnant women and is associated with adverse pregnancy outcomes.[32] Complications can include significant maternal end-organ damage, development of preeclampsia, placental abruption, intrauterine growth restriction, oligohydramnios, stillbirth, and indicated preterm delivery with associated complications of prematurity.[32]

The patient returns at 24 weeks and blood pressures range from a systolic of 142 to 149 mm Hg with diastolics of 82 to 98 mm Hg. Her laboratories are normal and she is asymptomatic. Fundal height is 23 cm and fetal heart tones are in the 140s by Doppler.

The NEXT step in her management would be

A. Initiation of oral labetalol
B. Initiation of oral lisinopril
C. Admission to the antepartum unit for administration of intravenous hydralazine
D. Continued monitoring of blood pressures and increased frequency of visits

Discussion

The correct answer is **D**. With the highest documented blood pressure of 152/97 mm Hg she is not yet at the point of requiring medication. Current recommendations are that blood pressure medication be initiated in a patient with chronic hypertension when maternal diastolic values are consistently above 100 mm Hg. Labetalol and methyldopa are typical first-line medications used for the treatment of chronic hypertension in pregnancy and have excellent efficacy and safety profiles. The frequency of her visits should be increased to every 1 to 2 weeks. Consideration could also be given to having the patient check her blood pressures daily in the community, record the values, and present for evaluation if her blood pressure is consistently elevated above her usual baseline. Lisinopril is an ACE inhibitor; this category of antihypertensives is associated with fetal renal abnormalities, oligohydramnios, and intrauterine growth restriction and is not used during pregnancy. IV hydralazine is usually reserved for markedly elevated BPs of 160 to 170/100 to 110 mm Hg in the inpatient setting.

The patient has had a relatively uncomplicated prenatal course but presents to Labor and Delivery at 33 weeks with blood pressures of 185 to 196/110 to 117 mm Hg. She is admitted for fetal monitoring, blood pressure control, and antenatal steroids. Ultrasound shows the fetal weight is <10th percentile and a biophysical profile of 10/10. A 24-hour urine is collected for protein and results in a value of 5,600 mg. Her complete blood count is normal but the chemistry panels show her liver enzymes are becoming elevated.

What is the MOST likely diagnosis in this scenario?
A. Chronic hypertension
B. Mild preeclampsia
C. Severe preeclampsia
D. HELLP (hemolysis, elevated liver enzymes, low platelets) syndrome

Discussion

The correct answer is **C**. With the laboratory abnormalities present, including proteinuria and elevated liver enzymes, the clinical picture suggests that the patient's chronic hypertension has progressed to become preeclampsia. The patient's blood pressures are substantially elevated above her usual baseline, her laboratories now have abnormalities and the fetus is growth restricted. In this case severe preeclampsia is present. Mild preeclampsia is defined as blood pressures consistently >140 mm Hg systolic or >90 mm Hg diastolic. Severe preeclampsia is diagnosed if one or more of the following criteria are present: blood pressure ≥160 mm Hg systolic or 110 mm Hg diastolic on two occasions 6 hours apart, proteinuria of 5 g or higher on a 24-hour urine, oliguria of <500 mg in 24 hours, cerebral or visual disturbances, pulmonary edema or cyanosis, epigastric or right upper quadrant pain, impaired liver function, thrombocytopenia, or intrauterine growth restriction.[33] HELLP syndrome involves hemolysis, elevated liver enzymes, and low platelets and is a variant of preeclampsia that may develop without markedly elevated blood pressure and proteinuria. Since the patient's CBC is normal and there

is no evidence of hemolysis by elevated bilirubin on her chemistry, HELLP is less likely than severe preeclampsia.

The patient has been managed on Labor and Delivery and has been stable. At 34 weeks her liver enzymes continue to rise and she now reports a severe headache that does not respond to medications. Blood pressures are again in the180 to 190/90s to 110 mm Hg and are difficult to control.

The NEXT step in her management is
A. Control of maternal blood pressure, initiation of magnesium sulfate, and induction of labor
B. Initiation of magnesium sulfate and weekly laboratories
C. Immediate delivery by c-section
D. Discharge home with close follow-up

Discussion

The correct answer is **A**. With worsening laboratories and symptoms of a severe headache, the maternal status is deteriorating. Maternal blood pressures should be controlled with IV medication, usually hydralazine, to keep blood pressure <160/110 mm Hg. Magnesium sulfate should be started for maternal seizure prophylaxis. Due to the elevated maternal blood pressure, change in maternal laboratories and symptoms, intrauterine growth restriction, and oligohydramnios delivery should be considered. There is currently no indication for immediate c-section, but if labor induction is prolonged or maternal/fetal status deteriorates during the induction then c-section should be considered. Severe preeclampsia can be managed expectantly if a stable patient is remote from term or to allow for the administration of antenatal steroids. In this patient, steroids have been administered, maternal blood pressures remain elevated, and she is now reporting a symptom of CNS involvement (headache) and chronic placental insufficiency exists as evidenced by fetal growth restriction. Since delivery is the "cure" for preeclampsia it should be considered in this patient for both maternal and fetal indications. Expectant management would not be the best option in light of maternal and fetal compromise at a gestational age of 34 weeks.[33]

Objectives

1. Recognize and distinguish between the various types of hypertensive diseases during pregnancy
2. Understand risk for the mother and fetus in pregnancies complicated by hypertension
3. Understand recommendations for monitoring pregnancies complicated by hypertension

CASE 15

A slightly obese 28-year-old patient at 16 weeks' gestation comes to your office for a prenatal visit. She has a history of gestational hypertension. Her obstetric history is significant for a first-trimester loss followed by a term vaginal delivery. Her last two pregnancies resulted in vaginal deliveries following the onset of spontaneous labor at 34 and 32 weeks, respectively.

What is her MOST significant risk factor for preterm birth in this pregnancy?
A. Previous preterm birth
B. Previous first-trimester loss
C. Obesity
D. Maternal age <30 years

Discussion

The correct answer is **A**. There are several identifiable risk factors for preterm (<37 weeks) birth, which complicates about 12% births in the United States.[34] These include a previous spontaneous preterm birth, maternal lifestyle factors such as smoking or substance abuse, maternal prepregnancy weight of <50 kg, maternal age <19 years or >35 years, race, low socioeconomic status, vaginal bleeding, stress, family history of preterm birth, and limited prenatal care. Of these, a previous preterm birth is the most important risk factor, which increases the risk of another preterm delivery by 3–5 fold.

Which of the following SHOULD be considered to reduce her risk of another preterm birth?
A. Placement of cervical cerclage at 18 weeks
B. Serial evaluations of cervical length by transvaginal ultrasound starting at 24 weeks
C. Modified bed rest with bathroom privileges starting 2 weeks prior to her earlier preterm delivery
D. Initiation of 17-alpha-hydroxyprogesterone caproate injections as soon as possible

Discussion

The correct answer is **D**. Progesterone injections have been shown in several well-conducted randomized controlled trials to prevent recurrent preterm delivery. The mechanism of action is not clear. These injections are given weekly starting around 16 weeks and conclude at 34 to 36 weeks. A cerclage may be utilized in the setting of cervical insufficiency, which is painless cervical dilatation followed by delivery during the second trimester. A history of cervical insufficiency may be an indication for cerclage in a subsequent pregnancy; preterm labor is not. Bed rest has not been demonstrated to prevent preterm labor and is disruptive to a patient's lifestyle. It may also put her at risk for a thromboembolic event if appropriate prophylactic measures such as sequential compression devices or heparin are not used. Serial cervical lengths by transvaginal ultrasound may be useful for diagnosing a shortened cervix (<2.5 cm) and determining who may benefit from cerclage but cervical length measurements for this purpose typically begin at 13 to 16 weeks.[35]

The patient presents to Labor and Delivery at 29 weeks complaining of contractions. Her cervix is dilated 3 cm. Ultrasound shows that the fetus is cephalic with an appropriate weight and amniotic fluid index. When placed on the monitor the fetal tracing is reassuring and contractions are regular occurring every 2 minutes.

Which of the following SHOULD be considered?
A. Initiation of a tocolytic agent and antenatal steroids
B. Ultrasound evaluation of the cervical length and antibiotics
C. Placement of cervical cerclage
D. Expectant management and preparation for imminent vaginal delivery

Discussion

The correct answer is **A**. In a patient with a history of preterm births at 34 and 32 weeks who presents at 29 weeks with a convincing picture of preterm labor, delivery may be imminent. Expectant management is most likely to result in a vaginal delivery. Efforts should be made to prolong the pregnancy for at least 48 hours to allow for the administration of antenatal steroids in a 29-week fetus.[36] Nifedipine and magnesium sulfate may be considered as tocolytic agents. Digital cervical examination would provide important information on cervical dilation and effacement, but ultrasound evaluation would not provide much additional information at 29 weeks. Since membranes are not ruptured antibiotics are not indicated.

Objectives

1. Identify risk factors for preterm birth
2. Know recommended treatment and management strategies to decrease the risk of preterm birth
3. Know current guidelines for management of pregnancies complicated by preterm labor

CASE 16

A 32-year old at 30 weeks presents to Labor and Delivery with the complaint of persistent leakage of fluid from her vagina. She has no other complaints and reports good fetal movement. Her prenatal course has been uncomplicated and her two previous children were born vaginally. Speculum examination shows a large pool of amniotic fluid in the vaginal vault. The cervix appears closed visually. Ultrasound shows the fetus is cephalic, fetal weight is appropriate for gestational age, and the amniotic fluid index is 3 cm. Fetal heart tracing is reassuring.

After the patient is admitted for preterm premature rupture of membranes (PPROM), what is the most appropriate next step in her management?
A. Immediate induction of labor due to ruptured membranes
B. Administration of subcutaneous terbutaline to prevent contractions
C. Administration of antenatal steroids and antibiotics
D. Collection of a fetal fibronectin sample

Discussion

The correct answer is **C**. The presence of a large pool of amniotic fluid on speculum examination and the low amniotic fluid index by ultrasound, along with the patient's complaint of leakage of fluid, confirm the diagnosis of ruptured membranes. At a gestational age of 30 weeks, antenatal steroids should be administered to enhance fetal lung maturity. Steroids are typically given between 24 and 34 weeks if there is evidence of preterm labor and delivery is thought to be likely within the next 7 days. Antibiotics would also be recommended to increase latency; a typical regimen would involve ampicillin and erythromycin.[37] Immediate delivery is not indicated because the mother is stable and the fetus shows no signs of distress. Delivery should be delayed to allow for the administration of antenatal steroids unless there is evidence of maternal or fetal compromise. Terbutaline is a beta-adrenergic agonist that can be used as a tocolytic agent. The use of a tocolytic agent when PPROM is present is controversial, but since this patient is not contracting and her cervix is not dilated there is no indication for a tocolytic. If a tocolytic agent were to be needed, terbutaline might not be the best choice due to its maternal side effects, including increased risk for pulmonary edema and tachycardia. Magnesium sulfate or oral nifedipine might be more appropriate tocolytic agents. Fetal fibronectin is a glycoprotein produced by the chorionic membranes and should not be present in cervical secretions between 24 and 34 weeks. Its presence in the vagina during this period has been associated with preterm labor and delivery. The vagina and cervix can be swabbed for its presence at the time of speculum examination. However, a fetal fibronectin sample should not be obtained under the following circumstances: recent vaginal examination, recent sexual activity, vaginal bleeding, or ruptured membranes because the false-positive rate of the test may be increased.

The patient has been stable following admission and fetal testing reassuring. At 33 weeks the patient begins to complain of abdominal pain. The uterus is tender to palpation. Maternal and fetal tachycardia are noted. Chorioamnionitis is diagnosed.

What should be the NEXT step in management?
A. Additional course of antibiotics to delay delivery until 34 weeks
B. Amniocentesis to confirm chorioamnionitis
C. Ultrasound to assess the amniotic fluid volume
D. Induction of labor

Discussion

The correct answer is **D**. Once chorioamnionitis is suspected, delivery is recommended regardless of gestational age. Chorioamnionitis is a clinical diagnosis based on the findings of uterine tenderness and maternal and fetal tachycardia. Other suggestive findings include maternal fever, foul-smelling vaginal discharge, and elevated maternal white blood cell count. Delivery should not be delayed until 34 weeks due to increased risk for maternal and/or fetal infection. Amniocentesis is not indicated due to the strong clinical picture of infection. If amniocentesis were needed to confirm the diagnosis, the fluid would be sent for Gram stain, culture, and interleukin-6 if available. Interleukin-6 has been shown to be a particularly useful amniotic fluid marker for chorioamnionitis but few facilities have assays available to test for its presence. Since rupture of membranes has been confirmed previously, there would be no strong indication to measure amniotic fluid again since it will not change management. Ultrasound might, however, be considered to confirm that the fetus has remained cephalic. Once this is confirmed then induction of labor should be considered as there appears to be no indications for cesarean section.

Helpful Hint: Although magnesium sulfate has fallen out of favor for use as a tocolytic agent due to its lack of efficacy in preventing preterm birth, it is gaining popularity again as an agent which may serve as a neuroprotectant for preterm babies. There is evidence to suggest that if magnesium sulfate is given before an anticipated early preterm birth, the risk of cerebral palsy in infants who survive is reduced.[38,39] The most efficacious treatment protocol has not yet been identified. A frequently used regimen involves administering a 6-g magnesium bolus intravenously over 20 to 30 minutes followed by continuous infusion at 2 g/h. The medication is discontinued if delivery has not occurred within 12 hours. It may be restarted if the patient again shows evidence of preterm labor.

Objectives

1. Know guidelines for expectant management of pregnancies complicated by premature rupture of membranes
2. Understand the role of tocolytic in the management of pregnancies complicated by premature and prolonged rupture of membranes
3. Recognized clinical signs and symptoms of chorioamnionitis
4. Know recommendations for delivery management in pregnancy complicated by chorioamnionitis

(intrauterine growth restriction with nonreassuring testing) may mandate delivery before 39 weeks none of these conditions appear to be present for this patient. There is no obstetric indication to schedule delivery at 38 weeks. Most providers would not allow a well-dated pregnancy to proceed to 43 weeks but would plan for delivery at 41 to 42 weeks with some form of antenatal testing such as weekly biophysical profiles during that time to ensure fetal well-being.

Helpful Hint: Monitoring the indications for induction or scheduled c-section less than 39 weeks' gestation has become an important quality-improvement metric in many labor and delivery units. As a result the number of nonindicated deliveries prior to 39 weeks has decreased dramatically. This has resulted in the reduction of neonatal complications associated with late preterm birth.[41]

CASE 17

A patient presents to Labor and Delivery at 37 weeks complaining only of irregular contractions. This is her second pregnancy and dating is by a 15-week ultrasound. Her pregnancy has been uncomplicated. Her cervix is closed and not effaced on examination. Today's ultrasound shows that the fetus is cephalic with a gestational-age appropriate weight. The amniotic fluid index is normal and the biophysical profile is 10/10.

She requests induction today so that she may join her family for a vacation in 2 weeks.

Her induction SHOULD
A. Take place today at patient's request
B. Be scheduled at 38 weeks
C. Be deferred to allow for onset of spontaneous labor
D. Be scheduled at 43 weeks if spontaneous labor has not occurred

Discussion

The correct answer is **C**. With no maternal or fetal indications present and no evidence that the patient is in labor there is no indication to begin her induction today. When no indications for delivery exist patients and providers should be encouraged to await the onset of spontaneous delivery. Awaiting spontaneous labor will provide the best chance for vaginal delivery. Social inductions, or those scheduled for patient or provider convenience, are discouraged and should not be scheduled prior to 39 weeks.[40] Although certain maternal conditions (diabetes, HIV, chronic hypertension) or fetal conditions

CASE 18

A 24-year-old patient presents to your office at 42.1 weeks' gestation by a 19-week ultrasound. She has no complaints and her pregnancy has been uncomplicated. Ultrasound reveals a singleton fetus in cephalic presentation with an appropriate weight. The amniotic fluid index is 2.8 cm. Her examination is negative for rupture of membranes and her cervix is dilated 1 cm with minimal effacement.

What should be the NEXT step in her management?
A. Induction of labor now
B. Schedule c-section within a week
C. Repeat ultrasound in 2 to 3 days to recheck fetal weight and amniotic fluid index
D. Amniocentesis to confirm fetal lung maturity

Discussion

The correct answer is **A**. Labor induction should be offered today due to her postterm pregnancy with oligohydramnios. A postterm pregnancy is one that has exceeded 42 weeks and is associated with complications such as stillbirth, macrosomia, shoulder dystocia, fetal distress in labor, obstetric trauma, and postpartum hemorrhage.[42] Oligohydramnios at term is associated with meconium staining of the amniotic fluid, abnormal fetal heart rate tracings and lower Apgar scores. There would be no value in performing a follow-up ultrasound to recheck the weight and AFI. Postdate pregnancies are also associated with an increased risk for c-section delivery, but vaginal delivery should be attempted if there are no contraindications such as breech presentation. This patient had dating by ultrasound performed at <20 weeks assuring her gestational age so amniocentesis would not be needed to confirm FLM before delivery.

The patient agrees to induction of labor today.

Which of the following would NOT be an appropriate cervical ripening agent?

A. Prostaglandin E1 analog such as misoprostol (Cytotec)
B. Intracervical prostaglandin E2 gel such as Cervidil®
C. Oxytocin alone
D. Foley bulb placed through the cervical canal with oxytocin started at time of placement

Discussion

The correct answer is **C**. Any of the other agents listed above would be appropriate cervical ripening agents.[43] Choice of agent to use would depend in part on the availability of each on the labor and delivery unit. Misoprostol is frequently used due to its effectiveness, very low cost, and stability at room temperature. When compared with intracervical prostaglandin E2 gel, misoprostol has been associated with increased rate of vaginal delivery within 24 hours but also with an increase in meconium-stained fluid and uterine tachysystole. Foley bulb placement, which mechanically dilates the cervix, and concurrent administration of oxytocin has a similar rate of vaginal delivery as does misoprostol. Since her cervix is dilated 1 cm it should be possible to place a foley. Oxytocin alone does not perform effectively as a cervical ripening agent. Cervical ripening by another agent should precede use of oxytocin to enhance its effectiveness as a uterine stimulant once the cervix has begun to dilate and efface.

Misoprostol was selected as the cervical ripening agent and when her cervix was 2 cm dilated and 50% effaced oxytocin was started since no contractions were noted. Her epidural provides adequate pain relief.

She is now 7 cm dilated and 80% effaced. An intrauterine pressure catheter is in place and she has an adequate contraction pattern. The oxytocin dosage has been maximized at 30 μ/min. Five hours later her cervix is unchanged.

The NEXT most appropriate step in her management is

A. Plan for delivery by c-section
B. Continue to increase the oxytocin to a maximum dose of 60 μ/min
C. Continue current management
D. Discontinue the oxytocin to allow her own contractions to work more effectively

Discussion

The correct answer is **A**. The patient is contracting adequately as assessed by an intrauterine pressure catheter and is on the typical maximum dose of oxytocin. Since there has been no cervical change in 5 hours, arrest of labor is diagnosed. Arrest occurs when there has been no cervical change in more than 2 to 4 hours with an adequate contraction pattern. C-section should be the next step in her delivery plan. Continuing to increase the oxytocin or continuing at its current dose would be unlikely to result in vaginal delivery. Discontinuing oxytocin to allow her own contractions to work more effectively would also be unlikely to have any benefit since oxytocin was needed to stimulate contractions.

Objectives

1. Know recommendations for induction of labor near-term gestation
2. Know recommendations for the management for postterm pregnancies

CASE 19

The medical students and residents have started a new rotation and the pediatric intern has questions about changes in maternal blood volume during pregnancy and how this relates to the developing fetus.

Which of the following is NOT a normal maternal physiologic adaptation to pregnancy?

A. Increased maternal cardiac output, increased blood volume, and increased respiratory rate
B. Decreased arterial blood pressure and decreased systemic vascular resistance
C. Increased hematocrit and decreased white blood cell count
D. Increased hyperventilation with mild respiratory alkalosis

Discussion

The correct answer is **C**. The adaptations that the maternal body makes to an ongoing gestation are remarkable.[44] They start essentially at the time of conception, continue throughout pregnancy, and are usually reversible after completion of the pregnancy. These adaptations are necessary for the development and maintenance of a pregnancy and are well tolerated by a healthy pregnant woman. All of the above changes in the cardiac and respiratory system occur to accommodate the development and functioning of the placenta and the growth of the fetus. Plasma volume increases by about 47% during a healthy pregnancy and the red blood cell mass by only 17%, so there is actually a decrease in maternal hemoglobin due to this dilutional effect of increased plasma volume. The white blood cell count is often slightly increased due to an increase in the production of neutrophils.

Objectives

1. Recognize changes in fluid volume and blood volume during pregnancy
2. Know physiologic changes in cardiorespiratory status during pregnancy
3. Know changes in hematologic parameters during pregnancy

CASE 20

A 34-year-old-woman at 32 weeks' gestation is a restrained passenger in the back seat of a car involved in a high-speed collision. The patient reports severe abdominal pain and has bruising on her abdomen secondary to the seatbelt but is otherwise stable. Initial x-rays, CAT scans, and abdominal ultrasound show no significant maternal injury. No fetal heart tones are heard.

The most common cause of fetal death in a mother who survives in this scenario is
A. Direct fetal injury
B. Placental abruption
C. Uterine rupture
D. Maternal pelvic fracture

Discussion

The correct answer is **B**. Placental abruption may occur in up to 2% of women who suffer abdominal trauma. Abruption may be difficult to diagnosis because occult bleeding but not vaginal bleeding may occur. Most women in an automobile accident will have monitoring for fetal heart rate and uterine contractions as well as ultrasound evaluation of the fetus and uterus. Abruption may not be immediately obvious by ultrasound and other methods of evaluating abruption such as coagulation studies usually do not have adequate sensitivity. Placental abruption is more likely to be detected by uterine and fetal monitoring. Uterine contractions may be a sign of abruption. Abruption, which usually results from shearing action of the placenta from the uterine wall when rapid deceleration occurs, often presents by base-

line tachycardia, decreased variability, and late decelerations on the fetal tracing.[51] This patient is complaining of abdominal pain and has bruising on her abdomen. Placental abruption should be suspected. Direct fetal trauma and uterine rupture would be less likely in a woman whose evaluation thus far shows no significant maternal injury. Maternal pelvic fractures are not usually associated with fetal death. Studies and diagnostic modalities that would be used in the evaluation of a nonpregnant patient following a significant injury should not be withheld if indicated since maternal well-being is paramount to the well-being of the fetus.

CASE 21

A 31-year-old patient presents at 38 weeks complaining of decreased fetal movement. She has no other complaints. This is her fourth pregnancy and it has been uncomplicated. She has been compliant with prenatal visits. A recent ultrasound showed a normally grown fetus with adequate amniotic fluid volume and normal anatomy. Ultrasound performed now confirms an intrauterine fetal demise (IUFD).

What is LIKELY to be the cause of this demise?
A. Placental abruption
B. Undiagnosed maternal diabetes
C. Poorly controlled maternal hypertension
D. Unexplained IUFD

Discussion

The correct answer is **D**. IUFD is a devastating event that occurs in about 1 in 160 pregnancies.[45] A recent evaluation of fetal deaths noted that in almost 66% of cases no cause is determined.[46] Since the patient had no other complaints such as abdominal pain or vaginal bleeding placental abruption would be unlikely. Maternal diabetes and hypertension are possible causes of IUFD but since this patient has had adequate prenatal care these maternal complications would have been recognized and treated. In determining the etiology of a demise a careful review of maternal, family, and obstetric history is important. Although the optimal workup for an IUFD has not been clearly elucidated, amniocentesis for karyotype and infection prior to delivery of the fetus, fetal autopsy, Kleihauer-Betke test for maternal–fetal hemorrhage and placental and umbilical cord evaluation by a qualified perinatal pathologist are among the most important procedures recommended.[45] Testing for other etiologies such as diabetes or antiphospholipid antibody syndrome will depend on the clinical situation. Patients often decline amniocentesis and autopsy and the provider should provide counseling on the value of these tests. Despite these tests, the etiology of the demise may remain unclear.

CASE 22

Last year you cared for a family who experienced a second-trimester loss. The mom is 32 years of age and has a history of two first-trimester and two second-trimester losses. She contacts you to seek advice and you recommend that she be evaluated by a maternal fetal medicine specialist for preconceptual counseling. During the subsequent evaluations she was diagnosed with antiphospholipid antibody (APA) syndrome by laboratory and clinical criteria. She wants to attempt a pregnancy.

Which medication regimen will likely be recommended for her?
A. Prednisone and Plaquenil
B. Low-dose aspirin and heparin
C. Prednisone alone
D. Weekly intravenous immunoglobulin

Discussion

The correct answer is **B**. Antiphospholipid antibody syndrome is an autoimmune disorder that affects women more than men. To diagnosis this syndrome a patient must meet both clinical and laboratory criteria. Clinical criteria include venous thrombolic events of arterial, venous or small vessels of any organ or tissue and adverse pregnancy outcomes, including fetal loss, placental insufficiency or abruption, intrauterine growth restriction, and severe preeclampsia. Laboratory criteria include the presence of anticardiolipin antibodies, lupus anticoagulant, and anti-beta-2 glycoprotein 1 antibodies. The combination of heparin and low-dose aspirin started in the first trimester once a viable pregnancy has been confirmed has been shown to reduce recurrent pregnancy loss.[47] If the patient does not have a history of vascular thrombosis then prophylactic dosing of heparin should be utilized. If vascular events are present, then a therapeutic dose should be used. The regimen should be continued through the 6-week postpartum period since the increased risk for thromboembolism appears to remain throughout this period.[48] Although the other medications listed as alternatives have been used to treat APA syndrome, low-dose aspirin and heparin are the

current medications recommended for the treatment of pregnant women. Complications of this syndrome include intrauterine growth restriction, severe preeclampsia, and fetal loss.

Objectives

1. Know potential causes of intrauterine fetal demise
2. Know recommended follow-up care and management after a fetal loss
3. Recognize clinical features of antiphospholipid antibody syndrome
4. Know recommended treatment regimen for pregnant women with antiphospholipid antibody syndrome

CASE 23

A 19-year old with a term pregnancy presents to Labor and Delivery with the complaint of frequent contractions and decreased fetal movement. She is placed on the monitor and contractions are noted to be occurring every 2 to 3 minutes.

The nurse caring for the patient tells you that the fetal heart rate tracing is Category 1 on ACOG's scale of I to III. This means
A. The fetal heart rate tracing is normal and predictive of normal fetal acid–base status
B. The fetal heart rate tracing is abnormal and immediate intervention is required
C. The fetal heart rate tracing is changing between categories and fetal status cannot be determined
D. None of the above are correct

Discussion

The correct answer is **A**. In 2008 guidelines were proposed by a group of experts for the interpretation of electronic fetal monitoring after a review of the systems in place worldwide and in the United States.[49,50] They proposed a three-tier system for the categorization of fetal tracings. A Category I tracing is normal. There is a baseline rate of 110 to 160 bpm; variability in the fetal heart rate is moderate (6–25 bpm); there are no late or variable decelerations in the fetal heart rate, although early decelerations may be present or absent; and accelerations of the fetal heart rate may be present or absent. Since there are no abnormalities noted in the tracing no immediate intervention is indicated. Although the fetal heart rate pattern may change between categories, there is no indication that this is occurring at the present time.

The patient begins active labor and after several hours has spontaneous rupture of membranes with meconium noted. The nurse tells you that the fetal tracing now shows no variability in the fetal heart rate and deep recurrent variable decelerations.

The tracing can now be described as
A. Category I
B. Category II
C. Category III
D. Cannot be described with this classification system

Discussion

The correct answer is **C**. A Category III tracing includes either absent baseline fetal heart rate variability with recurrent late decelerations, recurrent variable decelerations, or bradycardia; or may demonstrate a sinusoidal pattern. Since the tracing now has absent fetal heart rate variability and recurrent variable decelerations, it is considered Category III. Category I tracings are described above. A Category II tracing includes all fetal heart rate tracings that cannot be categorized as Category I or III. Category II tracings may have an abnormal baseline rate with bradycardia or tachycardia; baseline variability may be minimal or absent with no recurrent decelerations; baseline variability may be marked; there is absence of accelerations after fetal stimulation; periodic or episodic decelerations may be present. Most fetal heart rate tracings can be described with this classification system.

In light of the Category III tracing, which of the following would be appropriate during the initial evaluation?
A. Change in maternal position to the left or right side to reduce compression of vena cava and improve uteroplacental blood flow
B. Check maternal blood pressure and correct hypotension if present
C. Perform cervical examination to check for umbilical cord prolapse, descent of fetal head, or rapid cervical change
D. Assess maternal contraction frequency and duration for uterine tachysystole
E. All of the above would be appropriate

Discussion

The correct answer is **E**. All of the above maneuvers could be considered to improve a nonreassuring fetal tracing. Improvement in uterine blood flow by relief of vena caval compression often occurs with a change in maternal position, particularly if the nonreassuring tracing has occurred while the mother is on her back. If maternal hypotension is present and due to regional anesthesia, it may be treated by volume expansion, ephedrine, or both. Umbilical cord

prolapse or rapid descent of the fetal head or rapid cervical change can result in ominous fetal tracings. Cord prolapse is a true obstetric emergency and requires immediate elevation of the fetal head by a provider's hand in the vagina and c-section delivery. Rapid descent of the fetal head or cervical change should be identified as a cause of the nonreassuring tracing and careful monitoring of the patient's labor undertaken. If delivery is not imminent and the tracing does not improve, delivery by c-section may need to be considered. When uterine tachysystole occurs uterine blood flow is reduced and may be associated with a Category III tracing. A uterine relaxant such as terbutaline, a beta-agonist, may be administered quickly and improve uterine blood flow. One study found that up to 98% of cases where tachysystole caused the nonreassuring tracing will respond to treatment with beta-agonist. If no correctable cause is found or treatment of the presumed cause fails to improve a Category III tracing, then delivery should be expedited.

Objective

1. Know importance of fetal heart rate–tracing monitoring and its role in the active management of labor

CASE 24

An 18-year-old presents for prenatal care at 16 weeks. Her physical examination is normal and fundal height is consistent with gestational age. Her prenatal laboratories are normal with the exception of a positive rapid plasma regain test, which is a nonspecific test for syphilis. The confirmatory test for syphilis is also positive. Titers are 1:64. The patient has never been tested for syphilis prior to this pregnancy and does not know when she might have contracted the disease.

The most appropriate treatment for her would be
A. Azithromycin orally for 7 days
B. Doxycycline orally for 21 days
C. Benzathine penicillin G intramuscularly weekly for 3 weeks
D. Ciprofloxacin orally for 14 days

Discussion

The correct answer is **C**. Syphilis is a sexually transmitted disease caused by the spirochete *Treponema pallidum*. This organism can cross the placenta to cause congenital infection.[52] Congenital syphilis can result in preterm delivery, fetal death, and fetal infection. In some cases syphilis may be suspected by ultrasound examination when a fetus shows ascites and hydrops or placentamegaly is present. Screening for syphilis should take place at the first prenatal visit by a nonspecific test for syphilis. If this test is positive, then a specific treponemal test should be performed. If this test is positive then the diagnosis of syphilis is confirmed. Syphilis progresses through stages and penicillin G is the treatment of choice for all stages. This patient is not sure when she contracted syphilis so the duration of disease is unknown. She should receive weekly injections of penicillin G for 3 weeks and titers followed. Treatment is considered adequate when serial titers fall fourfold over 6 months. If titers rise or do not fall as expected, then this should be considered a treatment failure or a new infection has occurred. The other medications listed have not been demonstrated to be effective in treatment of syphilis, and doxycycline and ciprofloxacin are not recommended for use in pregnant women due to potential detrimental fetal effects. In addition, penicillin G is the only medication proven to prevent congenital syphilis. If the patient is allergic to penicillin, then desensitization by an experienced provider followed by administration of penicillin should be considered.

CASE 25

A patient presents to your office for her initial prenatal visit at 32 weeks. She states she was recently diagnosed with acute hepatitis B infection. Her hepatitis panel shows hepatitis B core antibodies and immunoglobulin M (IgM) class are present; her liver enzymes are mildly elevated.

She asks what effect maternal hepatitis may have on her baby. Which of the following MAY occur?
A. Transmission to the fetus
B. Preterm labor
C. Chronic childhood infection
D. All of the above may occur

Discussion

The correct answer is **D**. Acute hepatitis B infection may occur in 1 to 2 per 1,000 pregnancies. In mothers who experience an acute HBV infection during pregnancy, up to 10% of fetuses may become infected if infection occurs during the first trimester, while up to 80% to 90% may be infected if infection occurs in the third trimester. Acute hepatitis B infections have been associated with spontaneous abortions in the first trimester and with preterm labor if the infection occurs in the third trimester.

Mother to infant transmission may account for some cases of chronic childhood infections.

Helpful Hint: The American College of Obstetricians and Gynecologists (ACOG) as well as the Centers for Disease Control (CDC) and Prevention recommend routine screening for hepatitis B for all women at their first prenatal visit.[53,54] Screening based only on risk factors may miss a large proportion of infected women. Repeat hepatitis testing should occur later in pregnancy and in the postpartum period for seronegative women with risk factors such as intravenous drug use or numerous sexual partners. The hepatitis vaccination as well as hepatitis immune globulin is safe to use in pregnancy. Seronegative women with risk factors such as hepatitis B positive household contacts should receive the vaccination as well as the hepatitis immune globulin. This combination of active and passive immunization may prevent horizontal and vertical transmission of hepatitis B. Both ACOG and CDC recommend that newborns whose mothers are hepatitis B carriers receive combined immunoprophylaxis consisting of HBIG and hepatitis B vaccine in the immediate newborn period.[53,54]

Objectives

1. Know recommendations for the management of hepatitis infection during pregnancy
2. Know recommendations for the management of syphilis infection during pregnancy

CASE 26

A patient comes for a routine prenatal visit at 34 weeks. She has had one vaginal delivery followed by two low-transverse cesarean sections, the first for breech presentation followed by elective repeat.

You counsel her on all of the following aspects of vaginal birth after cesarean section (VBAC) EXCEPT
A. Increased blood loss with vaginal delivery
B. Uterine rupture
C. Possible hysterectomy for adherent placenta
D. Higher likelihood of successful VBAC than if cesareans were performed for failure to progress in labor

Discussion

The correct answer is **A**. VBAC remains a viable option for carefully selected patients in facilities equipped to handle emergency c-sections.[55] Vaginal births are usually associated with less, not more, blood loss than a c-section.

Uterine rupture may occur in <1% of patients who have had previous low-transverse c-sections. If this patient has had a classical c-section where a vertical incision is made on the uterus, a VBAC would not be offered to her due to the higher risk of uterine rupture. With two previous c-sections the risk for abnormal implantation of the placenta is about 11% if a placenta previa is present. Evaluation of the placenta by ultrasound is recommended. If abnormal placentation is suspected, the patient should be counseled very carefully on the possible need for blood transfusions and hysterectomy if life-threatening bleeding occurs. Since this patient has had a vaginal delivery and c-sections were performed for nonrecurring events, her likelihood of a successful VBAC may be as high as 60% to 70%.

Helpful Hint: The c-section rate in the United States is about 32%; many of these c-sections are repeat surgeries. Each uterine incision may damage the myometrium and increase the risk of abnormal placentation in subsequent pregnancies. The incidence of placenta accreta has increased from 1 in 4,027 pregnancies in the 1970s to 1 in 533 pregnancies in 2002.[56] Placental abnormalities include placenta previa, placenta accreta, placenta increta and placenta percreta. A placenta previa occurs when the placenta completely covers the cervical os. Vaginal delivery is not recommended since massive hemorrhage may occur. Accreta, increta, and percreta describe various degrees of abnormal implantation into the uterine wall and, in the case of percreta, through the uterus itself to potentially involve pelvic structures such as large pelvic blood vessels. Hysterectomy and in many cases other additional procedures such as bowel resection may be required as lifesaving measures along with blood transfusions. Whether the patient undergoes a cesarean section or wishes to attempt a VBAC, she should undergo meticulous counseling on the possibility of abnormal placentation and treatment needed if this complication is encountered. Each c-section appears to increase the risk for this complication in the next pregnancy. Providers and patients should strive to avoid unnecessary c-sections.

Objectives

1. Identify potential complications associated with an attempted vaginal birth after cesarean section
2. Know risk for abnormal placentation associated with history of previous cesarean section

REFERENCES

1. Landon MB, Gabbe SG. Gestational diabetes mellitus. *Obstet Gynecol*. 2011;118(6):1379–1393.

2. White P. Classification of obstetric diabetes. *Am J Obstet Gynecol*. 1978;130:228–230.

3. American College of Obstetricians and Gynecologists. Ultrasonography in pregnancy. ACOG Practice Bulletin No. 101. *Obstet Gynecol*. 2009;113:451–461.

4. American College of Obstetricians and Gynecologists. Antepartum fetal surveillance. ACOG Practice Bulletin No. 82. *Obstet Gynecol*. 2007;109:1233.

5. Casey BM, Leveno KJ. Thyroid disease in pregnancy. *Obstet Gynecol*. 2006;108:1283–1292.

6. Leung AS, Millar LK, Koonings PP, et al. Perinatal outcome in hypothyroid pregnancies. *Obstet Gynecol*. 1993;81(3):349–353.

7. Haddow JE, Palomaki GE, Allan WC, et al. Maternal thyroid deficiency during pregnancy and subsequent neuropsychological development of the child. *N Engl J Med*. 1999;341(8):549–555.

8. American College of Obstetricians and Gynecologists. Clinical management guidelines for obstetrician-gynecologists. ACOG Practice Bulletin No. 37. Thyroid disease in pregnancy. *Obstet Gynecol*. 2002;100(2):387–396. Reaffirmed 2013.

9. Moise KJ. Management of rhesus alloimmunization in pregnancy. *Obstet Gynecol*. 2002;100:600–611.

10. American College of Obstetricians and Gynecologists. Management of alloimmunization during pregnancy. ACOG Practice Bulletin No. 75. *Obstet Gynecol*. 2006;108(2):457–464. Reaffirmed 2014.

11. Liley AW. Liquor amnii analysis in management of pregnancy complicated by rhesus sensitization. *Am J Obstet Gynecol*. 1961;82:1359–1370.

12. Queenan JT, Thomas PT, Tomai TP, et al. Deviation in amniotic fluid optical density at a wavelength of 450 nm in Rh isoimmunized pregnancies from 14 to 40 weeks gestation. *Am J Obstet Gynecol*. 1993;168(5):1370–1376.

13. Morse K, Williams A, Gardosi J. Fetal growth screening by fundal height measurement. *Best Pract Res Clin Obstet Gynaecol*. 2009;23(6):809–818.

14. Resnick R. Intrauterine growth restriction. *Obstet Gynecol*. 2002;99:490–496.

15. American College of Obstetricians and Gynecologists. Fetal growth restriction. ACOG Practice Bulletin No. 134. *Obstet Gynecol*. 2013;121(5):1122–1133.

16. Centers for Disease Control and Prevention; Workowski KA, Berman SM. Sexually transmitted diseases treatment guidelines. *MMWR Recomm Rep*. 2006;55:1–94.

17. American College of Obstetricians and Gynecologists. Management of herpes in pregnancy. ACOG Practice Bulletin No. 82. *Obstet Gynecol*. 2007;109:1233.

18. Scott LL, Sanchez PJ, Jackson GL, et al. Acyclovir suppression to prevent cesarean delivery after first-episode genital herpes. *Obstet Gynecol*. 1996;87:69–73.

19. American College of Obstetricians and Gynecologists. Invasive prenatal testing for aneuploidy. ACOG Practice Bulletin No. 88. *Obstet Gynecol*. 2007;110:1179–1198.

20. American College of Obstetricians and Gynecologists. Screening for fetal chromosomal abnormalities. ACOG Practice Bulletin No. 77. *Obstet Gynecol*. 2007;109:217–227.

21. American College of Obstetricians and Gynecologists. Noninvasive prenatal testing for fetal aneuploidy. Committee Opinion No. 545. *Obstet Gynecol*. 2012;120:1532–1534.

22. Minkoff H. Human immunodeficiency virus infection in pregnancy. *Obstet Gynecol.* 2003;101:797–810.

23. Guay LA, Musoke P, Fleming T, et al. Intrapartum and neonatal single-dose nevirapine compared with zidovudine for prevention of mother-to-child-transmission (MTCT) of HIV-1 in Kampala, Uganda: HIVNET 012 randomised trial. *Lancet.* 1999;354:795–802.

24. World Health Organization. Consolidated guidelines on the use of antiretroviral drugs for treating and preventing HIV infection: Recommendation for a public health approach. Available online at http://www.who.int/hiv/pub/guidelines/arv2013/download/en/index.html. Accessed June 30, 2013.

25. Aminoff MJ. Neurologic disorders. In: Creasy RK, Resnik R, Iams JD, et al., eds. *Creasy and Resnik's Maternal-Fetal Medicine: Principles and Practice.* 6th ed. Philadelphia, PA: Elsevier Saunders; 2009.

26. Hull AD, Resnick R. Placenta previa, placenta accreta, abruptio placentae, and vasa previa. In: Creasy RK, Resnik R, Iams JD et al., eds. *Creasy and Resnik's Maternal-Fetal Medicine: Principles and Practice.* 6th ed. Philadelphia, PA: Elsevier Saunders; 2009.

27. American College of Obstetricians and Gynecologists. Multiple gestation: Complicated twin, triplet, and high-order multifetal pregnancy. ACOG Practice Bulletin No. 56. *Obstet Gynecol.* 2004;104:869–883.

28. Quintero RA, Morales WJ, Allen MH, et al. Staging of twin-twin transfusion syndrome. *J Perinatol.* 1999;19:550–555.

29. Pathak B, Sheibani S, Lee RH. Cholestasis of pregnancy. *Obstet Gynecol Clin North Am.* 2010;37:269–282.

30. American College of Obstetricians and Gynecologists. Update on carrier screening for cystic fibrosis. Committee Opinion No. 486. *Obstet Gynecol.* 2011;117:1028–1031.

31. American College of Obstetricians and Gynecologists. Carrier screening for fragile X syndrome. Committee Opinion No. 469. *Obstet Gynecol.* 2010;116:1008–1010.

32. American College of Obstetricians and Gynecologists. Chronic hypertension in pregnancy. ACOG Practice Bulletin No. 125. *Obstet Gynecol.* 2012;119:396–407.

33. American College of Obstetricians and Gynecologists. Diagnosis and management of preeclampsia and eclampsia. ACOG Practice Bulletin No. 33. *Obstet Gynecol.* 2002;99:159–167.

34. American College or Obstetricians and Gynecologists. Prediction and prevention of preterm birth. ACOG Practice Bulletin No. 130. *Obstet Gynecol.* 2012;120:964–973.

35. American College of Obstetricians and Gynecologists. Management of preterm labor. ACOG Practice Bulletin No. 127. *Obstet Gynecol.* 2012;119:1308–1317.

36. American College of Obstetricians and Gynecologists. Antenatal corticosteroid therapy for fetal maturation. Committee Opinion No. 475. *Obstet Gynecol.* 2011;117:422–424.

37. Mercer B. Premature rupture of membranes. In: Creasy RK, Resnik R, Iams JD, et al., eds. *Creasy and Resnik's Maternal-Fetal Medicine: Principles and Practice.* 6th ed. Philadelphia, PA: Elsevier Saunders; 2009.

38. Nelson KB, Grether JK. Can magnesium sulfate reduce the risk of cerebral palsy in very-low-birthweight infants? *Pediatrics.* 1995;95:263–269.

39. Rouse DJ, Hirtz DG, Thom E, et al. A randomized, controlled trial of magnesium sulfate for the prevention of cerebral palsy. *N Engl J Med.* 2008;359:895–905.

40. Clark S, Miller D, Belfort M, et al. Neonatal and maternal outcomes associated with elective term delivery. [Electronic Version]. *Am J Obstet Gynecol.* 2009;200(2):156.e1–156.e4.

41. Ramachandrappa A, Jain L. Health issues of the late preterm infant. *Pediatr Clin North Am.* 2009;56(3):565–577.

42. Resnik JL, Resnick R. Post-term pregnancy. In: Creasy RK, Resnik R, Iams JD, et al., eds. *Creasy and Resnik's Maternal-Fetal Medicine: Principles and Practice.* 6th ed. Philadelphia, PA: Elsevier Saunders; 2009.

43. American College of Obstetricians and Gynecologists. Induction of labor. ACOG Practice Bulletin No. 107. *Obstet Gynecol.* 2009;114:386–397.

44. American College of Obstetricians and Gynecologists. Critical care in pregnancy. ACOG Practice Bulletin No. 100. *Obstet Gynecol.* 2009;113:443–450.

45. American College of Obstetricians and Gynecologists. Management of stillbirth. ACOG Practice Bulletin No. 102. *Obstet Gynecol.* 2009;113:748–761.

46. Korteweg FJ, Erwich JJ, Timmer A, et al. Evaluation of 1025 fetal deaths: Proposed diagnostic workup. *Am J Obstet Gynecol.* 2012;206(1):53.e1–53.e12.

47. American College of Obstetricians and Gynecologists. Antiphospholipid syndrome. ACOG Practice Bulletin No. 132. *Obstet Gynecol.* 2012;120:1514–1521.

48. Bates SM, Greer JA, Pabinger I, et al. Venous thromboembolism, thrombophilia, antithrombotic therapy and pregnancy. American College of Chest Physicians Evidence-Based Clinical Practice Guidelines (8th Edition). *Chest.* 2008;133:844S–886S.

49. American College of Obstetricians and Gynecologists. Management of intrapartum fetal heart rate tracings. ACOG Practice Bulletin No. 116. *Obstet Gynecol.* 2012;116:1232–1240.

50. American College of Obstetricians and Gynecologists. Intrapartum fetal heart rate monitoring: Nomenclature, Interpretation, and General Management Principles. ACOG Practice Bulletin No. 106. *Obstet Gynecol.* 2009;114:192–202.

51. Cunningham FG, Leveno KJ, Bloom SL, et al. Critical care and trauma. In: *Wlliams Obstetrics.* 23rd ed. New York: The McGraw-Hill Companies; 2010.

52. Kellman TR, Dobson S. Syphilis. In: Remington JS, Klein JO, Wilson CB, et al., eds. *Infectious Diseases of the Fetus and Newborn Infant.* 7th ed. Philadelphia, PA: Elsevier Saunders; 2010.

53. American College of Obstetricians and Gynecologists. Viral hepatitis in pregnancy. ACOG Practice Bulletin No. 86. *Obstet Gynecol.* 2007;110:941–956.

54. Mast EE, Margolis HS, Fiore AE, et al. A comprehensive immunization strategy to eliminate transmission of hepatitis B virus infection in the United States: recommendations of the Advisory Committee on Immunization Practices (ACIP) part 1: immunization of infants, children, and adolescents. *MMWR Recomm Rep.* 2005;54(RR-16):1–31.

55. American College of Obstetricians and Gynecologists. Vaginal birth after previous cesarean delivery. ACOG Practice Bulletin No. 115. *Obstet Gynecol.* 2010;116:450–463.

56. American College of Obstetricians and Gynecologists. Placenta accreta. Committee Opinion No. 529. *Obstet Gynecol.* 2012;120:207–211.

Chapter 2
NORMAL NEWBORN CARE
Christel Biltoft, MD

CASE 1

You are called to a term vaginal delivery at 39 weeks' gestation because of meconium-stained amniotic fluid. The baby is brought to the warmer apneic with a heart rate of 60 beats per minute. The baby is intubated and suctioned. No meconium is recovered or visualized below the cords. Baby's mouth and nares are suctioned for meconium secretions. The baby grimaces with suctioning. While drying and stimulating the baby, you note that the baby holds its extremities in flexion. The heart rate is still less than 100 bpm. Baby is given positive pressure ventilation (PPV) for 1 minute. The baby's heart rate increases to over 100 bpm. By 3 minutes of life the baby starts to cry and becomes pink. By 5 minutes of life the baby is moving all extremities, cries intermittently, sneezes, and is pink centrally with blue extremities.

According to the latest neonatal resuscitation guidelines, which of the following is NOT an indication for endotracheal tube placement?
A. Initial endotracheal suctioning of nonvigorous meconium-stained newborns
B. If bag-mask ventilation is ineffective or prolonged
C. Baby born with congenital diaphragmatic hernia
D. All meconium-stained newborns

Discussion

The correct answer is **D**. The current 2010 American Heart Association guidelines for cardiopulmonary resuscitation and emergency cardiovascular care recommend endotracheal intubation for initial suctioning of nonvigorous meconium-stained newborns. Endotracheal intubation is no longer recommended for all meconium-stained newborns. Other indications for endotrachial intubation during resuscitation include, if the baby requires chest compressions during resuscitation, if bag-mask ventilation is ineffective, and for special resuscitation circumstances, such as congenital diaphragmatic hernia.[1]

True or False: Neonatal resuscitation should always be initiated with 100% oxygen.
A. True
B. False

Discussion

The correct answer is **B**. Appropriate oxygen administration during neonatal resuscitation is an important consideration since it is now known that excessive oxygenation is not only unnecessary but is actually harmful to the newborn. Recent studies have demonstrated that oxyhemoglobin saturation may normally remain in the 70% to 80% range for several minutes following birth in the healthy term newborn. The current 2010 American Heart Association guidelines for cardiopulmonary resuscitation and emergency cardiovascular care recommend the goal of resuscitation be an oxygen saturation value in the interquartile of the preductal saturations (measured by pulse oximetry) for the specific minute of life after birth of the newborn. It is recommended that these targets be achieved by initiating resuscitation with air or a blended oxygen and titrating the oxygen concentration to the target range. If the baby is bradycardic (heart rate <60 bpm) after 90 seconds of resuscitation, oxygen concentration should be increased to 100% until recovery of a normal heart rate.[1]

Which statement is true regarding the Apgar score?

A. Apgar scores are accurate predictors of specific neurologic outcomes, particularly with regard to cerebral palsy

B. Low Apgar scores at 5 minutes of life are necessary to give a diagnosis of perinatal asphyxia

C. Apgar scores are not affected by gestational age or resuscitation efforts

D. The Apgar score gives useful information about the transition of the baby from intrauterine to extrauterine life and the response to resuscitation

Discussion

The correct answer is **D**. The Apgar score was first established in 1952 by Dr. Virginia Apgar. The scoring system is a simple and efficient way to communicate the status of a newborn at delivery and the response to resuscitation. It is not an accurate predictor of specific neurologic outcome, particularly in the term newborn. While low Apgar scores at 5 minutes of life in a newborn might suggest neurologic compromise, 75% of babies with cerebral palsy had a normal Apgar score at 5 minutes of life.[2] A low Apgar score is neither necessary nor sufficient to make the diagnosis of perinatal asphyxia. Many factors can affect the Apgar score. For example, tone, color, and reflex irritability are all affected by prematurity. Other factors that affect the Apgar score are maternal medications, birth trauma, congenital anomalies, and resuscitation efforts. Resuscitation efforts should not be delayed until the 1-minute Apgar for a baby in distress. While continued Apgar scoring beyond 10 minutes is important during resuscitation efforts, the Apgar score cannot be interpreted the same as a baby with spontaneous respirations. Careful documentation of all resuscitation procedures is needed to accurately assign and interpret Apgar scores.[2,3]

Objectives

1. Understand basic principles of neonatal resuscitation
2. Understand how to generate the Apgar
3. Understand rationale and meaningful use of the Apgar score

CASE 2

You review the prenatal records of a new admission. A baby boy was born via normal standard vaginal delivery (NSVD) at term to a 15-year-old primigravida mother. Her prenatal records are Group B streptococcus (GBS) negative, hepatitis B surface antigen (HBsAg) negative, human immunodeficiency virus (HIV) negative, rubella immune, rapid plasma reagin (RPR) negative, *Neisseria gonorrhoeae* negative, and *Chlamydia trachomatis* positive in the first trimester. The *C. trachomatis* infection was treated and subsequent test of cure was negative.

What is the most appropriate course of action with regard to this baby's risk of neonatal chlamydial infection?

A. Ensure that proper eye prophylaxis with 0.5% erythromycin ointment is applied immediately

B. Start treatment with oral erythromycin

C. Ask the mother's obstetrician if any further testing for *C. trachomatis* was done in the third trimester

D. Test of cure was negative in the first trimester, so you have no concerns at this time

Discussion

The correct answer is **C**. *C. trachomatis* is the most common sexually transmitted disease, especially common in sexually active teenagers.[4] This mother should have been tested again in the third trimester, close to her delivery date because of her increased risk of repeating *C. trachomatis* infection. While topical ophthalmic erythromycin is effective prophylaxis against gonococcal conjunctivitis, it is not as effective in preventing chlamydial conjunctivitis. There is a high rate of neonatal transmission with *C. trachomatis* infection with about 50% of babies born vaginally to a mother with an active *C. trachomatis* infection becoming infected. Conjunctivitis occurs in 25% to 50% of the infected babies and pneumonia in 5% to 20%. Despite the high rate of transmission, prophylactic treatment with oral erythromycin for newborns born to mothers with active *C. trachomatis* infection is not universally recommended.[5] Close follow-up for signs and symptoms for chlamydial disease with prompt treatment as indicated is recommended. Some experts recommend prophylactic treatment if compliance with follow-up cannot be assured.

Which of the following are NOT causes of neonatal ophthalmia?

A. *Staphylococcus aureus*

B. Herpes simplex virus (HSV)

C. Chemical irritant, "sterile" conjunctivitis from prophlylaxis

D. Respiratory syncytial virus

Discussion

The correct answer is **D**. Neonatal ophthalmia is defined as conjunctival infection within the first 4 weeks of life. *C. trachomatis* accounts for about 40% of neonatal conjunctivitis. Gonococcal infection is a more severe infection but only accounts for 1% of cases. The remaining 50% of cases are from a variety of bacteria acquired from the skin, the gastrointestinal tract and the respiratory tract. *S. aureus* is a common cause of nosocomial acquired conjunctivitis, usually acquired in the nursery.[6] Respiratory syncytial virus is not a known pathogen for conjunctivitis. HSV is a rare, but severe cause of neonatal ophthalmia. Chemical or sterile conjunctivitis can be distinguished from an infectious cause by the timing of the presentation. Chemical irritant conjunctivitis occurs hours after birth at the time of contact and improves after 24 to 48 hours of life. Gonococcal conjunctivitis presents between 24 and 48 hours of life. Chlamydial conjunctivitis usually presents in the first 5 to 7 days of life. Prophylaxis with 0.5% of erythromycin ointment applied within 1 hour of delivery is highly effective at preventing bacterial, nonchlamydial conjunctivitis.[6,7]

Which of the following organisms of ophthalmia neonatorum is known to penetrate intact corneal epithelium, resulting in corneal scarring, ocular perforation, and blindness?
A. *N. gonorrhoeae*
B. *C. trachomatis*
C. *S. aureus*
D. Herpes simplex virus

Discussion

The correct answer is **A**. *N. gonorrhoeae* is a gram-negative diplococcus that, if left untreated, can penetrate the corneal epithelium. Since the implementation of universal ocular prophylaxis at birth, blindness due to gonococcal ophthalmia neonatorum has become rare in the United States.[8] All newborns born to a mother with a known gonococcal infection must be given prophylaxis with an intramuscular injection (IM) of ceftriaxone and followed closely for the development of disseminated disease, including ophthalmia neonatorum and meningitis. *C. trachomatis* conjunctivitis is a relatively mild and self-limited disease. It presents with eyelid edema, a papillary conjunctival response and pseudomembrane formation. Repeated and chronic chlamydial eye infection, however, can cause trachoma, a leading cause of blindness in the developing world. *S. aureus* conjunctivitis usually is acquired in the newborn nursery and can lead to abscess formation. Herpes simplex virus is usually associated with vesicular lesions. It can lead to severe herpetic keratitis and keratouveitis.[7]

Objectives

1. Identify common causes of neonatal ophthalmia
2. Understand distinguishing factors in clinical presentation for common causes of neonatal ophthalmia
3. Understand appropriate treatment options for common causes of neonatal ophthalmia

CASE 3

The next baby you examine looks small to you but is vigorous and appears symmetrically grown and has normal amounts of subcutaneous fat. You are in the mother's room and learn that she and the father are from Nepal. They have lived in the United States for 10 years. This is their third child. The father works as a teacher. Both parents have short stature. The birth history is unremarkable: term, NSVD, all prenatal records with normal results. You examine the growth chart: weight 2,400 g (9th percentile) and head circumference 31.5 cm (10th percentile). Examination of the neuromuscular maturity and physical maturity is consistent with a gestation of 39 weeks. The vital signs are HR 145, RR 45, temperature is 36.4°C, and glucose is 55.

What is a correct statement about this newborn with regard to its intrauterine growth?
A. Small for gestational age (SGA)
B. Intrauterine growth retarded (IUGR)
C. Late premature
D. Normal growth

Discussion

The correct answer is **A**. SGA is defined as a birth weight <10th percentile. This baby is just on the borderline of being classified as SGA. The baby's head is also small but of normal size. The head and body are relatively in proportion, thus this baby can be further categorized as symmetrical SGA. The baby may be late premature but with a Ballard examination and approximate gestational age of 37 to 38 weeks, SGA is the better answer. IUGR refers to the baby who did not meet its growth potential in utero. This could be from genetic or environmental factors that affect the fetus or the placenta. IUGR implies pathology and is a risk factor for neonatal morbidity and mortality. SGA is a descriptive term of where the baby plots on a growth chart and does not necessarily imply pathology; the baby may simply be constitutionally small. There is evidence that SGA is a risk factor for morbidity that increases with severity, with the babies born in less than the third percentile (severe SGA) at highest risk.[9–11]

What are some of the common complications with term babies who are born SGA?
A. Poor feeding, low tone, and temperature instability
B. Weight loss, fever, and hypernatremia
C. Jitteriness, sneezing, and yawning
D. Temperature instability, hypoglycemia, and polycythemia

Discussion

The correct answer is **D**. A baby born at term but SGA will likely have normal tone and the neuromuscular maturity needed for easy feeding, but because of low subcutaneous fat stores may have difficulty maintaining its temperature. Hypoglycemia from inadequate glycogen stores is sometimes seen with SGA babies, particularly those who suffer from severe SGA or IUGR with head sparing. Symmetric IUGR is thought to occur early in gestation (e.g., chromosomal defects and first trimester infections), while asymmetric (head sparing) IUGR occurs later in gestation and is more likely to be related to maternal complications of pregnancy (gestational hypertension). The majority of liver glycogen storage also occurs late in gestation. The liver of an asymmetrical IUGR baby may have inadequate glycogen storage for the glucose metabolism demands of the relatively large brain. Babies with asymmetrical IUGR are also at risk for polycythemia secondary to fetal hypoxia that leads to increased erythropoietin production. Polycythemia can contribute to hypoglycemia, hyperbilirubinemia, and necrotizing enterocolitis.[12] The late-premature baby may not have the physiologic maturity to coordinate suck, swallow, and breathing and may have difficulty with feeding. Prematurity is also a risk factor for temperature instability and hypoglycemia. Weight loss, fever, and hypernatremia are all unusual symptoms. Dehydration is a known cause of mild fever, typically in an exclusively breastfed baby. Sepsis or a viral infection such as HSV would need to be considered, as well. Jitteriness, sneezing, and excessive yawning are signs of opiate withdrawal.

A baby whose birthweight is >90th percentile is considered large for gestational age (LGA). These newborns are at risk for polycythemia, hypoglycemia, birth injuries, and respiratory distress at birth. These children should be monitored for neonatal complications.

Which of the following is NOT a mechanism of heat loss in the newborn?
A. Evaporative losses from skin and lungs
B. Radiation of heat away from the baby to cooler distant objects
C. Convection of heat from the skin to the cooler air
D. Conduction of heat from the skin to the cooler air

Discussion

The correct answer is **D**. All babies are susceptible to hypothermia at birth as they emerge wet from the warm intrauterine environment to the much colder extrauterine environment. In addition to this large temperature gradient, babies have a relatively large surface area to body weight. Generation of heat is related to body weight and heat loss is related to surface area. The neonate loses heat by four main mechanisms, listed in order of significance in the typical term delivery: evaporation of water and heat from the large surface area of the skin and the lungs; radiation of heat through electromagnetic radiation in the infrared spectrum from the neonate's skin to the cooler objects nearby but not touching the baby, such as the nursery walls; convection of heat from the skin surface to the cooler air; conduction of heat transferred from the skin to the cooler objects touching the baby, such as the table or blankets.[13] In the usual delivery room situation, a newborn drops its core temperature 2 to 3°C, which corresponds to about 200 kcal/kg.[14] It is critical for a newborn to be dried properly, fitted with a hat and placed skin-to-skin with mother or kept under a radiant warmer. The term baby will respond to cold stress by shunting warm blood to the core via vasoconstriction in dermal arterioles, which also results in an insulating fat layer between the core and the exposed skin. The baby will generate heat by increasing its metabolic rate and by oxidation of brown fat stores. A low–birth-weight or premature baby has limited subcutaneous white fat for insulation and may have limited brown fat for thermogenesis. The maintenance of body heat in a newborn is important because hypothermic stress can cause a cascade of complications, including hypoglycemia, metabolic acidosis, hypoxia, and neurologic depression.[15]

Objectives

1. Understand the differences between SGA, AGA, and LGA
2. Understand specific complications associated with being SGA or AGA that require additional monitoring in the immediate neonatal period
3. Understand basic principles of thermoregulation

CASE 4

The nurse informs you that one of the babies failed its discharge hearing screen. She also tells you that the mother has questions about the newborn blood spot test and discharge screening for heart disease.

What are the current recommendations regarding follow-up for the newborn who fails the newborn hearing screen?
A. Audiology and medical evaluation before 3 months of age
B. If the baby does not have other risk factors for hearing loss, the baby can be watched clinically for signs of hearing impairment
C. Refer the baby for genetic testing
D. Audiology and medical evaluation before 6 months of age

Discussion

The correct answer is **A**. The prevalence of any form of hearing loss is thought to be 1 to 6/1,000 newborns. Hearing loss, even mild forms, is known to cause linguistic and cognitive impairment.[16] If hearing loss is diagnosed and treatment started before 6 months of age, much of the morbidity associated with hearing loss can be prevented. Babies with hearing loss can appear developmentally normal with age appropriate smiling, cooing, and babbling.[17] The current AAP endorsement of the Joint Committee on Infant Hearing Detection recommends: (1) Universal hearing screening at birth and no later than 1 month of age. (2) Follow-up of all failed hearing screening with definitive diagnosis no later than 3 months of age. (3) Interventions as needed no later than 6 months of age for those with confirmed abnormal results.[18] Instructions for follow-up audiological screening should be provided at hospital discharge.

Most newborn hearing screening programs consist of a two-staged approach. First, hearing screening is conducted by evoked otoacoustic emission (OAE) testing, followed by auditory brainstem response (ABR) testing for all newborns who fail the OAE testing. OAE testing detects the generated sounds from the cochlea in the response to clicks and tones. The OAE emissions acoustic signals generated within the cochlea travel in a reverse direction through the middle ear space and tympanic membrane out to the ear canal. The signals are detected with a very sensitive microphone/probe system place in the external ear canal. The OAE tests the peripheral auditory system extending to the outer cochlear hair cells. The ABR detects nerve signals obtained from surface electrodes. The nerve signals are generated in the cochlea, auditory nerve, and brainstem in response to acoustic stimuli delivered via an earphone. The ABR provides information regarding the peripheral auditory system, the eighth nerve, and the brainstem auditory pathway. Accuracy of both hearing testing improves with age as the middle ear fluid clears and with improved tympanic membrane mobility. While parents can be reassured that many failed hearing screenings are not confirmed on further evaluation, it must be emphasized that further evaluation is of critical importance.

True or False: A failed ABR can be retested using OAE hearing screen
A. True
B. False

Discussion

The correct answer is **B**. While a "failed" OAE can be rescreened with ABR and considered a "pass," the reverse is not true. The OAE test does not quantify hearing loss or hearing threshold level, nor does it assess the integrity of the neural transmission of sound from the eighth nerve to the brainstem. A "fail" OAE test only implies hearing loss of more than 30 to 40 dB (the range for mild hearing loss) or that the middle ear status is abnormal. A "failed" ABR implies a hearing level of worse than 40 dB or that the middle ear status is abnormal. A "failed" ABR and "passed" OAE is evidence of auditory neuropathy/dyssynchrony.[18]

True or False: If a newborn has risk factors for hearing loss but passes the newborn hearing screen, no further audiology evaluation is necessary
A. True
B. False

Discussion

The correct answer is **B**. Babies born with known risk factors for progressive or delayed hearing loss, regardless of the newborn hearing screening results, should have continued developmental assessment of hearing and a specific audiology assessment at least once by 24 to 30 months of age.[16]

Which of the following is most commonly found during newborn screening prior to discharge?
A. Hearing loss
B. Primary congenital hypothyroidism
C. Sickle cell hemoglobinopathies
D. Phenylketonuria

Discussion

The correct answer is **A**. Hearing loss is the most common problem screened for with over 5,000 cases identified through newborn hearing screen each year. Detecting hearing loss in the newborn period helps with early intervention and the reduction of morbidity associated with hearing loss, including delayed language acquisition and low educational attainment. Of the 29 different metabolic, endocrine, and hematologic problems screened for by the Newborn Screen blood spots, congenital hypothyroidism is most commonly identified, followed by sickle cell hemoglobinopathies, and cystic fibrosis. Each year, 1 in 2,000 births is diagnosed with congenital hypothyroidism.[19]

What are the current recommendations for screening for congenital heart disease before discharge?
A. Screening should be performed before 24 hours of life
B. A negative screening is defined as one extremity with >95% oxygen saturation
C. Oxygen saturations should be obtained in the right hand and one foot
D. A pulse oximetry screening of <90% saturation should be repeated in 1 hour

Discussion

The correct answer is **C**. The AAP gave a written endorsement for the pulse oximetry screening for critical congenital heart disease in 2012. The current recommendations are for healthy, asymptomatic newborns: Screening should not be performed until 24 hours of life or as late as possible if early discharge is planned. Oxygen saturations should be obtained in the right hand and one foot. A pulse oximetry reading of >95% in either extremity with a <3% absolute difference between the upper and lower extremity would be considered a negative screen, with no further screening recommended. An initial screen between 90% and 95% or >3% difference in upper and lower extremities should be repeated in 1 hour to reduce the number of false-positive screenings. A pulse oximetry reading <90% is a positive screen and should receive immediate evaluation with cardiology consult and echocardiogram.[20,21]

Objectives

1. Understand current recommendations for routine hearing screening in all newborns
2. Understand appropriate follow-up for newborns with an abnormal screening evaluation
3. Understand the differences between different modalities to evaluate hearing status in a newborn
4. Understand current recommendations for pulse oximetry screening in all newborns prior to hospital discharge

CASE 5

You are called to a scheduled, repeat cesarean delivery of a term male infant at 38 weeks' gestation. Mother's prenatal history is significant for mild gestational diabetes that is diet controlled. The baby is delivered apneic but recovers with resuscitation. Apgars are 3 and 7 at 1 and 5 minutes of life. He weighs 4,000 g. One hour later, the nurse calls you to tell you the baby is breathing 70 breaths per minute, but without retractions or nasal flaring and is pink. The pulse oximetry reading is 97% on the left foot. The nurse had already determined that the baby was LGA and had obtained a blood glucose level at birth and just prior to your examination of the baby. The initial blood glucose was 70 mg/dL and the next was 50 mg/dL.

Elective cesarean birth for term and late-preterm infants increases the risk of all of the following, except
A. Pulmonary hypertension
B. Transient tachypnea of the newborn (TTN)
C. Respiratory distress syndrome
D. Polycythemia

Discussion

The correct answer is **D**. There has been a significant increase in cesarean deliveries rates with nearly a third of newborns delivered via cesarean section. The increase of cesarean deliveries has major implications because of the increased morbidity for both mother and newborn. Specifically, elective cesarean delivery is associated with increased risk of respiratory morbidity in the term and the late-preterm newborn, including mild-to-severe TTN, respiratory distress syndrome, and persistent pulmonary hypertension. TTN after elective cesarean delivery accounts for a major portion of term newborn special care and neonatal intensive care unit admissions, which has implications both for the health of the baby but also increased medical costs.[22] The respiratory complications that occur with elective cesarean delivery are thought to be due to truncation of important physiologic processes that occur in the final weeks of gestation and during spontaneous labor. A surge in endogenous steroids and catecholamines occurs late in gestation and during spontaneous labor and vaginal delivery that are important for the final maturation of the lung alveoli and for effective clearance of fetal fluid.[23] The morbidity associated with elective cesarean delivery decreases with advancing gestational age, with the lowest risk among newborns born between 38 and 40 weeks' gestation.[22–26]

Polycythemia is not directly related to cesarean delivery. Acute and chronic fetal hypoxia increases the risk for neonatal polycythemia and hyperviscosity. Fetal hypoxia increases the production of erythropoietin by the fetal kidneys that in turn increases red blood cell mass. Causes of chronic fetal hypoxia include poorly controlled maternal diabetes, fetal hyperthyroidism, maternal smoking, and any cause of intrauterine growth restriction. Perinatal asphyxia is a cause of acute fetal hypoxia, leading to polycythemia. A placental blood transfusion from delayed cord clamping and stripping of the umbilical cord also causes polycythemia and hyperviscosity. Symptoms of polycythemia include ruddiness, hypoglycemia, jitteriness, tachypnea, jaundice, lethargy, and vomiting.[27]

Which of the following is NOT a risk factor for the LGA newborn?
A. Transient hypoglycemia
B. Shoulder dystocia
C. Cesarean delivery
D. Hypothermia

Discussion

The correct answer is **D**. An infant whose birthweight is >90th percentile for gestational age is considered large for gestational age (LGA) and is at risk for multiple complications after birth. The baby born LGA, particularly with documented maternal gestational diabetes mellitus, is at risk for transient hypoglycemia because of a relative hyperinsulinemia. Transient hypoglycemia is defined as hypoglycemia that resolves after 24 hours and up to 7 days after birth. Any hypoglycemia that persists after 24 hours of life should be investigated for a persistent cause such as congenital hyperinsulinism.[28] There is a physiologic decline in blood glucose level at birth that occurs in all newborns as they transition to extrauterine life with the nadir at about 1 hour after birth. The healthy term newborn will then start to compensate with extrauterine adaptations by producing alternative fuels including ketone bodies that are released from fat and by demanding exogenous glucose from feeds. The severity of newborn hypoglycemia that occurs from maternal gestational diabetes is variable, depending on the extent of mother's glycemic control and disease burden. Current recommendations to screen for neonatal hypoglycemia in the asymptomatic, term IDM and LGA infant is to feed by 1 hour of life, test glucose level 30 minutes after first feed and, if within normal range, continue to follow glucose levels before each feed for the first 12 hours of life.[29]

LGA is a risk factor for cesarean delivery and for cephalopelvic disproportion, leading to possible shoulder dystocia if born vaginally. The LGA newborn is not at increased risk for hypothermia, but all newborns are susceptible to heat loss and have limited ways to generate heat.

Objectives

1. Define criteria for diagnosis of large for gestational age (LGA) infant
2. Understand specific risk for complications after delivery for LGA infants
3. Understand delivery complications commonly seen in newborns who are LGA

CASE 6

While examining a baby for discharge, the mother asks you when is the best time to start formula because she has heard that breast milk does not contain enough vitamin D for the baby.

What are the current recommendations for feeding the healthy newborn?
A. Exclusive breastfeeding for 2 months, with continuation of breastfeeding for 6 months
B. Exclusive breastfeeding for 4 months, with continuation of breastfeeding for 9 months
C. Exclusive breast feeding for 6 months, with continuation of breastfeeding for at least 12 months
D. Exclusive breastfeeding for 12 months of age, with continuation of breastfeeding for 24 months

Discussion

The correct answer is **C**. Breastfeeding is the normative standard for human infant feeding. The American Academy of Pediatrics (AAP) recommends exclusive breastfeeding, unless there is a medical contraindication present, until the infant is about 6 months old, followed by introduction of complementary foods at about 6 months of age, while breastfeeding is continued until the baby is at least 12 months old. Breastfeeding can continue beyond 12 months of age as long as it is mutually desired by both the mother and the baby.[30]

Which of the following describes the constituents of human colostrum?
A. High casein/whey ratio, butter fat and volatile fatty acids, lactose, and high phosphorus content
B. High whey/casein ratio, taurine, high fat content, absorbable triglycerides, lactose, high vitamin C content, immunoglobulins (Igs), cytokines, growth factors, lysozyme, and lactoferrin

C. High whey/casein ratio and overall high protein content, high Ig levels and immunologically competent mononuclear cells (leukocytes), and high fat-soluble vitamin and mineral content

D. Demineralized whey protein, lactose and corn syrup, palm oil, and high vitamin D and vitamin K content

Discussion

The correct answer is **C**. After birth, breastfeeding is the continuation of the mother–baby dyad that occurs prenatally via the placenta. In utero, the mother provides the optimal nutrition to support fetal growth and immunologic protection via transplacental transfer of nutrients and immunologic factors. After birth, both of these processes continue via breast milk. Human colostrum has high levels of secretory Ig A that is specific to the mothers environment and, thus, specifically protective for her newborn. There are also high levels of maternal leukocytes (macrophages, T cells, stem cells, and lymphocytes) as well as other infection protective components such as lactoferrin. Colostrum differs from mature human milk by having a higher protein to fat content and a high fat-soluble vitamin and mineral content. As human mature milk matures, there is a higher fat content and a higher water-soluble vitamin content, such as high levels of vitamin C which is an important antioxidant and also enhances the bioavailability of iron and calcium. The immunologic components also change with more IgG and IgM present. Human milk also promotes the development and maturation of the infant's immune system through numerous bioactive components, including cytokines, growth factors, lysozyme, and complex human milk oligosaccharides. In addition to enhancing immunologic development, human milk contains growth factors that have wide-ranging effects on the intestinal tract, vasculature, nervous system, and endocrine system.[31] It is known that breastmilk helps prevent many diseases and preterm complications including infectious diarrhea, otitis media, allergies, and necrotizing enterocolitis (Table 2-1). Cow milk differs from human milk in that it contains a much higher casein/whey ratio and overall too high of a solute content for human infants, specifically with high sodium and phosphorus content. Cow milk has volatile fatty acids thought to cause steatorrhea in human newborns. Cow milk also lacks specific amino acids important for human brain development, such as taurine. Infant cow milk-protein formula is highly modified cow milk and contains corn syrup and palm oil, as well as many vitamins. While it does support infant growth, it does not contain any of the immunologic or other growth factor benefits of breast milk.[31–34]

TABLE 2-1.   Conditions Associated with Not Breastfeeding

Among full-term infants
Acute ear infection (otitis media)
Eczema (atopic dermatitis)
Diarrhea and vomiting (gastrointestinal infection)
Hospitalization for lower respiratory tract diseases in the first year
Asthma
Childhood obesity
Type 2 diabetes mellitus
Acute lymphocytic leukemia
Acute myelogenous leukemia
Sudden infant death syndrome
Among preterm infants
Necrotizing enterocolitis

Adapted with permission from U.S. Department of Heatlh and Human Services. *The Surgeon General's Call to Action to Support Breastfeeding.* Washington, DC: U.S. Department of Heatlh and Human Services, Office of the Surgeon General; 2011.

Which of the following statements is true regarding the current recommendation for vitamin D supplementation?

A. All term and late-preterm newborns need vitamin D supplementation started at birth regardless of feeding method at discharge

B. The health benefit of vitamin D supplementation in formula is superior to breast milk after the colostrum is gone and, thus, formula should be encouraged

C. Vitamin D supplementation is needed for both breast milk and formula fed babies but not until the baby is 1-month old

D. Sunlight exposure is the preferred way for newborns to receive vitamin D, regardless of feeding method

Discussion

The correct answer is **A**. The AAP recommends all term and late-preterm babies be given 400 IU daily of vitamin D supplementation, starting on the day of discharge, regardless of feeding method. While formula does contain adequate vitamin D levels, the baby needs to consume at least 1 L a day to ensure adequate vitamin D intake. The average formula fed baby consumes about 1 L a day of formula at about 1 month of age. The newborn skin is particularly sensitive to the damaging effects of ultraviolet (UV) light in sunlight. Newborn babies should not be placed in direct sunlight. Avoidance of sun at peak UV exposure times, sun protective clothing, hat, and sunglasses are recommended to protect against UV radiation exposure in infancy.[35,36]

Which of the following is NOT a contraindication to breastfeeding in the United States of America?
A. Maternal HIV infection
B. Maternal Hepatitis B infection
C. Maternal cocaine use
D. Maternal statin use

Discussion

The correct answer is **B**. Maternal Hepatitis B infection is not a contraindication to breastfeeding and the mother may begin breastfeeding right from birth. However, the baby must receive the Hepatitis B vaccine and HBIG within 12 hours of life. The mother needs to be educated on the critical importance of her infant completing the Hepatitis B vaccine series at the recommended scheduled intervals. In the developed world, maternal HIV infection is a contraindication to breastfeeding. In the developing world however, maternal HIV is not a contraindication to breastfeeding, as the benefits of breastfeeding outweigh the risks in such circumstances. Other contraindications are illicit drug use, large quantities of alcohol, chemotherapy agents, and statins.[30,37]

Objectives

1. Understand "best practice" guidelines for the initiation of breastfeeding in newborns
2. Identify the constituents of breast milk
3. Understand the contraindications for human milk feeding
4. Understand the use of vitamin D supplementation in the breastfed newborn

CASE 7

The next day, a new mother asks to speak to you regarding circumcision. She heard that the AAP is now recommending universal circumcision. She does not want to circumcise her infant and would like your opinion.

Which response best describes the current AAP policy statement on circumcision?
A. The current AAP policy statement on circumcision states that although the health benefits of circumcision outweigh the potential risks of the procedure, the health benefits are not great enough to recommend routine circumcision for all male newborns

B. The AAP now recommends routine circumcision for all male newborns as a strategy to prevent the spread of HIV in the United States
C. The AAP states that circumcision is effective in preventing some sexually transmitted diseases (STI), including HIV, HSV, syphilis, gonorrhea, and chlamydia
D. The AAP states that circumcision reduces the risk of urinary tract infections (UTIs) in male infants in the first 2 years of life

Discussion

The correct answer is **A**. The current AAP policy on circumcision states that the health benefits of newborn male circumcision outweigh the risks, the procedure's benefits justify access to this procedure for families who choose it, and the procedure warrants third-party reimbursement. Specific benefits of male circumcision stated in the AAP policy statement, include prevention of UTI, penile cancer and transmission of some STIs, specifically HIV. The AAP policy, however, also states that the health benefits are not great enough to recommend routine circumcision for all male newborns. While there is evidence that circumcision reduces the risk of UTIs in the first year of life, the risk of developing a UTI for male infants is about 1%, which translates to 100 circumcisions needed to be performed to prevent one UTI. The benefit of circumcision to prevent UTI is best for those infants at high risk for UTIs, for example, those with urinary tract anomalies. Penile cancer is reduced with circumcision, but penile cancer is a very rare form of cancer, with an incidence of 0.58 cases for 100,000 individuals. Circumcision decreases the risk of heterosexual acquisition of HIV, with the strongest evidence coming from HIV endemic Africa. Circumcision does not reduce the transmission of chlamydia or gonorrhea and there is conflicting data whether it reduces the transmission of syphilis. The AAP emphasizes that parents ultimately should decide whether circumcision is best for their male child.[38,39]

Objectives

1. Understand the current AAP guidelines regarding circumcision
2. Understand risks and benefits of circumcision
3. Understand parental role in decision making prior to circumcision

Helpful Tip: The terms sexually transmitted disease (STD) is often used interchangeably with the term sexually transmitted infection (STI). Use of the term "disease" implies that the person has identifiable symptoms typically associated with the infection. In many cases, patients are asymptomatic yet have documented infection, hence the term sexually transmitted infection.

CASE 8

You are asked to come evaluate the arm of a newborn baby boy. The baby was born to a primigravida mother via vacuum-assisted vaginal birth, at 38 weeks' gestation. The birth weight is 4,025 g. The Apgar scores are 7 and 8. Mother's prenatal labs are all normal. On examination the baby is pink and alert. Head has significant molding. The baby is in a flexed position, except that baby keeps the right arm extended. The baby has an asymmetrical Moro reflex. Right hand grasp is intact. You suspect a brachial plexus injury (BPI) and decide to order a radiograph to confirm that there is not a clavicular fracture.

Which brachial plexus nerves are most commonly injured in a BPI?
A. C5 through T1
B. C5 through C6
C. C5 through C7
D. C8 through T1

Discussion

The correct answer is **B**. Neonatal BPI encompasses a spectrum of injuries involving cervical and upper thoracic nerves (C5 through T1) (Fig. 2-1). The peripheral nerves originating from the plexus innervate the muscle groups of the shoulder, upperarm, forearm, and hand. Traction injury to these nerves can leave varying degrees of paralysis to the affected upper and lower arm and hand. In severe BPIs, the phrenic nerve, comprised of fibers from C3 through C5, and the sympathetic fibers of

T1 are also affected. Injury to the phrenic nerve causes ipsilateral diaphragmatic paralysis and injury to the sympathetic fibers of T1 cause Horner syndrome (ipsilateral miosis, partial ptosis, and anhidrosis).

BPI occurs in approximately 1.5 in 1,000 live births.[40] Shoulder dystocia of a macrosomic newborn is the most common antecedent scenario for BPIs. Shoulder dystocia occurs when the shoulder (usually the anterior shoulder) is impacted against the pubic symphysis of the mother. It is important to note the majority of infants with a history of shoulder dystocia do not have BPIs. Although macrosomia is a risk factor for shoulder dystocia, most macrosomic babies do not have a history of shoulder dystocia. About 26% to 64% of babies born with a BPI have a history of shoulder dystocia. The etiology of BPI is multifactorial with intrauterine position and mechanical forces during labor implicated as potential causes of BPI. Risk factors for BPI are macrosomia, multiparous pregnancies, previous deliveries resulting in BPP, prolonged labor, breech delivery, assisted delivery (vacuum or forceps), cephalopelvic disproportion, gestational diabetes, and shoulder dystocia.[41] BPI can present with a range of severity from minimal stretching of the nerves to complete avulsion of the nerves from the spinal cord.

Injury to the upper trunk of the plexus, C5 through C6, accounts for 50% of BPIs.[42] This injury is called classic Erb palsy. The shoulder muscles for abduction and external rotation are weakened; the infant keeps the affected arm, thus, adducted and internally rotated. The elbow is held in extension and pronation. If C5 through C7 are involved, the hand will also be weakened. The newborn will keep the shoulder adducted and internally rotated; the elbow will be extended and pronated. The wrist and fingers will be kept in slight extension, resulting in the clinical appearance is of a "waiters tip." Injury to the lower trunk of the plexus, C8 through T1, is known as Klumpke palsy and is rare, accounting for 1% of cases. Total plexus injury accounts for about 10%, results in a flail arm. Bilateral injury occurs in 10% to 20% of cases, usually as a result of breech delivery.

Once injury to the brachial plexus is suspected, it is important to perform a thorough neurological examination to accurately describe the extent of the injury. The diagnostic sign for any BPI is an asymmetrical Moro reflex. In Erb palsy, the Moro and tonic neck clonic reflexes are asymmetric, the biceps reflex is absent, but the hand grasp is present. In Klumpke palsy, the biceps reflex is present, but the hand grasp reflex is absent. A flaccid arm without any reflexes throughout indicates total plexus injury. The infant should be examined closely for asymmetrical respiratory movements or respiratory distress that would indicate possible phrenic nerve injury. Signs for Horner syndrome should be

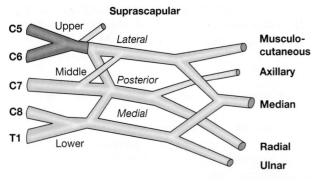

FIGURE 2-1. A simplified schematic diagram of the brachial plexus shows the spinal nerves from which it normally arises, the trunks (upper, middle, and lower), cords (lateral, posterior, and medial), and the major nerves of the forearm and shoulder. The shaded area, including the C5 and C6 spinal nerves and the upper trunk, signifies the portion of the plexus affected in the most common pattern of injury, Erb palsy. (Reproduced with permission from Piatt JH Jr. Birth injuries of the brachial plexus. *Clin Perinatol.* 2005;32(1):39–59.)

carefully assessed. The sympathetic nerve runs along the proximal T1 nerve root and involvement with the sympathetic nerve is a strong indicator of nerve avulsion. Torticollis can be present and may lead to plagiocephaly.

Management of an infant who has a BPI requires gentle handling of the affected limb to avoid additional trauma. The shoulder should be supported when picking up the baby; swaddling the baby before picking up is helpful. Radiographs to rule out fracture of the clavicle or humerus are indicated. Infants should be referred for physical therapy beginning 7 to 10 days after birth.

The prognosis for spontaneous recovery depends on the severity of the injury. Injury can be very severe from complete avulsion of the nerve root from the spinal cord, axonal rupture with or without disruption of the nerve sheath, or stretch injury to the nerve sheath alone. The most common injury is neuropraxia which involves stretch injury to the nerve sheath. Neuropraxia to the upper trunk only, C5 through C7, will spontaneous recover in approximately 75% to 90% of cases. Infants that do not recover spontaneously from a BPI are at risk for developing bony deformities and joint contractures, in addition to functional limitations.[43] Onset of recovery within 2 to 4 weeks of the injury is a favorable prognostic sign. Referral to a center specialized in BPI is indicated for those with severe injury and delayed recovery of function.

Which of the following is NOT associated with BPI?
A. Torticollis
B. Facial nerve injuries
C. Laryngeal nerve injuries
D. Fractures of clavicle and humerus
E. All of the above are associated with BPI

Discussion

The correct answer is **E**. Torticollis, facial nerve paralysis, laryngeal nerve injures, and fractures of clavicle and humerus are all known birth injuries. The mechanisms of injury (e.g., abnormal intrauterine posture, prolonged labor, and instrument-assisted delivery) can be similar and thus more than one injury is a common finding. Torticollis from sternocleidomastoid muscle contracture and a pain response by turning away from the injured shoulder are rather common findings in BPI. If not noticed and managed properly it can lead to plagiocephaly. Radiographs need to be obtained to assess for fractures in all infants with BPI. Traumatic facial nerve injuries are relatively common in the perinatal period, with or without associated BPI. Laryngeal nerve injury is usually from abnormal intrauterine posture and can affect swallowing or breathing (e.g., stridor). Laryngeal nerve injury is associated with both BPI and facial nerve paralysis.[44,45]

Which of the following is NOT on the differential diagnosis for facial paralysis?
A. Hypoxic ischemic encephalopathy
B. Mobius syndrome
C. Hypoplasia of the depressor anguli oris muscle
D. Down syndrome

Discussion

The correct answer is **D**. Facial nerve paralysis is a fairly common birth injury. While forceps-assisted delivery is a known risk factor for facial nerve palsy, most affected infants do not have a history of forceps delivery. Intrauterine pressure on the facial nerve by the sacral promontory is a likely mechanism for compression of the peripheral portion of the seventh nerve as it exits the stylomastoid foramen. This is further supported by the fact that the majority of facial nerve palsies are left sided and the most usual intrauterine position is left occiput anterior. The prognosis is good with spontaneous full recovery usually by 2 weeks of age.[44]

Peripheral facial nerve injury will involve the upper and lower face. The infant will have the following deficits on the ipsilateral side: unable to wrinkle the forehead while crying, inability to completely close the eye, the nasolabial fold will be flattened, and the mouth will be pulled to the unaffected side during crying. Other signs of external trauma such as lacerations and bruising may be present. Central lesions such as in hypoxic ischemic encephalopathy and intracranial contusions will not involve the upper face and frequently have other intracranial signs and symptoms. Mobius syndrome usually presents with bilateral facial weakness from hypoplasia of the seventh nerve nucleus. It is also associated with paralysis of the abducens nerve. Infants with congenital hypoplasia of the depressor anguli oris muscle will have an asymmetrical cry but no flattening of the nasolabial fold, abnormal eye closing, or forehead involvement. It is associated with other anomalies, specifically heart defects. Down syndrome is not more commonly associated with facial nerve paralysis.[44,45]

The next day at about 24 hours of life, you notice a well-circumscribed soft mass at the right parietal skull of the newborn. It does not cross the sagittal suture.

What is the best diagnosis for the described soft tissue injury?
A. Caput succedaneum
B. Cephalohematoma
C. Subgaleal bleed
D. Displaced skull fracture

Discussion

The correct answer is **B**. The baby has likely acquired a cephalohematoma from the vacuum-assisted delivery. Caput succedaneum occurs from serosanguinous fluid collecting above the periosteum. The caput succedaneum crosses the midline and suture lines. It is usually located on the occiput at the presenting part of the fetal cranium during delivery. They are present from birth and resolve quickly over the next 24 to 48 hours without any further complications. The cephalohematoma is a hematoma that forms from rupture of blood vessels between the skull and the periosteum. The cephalohematoma usually develops over 12 to 24 hours after birth and are usually located on the parietal skull. The slow resorption of the hematoma over the next days to weeks can lead to complications of hyperbilirubinemia. Most cephalohematomas resolve completely in 3 to 4 weeks, but some will persist due to ossification that may not resolve for 3 to 6 months. Rarely the ossification will require surgical excision. About 5% of cephalohematomas are associated with an asymptomatic linear skull fractures. Risk factors for cephalohematomas are instrument-assisted delivery and prolonged rupture of membranes.[46]

The subgaleal hemorrhage is often associated with a history of an instrument-assisted deliver, especially multiple attempts at vacuum-assisted delivery. The vacuum trauma can cause skull fracture and rupture of the emissary veins that bridge the subdural and subgaleal spaces. The bleeding into this potential space can cause hypovolemic shock. Like the developing cephalohematoma, the subgaleal hemorrhage enlarges over 12 to 24 hours after birth. Unlike the cephalohematoma, the subgaleal hemorrhage mass is fluctuant and crosses suture lines. It is usually gravity dependent and shifts with changing position. A fluid wave may be present.[47]

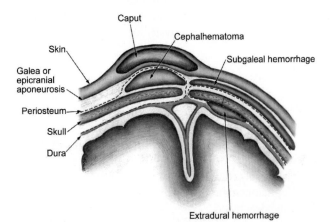

FIGURE 2-2. Location of Caput, Cephalohematoma and Subgaleal Hemorrhage in newborn.

Objectives

1. Identify the different types of brachial plexus injury
2. Identify risk factors associated with brachial plexus injury in the newborn
3. Identify factors that affect prognosis in newborns with brachial plexus injury
4. Differentiate between a caput, cephalohematoma, and subgaleal hemorrhage
5. Explain the natural history of a caput, cephalohematoma, and subgaleal hemorrhage

CASE 9

You are called to a delivery of a 25-year-old primigravida mother who desires a "natural birth." She hands you her birthing plan and states that she wants nothing but exclusive breastfeeding for her baby. She does not want vitamin K given via intramuscular injection (IM), but requests oral vitamin K to be given. She also requests that no erythromycin eye ointment be applied or hepatitis B vaccine be given. You review her prenatal records. She has had no prenatal complications. She has no chronic illnesses and does not take any medications. Her membranes ruptured at home 10 hours ago. Her prenatal labs are GBS negative, Hepatitis B negative, HIV negative, rubella immune, RPR negative, and GC/Chl negative. She is at term at 39 weeks' gestation. The baby boy is born vigorous and crying. You assign Apgar scores of 9 and 9. He weighs 3,400 g. You give the baby to mother who latches and starts breastfeeding immediately. Mother seems exhausted but happy and father is thrilled.

Vitamin K given at birth helps prevent all of the following, except

A. Cephalohematoma and intra-abdominal bleeding at birth in a baby born to a mother taking carbamazepine
B. Melanotic stools in the first few days after birth and bleeding from the circumcision site in an exclusively breastfeed baby with insufficient milk intake
C. Intracranial bleed at 1 month of age in an otherwise well exclusively breastfed baby
D. Rickets in the African-American exclusively breastfed baby

Discussion

The correct answer is **D**. Vitamin K is an important factor for normal clotting. Newborns are all born with low vitamin K stores because there is limited transplacental transfer of vitamin K, and vitamin K has a short half-life, about 17 hours. The stores a baby gets become depleted quickly. Breast milk does not contain much vitamin K, making exclusively breastfed babies particularly vulnerable to vitamin K deficiency. Although vitamin K deficiency bleeding (VKDB), once called hemorrhagic disease of the Newborn, is not common in an otherwise healthy baby without major risk factors, such as gestation less than 33 weeks or a mother taking vitamin K inhibiting drugs, when it occurs, the morbidity and mortality are high. There are three types of VKDB: (1) Early VKDB occurs during the first 24 hours of life and is usually due to a mother taking medications that inhibit vitamin K, such as antiepileptics. Drugs leading to early VKBD are carbamazepine, phenytoin, barbiturates, isoniazid, rifampicin, cephalosporins, and warfarin.[42] The bleeding can be severe, including large cephalohematoma, intra-abdominal bleeding, and intracranial bleeds. (2) Classic VKBD occurs in the first week of life and tends to not be as severe. Classic VKBD is thought to be due to insufficient feeding. The clinical signs include dark melanotic stools, nose bleeds, bloody vomit, and bleeding from the circumcision site and umbilical stump. The incidence of VKDB in the first week of life is reported to be 0.25% to 1.7%.[43] (3) Late VKDB occurs in infants 2 to 12 weeks after birth and occurs in exclusively breastfed infants who have received no or inadequate vitamin K prophylaxis and in babies with malabsorptive diseases such as cystic fibrosis and biliary atresia. Late VKDB presents with severe bleeding, 50% with intracranial bleeding and a 20% mortality rate. The rate of late VKDB is 4.4 to 7.2 per 100,000 births.[48–50]

Prophylaxis with IM injection of 1 mg of vitamin K given at birth is effective in preventing all forms of VKDB and has been the standard of care since 1961 in the United States. A single dose of 1 mg of oral vitamin K will prevent classic VKDB but not late VKBD. Special consideration needs to be taken into the optimal dosing regimens and duration of oral vitamin K to prevent late VKBD. Currently in the United States, no oral vitamin K preparation is licensed for neonatal prophylaxis.[50,51] Babies who are given greater than 50% of feedings from formula receive sufficient amounts of oral vitamin K and may not need supplementation.

What is the current viewpoint of the AAP regarding the controversy of IM vitamin K prophylaxis and childhood cancer risk?

A. In a revised policy statement made in 2003, AAP continued to recommend the 1 mg IM injection of vitamin K at birth. Vitamin K prophylaxis is known to prevent life-threatening disease and the likelihood of increased risk of childhood cancer from vitamin K prophylaxis is unproven and unlikely

B. There has been no increased risk of childhood cancer since the first use of IM vitamin K prophylaxis in 1961. Regardless, the AAP recommends oral administration of vitamin K, 2 mg at birth and 1 mg at weeks 1 and 4 for all babies

C. Childhood leukemia rates have increased significantly since the standard practice of IM vitamin K use, prompting many countries to adopt oral vitamin K prophylaxis

D. In a revised policy statement made in 2003, AAP recommends either the single administration of 1 mg IM injection of vitamin K at birth or a single oral administration of 2 mg of vitamin K for the prevention of leukemia

Discussion

The correct answer is **A**. The AAP recommends that all newborns received a single IM dose of 0.5 to 1 mg of vitamin K. Vitamin K prophylaxis is known to prevent life-threatening disease and the likelihood of increased risk of childhood cancer from vitamin K prophylaxis is unproven and unlikely. The AAP does support further research and development of an oral formulation that is licensed for use in the United States.[49]

Objectives

1. Understand the clinical presentation of vitamin K deficiency bleeding (VKDB) in the newborn
2. Identify risk factors associated with an increased risk of VKDB
3. Understand AAP recommendations for vitamin K supplementation in the newborn
4. Identify medications commonly associated with vitamin K deficiency

CASE 10

On the day of discharge, a baby has lost 6% of his body weight and has a transcutaneous bilirubin level of 8 at 42 hours of life. You review the mother's prenatal records and confirm that the mother's blood type is A+. The baby was born term to a primigravida mother via NSVD and all prenatal labs were normal. The baby is being exclusively breastfed. The baby has passed stool three times and urinated five times since birth. On examination the baby is slightly fussy but consoles easily by sucking on your finger. The mother says she has been putting the baby to the breast every 2 hours and that she is exhausted. She reports that the baby seems to latch on easily but that her nipples are sore and tender from such frequent feeding. The mother starts to cry and asks you if she's doing something wrong. The rest of the examination of the baby appears normal except for jaundice in the face and upper chest, the legs and abdomen are of normal color.

What is the most likely cause of this baby's jaundice?
A. Breastfeeding insufficient milk jaundice
B. Breast milk jaundice
C. Normal physiologic jaundice
D. ABO incompatibility hemolysis

Discussion

The correct answer is **C**. Jaundice is very common, 60% of all term newborns and 80% of all preterm newborns will have jaundice. The fact that so many babies become jaundiced speaks to the fact that the newborn is still transitioning to extrauterine life for days to weeks after birth. Newborn babies become jaundiced within the first few days of life because of increased production of unconjugated bilirubin and a limited ability to conjugate and excrete it. Unconjugated bilirubin comes from the degradation of heme, mostly from hemoglobin that is released during the breakdown of senescent or hemolyzed red blood cells. Newborns have an elevated hematocrit level and increased red blood cell volume per body weight. In addition, the fetal red blood cells have a shorter half-life, leading to a fast turnover of a large amount of hemoglobin. Heme is degraded by the enzyme heme oxygenase. Biliverdin, carbon monoxide, and iron are released in this process. Biliverdin is then converted to the lipophilic molecule unconjugated bilirubin via bilirubin reductase. The unconjugated bilirubin is then transported in the blood bound to albumin to the liver for conjugation to a water-soluble state for excretion.[52]

Unconjugated bilirubin is a lipophilic molecule that, during fetal life, crosses the lipid membranes of the placenta for maternal hepatic conjugation and excretion. Once the baby is born, the baby must rely on its own liver conjugation system to convert unconjugated bilirubin to the water-soluble form of bilirubin, a process that is not fully functioning for the first few days after birth. The process of eliminating bilirubin begins by transporting unconjugated bilirubin bound to albumin to the liver. In the liver, bilirubin is conjugated with glucuronic acid by the enzymes uridine diphosphate and monophosphate glucuronosyltransferase to make the water-soluble molecules monoglucuronide and diglucuronide. These bilirubin glucuronides are then eliminated in the bile.[52] The glucuronosyltransferase enzymes are only at 1% of adult levels at birth but reaches adult levels by 2 weeks of life.[53] In addition to the immature liver enzyme activity, glucuronidase enzymes present in bacteria in the gut deconjugate the bilirubin glucuronides back to the lipophilic state for enterohepatic circulation. The increased production of unconjugated bilirubin, the limited ability for liver conjugation, plus the enterohepatic circulation of bilirubin leads to the common finding of physiologic jaundice of the newborn. Physiologic jaundice is not visible before 24 hours of life, peaks on day 4 of life in a term newborn and declines slowly over the next week or two. This process can be exacerbated if the baby is not taking sufficient feeds and is not passing stool, as in some exclusively breastfed babies who are not getting sufficient quantities of breast milk. There are poorly understood properties of breast milk that are thought to inhibit conjugation that and perhaps slow gut motility that can cause exclusively breastfed newborn to have prolonged jaundice up to 3 weeks of age.[54] These babies are otherwise thriving. Any baby that remains jaundiced at 3 weeks of age warrants further investigation of the etiology of the jaundice.

You discuss the physiology of jaundice in the newborn and relay her fears that she is doing something wrong.

What is the recommended time frame for follow-up with this newborn?
A. Within 48 hours
B. In 1 week
C. In 2 weeks
D. At 1 month of age

Discussion

The correct answer is **A**. The AAP recommends that all term newborn babies be examined in the first few days after discharge to assess infant well-being and the presence or absence of jaundice. Timing of the follow-up visit is based on risk factors for developing hyperbilirubinemia and other criteria. Nomograms based on gestational age, hour of age, and serum bilirubin level have been established by the AAP and Center for Disease Control to help determine the risk of developing hyperbilirubinemia. For a term baby, without additional risk factors, discharged before between 24 and 47.9 hours of life, the AAP guidelines recommend that the baby be re-evaluated by 96 hours of age. The AAP does not recommend that late-preterm babies be discharged before 48 hours of life. Follow-up for all late-preterm newborns should be within 2 days.[55,56]

Which one factor below is NOT a risk factor for severe hyperbilirubinemia?
A. Exclusively breastfed
B. European descent
C. Sibling with history of hyperbilirubinemia
D. Born at 36 weeks' gestation

Discussion

The correct answer is **B**. European descent is not a known risk factor for hyperbilirubinemia, but babies of Asian descent are at increased risk for hyperbilirubinemia. Exclusive breastfeeding, late-preterm delivery, sibling with history of hyperbilirubinemia, and ABO incompatibilities are all risk factors for severe hyperbilirubinemia.[57]

Is it appropriate for you to encourage the father to give formula feeds at this time?
A. Yes, the baby shows signs of dehydration and requires formula supplementation
B. Yes, formula feeds will help this mother rest, and there is no evidence that bottle feeds within the first days of life impedes breastfeeding
C. No, this baby is not showing any abnormal signs of dehydration or insufficient intake at this time. However, a detailed history from the mother should be taken and a physical examination of mother's breasts and of the latch of the baby on the breast should be performed to assess that the feeds are progressing as they should. Ongoing breastfeeding support is needed
D. No. There are no abnormal signs of dehydration. Breast soreness and feeling tired are normal. No intervention or follow-up is needed at this time

Discussion

The correct answer is **C**. Unless medically necessary, it is not recommended to introduce bottle feeds of any kind to an otherwise healthy term baby before breastfeeding is fully established, at approximately 2 weeks after birth. It is important to take a detailed history and physical examination of mother's breast and baby before discharging an exclusively breastfed baby to ensure that the feedings are progressing properly. The history should include: (1) Mother's medical history, such as a history of breast surgery or hypothyroid disease. (2) Obstetric history, such as hemorrhage that could indicate Sheehan syndrome. (3) Mother's current medications. Examine mother's breasts for fullness and the ability to express colostrum. Ask her if she notice changes in her breasts during pregnancy. Encourage the mother by telling her that breast changes during pregnancy indicate that her body has been preparing for breastfeeding. In the first half of pregnancy the ductal tree in the breast tissue proliferates and more lobules form. In the second half of pregnancy, the alveoli get distended from accumulating colostrum.[33] Examine the nipple to look for shapes that may impact breastfeeding, such as inverted or retractile nipples. See if the nipples look bruised or misshapen from improper latch. Ask to watch a feed to assess latch and listen for swallows. Order a lactation consult before discharge to get help with complicated situations such as inverted nipples or to provide ongoing support in the hospital and to arrange for timely and supportive breastfeeding outpatient follow-up.[30]

While breastfeeding is not a major factor in the initial colostrum production, ongoing lactogenesis is directly linked to the baby suckling at the breast and the emptying of the milk ducts. Prolactin is the active hormone in the activation of mammary glands to produce breast milk. Once the placenta is delivered, the inhibitory hormones of progesterone and estrogen levels drop and the anterior pituitary increases prolactin levels. Suckling on the areola activates nerve endings to send signals to the posterior pituitary for the release of oxytocin. Oxytocin causes the myoepithelial cells surrounding the milk-filled alveoli to contract, allowing for the milk letdown reflex to occur.[33] To establish breastfeeding, 8 to 12 feeds every 24 hours are necessary. It is common for the mother's nipples to become sore from such frequent feedings, which is why it is imperative that meticulous attention be given to the baby's latch. Giving unnecessary formula feeds can interfere with establishing breast milk production and from establishing the proper breastfeeding latch techniques. Giving formula without a medical indication may unnecessarily cause undesirable effects such as changes in the gut flora and impeding the transfer of immunologically active factors present in breast milk. The father has an active and important role in helping establish and support breastfeeding. He can ensure that mother eats and drinks properly and that she has easy access to healthy food and drink choices. He can be responsible for holding, changing, and dressing the baby—events that also occur on a frequently recurring basis. He can be responsible for daily household chores so that mother can rest and recuperate when the baby is sleeping.

Which is NOT an indication of a baby at risk for insufficient feedings from unsuccessful breastfeeds?
A. 10% weight loss at 48 hours of life
B. One stool and one urine since birth at 60 hours of life
C. Lethargic, sleepy baby with dry mucous membranes
D. A baby that demands feeds 12 times a day

Discussion

The correct answer is **D**. In the healthy, normal pregnancy, the body is primed and ready for breastfeeding as soon as the baby is born. For the first hour after birth, the baby is quiet and alert; this time is known as the "golden hour." The healthy term baby, if given to mother right away, will frequently latch and suckle successfully and should be allowed to do so. After the "golden hour," the baby and mother frequently become drowsy. It is not uncommon for the baby to not eat much after the "golden hour" in the first 12 hours of life. This sleepiness and seeming disinterest in eating can be anxiety provoking for parents and healthcare staff members. Most healthy, term babies have sufficient glycogen stores to keep glucose levels in a normal range. Random glucose monitoring is not necessary for healthy, term infants. Careful attention needs to be taken in the birth history to rule out risk factors that may cause the baby to be at risk for illness. The vital signs need to be monitored to also help detect illness in the baby. After the sleepy phase, the baby will then feed very often, frequently in a cluster for the next 24 to 48 hours of life. It is normal and necessary for a baby to feed 8 to 12 times a day from the breast to establish adequate breast milk production and to provide sufficient breast milk intake for the infant. Urine and stool output are important determinates in the adequacy of breast feeds, particularly after the first 24 hours of life. Over 95% of babies will urinate within the first 24 hours of life and over 95% will have passage of at least one meconium stool within in 48 hours of life, regardless of feeding method. Ongoing and increasing numbers of stools and urine suggest adequate intake. At 3 to 5 days of life the baby should have at least 3 to 5 urine diapers a day and 3 to 4 stools a day.[58–60] No red urate crystal urine should be seen after the third day, and the stool should be transitional and lighter in color after the third day of life. Babies should not lose more than 7% of its birth weight at 3 days of life.[30] Before discharge, the breastfeeding needs to be observed by a trained staff member to assess for proper latch, evidence of breast changes, milk production via relative ease of manual expression of colostrum, and milk transfer by listening for audible swallows. Many babies are discharged before some of these events can be assessed fully, making educating the parents and establishing close outpatient follow-up essential to the discharge process.

Objectives

1. Understand common causes of hyperbilirubinemia in the newborn
2. Understand the difference between physiologic jaundice and abnormal bilirubin production
3. Understand the relationship between feeding, fluid, and electrolyte balance and risk for hyperbilirubinemia
4. Understand normal bilirubin production in the newborn
5. Identify clinical factors associated with and increased risk of developing hyperbilirubinemia

CASE 11

A mother comes to the emergency room in labor at 35 weeks' gestation and delivers immediately. Intrapartum antibiotics are not administered. She is from out-of-state and does not have a copy of her prenatal records. She denies any known abnormalities with her prenatal records but admits that she did not go very often. The baby is vigorous and crying. Apgar scores of 8 and 8 are given. The baby weighs 2,500 g and has the appearance of a late-premature infant. Mother reports her "water broke" a few hours ago. Hepatitis B vaccine is given. Vitamin K prophylaxis and erythromycin ointment is applied. STAT prenatal labs are obtained from the mother.

What is the recommended clinical management of the well-appearing late-preterm newborn whose mothers received inadequate GBS prophylaxis?

A. Well-appearing infants do not routinely require further diagnostic evaluation or special observation
B. Well-appearing infants born less than 37 weeks' gestation whose mothers did not received adequate intrapartum GBS prophylaxis do not routinely require further diagnostic evaluation, but should be observed for ≥48 hours
C. All newborns born less than 37 weeks' gestation, regardless of intrapartum antibiotic use, should undergo full diagnostic evaluation and treatment pending cultures results with observation for ≥48 hours
D. Well-appearing infants born less than 37 weeks' gestation without adequate intrapartum GBS prophylaxis should undergo limited evaluation and observation for ≥48 hours

Discussion

The correct answer is **D**. Universal screening for GBS colonization at 35 to 37 weeks' gestation and intrapartum prophylaxis has been highly successful in reducing the burden of neonatal GBS disease. Nonetheless, GBS infection is still the leading cause of early-onset sepsis in the newborn period. Early-onset GBS disease is defined as occurring in the first week of life. While neonatal GBS disease rates are down substantially, maternal colonization rates are stable, indicating the ongoing need for careful assessment of GBS risk factors before and during labor. Babies born with clinical signs of neonatal sepsis or whose mothers have signs of chorioamnionitis are at particularly high risk for GBS infection and require immediate treatment and a thorough evaluation. Babies who appear vigorous and healthy and whose mothers appear well may still be at risk for GBS disease. The Center for Disease Control and Prevention (CDC) has specific diagnostic and observation guidelines for the well-appearing newborn born with GBS risk factors (Fig. 2-3).[61] Maternal colonization with GBS is the primary risk factor for early-onset GBS disease. Risk factors

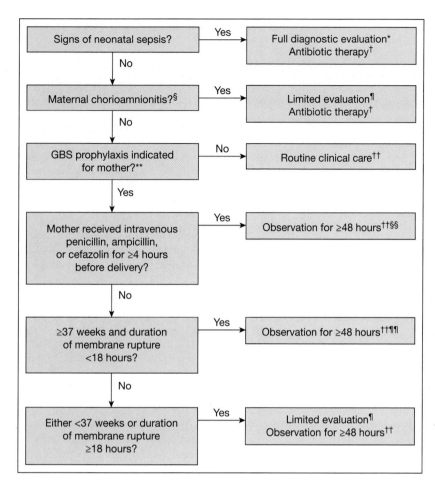

* Full diagnostic evaluation includes a blood culture, a complete blood count (CBC) including white blood cell differential and platelet counts, chest radiograph (if respiratory abnormalities are present), and lumbar puncture (if patient is stable enough to tolerate procedure and sepsis is suspected).

† Antibiotic therapy should be directed toward the most common causes of neonatal sepsis, including intravenous ampicillin for GBS and coverage for other organisms (including *Escherihia coli* and other gram-negative pathogens) and should take into account local antibiotic resistance patterns.

§ Consultation with obstetric providers is important to determine the level of clinical suspicion for chorioamnionitis. Chorioamnionitis is diagnosed clinically and some of the signs are nonspecific.

¶ Limited evaluation includes blood culture (at birth) and CBC with differential and platelets (at birth and/or at 6–12 hours of life).

** See table 3 for indications for intrapartum GBS prophylaxis.

†† If signs of sepsis develop, a full diagnostic evaluation should be conducted and antibiotic therapy initiated.

§§ If ≥37 week's gestation, observation may occur at home after 24 hours if other discharge criteria have been met, access to medical care is readily available, and a person who is able to comply fully with instructions for home observation will be present. If any of these conditions is not met, the infant should be observed in the hospital for at least 48 hours and until discharge criteria are achieved.

¶¶ Some experts recommend a CBC with differential and platelets at age 6–12 hours.

FIGURE 2-3.   Algorithm for secondary prevention of early-onset group B streptococcal (GBS) disease among newborns. (Reproduced with permission from Verani JR, McGee L, Schrag SJ, et al. Prevention of perinatal group B streptococcal disease—revised guidelines from CDC, 2010. *MMWR Recomm Rep.* 2010;59(RR-10):1–36.)

TABLE 2-2. Indications and Nonindications for Intrapartum Antibiotic Prophylaxis to Prevent Early-Onset Group B Streptococcal (GBS) Disease

INTRAPARTUM GBS PROPHYLAXIS INDICATED	INTRAPARTUM GBS PROPHYLAXIS NOT INDICATED

• Previous infant with invasive GBS disease
• GBS bacteriuria during any trimester of the current pregnancy[a]
• Positive GBS vaginal–rectal screening culture in late gestation[b] during current pregnancy[a]
• Unknown GBS status at the onset of labor (culture not done, incomplete, or results unknown) and any of the following:
  • Delivery at <37 weeks' gestation[c]
  • Amniotic membrane rupture ≥18 hours
  • Intrapartum temperature ≥100.4°F (≥38.0°C)
  • Intrapartum NAAT[d] positive for GBS
	• Colonization with GBS during a previous pregnancy (unless an indication for GBS prophylaxis is present for current pregnancy)
	• GBS bacteriuria during previous pregnancy (unless an indication for GBS prophylaxis is present for current pregnancy)
	• Negative vaginal and rectal GBS screening culture in late gestation[b] during the current pregnancy, regardless of intrapartum risk factors
	• Cesarean delivery performed before onset of labor on a woman with intact amniotic membranes, regardless of GBS colonization status or gestational age

NAAT, nucleic acid amplification tests.

[a]Intrapartum antibiotic prophylaxis is not indicated in this circumstance if a cesarean delivery is performed before onset of labor on a woman with intact amniotic membranes.

[b]Optimal timing for prenatal GBS screening is at 35–37 weeks' gestation.

[c]If amnionitis is suspected, broad-spectrum antibiotic therapy that includes an agent known to be active against GBS should replace GBS prophylaxis.

[d]NAAT testing for GBS is optional and might not be available in all settings. If intrapartum NAAT is negative GBS but any other intrapartum risk factor (delivery at <37 weeks' gestation, amniotic membrane rupture at ≥18 hours, or temperature ≥100.4°F [≥38.0°C]) is present, then intrapartum antibiotic prophylaxis is indicated.

Reproduced with permission from Verani JR, McGee L, Schrag SJ, et al. Prevention of perinatal group B streptococcal disease–revised guidelines from CDC, 2010. *MMWR Recomm Rep.* 2010;59(RR-10):1–36.

for the newborn born to a mother with unknown GBS status at onset of labor include maternal history of prolonged rupture of membranes, premature delivery before 37 weeks' gestation and maternal fever. All mothers with GBS risk factors should receive intrapartum prophylaxis (Table 2-2). Adequate intrapartum prophylaxis is considered ≥4 hours of an appropriate intravenous antimicrobial agent prior to delivery. For the nonallergic mother, penicillin remains the drug of choice for GBS prophylaxis. The premature newborn is at increased risk for GBS disease, particularly if the mother is colonized with GBS. Frequently GBS screening results are not available at the time of a premature birth. The CDC recommends that all mothers with the onset of labor before 37 weeks' gestation, with unknown GBS status, should be screened and given intrapartum antibiotic prophylaxis. The current recommendations for a well-appearing preterm infant born whose mother did not receive adequate intrapartum prophylaxis is a limited evaluation that includes complete blood count (CBC) differential, platelet count, and blood culture as well as in-hospital observation for clinical signs of sepsis for ≥48 hours after birth.

What are the current recommendations for the well-appearing late-preterm newborn whose mother received adequate GBS prophylaxis?

A. Well-appearing infants born less than 37 weeks gestation, regardless of adequate maternal intrapartum GBS prophylaxis, must undergo limited evaluation and observation for ≥48 hours

B. A newborn at any gestation who is well appearing and whose mother received adequate intrapartum GBS prophylaxis, should have a blood culture drawn before discharge, does not need further diagnostic evaluation and can be discharged at any time after 24 hours of birth if all other discharge criteria have been met, ready access to medical care is available and a person is present to comply fully with home observation instructions

C. A well-appearing newborn with a gestation of 35 to 36 weeks whose mother received adequate intrapartum GBS prophylaxis does not routinely need further diagnostic evaluation but should be observed in the hospital for 48 hours

D. Well-appearing infants born less than 37 weeks' gestation whose mother received adequate intrapartum GBS prophylaxis should undergo full evaluation and should start antimicrobial therapy until blood culture results are known

Discussion

The correct answer is **C**. Intrapartum antibiotic prophylaxis is very effective in preventing GBS disease in babies born to colonized mothers. The signs of clinical sepsis are often difficult to detect in a preterm newborn. The current recommendation for well-appearing late-preterm babies whose mother received intrapartum prophylaxis is no routine diagnostic evaluation but observation in the hospital for 48 hours for signs of clinical sepsis. The well-appearing term infant whose mother received adequate intrapartum antibiotic prophylaxis, observation for 48 hours is recommended, but continued observation at home after 24 hours in the hospital is acceptable. Early discharge of a term newborn with observation at home is acceptable after 24 hours after delivery if all other discharge criteria have been met, ready access to medical care is available and parents agree to comply fully with home observation instructions and return for follow-up with the primary care provider.[61]

How does a history prolonged rupture of membranes effect the clinical management of well-appearing babies whose mothers had an indication for GBS prophylaxis, but did not receive adequate GBS prophylaxis?

A. Regardless of gestational age, all well-appearing babies with a maternal history of prolonged rupture of membranes and whose mother did not receive adequate IAP should have a limited evaluation and observation in the hospital for 48 hours
B. Late-preterm babies with a maternal history of prolonged rupture of membranes and whose mother did not receive adequate IAP require limited evaluation and observation for at least 48 hours, but term babies with a similar history require only observation for 48 hours
C. Regardless of gestational age, all babies with a maternal history of prolonged rupture of membranes and whose mother did not receive adequate IAP require only observation for at least 48 hours
D. Babies born at term with a maternal history of prolonged rupture of membranes and whose mother did not receive adequate IAP require limited evaluation and discharge at 24 hours is recommended

Discussion

The correct answer is **A**. The risk for early-onset neonatal GBS sepsis in the newborn born to a mother with an indication for GBS prophylaxis who does not receive adequate IAP is stratified according to gestational age and length of rupture of membranes. The well-appearing term newborn without a maternal history of prolonged rupture of membranes whose mother did not receive adequate IAP requires in-hospital observation for signs of clinical sepsis for 48 hours, but not necessarily laboratory evaluation. The well-appearing term newborn with a history of maternal prolonged rupture of membranes and inadequate IAP and all well-appearing preterm newborns whose mothers did not receive adequate IAP require a limited evaluation and in-hospital observation for 48 hours.

Objectives

1. Understand recommendations for evaluation and management of newborns born to mothers with a known history of GBS colonization during pregnancy
2. Understand recommendations for evaluation and management of newborns born to mothers with unknown GBS status at delivery
3. Understand how management strategy is modified by the presence of risk factors including premature birth and prolonged rupture of membranes

CASE 12

You get a call from the laboratory that a mother's HBsAg is positive. Prenatal labs were drawn because the mother came in labor without her prenatal labs available. The mother's prenatal laboratory results come back at 17 hours after birth. The rapid HIV test is negative and RPR nonreactive. The mother denies knowing that she was positive for Hepatitis B. She also denies using intravenous drugs.

What percentage of newborn babies born to mothers who are HBsAg positive and Hepatitis e antigen positive will become infected with Hepatitis B, if prophylaxis is not given?

A. 10%
B. 20%
C. 30%
D. 90%

Discussion

The correct answer is **D**. Hepatitis B virus (HBV) is a small double-stranded DNA virus with many antigen markers present. When the HBsAg is present in the blood it means that the person is infectious. The Hepatitis e antigen is a marker for high viral titers. About 90% of newborns will become infected if the mother is Hepatitis surface antigen and Hepatitis e antigen positive. The transmission rate is about 10% if the mother is only positive for the surface antigen. The Hepatitis surface antibody is a marker for previous infection and life-long immunity or vaccination against the HBV. Much of the world (45%) is endemic for HBV infection, defined as 8% of the population or more are chronic carriers for Hepatitis B. The United States has a low prevalence of chronic carriers for Hepatitis B. Hepatitis B infection is often associated with at risk behaviors, such as multiple sexual contacts and IV drug use. Chronic infection is responsible for much of the morbidity and mortality associated with Hepatitis B infection, including chronic hepatitis, hepatocellular carcinoma, cirrhosis of the liver, and premature death.[37]

What percentage of newborn babies who acquire Hepatitis B from birth develop chronic infection?
A. 10%
B. 20%
C. 30%
D. 90%

Discussion

The correct answer is **D**. Nearly all newborns infected with Hepatitis B will develop chronic infection (Fig. 2-4). Thankfully perinatal exposure prophylaxis is available, with the Hepatitis B vaccine and Hepatitis B immunoglobulin (HBIG).[37]

What are the current recommendations for Hepatitis B perinatal exposure prophylaxis for the newborn whose mother is known to be positive for the HBsAg?
A. Give Hepatitis B vaccine and HBIG within 7 days
B. Give Hepatitis B and HBIG 12 to 24 hours afterbirth at separate injection sites, followed by completion of a 3-dose vaccine series
C. Give Hepatitis B vaccine and HBIG at separate injection sites before discharge
D. Give Hepatitis B vaccine within 12 hours of birth and HBIG at day 7 after birth

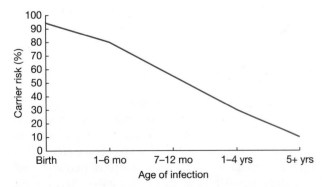

FIGURE 2-4. Risk of chronic HBV carriage by age of infection. (Reproduced with permission from Centers for Disease Control and Prevention. Epidemiology and Prevention of Vaccine-Preventable Diseases. Atkinson W, Wolfe S, Hamborsky J, eds. 12th ed., second printing. Washington DC: Public Health Foundation; 2012.)

TABLE 2-3. Effectiveness of Postexposure Prophylaxis in Preventing Perinatal Transmission of Hepatitis B virus (HBV) Infection[56]

POSTEXPOSURE PROPHYLAXIS	EFFECTIVENESS (%)
Hepatitis B vaccine + HBIG	85–95
Hepatitis B vaccine alone	70–95

Given within 12 hours after birth, followed by completion of 3-dose hepatitis B vaccine series.

Discussion

The correct answer is **B**. Postexposure prophylaxis with Hepatitis B vaccine and HBIG is very effective at preventing both acute and chronic HBV infection. Studies have shown that the Hepatitis B vaccine if given within 12 hours of life is about 70% to 95% effective in preventing newborn infection. If both the Hepatitis B vaccine and HBIG are given 12 to 24 hours after birth, the efficacy is about 85% to 95% protective (Table 2-3). The current recommendation from the CDC for prophylaxis for a newborn whose mother is known to be Hepatitis B positive is to give Hepatitis B vaccine and HBIG within 12 hours of life at separate injection sites. If the Hepatitis B vaccine status of the mother is unknown the current recommendation is for the newborn to receive Hepatitis vaccine B within 12 hours of life and mothers Hepatitis status to be tested as soon as possible. If the mother is found to be positive, HBIG should be administered immediately, up to 7 days after birth. The current recommendations for infants born to mothers whose HBsAg is known to be negative, is for the Hepatitis B vaccine to be given before discharge from the birthing hospital.

It is important to emphasize to the mother who is Hepatitis B positive that it is critically important that her newborn complete the 3-dose Hepatitis B vaccine series at the recommended scheduled intervals, with the third dose no later than 6 months of age. The initial birth vaccine and HBIG give passive and humoral protection for the short term, but does not offer long-term immunity. The newborn is at continued risk for infection by interpersonal contact with the infected mother. Hepatitis is known to be transmitted from household contact, such as sharing utensils, toothbrushes, and eating after someone. Infants and children need long-term protection by completing the Hepatitis B vaccine series. The newborn with perinatal exposure should have HBsAg testing performed between 9 and 18 months of age.[37]

What are the recommendations for perinatal exposure prophylaxis for the preterm newborn whose birth weight is less than 2,000 g and whose mother's Hepatitis B status is unknown?

A. Give Hepatitis B vaccine within 12 hours of birth and HBIG within 7 days once the mother's Hepatitis B status is known

B. Give the Hepatitis B vaccine at 1 month of age. HBIG is not recommended in the preterm newborn born less than 2,000 g

C. Give the Hepatitis B vaccine within 12 hours of birth, but repeat at 1 month of age HBIG is not recommended in the preterm newborn born less than 2,000 g

D. Give Hepatitis B vaccine and HBIG within 12 hours of birth at separate injection sites and repeat the Hepatitis B vaccine at 1 month of age

Discussion

The correct answer is **D**. The preterm baby weighing less than 2,000 g at birth has a reduced response to the Hepatitis B vaccine. The current recommendation by the Advisory Committee on Immunization Practices for the preterm newborn whose birth weight is less than 2,000 g and whose mother's Hepatitis B status is unknown is to give Hepatitis B vaccine immediately within 12 hours of birth. If mother's hepatitis B status cannot be determined within 12 hours after birth, HBIG should also be given within 12 hours of birth at a separate injection site. The Hepatitis B vaccine prophylaxis given to the preterm weighing less than 2,000 g should not be considered the first dose of the vaccine series and needs to be repeated at 1 month of age. If the mother of the preterm newborn weighing less than 2,000 g is known to be negative for Hepatitis B, the Hepatitis B vaccine should be first given at 1 month of age.[37]

Objectives

1. Understand risk for perinatal transmission of Hepatitis B in mothers with active infection
2. Understand recommended timing for administration of Hepatitis B vaccine based on birth weight
3. Understand indications for prophylaxis to decrease the risk of perinatal transmission of Hepatitis B infection

CASE 13

A baby girl was born at 36 weeks' gestation via spontaneous vaginal delivery. The baby weighs 2,500 g. The mother is 36 years old and this is her third baby. The mother's prenatal labs are all within normal limits, including a negative GBS screen. The baby is vigorous at birth. The Apgar scores are 8 at 1 minute of life and 8 at 5 minutes of life. The baby suckles right away on the mother's breast in the delivery room. In the nursery, vital signs are heart rate 156 bpm, respiratory rate 70 bpm, temperature 36.4°C, pulse oximetry is 97%. The glucose level is 47 mg/dL. Breath sounds are equal and clear bilaterally. There is no nasal flaring and no retractions. Heart sounds are normal with no murmur. Baby is pink with good femoral pulses. Tone is consistent with a baby born at 36 weeks.

Late-preterm birth increases the risk for all of the following, except

A. Hypoglycemia
B. Respiratory distress syndrome
C. Pulmonary hypertension
D. Meconium aspiration

Discussion

The correct answer is **D**. The preterm birth rate in the United States is currently 11.7% of all births.[62] Late-preterm births, defined as 34 0/7 to 36 6/7, represent a significant proportion (71% in 2010) of the preterm births. The late-term preterm baby is physically and metabolically immature and should not be treated like a term newborn. Late-preterm babies have significantly more morbidity and mortality than the term newborn. They make up a significant proportion of neonatal intensive care and specialty care admissions and are increased risk for rehospitalization after discharge. The neonatal mortality rate for the late preterm is 4.6 times higher than for a term gestation.[56] Common complications for the late-preterm newborn are hypothermia, hypoglycemia, respiratory distress, TTN, apnea, feeding difficulties, jaundice, and increased susceptibility for infections.[13] Gestational age, maternal morbidity, intrauterine growth restriction, and mode of delivery are all important factors for the late-preterm newborn's risk for severe complications. For example, cesarean delivery greatly increases the risk for respiratory distress including respiratory distress syndrome, "malignant" TTN, and pulmonary hypertension.[23,24,63]

What is the most likely cause for the baby's elevated respiratory rate?

A. Sepsis
B. Hypoglycemia
C. Pneumothorax
D. TTN

Discussion

The correct answer is **D**. At birth, the newborn must go through a rapid transition from the fluid-filled fetal lungs to air-filled lungs. The fetal lungs start preparing for this change in the last weeks of gestation. From 34 to 37 weeks' gestation, terminal respiratory units of the lung are evolving from alveolar saccules lined with both cuboidal type II and flat type I epithelial cells (terminal period) to mature alveoli lined primarily with extremely thin type I epithelial cells (alveolar period). The process of developing the alveolar period allows for the next major transition to occur smoothly at birth, which is the switch from chloride secreting channels to sodium absorbing channels. In addition to lung maturity continuing during final weeks of gestation, labor itself is important for the success of newborn fetal lung fluid clearance. The late-preterm newborn born via cesarean delivery without labor is a particular risk for respiratory distress and admission to the NICU. Since this newborn does not have risk factors for sepsis, examination is normal with breath sounds heard equally bilaterally, no hypoxia and the glucose value is within normal range, the most likely cause of the mild tachypnea is delayed clearance of fetal lung fluid. The baby needs continued monitoring. The CXR and septic screen should be considered.[13,23,26]

What are the current recommendations for monitoring the glucose levels for an asymptomatic late-preterm newborn?

A. No routine screening for glucose homeostasis is necessary in an asymptomatic late-preterm newborn
B. Screening for postnatal glucose homeostasis should be initiated for at least the first 24 hours of life for the late-preterm newborn
C. Screening for postnatal glucose homeostasis should be initiated for at least the first 12 hours of life for the late-preterm newborn
D. Only LGA infants born to mothers with diabetes (IDM) and SGA or require routine screening for postnatal glucose homeostasis in the asymptomatic late-preterm newborn

Discussion

The correct answer is **B**. Glucose homeostasis is one of the major transitions that the newborn must makes from the intrauterine to the extrauterine life. In the healthy intrauterine environment, the baby relies almost entirely on maternal glucose for its metabolic demands. The fetal glucose level stays at about 70% of the mother's glucose level. In the healthy fetus very little endogenous gluconeogenesis occurs. The healthy fetus is in a state of energy storage with a high insulin/glucagon ratio. High insulin and cortisol levels in the third trimester promote hepatic glycogen storage and lipid storage and inhibit lipolysis. The majority of hepatic glycogen storage and subcutaneous fat stores are made during the third trimester. At birth, there is sudden discontinuation in maternal glucose transfer. The

baby must shift to a high glucagon/insulin ratio for endogenous gluconeogenesis. This shift from energy storage to glucose consumption is thought to be triggered by the catecholamine and glucagon surge that occurs at delivery. The catecholamine surge stimulates glucagon secretion, causing the state of high glucagon/insulin ratio and the subsequent release of glucose from glycogen stores. In the term, healthy newborn, there is usually a physiologic nadir at 1 hour of life, as the counter regulatory system is shifting from insulin to glucagon secretion. The term newborn usually has no trouble with feeding to help stabilize its glucose levels as the metabolic processes adapt to extrauterine life. The late-preterm baby is at risk for developing hypoglycemia because it has limited glycogen stores, a more immature counter regulatory system, and is more immature with feeding. It is therefore recommended that all late-preterm newborn babies have glucose monitored for the first 24 hours of life.[13,28,29] The IDM babies are at risk for transient hypoglycemia because of induced hyperinsulinemia and diminished glucagon responses. The term asymptomatic IDM baby should have glucose homeostasis monitored for at least the first 12 hours of life. Other babies at risk for transient hypoglycemia include SGA, LGA, intrauterine growth restricted, postdated, and stressed infants (e.g., hypothermia).

What is the definition of hypoglycemia in the newborn, a serum glucose level?

A. ≤20 mg/dL
B. ≤30 mg/dL
C. ≤40 mg/dL
D. None of the above are correct

Discussion

The correct answer is **D**. The exact cut off point for normal glucose level is not known, because it depends on the individual clinical scenario. One generally accepted definition for hypoglycemia in the asymptomatic newborn is a serum glucose concentration of <47 mg/dL.[29] The glucose levels should rise after the physiologic nadir at 1 hour of life and stabilize by 12 hours of life. For example, a level of 45 mg/dL might be considered acceptable in a term newborn at 1 hour of life but would not be considered normal at 24 hours of life.

There is no absolute definition for hypoglycemia or known level at which brain damage will occur. It is known, however, that the newborn brain is vulnerable to shifts in glucose levels. This is because of the relative large brain size to the rest of the body. A majority of all glucose metabolism occurs in the brain in a newborn. The newborn utilization rate is 5 to 8 mg/kg/min—a rate 3 to 4 times that of adults.[28] The newborn brain has limited ability to use or create other substrates other than blood glucose. Although, the exact level at which brain damage occurs is not known, it is known that persistent hypoglycemia, defined as less than 40 mg/dL, for more than a few hours will likely lead to brain damage. If the baby is otherwise ill and stressed, its metabolic rate may be higher and relative hypoglycemia may have deleterious effects on the brain at higher glucose levels.[28,29] Clinical signs for hypoglycemia include tachypnea, apnea, tachycardia or bradycardia, jitteriness, lethargy, weak suck, temperature instability, and seizures.

Which is NOT a cause of temperature instability in the late-preterm newborn?
A. Limited brown fat for insulation
B. Large surface area to body weight
C. Inadequate glycogen stores
D. Inability to shiver

Discussion

The correct answer is **C**. Birth is a dramatic change in the ambient temperature for the newborn baby. The late-preterm newborn may not have the adaptations necessary for adequate thermoregulation. The late preterm has a large surface area to body weight. Surface area is directly related to heat loss and body weight is directly related to heat generation. The late preterm may have limited brown fat stores for thermogeneration and limited white fat stores for insulation. Babies of any gestation do not have the ability to shiver for thermoregulation. In addition the late-preterm baby may have an immature hypothalamic response to cold stress.[13]

Which is NOT within the current recommendations for the discharge of the late-preterm newborn?
A. Discharge weight no more than 8% less than birth weight
B. Normal vital signs for at least 12 hours prior to discharge
C. Discharge bilirubin screen within normal limits
D. Established follow-up outpatient care in 24 to 48 hours, depending on clinical need

Discussion

The correct answer is **A**. The late preterm is a risk for rehospitalization. Thus, it is very important that the discharge criteria be evaluated closely for the late preterm. The current recommendation from the AAP is weight loss no less than 7% at 48 hours of life, and no more than 2% to 3% per day of life. It is also emphasized that the breastfeeding needs to be observed by trained personnel for adequacy. Sufficient urine and stool output needs to be documented. Timely follow-up, paying particular attention to jaundice is imperative. It is not uncommon

for the late-preterm baby to initially do well for the first 2 days of life, but after discharge begin to not feed well, lose excessive weight, and becomes jaundiced. Insuring adequate and close follow-up is a very important part of discharge planning for all late-preterm babies.[56]

What is the most common reason for readmission for the late-preterm baby?
A. Weight loss
B. Sepsis
C. Apnea
D. Jaundice

Discussion

The correct answer is **D**. The late-preterm newborn is a particular risk for developing hyperbilirubinemia and kernicterus is disproportionately prevalent among late-preterm newborns. The risk for hyperbilirubinemia is another example of the immature physiology of the late-preterm newborn. The delayed maturation and lower available concentrations of uridine diphosphate glucuronosyltransferase cause the late-preterm newborn to have a peak in bilirubin not until day 5 to 7 of life. In addition, the immature brain of the late preterm frequently causes difficulty with coordinating effective suck and swallowing, putting the baby at risk for dehydration and hyperbilirubinemia. The first born, late-preterm newborn who is exclusively breastfed is most at risk for developing hyperbilirubinemia, requiring hospital readmission.[56,57]

Other important discharge criteria for all newborns are that the newborn screen should be performed before discharge and that anticipatory guidance be given regarding sudden infant death syndrome (SIDS). Birth before 37 weeks' gestation is an important risk factor for SIDS.

Which is NOT a current recommendation for the prevention of SIDS?
A. Supine position for sleeping
B. Infant home monitors
C. Pacifier use
D. Breastfeeding

Discussion

The correct answer is **B**. Since the "Back-to-Sleep" educational campaign in 2002, deaths due to SIDS has declined significantly. However, in the past 5 years, while still lower than before, the rates have plateaued. SIDS is thought to be from the limited arousal functions in the newborn brain. Some of the current recommendations for SIDS prevention are supine position at sleep, baby in his/her own crib or bassinet that has met current safety standards, breastfeeding, pacifier use during sleep, no pillows or quilts in the crib, and no smoking in the same room as a sleeping baby. Routine use of infant apnea monitors like those used for infants who have had an apparent life-threatening event are not recommended as a strategy for preventing SIDS.[64]

Objectives

1. Understand recommendations for evaluation and management of the late-preterm infants after birth
2. Understand potential morbidity associated with late-preterm birth
3. Understand common reasons for hospital readmission for late-preterm infants after birth
4. Understand discharge criteria for late-preterm infants
5. Understand risk for SIDS among late-preterm infants

CASE 14

You are called by the nurse about a baby who appears jaundiced. The transcutaneous bilirubin measurement was 8 at 12 hours of life. The total serum bilirubin level is 8.4 mg/dL. The African-American baby boy was born at 39 weeks' gestation to a G3P3 mother via NSVD. The prenatal labs were all normal. The Apgar scores were 9 and 9. The birth weight was 3,600 g. The mother's blood type is O+ and the baby's blood type is B+. You confirm that the direct Coombs test was weakly positive from the cord blood serum. The cord blood bilirubin level was essentially normal at 2.5 mg/dL. You examine the baby. He looks jaundiced but otherwise is vigorous and well appearing. You explain to the mother that the baby has hyperbilirubinemia and will require immediate intensive phototherapy and potentially some other therapies. The mother tells you that all her babies where "under lights" before going home. The baby is exclusively breastfeed. You tell the mother that you will make every effort to support her breastfeeding but that the baby will require some formula supplementation until the bilirubin problem is under control. The mother says she understands. Your first step is to determine if this is hemolytic jaundice. You order a CBC and reticulocyte count. The CBC is within normal limits. The reticulocyte count is mildly elevated at 6.5%. When determining the etiology of hyperbilirubinemia, it is important to get a direct and total bilirubin level. The total serum bilirubin level is now 9 mg/dL (4 hours later) and the direct bilirubin level is 0.4 mg/dL.

Which of the following accurately describes the positive direct Coombs test?
A. Agglutination is observed when antigenic RBCs are added to mother's serum
B. Agglutination is observed when antibody reagent binds to infant's RBCs
C. No agglutination is observed when antigenic RBCs are added to mother's serum
D. No agglutination is observed when antibody reagent binds to infant's RBCs

Discussion

The correct answer is **B**. The direct Coombs test is a test for antibody-mediated hemolysis. It is positive when agglutination (clumping or matrix forming) occurs when test antibody reagent binds to the patient's (frequently cord blood) RBCs. Like with any test, false positives and false negatives can occur. It is more accurate for Rh disease because the Rh antibodies bind more than Anti-A and Anti-B. The Coombs test is helpful in determining which newborn is at risk for developing hyperbilirubinemia secondary to antibody-mediated hemolysis. It does not replace the need for clinical examination for signs of jaundice with every assessment of the baby. Taking a family history is also very important. A history of a sibling with hyperbilirubinemia is an important risk factor.[65]

What percentage should the direct bilirubin level be of the total bilirubin level to make a diagnosis of unconjugated hyperbilirubinemia?
A. Less than 5%
B. Less than 10%
C. Less than 20%
D. Less than 50%

Discussion

The correct answer is **C**. The precise measurement of direct versus indirect bilirubin is assay and laboratory dependent. However, generally speaking, in unconjugated hyperbilirubinemia the direct bilirubin level should be less than 1 mg/dL or less than 20% of the total bilirubin level. Sepsis, UTIs, galactosemia, thyroid disorders, and biliary obstruction are all causes of conjugated hyperbilirubinemia.[55]

What is the most likely hemolytic cause of this baby's unconjugated hyperbilirubinemia?
A. ABO incompatibility
B. Rh sensitization
C. Glucose 6 phosphate dehydrogenase (G6PD) deficiency
D. Spherocytosis

Discussion

The correct answer is **A**. ABO incompatibility is the most common form of hemolytic jaundice. While about 20% of newborns are at risk for blood ABO incompatibility, the incidence of developing significant jaundice is 1:150 to 1:3,000, depending on the definition used. In most instances, the ABO incompatibilities do not cause severe jaundice, but there are exceptions. The mother who is O negative and who has been sensitized to a Rh positive baby is much more likely to have severe jaundice and hydrops fetalis (rare now, thanks to anti-D Ig). The A and B antigenic sites are weak on newborn red blood cell (RBC) membranes, so very little maternal anti-A or anti-B antibody binds to the neonatal RBC. In addition, there are A and B antigen receptors in multiple fetal tissues (not just on RBC membranes) that bind and remove the circulating maternal anti-A and anti-B antibodies. Unlike the Rh negative mother who must be first sensitized by a Rh positive fetus, the O positive mother can have anti-A and Anti-B antibodies during the first pregnancy. This is because of environmental sensitization from bacteria can induce maternal anti-A and anti-B antibodies, however most of the antibodies acquired are IgM and do not cross the placenta. The O–A incompatibility is the most common, but O–B can be more severe.[66]

G6PD deficiency is also an important consideration. G6PD deficiency is a sex-linked inherited disorder that disrupts antioxidant defense mechanisms. The enzyme G6PD is the primary catalyst for the hexose monophosphate pathway and causes the reduction of NADP to NADPH, which is important for antioxidant activity. The RBC membrane relies solely on G6PD as an antioxidant. Without sufficient quantities of NADPH, the RBC membrane is highly susceptibility to hemolysis secondary to oxidative stress. G6PD deficiency is common worldwide, particularly in populations in the Mediterranean and Middle East, Arabian Peninsula, Southeast Asia, and Africa. It is also occurs in about 15% of African Americans. A significant number of infants who develop kernicterus have G6PD deficiency. Of note, for reasons not fully understood, the reticulocyte count can be normal despite hemolysis secondary to G6PD deficiency. Evidence of increased bilirubin production secondary to hemolysis has been shown, however, in G6PD deficiency by elevated end-tidal carbon monoxide levels.[55,67,68]

Spherocytosis is a relatively rare inherited RBC membrane defect that can be difficult to diagnosis during the newborn period. Hemolysis secondary to ABO incompatibility can have a "spherocytosis" on the CBC secondary to a progressive reduction in the IgG-coated RBC membranes as they are cleared by the reticuloendothelial system.[66]

What is the most likely nonhemolytic disorder that may contribute to the baby's unconjugated hyperbilirubinemia?

A. Sepsis
B. Galactosemia
C. Gilbert syndrome
D. Crigler–Najjar syndrome type I

Discussion

The correct answer is **C**. Gilbert syndrome is a relatively common condition that can cause exaggerated neonatal jaundice due to decreased uridine diphosphate glucuronosyltransferase (UGT1A1) enzyme activity. It is due to a common polymorphism by the insertion of thymine-adenine (TA) repeats in the promoter gene of UGT1A1. Gilbert syndrome is thought to be a possible cause of hyperbilirubinemia in ABO incompatible newborns that have a negative Coombs test. The combination of G6PD deficiency and Gilbert syndrome can cause severe hyperbilirubinemia.[52,55,67,69]

Crigler–Najjar syndrome types I and II are both recessive disorders of the UGT1A1 enzyme. Crigler–Najjar type I is the more severe form, due to a mutation that causes a premature stop codon for UGT1A1 production. The affected newborn has essentially no UGT1A1 activity and is at extreme risk for developing hyperbilirubin encephalopathy. Crigler–Najjar type II is much less severe and may present with prolonged but mild jaundice. It is due to a mild deficiency in UGT1A1 enzyme production secondary to a homozygous missense mutation. Phenobarbital is both therapeutic and diagnostic for type II Crigler–Najjar syndrome, as phenobarbital will induce UGT1A1 activity and thus clear the hyperbilirubinemia of type II only.[70]

Galactose-1 phosphate uridyl transferase deficiency galactosemia usually does not present with hyperbilirubinemia within the first 24 hours of life, but can present in the first days to weeks. It is caused by the inability to metabolize galactose-1 phosphate. Breast milk and most formula contain large amounts of lactose which is converted into glucose and galactose. The accumulation of galactose-1 phosphate damages the kidneys, liver, and brain. Affected babies can present with any of the following: jaundice (may have conjugated component), hepatomegaly, hypoglycemia, vomiting, failure to thrive, seizures, or *Escherichia coli* sepsis.[71]

Sepsis can cause a mixed picture of hemolytic and nonhemolytic hyperbilirubinemia. Sepsis is unlikely in an otherwise well-appearing newborn. The birth and prenatal history as well as CBC and differential can help rule out sepsis as a cause of jaundice. Although severe hemolysis can cause a left shift; the reticulocyte count will be markedly elevated as well.[66]

Which of the following is the correct definition of intensive phototherapy?

A. Spectral irradiance of 30 μW/nm in the 460 to 490-nm bandwidth delivered to a maximum body-surface area

B. Spectral irradiance of 30 μW/nm in the <400-nm bandwidth delivered to a maximum body-surface area

C. Spectral irradiance of 30 μW/nm in the 380 to 800-nm bandwidth delivered to a maximum body-surface area

D. Spectral irradiance of 8 to 10 μW/nm in the 430 to 490-nm bandwidth delivered to a maximum body-surface area

Discussion

The correct answer is **A**. Phototherapy uses light energy to convert bilirubin to a photoisomer that is a more lipophilic molecule. The photoisomer (lumirubin) does not require hepatic glucuronidation for excretion into bile and urine. The visible white light spectrum ranges from 350 to 800 nm. Bilirubin absorbs light energy most strongly in the blue-green spectrum (460–490-nm wavelength). The

effectiveness of phototherapy depends on the wavelength of light energy and the irradiance (energy output) of the light source, as well as the total surface area exposed. Conventional (nonintensive) phototherapy lights (daylight, white or blue fluorescent tubes), deliver a spectral irradiance of 8 to 10 μW/nm in the 430 to 490-nm bandwidth. Intensive phototherapy should include use of special blue fluorescent lamps that will deliver 30 μW/nm in the 460 to 490-nm bandwidth. UV light (<400 nm) is to be avoided. Caution should be taken to protect the eyes and genitals. A self-limited, benign rash sometimes occurs.[72,73] The AAP has a nomogram to help guide when to initiate intensive phototherapy (see Fig. 2-5).[74]

Which is an absolute contraindication for phototherapy?

A. Congenital porphyria or a family history of porphyria

B. Combined cholestatic jaundice and unconjugated hyperbilirubinemia

C. Temperature instability

D. Exclusive breastfeeding

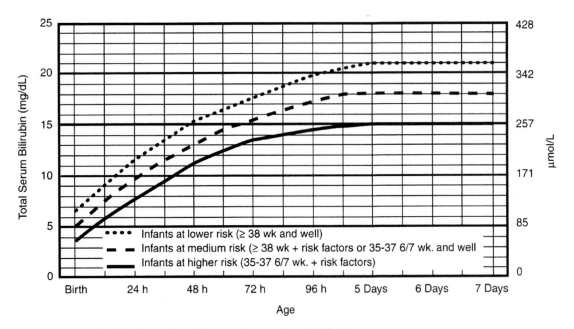

• Use total bilirubin. Do not subtract direct reacting or conjugated bilirubin.
• Risk factors = isoimmune hemolytic disease, G6PD deficiency, asphyxia, significant lethargy, temperature instability, sepsis, acidosis, or albumin < 3.0g/dL (if measured)
• For well infants 35-37 6/7 wk can adjust TSB levels for intervention around the medium risk line. It is an option to intervene at lower TSB levels for infants closer to 35 wks and at higher TSB levels for those closer to 37 6/7 wk.
• It is an option to provide conventional phototherapy in hospital or at home at TSB levels 2-3 mg/dL (35-50mmol/L) below those shown but home phototherapy should not be used in any infant with risk factors.

FIGURE 2-5. Nomograms for recommendation for treatment of hyperbilirubinemia in neonates. TcB, Transcutaneous bilirubin level; TSB, total serum bilirubin level; G6PD, glucose-6-phosphate dehydrogenase. (Reproduced with permission from American Academy of Pediatrics Subcommittee on Hyperbilirubinemia. Clinical practice guideline: Management of hyperbilirubinemia in the newborn infant 35 or more weeks of gestation. *Pediatrics.* 2004;114(1):297–316.)

Discussion

The correct answer is **A**. Known congenital porphyria, a family history of porphyria, and use of photosensitizing drugs are absolute contraindications for phototherapy. Severe blistering of the skin while under phototherapy can be first signs of congenital porphyria. Use of phototherapy with combined direct and indirect hyperbilirubinemia is not an absolute contraindication, but needs to be assessed carefully and on an individual basis. The bronze baby syndrome (grayish-brown discoloration of skin, serum, and urine) is frequently benign and reversible. Close attention to the baby's well-being while under phototherapy is needed, particularly regarding the baby's hydration status and temperature stability. Small- and late-preterm babies may require an isolate to help stabilize temperature while under phototherapy. It is important to help mothers continue lactation if breastfeeding needs to be temporarily interrupted during intensive phototherapy.[72,73]

Objectives

1. Identify common nonhemolytic causes of jaundice in the newborn
2. Identify common hemolytic disorders known to causes jaundice in the newborn
3. Understand the diagnostic evaluation of a newborn with jaundice
4. Understand principles of phototherapy
5. Identify known contraindications for use of phototherapy

REFERENCES

1. Kattwinkel J, Perlman JM, Aziz K, et al. Neonatal Resuscitation: 2010 American Heart Association Guidelines for Cardiopulmonary Resuscitation and Emergency Cardiovascular Care. *Pediatrics.* 2010;126(5):e1400–e1413.
2. American Academy of Pediatrics, Committee on Fetus and Newborn, American College of Obstetricians and Gynecologists, et al. The Apgar score. *Pediatrics.* 2006;117(4):1444–1447.
3. Casey BM, McIntire DD, Leveno KJ. The continuing value of the Apgar score for the assessment of newborn infants. *N Engl J Med.* 2001;344(7):467–471.
4. American Academy of Pediatrics. Chlamydia trachomatis. In: Pickerling LK, ed. *Red Book: 2012 Report of the Committee on Infectious Disease.* 29th ed. Elk Grove Village, IL: American Academy of Pediatrics; 2012:276–281.
5. Workowski KA, Berman S; Centers for Disease Control and Prevention (CDC). Sexually transmitted diseases treatment guidelines, 2010. *MMWR Recomm Rep.* 2010;59(RR-12):1–110.
6. American Academy of Pediatrics. Prevention of neonatal ophthalmia. In: Pickerling LK, ed. *Red Book: 2012 Report of the Committee on Infectious Disease.* 29th ed. Elk Grove Village, IL: American Academy of Pediatrics; 2012:880–881.
7. Rubenstein JB, Virasch V. Neonatal conjunctivitis (Ophthalmia Neonatorum). In: Yanoff M, Duker JS, eds. *Ophthalmology.* 3rd ed. St. Louis, MO: Mosby and imprint of Elsevier, Inc; 2008:231–232.
8. U.S. Preventive Services Task Force. Ocular prophylaxis for gonococcal ophthalmia neonatorum: Reaffirmation recommendation statement. *Am Fam Physician.* 2012;85(2):195–196.
9. Breeze AC, Lees CC. Prediction and perinatal outcomes of fetal growth restriction. *Semin Fetal Neonatal Med.* 2007;12(5):383–397.
10. Campbell MK, Cartier S, Xie B, et al. Determinants of small for gestational age birth at term. *Paediatr Perinat Epidemiol.* 2012;26(6):525–533.
11. McIntire DD, Bloom SL, Casey BM, et al. Birth weight in relation to morbidity and mortality among newborn infants. *N Engl J Med.* 1999;340(16):1234–1238.
12. Yu VY, Upadhyay A. Neonatal management of the growth-restricted infant. *Semin Fetal Neonatal Med.* 2004;9(5):403–409.
13. Raju TN. Developmental physiology of late and moderate prematurity. *Semin Fetal Neonatal Med.* 2012;17(3):126–131.
14. Carlo W. Maintenance of body heat. In: Kliegman R, ed. *Nelson Textbook of Pediatrics.* 19th ed. Philadelphia, PA: Elsevier Saunders; 2011:536–537.
15. Baumgart S. Iatrogenic hyperthermia and hypothermia in the neonate. *Clin Perinatol.* 2008;35(1):183–197.
16. Harlor AD Jr., Bower C. Hearing assessment in infants and children: Recommendations beyond neonatal screening. *Pediatrics.* 2009;124(4):1252–1263.
17. Gifford KA, Holmes MG, Bernstein HH. Hearing loss in children. *Pediatr Rev.* 2009;30(6):207–215.
18. American Academy of Pediatrics, Joint Committee on Infant Hearing. Year 2007 position statement: Principles and guidelines for early hearing detection and intervention programs. *Pediatrics.* 2007;120(4):898–921.
19. Centers for Disease Control and Prevention (CDC). CDC Grand Rounds: Newborn screening and improved outcomes. *MMWR Morb Mortal Wkly Rep.* 2012;61(21):390–393.
20. Mahle WT, Martin GR, Beekman RH, et al. Endorsement of Health and Human Services recommendation for pulse oximetry screening for critical congenital heart disease. *Pediatrics.* 2012;129(1):190–192.
21. Kemper AR, Mahle WT, Martin GR, et al. Strategies for implementing screening for critical congenital heart disease. *Pediatrics.* 2011;128(5):e1259–e1267.
22. Tita AT, Landon MB, Spong CY, et al. Timing of elective repeat cesarean delivery at term and neonatal outcomes. *N Engl J Med.* 2009;360(2):111–120.
23. Jain L, Eaton DC. Physiology of fetal lung fluid clearance and the effect of labor. *Semin Perinatol.* 2006;30(1):34–43.
24. De Luca R, Boulvain M, Irion O, et al. Incidence of early neonatal mortality and morbidity after late-preterm and term cesarean delivery. *Pediatrics.* 2009;123(6):e1064–e1071.
25. Hansen AK, Wisborg K, Uldbjerg N, et al. Risk of respiratory morbidity in term infants delivered by elective caesarean section: Cohort study. *BMJ.* 2008;336(7635):85–87.

26. Janer C, Pitkanen OM, Helve O, et al. Airway expression of the epithelial sodium channel alpha-subunit correlates with cortisol in term newborns. *Pediatrics*. 2011;128(2): e414–e421.

27. Sarkar S, Rosenkrantz TS. Neonatal polycythemia and hyperviscosity. *Semin Fetal Neonatal Med*. 2008;13(4):248–255.

28. Sperling MA, Menon RK. Differential diagnosis and management of neonatal hypoglycemia. *Pediatr Clin North Am*. 2004; 51(3):703–723, x.

29. Adamkin DH. Postnatal glucose homeostasis in late-preterm and term infants. *Pediatrics*. 2011;127(3):575–579.

30. Section on Breastfeeding. Breastfeeding and the use of human milk. *Pediatrics*. 2012;129(3):e827–e841.

31. Ballard O, Morrow AL. Human milk composition: Nutrients and bioactive factors. *Pediatr Clin North Am*. 2013;60(1):49–74.

32. Brandtzaeg P. The mucosal immune system and its integration with the mammary glands. *J Pediatr*. 2010;156(2 suppl): S8–S15.

33. Chandran L, Gelfer P. Breastfeeding: The essential principles. *Pediatr Rev*. 2006;27(11):409–417.

34. Johnson CL, Versalovic J. The human microbiome and its potential importance to pediatrics. *Pediatrics*. 2012;129(5): 950–960.

35. Lauer B, Spector N. Vitamins. *Pediatr Rev*. 2012;33(8): 339–351.

36. Wagner CL, Greer FR. Prevention of rickets and vitamin D deficiency in infants, children, and adolescents. *Pediatrics*. 2008;122(5):1142–1152.

37. Mast EE, Margolis HS, Fiore AE, et al. A comprehensive immunization strategy to eliminate transmission of hepatitis B virus infection in the United States: Recommendations of the Advisory Committee on Immunization Practices (ACIP) part 1: Immunization of infants, children, and adolescents. *MMWR Recomm Rep*. 2005;54(RR-16):1–31.

38. American Academy of Pediatrics Task Force on Circumcision. Circumcision policy statement. *Pediatrics*. 2012;130(3): 585–586.

39. American Academy of Pediatrics Task Force on Circumcision. Male circumcision. *Pediatrics*. 2012;130(3):e756–e785.

40. Walsh JM, Kandamany N, Ni Shuibhne N, et al. Neonatal brachial plexus injury: Comparison of incidence and antecedents between 2 decades. *Am J Obstet Gynecol*. 2011;204(4):23.

41. Sebastin SJ, Chung KC. Pathogenesis and management of deformities of the elbow, wrist, and hand in late neonatal brachial plexus palsy. *J Pediatr Rehabil Med*. 2011;4(2):119–130.

42. Ruchelsman DE, Pettrone S, Price AE, et al. Brachial plexus birth palsy: An overview of early treatment considerations. *Bull NYU Hosp Jt Dis*. 2009;67(1):83–89.

43. Marcus JR, Clarke HM. Management of obstetrical brachial plexus palsy: Evaluation, prognosis, and primary surgical treatment. *Clin Plast Surg*. 2003;30(2):289–306.

44. Uhing MR. Management of birth injuries. *Clin Perinato*. 2005;32(1):19–38, v.

45. Volpe J. *Injuries of Extracranial, Cranial, Intracranial, Spinal Cord, and Peripheral Nervous System, in Neurology of the Newborn*. Philadelphia, PA: Saunders, Elsevier Inc; 2008:959–985.

46. Guclu B, Yalcinkaya U, Kazanci B, et al. Diagnosis and treatment of ossified cephalhematoma. *J Craniofac Surg*. 2012;23 (5):e505–e507.

47. Doumouchtsis SK, Arulkumaran S. Head injuries after instrumental vaginal deliveries. *Curr Opin Obstet Gynecol*. 2006; 18(2):129–134.

48. Suskind DL. Nutritional deficiencies during normal growth. *Pediatr Clin North Am*. 2009;56(5):1035–1053.

49. American Academy of Pediatrics Committee on Fetus and Newborn. Controversies concerning vitamin K and the newborn. *Pediatrics*. 2003;112(1 pt 1):191–192.

50. Van Winckel M, De Bruyne R, Van De Velde S, et al. Vitamin K, an update for the pediatrician. *Eur J Pediatr*. 2009;168 (2):127–134.

51. Ipema HJ. Use of oral vitamin K for prevention of late vitamin k deficiency bleeding in neonates when injectable vitamin K is not available. *Ann Pharmacother*. 2012;46(6):879–883.

52. Dennery PA, Seidman DS, Stevenson DK. Neonatal hyperbilirubinemia. *N Engl J Med*. 2001;344(8):581–590.

53. Watchko JF, Lin Z. Exploring the genetic architecture of neonatal hyperbilirubinemia. *Semin Fetal Neonatal Med*. 2010; 15(3):169–175.

54. Soldi A, Tonetto P, Varalda A, et al. Neonatal jaundice and human milk. *J Matern Fetal Neonatal Med*. 2011;24 suppl 1:85–87.

55. American Academy of Pediatrics Subcommittee on Hyperbilirubinemia. Management of hyperbilirubinemia in the newborn infant 35 or more weeks of gestation. *Pediatrics*. 2004;114(1):297–316.

56. Engle WA, Tomashek KM, Wallman C, et al. "Late-preterm" infants: A population at risk. *Pediatrics*. 2007;120(6):1390–1401.

57. Maisels MJ, Bhutani VK, Bogen D, et al. Hyperbilirubinemia in the newborn infant ≥35 weeks' gestation: An update with clarifications. *Pediatrics*. 2009;124(4):1193–1198.

58. Gartner LM, Morton J, Lawrence RA, et al; American Academy of Pediatrics Section on Breastfeeding. Breastfeeding and the use of human milk. *Pediatrics*. 2005;115(2):496–506.

59. Holmes AV. Establishing successful breastfeeding in the newborn period. *Pediatr Clin North Am*. 2013;60(1):147–168.

60. Metaj M, Laroia N, Lawrence RA, et al. Comparison of breast- and formula-fed normal newborns in time to first stool and urine. *J Perinatol*. 2003;23(8):624–628.

61. Verani JR, McGee L, Schrag SJ. Prevention of perinatal group B streptococcal disease–revised guidelines from CDC, 2010. *MMWR Recomm Rep*. 2010;59(RR-10):1–36.

62. Martin JA, Hamilton BE, Ventura SJ, et al. Births: Final data for 2010. 2012 [updated Nov 3; cited 60 1]; 2012/06/08: Available from: http://www.cdc.gov/nchs/nvsr/nvsr61.

63. Ramachandrappa A, Rosenberg ES, Wagoner S, et al. Morbidity and mortality in late preterm infants with severe hypoxic respiratory failure on extra-corporeal membrane oxygenation. *J Pediatr*. 2011;159(2):192–198.e3.

64. Task Force on Sudden Infant Death Syndrome, Moon RY. SIDS and other sleep-related infant deaths: Expansion of recommendations for a safe infant sleeping environment. *Pediatrics*. 2011;128(5):1030–1039.

65. Zantek ND, Koepsell SA, Tharp DR, et al. The direct antiglobulin test: A critical step in the evaluation of hemolysis. *Am J Hematol*. 2012;87(7):707–709.

66. Geaghan SM. Diagnostic laboratory technologies for the fetus and neonate with isoimmunization. *Semin Perinatol*. 2011;35 (3):148–154.

67. Herschel M, Caldarelli L, Karrison T, et al. Isoimmunization is unlikely to be the cause of hemolysis in ABO-incompatible but direct antiglobulin test-negative neonates. *Pediatrics.* 2002;110(1 pt 1):127–130.

68. Kaplan M, Hammerman C. Glucose-6-phosphate dehydrogenase deficiency and severe neonatal hyperbilirubinemia: A complexity of interactions between genes and environment. *Semin Fetal Neonatal Med.* 2010;15(3):148–156.

69. Kaplan M, Hammerman C, Renbaum P, et al. Gilbert's syndrome and hyperbilirubinemia in ABO-incompatible neonates. *Lancet.* 2000;356(9230):652–653.

70. Carey RG, Balisteri WF. Inherited deficient conjugation of bilirubin In: Kliegman RM, Stanton BF, Schol NF, et al., eds. *Nelson Textbook of Pediatrics.* 19th ed. Philadelphia, PA: Saunders; 2011:1389–1390.

71. Kishnani PS, Chen, Y. Defects in galactose metabolism. In: Kliegman RM, Stanton BMD, et al., eds. *Nelson Textbook of Pediatrics.* 19th ed. Philadelphia, PA: Saunders; 2011:502.

72. Bhutani VK; Committee on Fetus and Newborn; American Academy of Pediatrics. Phototherapy to prevent severe neonatal hyperbilirubinemia in the newborn infant 35 or more weeks of gestation. *Pediatrics.* 2011;128(4):e1046–e1052.

73. Maisels MJ, McDonagh AF. Phototherapy for neonatal jaundice. *N Engl J Med.* 2008;358(9):920–928.

74. American Academy of Pediatrics Subcommittee on Hyperbilirubinemia. Clinical practice guideline: Management of hyperbilirubinemia in the newborn infant 35 or more weeks of gestation. *Pediatrics.* 2004;114(1):297–316.

Chapter 3
ASPHYXIA AND RESUSCITATION

Shilpa Vyas-Read, MD

This chapter contains a series of short vignettes that describe circumstances commonly encountered during efforts to resuscitate and stabilize a newborn infant. The principles of resuscitation overlap between cases, therefore we have provide a summary of chapter objectives that the reader should have mastered upon completing this chapter.

CASE 1

You are called to the delivery of a 28-year-old primigravid woman with a 35-week infant being born by cesarean section. The labor and delivery nurse calls out to you that mother has a history of chronic hypertension with super-imposed preeclampsia, and she is being delivered for blood pressures of 205/110, elevated liver enzymes, and low platelets. The mother's serologies, including GBS are negative, and rupture of membranes is at the time of delivery. The baby is brought to the warmer and positioned, suctioned, dried, and stimulated. He is noted to be pale, limp, and apneic and the baby's heart rate is 50 beats per minute.

This baby's cardiorespiratory compromise is most likely a result of

A. Surfactant deficiency and respiratory distress syndrome
B. Early-onset bacterial sepsis
C. Intrauterine asphyxia from placental abruption
D. Cyanosis from congenital heart disease

Discussion

The correct answer is **C**. The case describes a mother with HELLP syndrome, a serious condition consisting of hemolysis, elevated liver enzymes, and low platelets. The diagnosis of HELLP carries a maternal mortality risk of up to 24%, and the most common complication in mothers with HELLP syndrome is placental abruption followed by disseminated intravascular coagulation.[1] Infants born to mothers with placental abruption have a 15-fold higher risk in perinatal mortality, and may have increased morbidities including intraventricular hemorrhage, periventricular leukomalacia, and cerebral palsy.[2] The incidence of surfactant deficiency and respiratory distress syndrome at 35 weeks is approximately 4%, making choice A an unlikely choice.[3] Similarly, GBS negative status and intact amniotic fluid make early-onset sepsis an unlikely etiology for cardiorespiratory compromise in this infant. An infant with cyanotic congenital heart disease may be blue, rather than pale, and is often asymptomatic at the time of birth due to a patent ductus arteriosus.

CASE 2

You are called to an emergency cesarean section of a 40-week gestation. The fetal heart rate monitoring strip showed lack of variability for 1 hour followed by bradycardia to the 60s. The fetal heart rate did not improve with maternal repositioning or oxygen, and an emergency delivery was performed within 5 minutes. Following positive-pressure ventilation and endotracheal intubation in the delivery room, the infant is stabilized and a cord blood gas shows pH 6.6, pCO_2 76, PaO_2 14, and base deficit of –26.

Hypoxic-ischemic brain injury is most likely to develop after which of the following sequence of events?

A. Increased intranuclear calcium → Transcriptional modification of genes → Increased nitric oxide → Cerebral tissue hypoxia

B. Cerebral tissue hypoxia → Excitotoxic mechanisms → Increased intranuclear calcium → Cellular death
C. Inflammatory cytokine release from macrophages → Direct injury to neighboring cells → Cerebral tissue hypoxia → Increased intranuclear calcium
D. Free radical formation → Cerebral tissue hypoxia → Cellular death → Inflammatory cascades

Discussion

The correct answer is **B**. Cerebral tissue hypoxia depletes cells of adenosine triphosphate (ATP), which is needed for oxidative phosphorylation and energy balance. Lack of energy substrate leads to cellular breakdown, increased intracellular calcium and increased excitotoxic neurotransmitters, such as glutamate. Glutamate influx activates excitatory NMDA and AMPA receptors, which further increase intracellular calcium. Cellular function and signaling pathways are adversely affected by increased cellular and nuclear calcium, and the resultant-free radical formation, membrane injury, and nitric oxide generation ultimately lead to cellular necrosis and apoptosis.[4,5] Posthypoxic injury hypothermia has been shown in animal models to improve cerebral energy state, attenuate excitatory pathways, prevent nitric oxide production, and decrease neuronal apoptosis. For infants who have moderate-to-severe encephalopathy following hypoxic injury, therapeutic hypothermia (33.5°C for 72 hours) has been shown to decrease the risk of moderate-to-severe disability at both 18 to 22 months and 6 to 7 years of age.[6-8]

CASE 3

You are called to the cesarean section of a 42-week infant born through meconium-stained amniotic fluid. The prenatal course is unremarkable and an operative delivery is being performed for arrest of descent. As the infant is being brought to the radiant warmer, you notice that she is blue, apneic, and limp. You immediately intubate the infant and when the aspirator is attached, you notice particulate green meconium in the endotracheal tube. The bedside nurse calls out that the heart rate is 40 beats per minute, and you decide to proceed with resuscitation rather than attempt a second intubation. The infant requires positive-pressure ventilation for 3 minutes, but the heart rate, tone and color gradually improve. By 5 minutes, the infant is crying spontaneously, has good tone, a heart rate of 160 beats per minute, and is pink with oxygen saturations of 95% in the right hand.

Of the following statements, which one most closely reflects the next appropriate step in this infant's management?
A. Pass the infant to the mother to breastfeed, since initial bonding may have been interrupted by resuscitation
B. Order a sepsis evaluation on the infant and transition her to the postpartum room, since the reason for the initial respiratory depression is unclear
C. Arrange for frequent vital signs, intermittent pulse oximetry, and close observation of the infant, since meconium below the vocal cords may predispose the infant to meconium aspiration syndrome
D. Explain to the father that the baby aspirated meconium and detail the signs and symptoms of respiratory distress for which he should alert the postpartum nurse

Discussion

The correct answer is **C**. Meconium-stained amniotic fluid (MSAF) is noted in 10% to 15% of live birth due to intestinal peristalsis and anal sphincter relaxation in response to hypoxia, acidosis or infection.[9] Five percent of infants born through MSAF will develop meconium aspiration syndrome. Meconium aspiration syndrome is characterized by the development of respiratory distress in an infant shortly after delivery, with a history of MSAF and no other identifiable causes of respiratory distress (i.e., infection, pneumothorax, etc.). Chest x-rays of infants with meconium aspiration syndrome may show patchy alveolar infiltrates, areas of meconium plugging and subsequent atelectasis, and neighboring areas of hyperexpansion.[10] The Neonatal Resuscitation Program (NRP) currently recommends tracheal suctioning of nonvigorous infants, such as the one described in the scenario.[11] A nonvigorous infant is defined by poor tone, heart rate less than 100, and absent or irregular respiratory effort.[12] Conversely, the 2011 NRP guidelines recommend that infants who meet the criteria for "non-resuscitation" are not removed from the mother. Infants who require "non-resuscitation" demonstrate all of the following three characteristics: (1) term gestation, (2) crying or breathing, and (3) good muscle tone.[11,12] Although infection is a concern in infants with respiratory depression, and it may predispose the passage of meconium, it is not appropriate to transition this infant who required resuscitation directly to the mother's room following a sepsis evaluation without an observation period. Answer D is incorrect because the father should not be the primary evaluator of the infant's medical condition.

CASE 4

The pediatric resident who is working with you is preparing to attend the delivery of a male infant. The infant is estimated to be 1,815 g at 37 weeks, and is to be delivered by vaginal delivery in a few minutes. The resident is eager to know more of the expected perinatal and postnatal course for this infant.

Which of the following statements regarding this infant is *incorrect*?
A. This infant is at increased risk of perinatal asphyxia and death when compared with term infants in general
B. Very few of infants like this one will have caught up on growth in the first year of life
C. This infant is at risk for metabolic derangements, such as hypoglycemia, hypocalcemia, and increased energy requirements
D. Absent or reversed umbilical artery end-diastolic velocity and cerebral head sparing may be a sign of deterioration of placental function in infants such as this one

Discussion

The correct answer is **B**. The infant described in the scenario has experienced intrauterine growth restriction. Depending on whether the fetus is affected early or late in pregnancy and the etiology of the growth failure, the infant may have symmetric or asymmetric growth restriction. Symmetric growth restriction is defined by having a head circumference, weight, and height less than the third percentile for gestational age and growth failure typically occurs early in pregnancy. Symmetric growth restriction may be caused by genetic abnormalities, syndromes, congenital viral infections, some inborn errors of metabolism, and intrauterine drug exposures.[13] Asymmetrically affected fetuses will have poor weight gain, with relative sparing of length and head circumference. Impaired uteroplacental function and nutritional deficiencies are classically associated with asymmetric growth restriction.[13] Infants who are growth restricted have at least a sevenfold increase in mortality when compared with appropriately grown infants of similar gestational age. Because of chronic uteroplacental insufficiency and hypoxia, they are at increased risk for stillbirth and perinatal asphyxia compared with their term counterparts.[14] Metabolic abnormalities, such as hypoglycemia, hypocalcemia and increased energy requirements are common among growth-restricted infants. In addition, polycythemia and hypothermia are complications of chronic hypoxia and decreased adipose tissue storage. However,

over 80% of growth-restricted infants will catch up to normal growth within the first year of life.[14] Repetitive biophysical assessments and ultrasonographic evaluations, such as umbilical artery end-diastolic flow, are used to assess well-being when fetal growth restriction is suspected. Absent or reversed umbilical artery end-diastolic flow, cerebral head sparing, elevated venous Doppler indices, oligohydramnios, and abnormal biophysical profiles are all signs of worsening placental function and may help predict optimal timing of delivery.[15]

CASE 5

A 43-week infant is born to a mother with limited prenatal care by vacuum-assisted vaginal delivery. You are called by the labor and delivery nurse because the infant is 10 minutes old and is blue despite blow-by oxygen to the face. When you arrive, you note that the infant is lying with his arms and legs extended on the warmer. He is quiet and not moving unless stimulated on his back or heels. He is breathing but periodically has periods of apnea lasting 30 seconds during which he turns blue. On your examination, you cannot elicit a sucking reflex, but as you are removing the pacifier, he thrusts his tongue out for 2 minutes. The umbilical arterial cord gas is resulted while you are waiting for the transport isolette, and it shows a pH of 6.5 and a base deficit too large to calculate.

This baby's modified Sarnat stage of hypoxic-ischemic encephalopathy can best be described as
A. Mild encephalopathy
B. Moderate encephalopathy
C. Severe encephalopathy
D. This baby does not exhibit signs of encephalopathy

Discussion

The correct answer is **C**. The clinical features of each modified Sarnat stage for hypoxic-ischemic encephalopathy are listed in Table 3-1.[16]

This staging system is used to categorize the severity of hypoxic-ischemic encephalopathy in infants, and to aid in predictions about outcome.[17] Using this system of evaluation, neurologic outcomes at 2 to 5 years for infants with mild encephalopathy were all normal, whereas 25% infants with moderate encephalopathy and 76% of infants with severe encephalopathy were handicapped.[18] Need for chest compressions for over 1 minute, base deficit of over 16, and onset of respirations beyond 30 minutes enhance predictions of severe adverse outcomes.[19] This

TABLE 3-1. **Staging of Encephalopathy**

CLINICAL CHARACTERISTICS	MILD	MODERATE	SEVERE
Level of consciousness	Normal or hyperalert	Lethargy	Stupor or coma
Activity	Normal or increased	Decreased	None
Posture	Flexion	Distal flexion, complete extension	Decerebrate
Tone	Normal to increased	Hypotonia	Flaccid
Primitive reflexes	Suck strong	Suck weak	Suck absent
	Complete Moro	Incomplete Moro	Absent Moro
Autonomic nervous system	Pupils reactive to light	Pupils constricted	Pupils deviated, dilated, or nonresponsive to light
	Heart rate normal	Heart rate bradycardic	Heart rate variable
	Respirations regular	Respirations irregular	Respirations apneic

patient has extensor posturing, poor tone, no spontaneous activity, no suck, apnea, stupor, and presumed seizures. These clinical characteristics are consistent with severe encephalopathy.

Multiple randomized-controlled trials have been published in recent years that infants who have moderate-to-severe encephalopathy resulting from a perinatal event have decreased mortality and neurodevelopmental disability when they receive either selective head-cooling or whole-body hypothermia within 6 hours of delivery.[20,21]

CASE 6

A full-term neonate is transferred to your neonatal intensive care unit for evaluation for hypothermia. The Apgar scores in the medical record are listed as 0, 1, 2, 7 at 1, 5, 10 and 20 minutes, respectively. The father is at the bedside and wants to know what these numbers mean.

Which of the following statements regarding Apgar scores is *correct*?

A. Apgar scores should be used to guide resuscitative efforts.
B. Inter-observer variability among medical providers assigning Apgar scores is high so the scores have little predictive value.
C. Since the Apgar score improved in this infant over 20 minutes, he is at little risk for death or long-term neurodevelopmental disability.
D. The Apgar scores for this infant indicate a high probability for death or long-term neurodevelopmental disability.

Discussion

The correct answer is **D**. Apgar scores were designed by Virginia Apgar as a way to standardize neonatal assessment in the delivery room.[22] Newborns are scored from 0 to 2 in five categories, with a highest possible score of 10 (Table 3-2).

Although components of the Apgar score overlap with the signs that are used to guide neonatal resuscitation, assignment of the Apgar score should never delay or guide resuscitative efforts. The 5-minute Apgar score has been shown to be reflective of the effectiveness of resuscitation, and a low Apgar score (0–3) at 5 minutes confers a higher risk for death in term neonates.[22] For infants less than 30 weeks, a 5-minute Apgar score of less than 2 was associated with an increased likelihood of death within 12 hours and an 86% chance of death of neurodevelopmental impairment at 18 to 22 months.[23] Ten-minute Apgar scores of 0 to 2 for near-term infants have been associated with a 76% to 80% risk of death or moderate/severe disability at 18 to 22 months of age.[24] The infant in the scenario with low Apgar scores at 5 and 10 minutes would be expected to have an increased risk of death or moderate/severe neurodevelopmental disability as a toddler. Answer B would be incorrect because a recent survey of neonatologists who were shown resuscitation clips showed a close correlation in Apgar assignment between observers for term newborns, but not for infants less than 30 weeks.[25]

TABLE 3-2. **Assignment of Apgar Scores**

Category	0	1	2
Heart rate	0	<100 bpm	≥100 bpm
Respirations	0	Weak cry, hypoventilation	Good, crying
Tone	Limp	Some flexion of extremities	Active motion
Grimace	None	Grimace	Cry or active withdrawal
Color	Blue, pale	Body pink, extremities blue	Completely pink

CASE 7

A 29-week infant is born by urgent cesarean section due to concerns of poor variability on the fetal heart rate monitor tracing. After positioning the infant, suctioning the oropharynx, drying and stimulating the infant, the heart rate is reported as 20 beats per minute. Positive-pressure ventilation is begun, followed by chest compressions, but the heart rate remains less than 60 beats per minute. You decide to intubate the infant to secure the airway and to allow for endotracheal drug delivery. The intubation proceeds smoothly, but when the respiratory therapist applies a colorimetric capnometer to ensure placement in the trachea, no color change is noted.

What is the most appropriate next step in the management of this neonatal resuscitation?
A. Ensure that the endotracheal tube is in place by visualizing passage through the vocal cords and auscultating breath sounds
B. Immediately remove the endotracheal tube, continue positive-pressure ventilation, and reattempt intubation once the heart rate is over 60
C. Place an umbilical venous catheter and infuse 10 mL/kg of normal saline over 10 minutes
D. Place an umbilical venous catheter and administer 2 mEq/kg of sodium bicarbonate

Discussion

The correct answer is **A**. Colorimetric capnometers contain a pH-sensitive detector that change from purple to yellow with exposure to exhaled CO_2. Placing a colorimetric capnometer is an important tool that can be used in addition to the traditional signs of increasing heart, the presence of equal and bilateral breath sounds, the absence of breath sounds over the epigastrium, and improving color, to confirm tracheal intubation.[26] A positive colorimetric result confirms tracheal intubation, or, in rare circumstances, may result from contamination with intratracheal medication, gastric contents, or humidity.[26] Since color change relies on the production of alveolar CO_2, in cases of cardiopulmonary arrest, the colorimetric capnometer will be falsely negative.[27] Interestingly, since colorimetric capnometers were designed for usage in neonates over 2 kg and in pediatric patients, a false-negative result may occur in up to 30% of the time in infants less than 32 weeks.[28] In the infant in the scenario, who has profound bradycardia, a low cardiac output, impaired pulmonary blood flow, and decreased production of alveolar CO_2, the colorimetric capnometer may have limited utility. In this circumstance, direct visualization of endotracheal tube placement through the vocal cords, and evaluation of other signs of tracheal intubation (heart rate, color, breath sounds) should be assessed before removing the tube, as long as the intubator is skilled and confident of correct placement.

CASE 8

The obstetrician calls you to the operating room for the delivery of a 24-week infant, who is expected to be 510 g by fetal ultrasound. The mother has no significant prenatal history except for being admitted to the hospital with preterm cervical dilatation 8 days ago at which time she received a course of betamethasone. Today, she began having regular contractions and has progressed rapidly to an imminent delivery. As you are preparing the radiant warmer, you consider that this extremely low–birth-weight infant will likely have rapid heat loss and that some preparations should take place to prevent hypothermia.

Of the following options, which sequence of events most closely approximates those recommended by the NRP to prevent heat loss in extremely low–birth-weight neonates?

A. Place the infant on a warmed radiant warmer and exothermic mattress, dry and remove wet linens, and place a hat

B. Increase the temperature of the delivery room, place the infant on a warmed radiant warmer, dry and remove wet linens, and place a hat

C. Increase the temperature of the delivery room, place the infant on a warmed radiant warmer and an exothermic mattress, cover the infant with occlusive wraps, and place a hat

D. Increase the temperature of the delivery room, place the infant on a warmed radiant warmer, dry and remove wet linens, place a hat, and cover the infant with occlusive wraps

Discussion

The correct answer is **C**. Degrees of hypothermia range from mild (36–36.5°C), or moderate (32–35.9°C), to severe (<32°C).[29] In very low–birth-weight premature infants, even mild-to-moderate hypothermia has been associated with an increase in oxygen consumption and body metabolism, and cold stress may increase the risk of neonatal morbidity and mortality.[29–31] Heat transfer occurs through four physical mechanisms: (1) conduction, or the transfer of heat to a cold surface in contact with the infant; (2) convection, or transfer of heat to the cold air surrounding the infant; (3) evaporation, or the transfer of heat through water molecules into the air; (4) radiation, or the transfer of heat through electromagnetic energy to surfaces not in contact with the infant.

The extremely low–birth-weight neonate is particularly vulnerable to cold stress, given its high body surface area, immature skin, lack of brown fat, and narrow thermoneutral zone. Evaporation is the largest contributor to heat loss early after birth for premature infants, and several well-designed studies have shown that decreasing evaporative heat loss by placing infants in occlusive plastic coverings after birth augments admission temperature.[32–34] The use of an exothermic mattress in conjunction with occlusive wraps have been shown to further increase admission temperature over the use of wraps alone, but this combination may increase the likelihood of hyperthermia and infant temperatures should be carefully monitored.[35,36] The World Health Organization recommends keeping delivery/operating room temperatures minimally at 25°C, and a recent randomized trial documented the benefit of this approach on the prevention of neonatal hypothermia.[37] The 2010 Neonatal Resuscitation Program recommends the placement of infants less than 28 weeks in an occlusive plastic wrap up to the neck, immediately and without prior drying. Resuscitation measures can be performed through the occlusive wrap, and delivery room temperatures should be kept at 26°C.[11,38]

CASE 9

A 39-week male, born by vaginal delivery through clear amniotic fluid 1 minute ago, is limp, blue, and apneic. The intern, with whom you are conducting the resuscitation, has attempted repositioning, suctioning of the oropharynx, drying, and stimulating, but the infant has continued to be apneic with a heart rate of 90 bpm. The young doctor began positive-pressure ventilation, but she is now disturbed because it has been 30 seconds and she does not see adequate chest rise, improving pulse oximetry, or an increasing heart rate.

What is the sequence of steps that should be taken at this time to ensure that effective ventilation is being achieved?

A. Intubate the infant, increase the peak inspiratory pressure, and deep suction the trachea

B. Suction the mouth and nose of the infant, reposition the airway, open the mouth and, if these efforts fail, intubate the trachea

C. Suction the mouth and nose of the infant, open the mouth, increase the peak inspiratory pressure, and then check the mask

D. Check the mask; reposition the airway of the infant. If these measures fail, suction the mouth and nose, open the mouth, and increase the peak inspiratory pressure

Discussion

The correct answer is **D**. When adequate ventilation is being delivered to a depressed infant, the heart rate and pulse oximetry should improve with the first 5 to 10 breaths. In addition, chest movement should be observed by the resuscitator and equal breath sounds should be auscultated. In this scenario, attempts at ventilation are being made, but the heart rate, color, and chest rise are not improving. Before attempting intubation, several ventilation corrective measures should be performed to ensure optimal positive-pressure ventilation is occurring. These steps can be remembered through the use of the acronym, MR SOPA. The steps corresponding to the acronym are listed in Table 3-3.

TABLE 3-3.   **Ventilation Corrective Steps**

	CORRECTIVE STEPS	DETAILED EXPLANATION
M	Mask adjustment	An inadequate seal often occurs between the cheek and bridge of the nose. If air is escaping around the mask, apply pressure to the mask without pressing down hard on the infant's face.
R	Reposition the airway	Check to make sure that the infant is in a "sniffing" position and the neck is not flexed or hyperextended. In the correct position, the infant's nose will be as anterior as possible. A neck roll may be used to help maintain the correct position.
S	Suction the oropharynx	A blocked airway will prevent adequate ventilation. The infant's mouth and then nose ("M before N") may be suctioned if needed to clear the airway.
O	Open the mouth	An infant's nose is small and has a high resistance to airflow. Opening the mouth slightly and keeping the jaw forward may improve tracheal air entry.
P	Pressure increase	Increase the pressure gradually with every few breaths until adequate chest rise is observed and bilateral breath sounds are auscultated.
A	Airway alternative	If the above corrective steps do not improve signs of adequate ventilation, proceed with endotracheal intubation or placement of a laryngeal mask airway.

The ventilation corrective steps should be performed in the order they are listed above. The first two steps (MR) should be attempted first, as these measures will often improve ventilation. If not successful, the next two steps (SO) should be performed, with pressure increases and endotracheal intubation being reserved for those infants who do not respond to the initial four actions.[11]

CASE 10

The obstetrician calls you to the delivery of a 38-week infant for an emergent cesarean, who has had bradycardia to the 60s on the fetal monitor. Despite giving the mother oxygen and repositioning her, the heart rate remains in the 60s and is not recovering. As you prepare for resuscitation, you contemplate what you know about fetal circulatory response to asphyxia.

Which of the following statements about the fetal circulatory response to asphyxia is *incorrect*?
A. Increased catecholamines cause cerebral vasoconstriction, which increases cerebral vascular resistance but does not increase cerebral blood flow
B. Fetal blood flow is shunted preferentially toward the brain, heart, and adrenal glands, and away from peripheral organs, the kidney, and the intestines
C. Myocardial injury or cardiovascular dysfunction is evident in 20% of neonates following asphyxia
D. The amount of blood returning from the inferior vena cava that is shunted across the ductus venosus and the foramen ovale is increased during intrauterine hypoxia

Discussion

The correct answer is **C**. Severe fetal asphyxia has been demonstrated in animal models following as little as 4 minutes of uterine blood flow interruption. Following acute asphyxia, oxygen delivery to the brain falls, catecholamines surge, and cerebral reflex vasoconstriction occurs. Overall, cerebral blood flow remains constant, but flow to the brainstem is initially increased and oxygen extraction is augmented.[39] In addition to the brain, blood flow is directed to the heart and adrenal glands, at the expense of other organs, such as the lung, kidney, intestines, and muscle. Interestingly, a larger proportion of umbilical blood flow bypasses the liver through the ductus venosus and passes through the foramen ovale to the left ventricle, in order to preserve oxygen delivery to the heart and the brain.[39] Although these compensatory mechanisms will preserve blood pressure in the fetus initially, with prolonged asphyxia, mean arterial pressure, and cerebral blood flow will ultimately fall.[40] Consequently, myocardial injury and cardiovascular dysfunction are present in 50% to 80% of neonates following asphyxia.[41] Fetal acidemia with an umbilical arterial pH <7 confers the highest risk for neurologic injury.[40]

CASE 11

You are at the delivery of a full-term male infant, whose entire body and mucosa appear cyanotic at 2 minutes of life. The labor and delivery nurse is reaching for the flow-inflating bag so that she may deliver blow-by oxygen over the infant's nose and mouth.

Which of the following statements regarding the use of oxygen in the delivery room is *correct*?

A. Full-term infants may appear cyanotic for up to 10 minutes after birth, but preterm infants transition faster and should be pink by 5 minutes of life

B. Full-term neonates resuscitated with room air are more likely to survive than those who are resuscitated with 100% oxygen

C. Because of fetal hemoglobin, neonates will appear cyanotic, even when they have oxygen saturations of 85%

D. The in utero arterial partial pressure of oxygen (PaO_2) in the fetus is approximately one-tenth of the PaO_2 of the neonate in room air

Discussion

The correct answer is **B**. Fetal hemoglobin has a high affinity for oxygen, ensuring adequate uptake from the placenta. However, in utero, the PaO_2 ranges from 25 to 30 mm Hg and, following room air transition, the PaO_2 climbs rapidly to 80 to 90 mm Hg. This abrupt change in oxygen tension, coupled with the relative lack of antioxidant defense in infants, has prompted concern about the routine use of supplemental oxygen in the delivery room and its deleterious effects on the neonate.[42] Furthermore, recent investigations have shown that full-term infants may not reach oxygen saturations ≥85% until after 5 minutes of life, and those that are born by cesarean section may take several minutes longer to reach this goal.[43,44] Premature infants between 23 and 32 weeks of gestation may take up to 10 minutes to achieve oxygen saturations of ≥85%.[45] The recommended placement for a pulse oximeter probe is on the right hand, to monitor preductal saturations. Room air resuscitation in full-term infants is associated with less oxidative stress and resuscitation with initial oxygen concentrations less than 100% may protect against respiratory morbidities in infants born at less than 34 weeks.[46,47] Further, animal models demonstrate that changes in gene expression, apoptosis, and inflammatory pathways may be influenced by excessive oxygen exposure.[48–50] Given these data, the NRP recommends resuscitation of full-term infants with room air initially with increases in inspired oxygen if pulse oximetry is outside of the target saturation range, or if the heart rate remains unacceptable. For premature infants less than 32 weeks, the use of oxygen for resuscitation is recommended, and the percentage should be guided by the preductal pulse oximetry readings in the neonate.[38] Answer C is incorrect because fetal hemoglobin has a higher affinity for oxygen than adult hemoglobin. Cyanosis is not clinically apparent until 5 g/dL of hemoglobin is deoxygenated in the capillaries. Therefore, a neonate is likely to have lower oxygen saturations by pulse oximetry than an adult (<80%) before

TABLE 3-4. Target Preductal Oxygen Saturations for Neonates in the First 5 Minutes of Life

MINUTES OF LIFE	TARGET OXYGEN SATURATIONS (%)
1	60–65
2	65–70
3	70–75
4	75–80
5	80–85
10	85–95

appearing clinically cyanotic. The target oxygen saturations for neonates that are recommended by the NRP are listed in Table 3-4.[11]

CASE 12

The neonatal resuscitation team has been called to the emergency room for the anticipated delivery of a 30-week infant whose mother is unconscious and was just brought in by ambulance after a motor vehicle crash. Since the mother has profuse vaginal bleeding and the fetal heart rate is undetectable by monitor, the obstetricians have decided to proceed with an emergency cesarean section. As the leader of the neonatal resuscitation team, you are preparing for delivery, considering if the infant will require volume expansion, and debating which solutions you should request.

A. Which of the following statements regarding volume expansion is *incorrect*?

A. Given the clinical history, the need for additional providers may be anticipated and a call should be placed to request additional nursing, medical, or respiratory help

B. Given the clinical history of acute blood loss, after the initial steps of NRP are accomplished and the infant is intubated, 20 to 50 mL/kg of volume expanders should be administered through an umbilical venous line as fast as possible

C. Given the clinical history, the initial steps of NRP should be performed, an airway should be established, and the need for umbilical venous line placement and volume expansion should be anticipated

D. None of the above statements is incorrect

Discussion

The correct answer is **C**. The preterm infant in the scenario represents an example of a very high-risk delivery since the mother has sustained abdominal trauma and is likely having a placental abruption as a result. The infant's undetectable heart rate is a sign that he is hypoxic in utero and may have asphyxial injury from an interruption in uterine blood flow. Placental abruption is a leading cause of fetal loss following blunt maternal trauma, followed by preterm labor and fetal–maternal hemorrhage, with direct uterine trauma and uterine rupture being rare.[51] Although less than 1% of infants require extensive resuscitative measures at birth, one may anticipate that the prematurity, asphyxia, and potential volume loss in this infant will necessitate additional personnel and broad resuscitative efforts. The NRP recommends that one skilled person should be available at every delivery solely for the management of the newborn, and two skilled providers be available for high-risk deliveries. In some circumstances, additional personnel may be required to accomplish all resuscitative tasks in a timely manner.[11] In this scenario, several providers should be recruited to the emergency room prior to the delivery since extensive resuscitative efforts are expected.

Volume expansion is not routinely recommended for the depressed neonate, since hypovolemia is infrequently a cause of myocardial depression in asphyxiated infants. Further, a large volume load in the absence of adequate myocardial function has not been shown to improve blood pressure and may lead to pulmonary edema formation.[11,52–54] In this scenario, it is possible that fetal vessels may have been disrupted from shearing injuries sustained during the motor vehicle crash, and preparations for potential volume administration should be begun predelivery. Recommended solutions for volume expansion include (1) normal saline, (2) Ringer's lactate, or (3) O Rh-negative packed red blood cells.[11] The easiest route of administration in a newly born infant is IV, through an emergently placed umbilical venous catheter. Volume should be given in an initial dosage of 10 mL/kg, slowly over 5 to 10 minutes, since rapid volume administration may result in intracranial hemorrhage, particularly in preterm infants.[55] Another 10 mL/kg of volume may be administered if the infant does not respond to the first dose.

At delivery the infant is depressed and has poor respiratory efforts but responds to your initial resuscitation efforts. Due to the respiratory depression the infant is intubated but heart rate and perfusion improve quickly. The results of the cord blood gas are pH 6.8, pCO_2 95, pO_2 20, base deficit of –10. The resident asks if the patient is a candidate for hypothermia.

B. What is the most appropriate response to this question?
A. Whole-body cooling should be initiated as soon as possible
B. An MRI of the brain should be performed before initiating whole-body hypothermia in this preterm infants
C. Currently, data are not available to determine the safety or efficacy of whole-body or selective head-cooling in the preterm infants
D. Hypothermia should only be initiated in this patient if they develop clinical seizure activity

Discussion

The correct answer is **C**. Although this therapy has been shown to decrease the risk of death and/or moderate-to-severe neurodevelopmental impairment in term infants, this therapy has not been evaluated in preterm infants and should not be used in preterm infants. Further clinical trials to evaluate safety and efficacy will be need prior to extrapolation of this therapy to preterm infants.

CASE 13

The respiratory therapist reads you a cord blood gas result from a patient you just admitted to the neonatal intensive care unit following intubation in the delivery room for sustained apnea. The results of the cord blood gas are as follows pH 6.9, pCO_2 100, pO_2 20, base excess –5.

Which of the following statements regarding this cord blood gas is true?
A. The blood gas is a mixed arterial and venous sample
B. The blood gas demonstrates fetal respiratory acidosis
C. The blood gas demonstrates fetal mixed respiratory and metabolic acidosis
D. The blood gas is contaminated and cannot be interpreted

Discussion

The correct answer is **B**. Under normal circumstances, fetal tissues produce CO_2, which mixes with water and is converted to carbonic acid through the action of carbonic anhydrase on the fetal red blood cell. The carbonic acid is carried via the umbilical artery back to the placenta, where it is converted back to CO_2, diffuses across the placenta, and is ultimately excreted by the maternal lungs.[56] The normal range for cord umbilical arterial cord gas values are as follows: pH 7.15 to 7.38 (approximately ≤7.2), pCO_2 35 to 70 mm Hg (approximately ≤60), pO_2 11 to 25 mm Hg (approximately ≥20 mm Hg), base deficit −2 to −9 (approximately ≤10).[57] An acute interruption in placental function of less than 30 minutes duration may be accompanied by a rapid increase in pCO_2, as seen in the patient in the scenario.[58] Acidosis primarily affecting placental respiration and pCO_2 elimination is termed respiratory acidosis. If the asphyxial insult is not corrected or the infant is not delivered, a metabolic acidosis will develop over time. An umbilical *venous* cord gas sample is reflective of the maternal acid–base status, rather than the fetus, and the pO_2 in the umbilical vein is approximately 40 mm Hg. A clue that the cord blood gas may be a mixed venous sample is if the pO_2 is substantially higher than the 11 to 25 mm Hg expected for the umbilical artery. Our patient's pO_2 of 20 mm Hg eliminates that possibility.

The contribution of the respiratory component, or pCO_2, can be calculated by subtracting a normal cord pCO_2 of 50 mm Hg from the observed. In this case, 100 − 50 = 50 mm Hg. Since the pH is lowered 0.08 for every 10 mm Hg the pCO_2 is increased over normal, one may calculate for this patient that the pH should be 50/10 mm Hg or 5 × 0.08 = 0.4 less than the normal of 7.3. Therefore, our infant's pH of 6.9 is entirely attributable to the respiratory acidosis. If the pH is lower than that expected for a given pCO_2, a metabolic component must be present and hence, the patient would have a mixed respiratory and metabolic acidosis.[58] A number of factors may affect cord blood gas values. The altitude at which the mother resides, her smoking history and her parity have been associated with alterations of cord pH and pCO_2. Intrapartum factors, such as breech delivery, umbilical cord abnormalities and spinal anesthesia have also been associated with a lower cord pH at birth. Although mixture with heparin may lead to an acidosis on the cord gas, this type of contamination would result in metabolic acidosis.[56]

CASE 14

You are called to attend an elective repeat cesarean section of a 39-week female infant. The mother has no significant past medical or prenatal history. As you are waiting for the delivery, the mother begins to cry out. The anesthesiologist motions you over to her and states that she has just given IV fentanyl to the mother for pain control. One minute later, the infant is born and cries at the abdomen. Following positioning, drying and stimulating, the infant's respiratory effort is regular with good chest rise and a heart rate of 120 bpm. At 2 minutes of life, you notice the infant has irregular deep respirations, and you begin positive-pressure ventilation.

Which of the following is the most appropriate next step in the management of this infant?
A. Administer 0.1 mg/kg of naloxone intramuscularly and if the baby is breathing regularly, transition her to the newborn nursery
B. Place a pulse oximeter, position the airway in a "sniffing" position, and stimulate the infant's back and heels
C. Administer 0.2 mg/kg of naloxone intramuscularly and if the baby is breathing regularly, transition her to the neonatal intensive care unit for observation
D. Administer positive-pressure ventilation until respiratory effort improves or the infant is intubated

Discussion

The correct answer is **D**. Opioids are routinely used for the management of maternal pain, and are highly lipid-soluble and readily cross the placenta. If given within 4 hours of delivery, opioids may cause significant depression in the neonate, including poor suck, respiratory depression, and lethargy.[59] Naloxone, an opioid antagonist, had been previously used commonly to reverse the effects of intrapartum opioids in the neonate. The recommended dosage is 0.1 mg/kg and the route of administration may be endotracheal, intravenous, intramuscular, or subcutaneous. However, recent reviews of available evidence have demonstrated that safety data for the routine administration, particularly for routes other than IV, of naloxone is lacking, and that it has been associated with the development of pulmonary edema in older children.[60] Further, the administration of naloxone to infants of opioid-addicted mothers may precipitate withdrawal seizures. The most recent edition of the NRP has revised its recommendation for the use of naloxone to state, "administration of naloxone is not necessary as long as the baby can be adequately ventilated." It further states that naloxone may be considered in infants, like the one in our scenario, whose mother is not opioid-addicted and who has received a narcotic within 4 hours of delivery.[11] Answer A is incorrect because, even if the infant was breathing regularly following naloxone administration, it would be inappropriate to transition her to the newborn nursery since the half-life of the maternal opioid may be longer than the half-life of naloxone. The infant may become apneic several hours later in a setting in which she is not being monitored. Answer B is incorrect because an infant who does not initially respond to initial NRP steps such as positioning and stimulating is not likely to respond to repeated attempts at these maneuvers. If positioning and suctioning do not improve ventilatory drive within 30 seconds, supporting the ventilation of an apneic or ineffectively breathing infant with positive pressure, regardless of the etiology of the depression, is recommended.[11]

initial steps, the NRP recommends 30 seconds of warmth, drying, and stimulation. If the newborn does not resume spontaneous respiration and the heart rate is not over 100 bpm, the resuscitator should move quickly to the implementation of positive-pressure ventilation, since the infant is likely in a secondary apnea stage. Our infant in the scenario is in a stage of secondary apnea, since he continues to be apneic and bradycardic despite 30 seconds of tactile stimulation.

CASE 15

A 35-week infant has just been brought to the radiant warmer. He was positioned, warmed, dried, and stimulated for 30 seconds and his heart rate is auscultated at 80 beats per minute and he is not breathing.

The infant described in the scenario is in what stage of the physiological response to asphyxia?
A. Primary apnea
B. Secondary apnea
C. Tertiary apnea
D. Apnea of prematurity

Discussion

The correct answer is **B**. Approximately 90% of newborns will breathe spontaneously and require no assistance to transition from intrauterine to extrauterine life. Approximately 10% of newborns will require assistance to begin breathing following birth.[11] The first response of the hypoxia-exposed neonate is to alter respiratory movements.[61] In the 1960s, experiments in newborn rabbits immersed in nitrogen illustrated a biphasic response to hypoxia and these stages were later confirmed in newborn infants.[62] In the initial stage of primary apnea, respirations cease, heart rate begins to fall, but blood pressure remains relatively stable for several minutes. Tactile stimulation alone will induce the infant to begin regular respirations again, and no further resuscitation measures are needed. If the hypoxic insult is prolonged, however, the newborn enters a stage of secondary, or "terminal," apnea during which the respirations cease, the heart rate and blood pressures falls. There will be no response to tactile stimulation, and only positive-pressure ventilation will ensure a recovery of the heart rate, blood pressure, and survival.[62] When an infant is delivered, it is not possible to know which stage of apnea the infant is in, since he may have passed through primary apnea in utero. For this reason and since 90% of infants will respond to these

CASE 16

You are called emergently to the delivery room to assist in a neonatal resuscitation that is already underway. The infant was delivered 5 minutes ago to a 37-year-old primigravid mother by vaginal delivery. The infant was blue and apneic when placed on the radiant warmer, and was noted to have a heart rate of 40 beats per minute at 30 seconds. Effective positive-pressure ventilation was begun through a bag-and-mask, and when the heart rate continued to be less than 60 at 2 minutes, the senior resident intubated the infant and confirmed appropriate placement by auscultation of equal breath sounds and chest rise. A pulse oximeter has been placed on the right hand but is not reading an oxygen saturation or heart rate.

What is the most appropriate next step in the management of this critically ill infant?
A. Place an umbilical venous line and administer IV epinephrine
B. Begin chest compressions on the lower third of the sternum in a 5:1 cycle using the thumb technique
C. Begin chest compressions on the lower third of the sternum in a 3:1 cycle using the two-finger technique
D. Begin chest compressions on the lower third of the sternum in a 3:1 cycle using the thumb technique

Discussion

The correct answer is **D**. Chest compressions are indicated when the heart rate is less than 60, despite 30 seconds of effective positive-pressure ventilation. Since the majority of neonatal resuscitation (approximately 90%) will respond to ventilation, it is imperative that the resuscitator is confident that effective positive pressure is being applied. In this scenario, the resident has chosen to proceed with endotracheal intubation to secure an airway and has used clinical signs of appropriate endotracheal tube placement (equal breath sounds and chest rise) to ensure effective ventilation. The proper depth of insertion for an endotracheal tube is 6 cm + the weight (kg) of the infant. Using the infant in the scenario, if he is a 3-kg neonate, 9 cm is the depth of insertion, and this measurement represents the distance from the end of the endotracheal tube to the vermilion border of the upper lip. Other signs of appropriate endotracheal tube placement include increasing heart rate, improving oxygen saturations, vapor condensing in the tube, and direct visualization of the tube passing through the vocal cords.[11]

Less than 1% of the time, effective ventilation will not remedy a bradycardic infant. In this case, chest compressions are indicated. Chest compressions should occur in a 3:1 cycle, with three compressions for one ventilation breath. In 1 minute, 120 "events" should occur, 90 compressions and 30 breaths. At least two skilled personnel are required to administer chest compressions, one to perform the compressions and the other to provide ventilation. The person administering compressions should speak the rhythm "One-and-Two-and-Three-and-Breathe-and," loud enough for both people to hear, and should hold compressions during "Breathe-and" while ventilation is provided. The purpose of chest compressions is to provide aortic diastolic blood pressure or coronary perfusion with oxygenated blood to restore energy substrates in the hypoxic heart.[63] The thumb technique is preferred over the two-finger technique because it allows for better control of the depth of compression. Compressions should occur on the lower third of the sternum, just below the nipple line and above the xiphoid bone of the rib cage. The optimal depth of chest compressions is one-third of the anterior–posterior diameter of the chest. The heart rate should be evaluated every 45 to 60 seconds (instead of every 30 seconds as previously recommended) to avoid falls in coronary perfusion pressure and time lost in auscultation of the heart rate. If the heart rate increases to above 60 beats per minute, chest compressions may be discontinued.[11]

CASE 17

You are attending the delivery of a 27-week female infant whose mother was hospitalized last week for premature cervical dilatation at which time she received a course of betamethasone. The mother had spontaneous rupture of amniotic membranes this morning and progressed to vaginal delivery over the next few hours. At delivery, the infant is brought to the radiant warmer, covered in an occlusive wrap, and placed on an exothermic mattress.

The infant is crying spontaneously and has a heart rate of 140 beats per minute. Despite her regular respiratory effort and vigor, at 1 minute, the infant is still centrally cyanotic with moderate-to-severe intercostal and substernal retractions. Auscultation of the chest demonstrates decreased air entry bilaterally and pulse oximetry reads a saturation of 75%. You place the infant on continuous positive airway pressure (CPAP).

Which of the following statements regarding CPAP are incorrect?
A. CPAP is most effectively administered with a self-inflating bag
B. Positive end-expiratory pressure for CPAP delivery on a flow-inflating bag is controlled by an adjustable flow-control valve
C. The valve for adjustment of the positive end-expiratory pressure on a T-piece resuscitator is located on a positive end-expiratory pressure (PEEP) cap adjacent to the mask
D. CPAP is not indicated for infants with irregular respirations or apnea

Discussion

The correct answer is **A**. CPAP is a lung recruitment strategy used to establish functional residual capacity in newborns without subjecting them to the high pressures and large tidal volumes associated with mechanical ventilation. Several large randomized-controlled trials have compared CPAP administration with intubation and surfactant administration in extremely low–birth-weight infants and shown no increase in morbidities or mortality. However, no benefit has been established on the combined outcomes of death or bronchopulmonary dysplasia.[64–66] CPAP use may be appropriate in spontaneously breathing infants who require augmentation of positive end-expiratory pressure (PEEP), such as the neonate in the scenario. CPAP may not be used in infants who are apneic or have irregular respiratory drive, or those with a heart rate less than 100 bpm.[11]

A self-inflating bag inflates automatically without a compressed gas source. Unless the self-inflating bag is being squeezed, there is no gas or oxygen flow to the neonate. As such, it may not be used to deliver free-flow oxygen or CPAP. The self-inflating bag may be used to provide 90% to 100% oxygen to the infant if an oxygen reservoir is attached to the bag, and its spontaneous refill properties allow it to be used for positive-pressure ventilation in areas where a compressed gas source is not available. In contrast, a flow-inflating bag requires that gas source be flowing through the bag. Holding the bag in front of the infant's face will allow for blow-by oxygen delivery, but a good seal between the mask and the neonate's face is required to deliver inspiratory or end-expiratory pressure. The flow-inflating bag has a flow-control valve that is used to set the amount of PEEP. The disadvantages of a flow-inflating bag are that it requires experienced personnel for reliable use, and that it is possible to deliver very high pressures to the infant if the pressure manometer is not being carefully monitored. A T-piece resuscitator has the same abilities as a flow-inflating bag in that it may deliver free-flow oxygen, and in that inspiratory and expiratory pressure generation requires a good seal between the patient's face and the mask. It has the additional safety feature of a "dial in" peak inspiratory pressure, which avoids excessive unintentional pressures during resuscitation. However, increasing peak inspiratory pressure during resuscitation requires a manual mechanical adjustment on the T-piece resuscitator, and inspiratory time may be inadvertently prolonged by holding a finger over the PEEP cap for too long.[11]

CASE 18

A full-term infant is born to a multiparous mother with no significant prenatal history. The mother is group-B streptococcus negative and the amniotic fluid is clear and ruptured at delivery. Following delivery, the newborn cries vigorously, has good tone, and a heart rate of 150 beats per minute.

What is the chronologic sequence of circulatory events that lead to a successful transition after birth?

1. The foramen ovale closes due to the higher pressure in the left atrium compared with the right
2. Pulmonary vascular resistance drops once functional residual capacity is established and pO_2 increases
3. Functional closure of the ductus arteriosus occurs, separating the right and left ventricular circulation
4. Flow reversal in the ductus arteriosus leads to an increase in pulmonary venous return and left ventricular output

A. 2, 4, 3, 1
B. 2, 4, 1, 3
C. 2, 1, 4, 3
D. 2, 1, 3, 4

Discussion

The correct answer is **B**. The fetal circulation in utero is characterized by a small percentage (10–25%) of the cardiac output going to the pulmonary circulation.[67,68]

Oxygenated blood enters the fetus through the umbilical vein, passes into the liver, and is largely shunted into the inferior vena cava via the ductus venosus. The oxygenated blood from the ductus venosus enters the right atrium of the heart, and is "streamed" directly across the foramen ovale to the left atrium. This arrangement is useful in that it preferentially supplies oxygen to the brain and myocardium of the developing fetus. Of the small amount of blood from the inferior vena cava that traverses the right ventricle, the majority crosses the ductus arteriosus and either returns to the placenta via the umbilical artery or perfuses the lower body via the aorta.[11,67] Thus, although the right ventricle is the dominant contributor to cardiac output in the fetus, little right-sided blood flow enters the pulmonary circulation.

During labor, catecholamines surge and, the lung, which has previously been distended with fluid, begins to absorb lung liquid in preparation for birth. Fluid absorption prior to and around the time of birth is primarily accomplished through the action of ENaC channels, which allow for passive water clearance through the active uptake of sodium from the alveolar space.[69] In addition, vasodilators, such as prostaglandins and nitric oxide, are upregulated in preparation for the need for pulmonary vasodilation.[70] Following delivery, the newly breathing infant establishes a functional residual capacity through a net gain in inspiratory volume with each breath, and expiratory breaking maneuvers that increase end-expiratory pressure.[71] These changes, coupled with a more than doubled PaO_2, lead to the relaxation of the pulmonary vasculature and decreased lung resistance.[70] The removal of the placenta simultaneously increases systemic vascular resistance, and blood flow in the ductus arteriosus reverses from the right to left in utero flow, to a predominantly left to right flow pattern. Increased pulmonary blood flow leads to increased venous return and left atrial pressure, which closes the foramen ovale flap. As oxygen tension continues to increase and circulating prostaglandins decrease, functional closure of the ductus arteriosus commences. This functional closure of the ductus usually begins at 24 hours in the full-term neonate, but anatomic closure that involves fibrosis of the connection may take several months to achieve.[67]

CASE 19

You are anticipating the delivery of a 25-week male whose mother has been hospitalized for preeclampsia. She has been receiving magnesium sulfate, and the obstetrician has decided to proceed with a cesarean section due to severely elevated blood pressures that are refractory to medical treatment. You are considering what to request from the respiratory therapist for airway management.

What size endotracheal tube should you request for this preterm infant in the event that intubation is necessary?

A. It is best to weigh the baby first, and then decide
B. 2.0 mm
C. 2.5 mm
D. 3.0 mm

Discussion

The correct answer is **C**. The appropriate size for endotracheal tubes is determined by the weight of the baby. However, airway management should never be delayed in order to obtain a birth weight. Rather, it can be anticipated that infants less than 28 weeks (and 1,000 g) will require a 2.5-mm tube, 28 to 34 weeks (1,000–2,000 g) will require a 3.0-mm tube, 34 to 38 weeks (2,000–3,000 g) will require a 3.5-mm tube, and >38 weeks (>3,000 g) will require a 3.5–4.0-mm tube.[11] If endotracheal intubation is anticipated, supplies are needed for successful tube placement should be readily available in the delivery room. These supplies include the following: an appropriate size endotracheal tube, an appropriately sized blade (No. 1 for term newborns, No. 0 or No. 00 for preterm newborns), laryngoscope, carbon dioxide detector or monitor, waterproof tape or endotracheal tube holder, stethoscope, positive-pressure device, scissors, suction setup and catheters, pulse oximeter and probe, and an optional stylet.

CASE 20

You are attending the delivery of a 39-week infant whose prenatal ultrasounds have been concerning for micrognathia. At birth, the infant is limp, blue, and apneic. The heart rate is 80 beats per minute. The resuscitation team is attempting to provide positive-pressure ventilation, but is having difficulty achieving an adequate seal with the T-piece resuscitator. Breath sounds are difficult to auscultate and no chest rise is evident. The pulse oximeter is unable to detect an oxygen saturation or heart rate. Intubation is attempted three times, but vocal cord visualization is unsuccessful due to glossoptosis, a small oral opening, and a cleft palate.

What is the next most appropriate step in the airway management of this infant with Pierre-Robin sequence?

A. Place the infant in a prone position
B. Call for an emergency surgical consult for tracheostomy placement
C. Begin chest compressions while continuing to attempt intubation
D. Place a laryngeal mask airway to improve ventilation acutely

Discussion

The correct answer is **D**. Laryngeal mask airways are elliptical soft mask devices that can be used in patients in whom intubation is unsuccessful or positive-pressure ventilation with a bag-and-mask is unsuccessful. The NRP currently recommends considering the use of the laryngeal mask airway in four situations: (1) congenital anomalies of the face that prevent a good seal with a face mask; (2) anomalies of the mouth, tongue, pharynx, or neck that make vocal cord visualization difficult; (3) small mandibles or large tongues that may prevent ventilation or intubation; (4) ineffective ventilation with a bag-and-mask or T-piece resuscitator and an inability to successfully intubate.[11] A recent meta-analysis of available randomized-controlled trials has shown that laryngeal mask airways are safe in full-term infants, and that they can be inserted appropriately in the delivery room.[72] The safety of laryngeal mask airways has not been evaluated in very preterm infants (<32 weeks), and only the size-1 device is acceptable for use in newborns. Insertion of a laryngeal mask airway is accomplished by guiding the deflated soft cuff, with the aperture bar facing the infant's tongue, along the hard palate of the mouth until the tip nearly reaches the esophagus. The cuff may then be inflated with 4 mL of air to ensure a seal along the laryngeal opening, and the bag-and-mask or T-piece resuscitator may be attached to the airway tube. Proper placement may be confirmed by color change on the CO_2 detector, improved breath sounds and heart rate, adequate chest rise with breaths, and increasing oxygen saturations on pulse oximetry. The use of this device in special circumstances allows for a way to provide effective ventilation in a scenario in which it might otherwise not be possible.[11,72,73] Although prone positioning is a means of opening the airway for patients who have an obstruction due to glossoptosis, it requires that the patient have respiratory effort and would not be appropriate for the patient in the scenario. Although emergency tracheotomy is necessary in some patients with upper airway obstruction, it would be better to defer this procedure until the infant had been ventilated and had a stable heart rate. Answer C is incorrect because chest compressions are not indicated in an infant whose heart rate is 80 beats per minute.

CASE 21

A 42-week infant was just delivered through meconium-stained amniotic fluid. The fetal heart rate was 200 beats per minute prior to delivery, and the mother had spiked a temperature to 39 °C. The mother received antibiotics, and the obstetric team delivered the infant by urgent cesarean section. The infant has poor tone and no respiratory effort when she is brought to the radiant warmer. She is intubated for meconium, but none is noted below the vocal cords. Following positioning, warming, drying, and stimulating, her heart rate is announced as undetectable. Positive-pressure ventilation is begun, initially through a bag-and-mask and then through a successfully placed endotracheal tube. Chest compressions have now been started, because at 3 minutes of life, her heart rate is still undetectable with auscultation. An umbilical venous line is placed for intravenous access.

Which of the following statements regarding the use of epinephrine in neonatal resuscitation is true?
A. Endotracheal epinephrine at the higher dose of 0.05 to 0.1 mg/kg is more effective than 0.01 mg/kg of intravenous epinephrine
B. Intravenous epinephrine may escalated to doses as high as 0.03 mg/kg
C. Intraosseous delivery is the preferred route of epinephrine administration
D. In rare circumstances, if there is no response to high-dose epinephrine intravenously, a 1:1,000 concentration of epinephrine may be used

Discussion

The correct answer is **B**. Epinephrine administration is indicated when the heart rate is less than 60 beats per minute despite effective ventilation and 45 to 60 seconds of chest compressions. In neonatal resuscitation, the only concentration that is used is 1:10,000. The preferred route of epinephrine administration is intravenously. The intravenous epinephrine dose is 0.01 to 0.03 mg/kg, and the use of high-dose epinephrine is not recommended for intravenous administration.[73] Endotracheal epinephrine administration is variable in its absorption and efficacy, and much higher doses may be needed to achieve return of spontaneous circulation.[74,75] The NRP recommends that endotracheal epinephrine be considered only while intravenous access is being established, and that doses of 0.05 to 0.1 mg/kg be given for endotracheal administration. Intraosseous epinephrine administration may be considered for patients who are older and without intravascular access, such as those in outpatient settings and emergency departments. However, in the delivery room, the ease of umbilical venous catheter placement obviates the need for intraosseous lines.

CASE 22

You are called to the delivery room to evaluate a full-term male who is cyanotic at 10 minutes of life. The mother had no significant prenatal history, and the vaginal delivery was uneventful. On examination, the infant is crying vigorously, but his mucous membranes are blue. He has a heart rate of 120 beats per minute, and pulse oximetry is reading 65% in his right hand. On auscultation you note that the heart sounds can be heard predominantly in the right chest, and you question if you hear gurgling sounds over the left lower lung field. On closer inspection, the abdomen appears unusually flat and concave.

What is the next most appropriate step in the delivery room management of this infant?
A. Avoid oxygen and order an urgent echocardiogram and cardiology consult for the infant
B. Begin bag-and-mask ventilation with 100% oxygen to determine if oxygen saturations will improve
C. Transilluminate the chest while you ask a nurse to prepare for thoracentesis
D. Immediately intubate the infant and place a Replogle tube to decompress the stomach

Discussion

The correct answer is **D**. The baby in the scenario has congenital diaphragmatic hernia. The most common type of congenital diaphragmatic hernia is the Bochdalek type, which results from failure of the closure of the posterolateral portions of the diaphragm during development. Eighty-five percent of diaphragmatic hernias occur on the left side and 13% occur on the right. The defect in diaphragmatic closure allows abdominal contents to migrate into the thorax, impairing normal lung growth both on the ipsilateral and contralateral side of the defect.[76] The infant in the scenario is cyanotic due to the lack of normal lung development, and, potentially, from persistent pulmonary hypertension of the newborn due to hypoxia and abnormal pulmonary vascular development. Delivery room resuscitation maneuvers for infants with congenital diaphragmatic hernia center around limiting the accumulation of gas in the displaced intestines, which would further impair lung expansion and oxygenation. Positive-pressure ventilation is avoided and immediate intubation of the trachea is recommended to allow for airway management while restricting airflow into the intestines. In addition, a Replogle tube should be placed in order to decompress stomach air and contents.[11] Answer A is incorrect because, although an infant with congenital heart disease may appear cyanotic without work of breathing, and may have displaced cardiac sounds, the abdomen should not appear scaphoid and bowel sounds should not be heard in the chest. Answer B is incorrect. Positive-pressure ventilation is indicated for patients with low oxygen saturations that do not improve with blow-by oxygen or CPAP. However, in this scenario the infant has physical examination findings of congenital diaphragmatic hernia, and positive-pressure ventilation may increase bowel dilatation and worsen the respiratory status. Answer C is incorrect because, although a left pneumothorax could displace heart sounds to the right, the other physical examination findings make this diagnosis an unlikely possibility.

Objectives

1. Understand the basic principles of neonatal resuscitation
2. Understand appropriate response to the hypoxic newborn during neonatal resuscitation
3. Understand the differences in the types of equipment used to provide respiratory support in the newborn, including bag-and-mask ventilation, appropriate ETT sizes, and oral airway
4. Understand indications for volume expansion during neonatal resuscitation
5. Understand indications for use of medications during neonatal resuscitation
6. Describe features associated with hypoxic-ischemic encephalopathy and appropriate management
7. Describe Sarnat staging
8. Understand the physiologic changes that occur during the transition to extrauterine life
9. Identify maternal risk factors that are frequently associated with the need for advanced resuscitation after delivery
10. Understand mechanisms of heat loss in the neonate and describe prevention strategies to minimize heat loss during resuscitation

REFERENCES

1. Gasem T, Al Jama FE, Burshaid S, et al. Maternal and fetal outcome of pregnancy complicated by HELLP syndrome. *J Matern Fetal Neona*. 2009;22:1140–1143.

2. Han CS, Schatz F, Lockwood CJ. Abruption-associated prematurity. *Clin Perinatol*. 2011;38(3):407–421.

3. Mally PV, Hendricks-Munoz KD, Bailey S. Incidence and etiology of late preterm admissions to the neonatal intensive care unit and its associated respiratory morbidities when compared to term infants. *Am J Perinatol*. 2013;30(5):425–431.

4. Delivoria-Papadopoulos M, Mishra OP. Nuclear mechanisms of hypoxic cerebral injury in the newborn. *Clin Perinatol*. 2004;31:91–105.

5. Fatemi A, Wilson MA, Johnston MV. Hypoxic-ischemic encephalopathy in the term infant. *Clin Perinatol*. 2009;36: 835–858, vii.

6. Shankaran S, Laptook AR, Ehrenkranz RA, et al. Whole-body hypothermia for neonates with hypoxic-ischemic encephalopathy. *N Engl J Med*. 2005;353:1574–1584.

7. Azzopardi DV, Strohm B, Edwards AD, et al. Moderate hypothermia to treat perinatal asphyxial encephalopathy. *N Engl J Med*. 2009;361:1349–1358.

8. Shankaran S, Pappas A, McDonald SA, et al. Childhood outcomes after hypothermia for neonatal encephalopathy. *N Engl J Med*. 2012;366:2085–2092.

9. Wiswell TE. Handling the meconium-stained infant. *Semin Neonatol*. 2001;6:225–231.

10. Xu H, Calvet M, Wei S, et al. Risk factors for early and late onset of respiratory symptoms in babies born through meconium. *Am J Perinatol*. 2010;27:271–278.

11. American Heart Association and American Academy of Pediatrics. *Textbook of Neonatal Resuscitation*. 6th ed. AAP, 2011.

12. Kattwinkel J, Perlman JM, Aziz K, et al. Part 15: Neonatal resuscitation: 2010 American Heart Association Guidelines for Cardiopulmonary Resuscitation and Emergency Cardiovascular Care. *Circulation*. 2010;122:S909–S919.

13. Rosenberg A. The IUGR newborn. *Semin Perinatol*. 2008; 32:219–224.

14. Pallotto EK, Kilbride HW. Perinatal outcome and later implications of intrauterine growth restriction. *Clin Obstet Gynecol*. 2006;49:257–269.

15. Miller J, Turan S, Baschat AA. Fetal growth restriction. *Semin Perinatol*. 2008;32:274–280.

16. Shankaran S, Laptook AR, Tyson JE, et al. Evolution of encephalopathy during whole body hypothermia for neonatal hypoxic-ischemic encephalopathy. *J Pediatr*. 2012;160:567–572.e3.

17. Levene ML, Kornberg J, Williams TH. The incidence and severity of post-asphyxial encephalopathy in full-term infants. *Early Hum Dev*. 1985;11:21–26.

18. Levene MI, Sands C, Grindulis H, Moore JR. Comparison of two methods of predicting outcome in perinatal asphyxia. *Lancet*. 1986;1:67–69.

19. Shah PS, Beyene J, To T, et al. Postasphyxial hypoxic-ischemic encephalopathy in neonates: outcome prediction rule within 4 hours of birth. *Arch Pediatr Adolesc Med*. 2006;160:729–736.

20. Shah PS. Hypothermia: A systematic review and meta-analysis of clinical trials. *Semin Fetal Neonatal Med*. 2010;15:238–246.

21. Shankaran S. Therapeutic hypothermia for neonatal encephalopathy. *Curr Treat Options Neurol*. 2012;14:608–619.

22. Ehrenstein V. Association of Apgar scores with death and neurologic disability. *Clin Epidemiol*. 2009;1:45–53.

23. Wyckoff MH, Salhab WA, Heyne RJ, et al. Outcome of extremely low birth weight infants who received delivery room cardiopulmonary resuscitation. *J Pediatr.* 2012;160:239–244.e2.

24. Laptook AR, Shankaran S, Ambalavanan N, et al. Outcome of term infants using apgar scores at 10 minutes following hypoxic-ischemic encephalopathy. *Pediatrics.* 2009;124:1619–1626.

25. Bashambu MT, Whitehead H, Hibbs AM, et al. Evaluation of interobserver agreement of apgar scoring in preterm infants. *Pediatrics.* 2012;130:e982–e987.

26. Molloy EJ, Deakins K. Are carbon dioxide detectors useful in neonates? *Arch Dis Child Fetal Neonatal Ed.* 2006;91:F295–F298.

27. Bhende MS, Thompson AE. Evaluation of an end-tidal CO_2 detector during pediatric cardiopulmonary resuscitation. *Pediatrics.* 1995;95:395–399.

28. Schmolzer GM, Poulton DA, Dawson JA, et al. Assessment of flow waves and colorimetric CO2 detector for endotracheal tube placement during neonatal resuscitation. *Resuscitation.* 2011;82:307–312.

29. Laptook AR, Watkinson M. Temperature management in the delivery room. *Semin Fetal Neonatal Med.* 2008;13:383–391.

30. Laptook AR, Salhab W, Bhaskar B. Admission temperature of low birth weight infants: predictors and associated morbidities. *Pediatrics.* 2007;119:e643–e649.

31. Dollberg S, Hoath S. "Temperature regulation in preterm infants: Role of the skin-environment interface." *Neoreviews.* 2001;2:e282–e291.

32. Rohana J, Khairina W, Boo NY, et al. Reducing hypothermia in preterm infants with polyethylene wrap. *Pediatr Int.* 2011;53:468–474.

33. Mathew B, Lakshminrusimha S, Sengupta S, et al. Randomized controlled trial of vinyl bags versus thermal mattress to prevent hypothermia in extremely low-gestational-age infants. *Am J Perinatol.* 2012;30(4):317–322.

34. Vohra S, Roberts RS, Zhang B, et al. Heat loss prevention (HeLP) in the delivery room: A randomized controlled trial of polyethylene occlusive skin wrapping in very preterm infants. *J Pediatr.* 2004;145:750–753.

35. Simon P, Dannaway D, Bright B, et al. Thermal defense of extremely low gestational age newborns during resuscitation: exothermic mattresses vs polyethylene wrap. *J Perinatol.* 2011;31:33–37.

36. Singh A, Duckett J, Newton T, et al. Improving neonatal unit admission temperatures in preterm babies: Exothermic mattresses, polythene bags or a traditional approach? *J Perinatol.* 2010;30:45–49.

37. Jia YS, Lin ZL, Lv H, et al. Effect of delivery room temperature on the admission temperature of premature infants: a randomized controlled trial. *J Perinatol.* 2013;33(4):264–267.

38. Perlman JM, Wyllie J, Kattwinkel J, et al. Part 11: Neonatal resuscitation: 2010 International Consensus on Cardiopulmonary Resuscitation and Emergency Cardiovascular Care Science With Treatment Recommendations. *Circulation.* 2010;122:S516–538.

39. Jensen A, Garnier Y, Berger R. Dynamics of fetal circulatory responses to hypoxia and asphyxia. *Eur J Obstet Gynecol Reprod Biol.* 1999;84:155–172.

40. Perlman JM. Interruption of placental blood flow during labor: Potential systemic and cerebral organ consequences. *J Pediatr.* 2011;158:e1–e4.

41. Leone TA, Finer NN. Shock: A common consequence of neonatal asphyxia. *J Pediatr.* 2011;158:e9–e12.

42. Escobar J, Cernada M, Vento M. "Oxygen and oxidative stress in the neonatal period". *Neoreviews.* 2011;12:e613–e623.

43. Kamlin CO, O'Donnell CP, Davis PG, et al. Oxygen saturation in healthy infants immediately after birth. *J Pediatr.* 2006;148:585–589.

44. Mariani G, Dik PB, Ezquer A, et al. Pre-ductal and post-ductal O_2 saturation in healthy term neonates after birth. *J Pediatr.* 2007;150:418–421.

45. Wang CL, Anderson C, Leone TA, et al. Resuscitation of preterm neonates by using room air or 100% oxygen. *Pediatrics.* 2008;121:1083–1089.

46. Kapadia VS, Chalak LF, Sparks JE, et al. Resuscitation of preterm neonates with limited versus high oxygen strategy. *Pediatrics.* 2013;132:e1488–e1496.

47. Vento M, Saugstad OD. Oxygen supplementation in the delivery room: Updated information. *J Pediatr.* 2011;158:e5–e7.

48. Wollen EJ, Sejersted Y, Wright MS, et al. Transcriptome profiling of the newborn mouse brain after hypoxia-reoxygenation: Hyperoxic reoxygenation induces inflammatory and energy failure responsive genes. *Pediatr Res.* 2014;75:517–526.

49. Fanos V, Noto A, Xanthos T, et al. Metabolomics network characterization of resuscitation after normocapnic hypoxia in a newborn piglet model supports the hypothesis that room air is better. *BioMed Res Internat.* 2014;2014:731620.

50. Faa G, Fanos V, Fanni D, et al. Reoxygenation of asphyxiated newborn piglets: administration of 100% oxygen causes significantly higher apoptosis in cortical neurons, as compared to 21%. *BioMed Res Internat.* 2014;2014:476349.

51. Weintraub AY, Leron E, Mazor M. The pathophysiology of trauma in pregnancy: a review. *J Matern Fetal Neona.* 2006;19:601–605.

52. Boluyt N, Bollen CW, Bos AP, et al. Fluid resuscitation in neonatal and pediatric hypovolemic shock: a Dutch Pediatric Society evidence-based clinical practice guideline. *Intensive Care Med.* 2006;32:995–1003.

53. Wyckoff M, Garcia D, Margraf L, et al. Randomized trial of volume infusion during resuscitation of asphyxiated neonatal piglets. *Pediatr Res.* 2007;61:415–420.

54. Wyckoff MH, Perlman JM, Laptook AR. Use of volume expansion during delivery room resuscitation in near-term and term infants. *Pediatrics.* 2005;115:950–955.

55. Dykes FD, Lazzara A, Ahmann P, et al. Intraventricular hemorrhage: a prospective evaluation of etiopathogenesis. *Pediatrics.* 1980;66:42–49.

56. Thorp JA, Rushing RS. Umbilical cord blood gas analysis. *Obstet Gynecol Clin North Am.* 1999;26:695–709.

57. Druzin M, Peterson N. "Strip of the month: December 2012". *Neoreviews.* 2012;13:e736–e745.

58. Blickstein I, Green T. Umbilical cord blood gases. *Clin Perinatol.* 2007;34:451–459.

59. Benitz W, Druzin M. "Pharmacology review: Drugs that affect neonatal resuscitation". *Neoreviews.* 2005;6:e189–e194.

60. Guinsburg R, Wyckoff MH. Naloxone during neonatal resuscitation: acknowledging the unknown. *Clin Perinatol.* 2006;33:121–132, viii.

61. Alonso-Spilsbury M, Mota-Rojas D, Villanueva-Garcia D, et al. Perinatal asphyxia pathophysiology in pig and human: A review. *Anim Reprod Sci.* 2005;90:1–30.

62. Gupta JM, Tizard JP. The sequence of events in neonatal apnoea. *Lancet.* 1967;2:55–59.

63. Wyckoff M. "Neonatal cardiopulmonary resuscitation: Critical hemodynamics". *Neoreviews.* 2010;11:e123–e129.

64. Carlo WA. Gentle ventilation: The new evidence from the SUPPORT, COIN, VON, CURPAP, Colombian Network, and Neocosur network trials. *Early Hum Dev.* 2012;88(Suppl 2): S81–S83.

65. Wiswell TE. Resuscitation in the delivery room: lung protection from the first breath. *Respir Care.* 2011;56:1360–1367; discussion 1367–1368.

66. Gupta S, Sinha SK, Donn SM. Myth: Mechanical ventilation is a therapeutic relic. *Semin Fetal Neonatal Med.* 2011;16: 275–278.

67. Dyer A, Ikemba C. "Core concepts: Fetal cardiac physiology". *Neoreviews.* 2012;13:e583–e589.

68. Bry K. "Newborn Resuscitation and the Lung". *Neoreviews.* 2008;9:e506–e511.

69. Elias N, O'Brodovich H. "Clearance of fluid from airspaces of newborns and infants". *Neoreviews.* 2006;7:e88–e93.

70. Khonduri G. "Modulation of nitric oxide release in perinatal lung". *Neoreviews.* 2001;2:e61–e66.

71. Hooper S, te Pas A, Lewis R, et al. "Establishing functional residual capacity at birth". *Neoreviews.* 2010;11:e474–e483.

72. Schmolzer GM, Agarwal M, Kamlin CO, et al. Supraglottic airway devices during neonatal resuscitation: An historical perspective, systematic review and meta-analysis of available clinical trials. *Resuscitation.* 2013;84(6):722–730.

73. The International Liaison Committee on Resuscitation (ILCOR) consensus on science with treatment recommendations for pediatric and neonatal patients: neonatal resuscitation. *Pediatrics.* 2006;117:e978–e988.

74. Barber CA, Wyckoff MH. Use and efficacy of endotracheal versus intravenous epinephrine during neonatal cardiopulmonary resuscitation in the delivery room. *Pediatrics.* 2006; 118:1028–1034.

75. Wyckoff MH, Wyllie J. Endotracheal delivery of medications during neonatal resuscitation. *Clin Perinatol.* 2006;33: 153–160, ix.

76. Benjamin J, Bizzarro M, Cotten CM. "Congenital diaphragmatic hernia: Updates and outcomes". *Neoreviews.* 2011;12: e439–e452.

Embryology and Morphogenesis

CASE 1

A friend tells you that she is in her first trimester of a thus far uncomplicated pregnancy. There is no family history of congenital heart disease (CHD) in either her or her spouse. She reports that she is a copious consumer of caffeine and has a history of anxiety. She also had a urinary tract infection prior her knowledge of the pregnancy and was treated with two antibiotics. She is concerned about increased risk for anomalies.

Which of the following about the risk of CHD is NOT true?
A. High levels of caffeine intake (>800 g/day or eight cups of coffee) are associated with an increased risk of fetal cardiac valve abnormalities
B. Increased risk of CHD associated with the use of folate antagonists such as trimethoprim/sulfamethoxazole in the second trimester can be reduced with folic acid supplementation
C. Maternal ampicillin use has not been associated with an increased risk of congenital cardiac disease
D. Moderate intake (400 g/day) of caffeine in coffee, tea, or soda is not associated with an increased risk of CHD
E. Several case-control studies have not shown an increased risk of cardiac malformation after first-trimester maternal use of diazepam

Discussion

The correct answer is **A**. Multiple studies have not demonstrated an association between maternal caffeine intake and CHD, even at high doses. Few antibiotics have been well studied in pregnancy but maternal treatment with ampicillin and penicillin has not been shown to increase risk.[1] Tetrahydrofolate is necessary for the conversion of homocysteine to methionine and thus essential for Deoxyribonucleic acid (DNA) and Ribonucleic acid (RNA) synthesis. Intrauterine exposure to folic acid antagonists including methotrexate, trimethoprim/sulfamethoxazole, and sulfasalazine is associated with a number of specific birth defects, including neural tube, cardiovascular, and urinary tract malformations. Folic acid supplementation in women at increased risk or with prior antifolate exposure has been shown to attenuate these risks.[2] Since many pregnancies are unplanned or the increased risk is unknown, folic acid supplementation of grains has been undertaken in the United States and Canada, as well as other countries worldwide, with a reduction in the incidence of associated anomalies.[3]

Helpful Tip: The overall incidence of serious CHD is approximately 6/1,000 live births, although it is higher in high-risk populations. Of these only 1 to 2/1,000 will have critical CHD, requiring treatment or surgery in the first 30 days of life.[4]

Helpful Tip: Despite their rarity, cardiac defects are the most common congenital malformations leading to mortality.

CASE 2

You attend the delivery of an infant whose mother received limited prenatal care but did reportedly appear in triage visibly intoxicated on at least one occasion. The infant weighs just 1,950 g but examination is consistent with a 36 weeks' gestation. The head appears small and there are several minor facial dysmorphisms. The infant is pink and breathing comfortably in room air by 15 minutes of life.

What is the most common type of CHD you might find?
A. Tetralogy of Fallot (TOF)
B. Atrial septal defect (ASD)
C. Ventricular septal defect (VSD)
D. Ebstein anomaly
E. Patent ductus arteriosus (PDA)

Discussion

The correct answer is **C**. The infant described has features of fetal alcohol syndrome (FAS), which include growth restriction, microcephaly, short nose and smooth philtrum, joint abnormalities, small fifth fingers and fingernails, and irritability. Heart murmurs are frequent and often not associated with cardiac malformations. CHD is more frequent in infants with FAS, with the most common form being a VSD, ASD, TOF, and coarctation of the aorta (CoA) are also seen with decreasing frequency.[5,6] Ebstein anomaly is associated with intake of Lithium and use of marijuana. A PDA is common in preterm infants and also associated with maternal rubella exposure.

Helpful Tip: The location of a VSD can help predict the risk of a genetic syndrome. Membranous VSDs are more frequently associated with chromosomal anomalies than muscular VSDs.[7]

The infant is subsequently diagnosed with TOF and will need corrective surgery in the first 3 to 6 months of life. The mother states that she gave up alcohol once she knew for certain she was pregnant and wonders if this is related to her prior intake.

She asks when such an abnormality occurs in cardiac development?
A. Embryonic day 21
B. Embryonic day 28
C. Embryonic day 35
D. Embryonic day 45
E. Embryonic day 58

Discussion

The correct answer is **D**. The normal cardiac outflow tract develops following rightward heart looping that occurs on day 28 and places the primitive outflow tissues next to the endocardial cushions.[8] The atrioventricular septum forms at day 35 and separates the right and left side of the heart. The conotruncus arises primarily from the right ventricle and then shifts to the left, becoming the aortopulmonary trunk also at day 35. The conotruncal septum arises from mesenchymal cells and creates the primitive aorta and pulmonary arteries. Failure of this process will result in truncus arteriosus (TA). The primitive aorta communicates with the right ventricle and the pulmonary outflow tract with the left, so rotation is necessary for proper connection and function. Failure of rotation (day 42) results in the development of transposition of the great arteries (TGA), while incomplete rotation (day 45) will result in TOF. The normal positioning places the pulmonary artery rightward and ventral while the aorta is dorsal and leftward.

The cells that form the distal conotruncal septum originate from which population of cells?
A. Mesenchymal cells derived from primitive endocardium (cushions) through epithelial-to-mesenchymal transformation (EMT)
B. Cardiac mesodermal cells from the primitive streak
C. Neural crest derived mesenchymal cells from the hindbrain
D. Local recruitment of differentiating myocytes in the developing coronary artery system
E. Coelomic mesenchyme originating from the septum transversum

Discussion

The correct answer is **C**. The embryonic heart is formed from cells of several different embryonic lineages and development is dependent on a number of cell–cell interactions and cellular transformation. It is the first organ to form in vertebrates, shortly after gastrulation (day 20) and begins contracting at day 23. The majority of heart tissue arises from mesodermal cells from the primitive streak which migrate to form the first heart field or cardiac crescent.[8] The primitive heart tube elongates and eventually undergoes looping. The endocardial and myocardial layers develop and become segmented into the atria, atrioventricular valve, ventricle, and the outflow tract. In the extracellular matrix tissue between the endocardial and myocardial layers, mesenchymal cells from the endocardium undergo EMT and begin to form the atrioventricular cushions, which become the atrioventricular valves, and the proximal outflow tract. This is mediated by multiple signaling factors including the TGF-β family, bone morphogenetic proteins (BMP 2, 4), and vascular endothelial growth factor (VEGF). Coelomic mesenchyme develops into the proepicardial organ then migrates to the heart to form the epicardium.

Neural crest cells migrate from the hindbrain, across the pharyngeal arches, into the early distal outflow tract. They settle in truncal cushions, then grow, and fuse to form the aortopulmonary septum, separating the systemic and pulmonary circulations.[9] They are also necessary for aortic arch formation. Other neural crest cells migrate throughout the body to form the peripheral nervous system, adrenal glands, and melanocytes. The development of the cardiac conduction system is poorly understood and was once thought to be derived from neural crest cells, but recently studies have shown that conducting cells are recruited from myocytes in the coronary artery system.

In addition to fetal alcohol exposure, many other exposures frequently result in abnormalities of the cardiac outflow tract. Which of the following is NOT associated?
A. Retinoic acid exposure
B. Lithium exposure
C. Maternal influenza
D. Pregestational diabetes
E. Pesticide exposure

Discussion

The correct answer is **B**. The complexity of outflow tract development causes it to be a common form of CHD and many in utero exposures are associated with disruption of this complex signaling cascade.[10] A variety of conotruncal abnormalities may arise depending on the nature and timing of the insult, including TOF, double outlet right ventricle (DORV), TGA, and TA. Pregestational maternal diabetes is associated with a number of congenital heart malformations including conotruncal defects and TGA, outflow tract defects, and hypoplastic left heart syndrome (HLHS).[11,12] An association is sometimes seen with CHD and purely gestational diabetes, but some of these cases may represent undiagnosed type 2 diabetes in women prior to pregnancy. Good glycemic control can substantially decrease this risk, though the mechanism is unknown. Maternal phenylketonuria is also associated with a six-fold increased risk of CHD.

Maternal infection in the first trimester also increases the risk of cardiac malformation. Of these, rubella is the most well-known, but any maternal febrile illness increases the risk of heart disease in the developing fetus. Influenza specifically is associated with right-and left-sided obstructive lesions in addition to conotruncal defects, tricuspid atresia, and coarctation. The mechanism by which abnormalities develop is unclear and it is currently unknown whether fever itself, in the absence of illness, is teratogenic.

Multiple known cardiac teratogens also exist including therapeutic drugs, recreational drugs, and environmental toxin exposures. Maternal use of vitamin A derivatives for acne treatment or excess vitamin A exposure causes CHD and other central nervous system and craniofacial abnormalities. Vitamin A has a role in regulating neural crest cell development and migration, leading to these abnormalities.[1,12] Other medications with definitively increased risk of congenital heart malformation include thalidomide, nonsteroidal anti-inflammatory medications, and trimethoprim-sulfamethoxazole, a folate antagonist. Many other medications have a potential risk. A number of occupational exposures have also been associated with CHD. Mothers working in the agricultural industry have an increased risk of conotruncal defects. Organic solvent exposure leads to a wide variety of anomalies.

Characteristic anomalies are associated with some antiepileptic drugs (hydantoin, valproic acid) but an increased frequency of malformations is also documented in epileptic women not taking medication.[13] Maternal lithium use is classically associated with Ebstein abnormality rather than outflow tract malformations and more recent data shows this risk may have been overstated.[1]

Helpful Tip: A glycosylated hemoglobin level (HgbA1c) is indicative of the degree of glucose control. A first-trimester HgbA1c level of >10% is indicative of poor control and almost one-third of these infants will have fetal malformations.[14]

CASE 3

A mother presents in labor at an estimated 39 weeks by LMP. She reports she has recently emigrated from Guatemala and not been able to afford prenatal care since arrival. She had two prenatal visits prior to arrival in the US. She is unsure which prenatal labs were sent and did not receive any recent vaccinations. The infant is delivered vaginally, is breathing spontaneously at delivery, pink, and weighs 2,100 g. In addition to his small size, you notice a smaller than expected head with small eyes and cloudy corneas. On further examination you note a protuberant abdomen with a liver palpable 4 cm below the costal margin. There are multiple purpuric areas seen on the chest and shoulders. The infant is admitted to the NICU for observation. The following day, a murmur is noted.

What type of CHD is most characteristic for this infant?

A. Pulmonary atresia (PA)
B. DORV
C. VSD
D. CoA
E. PDA

Discussion

The correct answer is **E**. This infant has clinical and historical features consistent with congenital rubella syndrome (CRS). CRS is often a severe illness causing growth restriction, chorioretinitis, cataracts, hearing loss, hepatosplenomegaly, and thrombocytopenia as well as heart disease. Extramedullary hematopoiesis visible in the skin causes the characteristic blueberry muffin rash, but this can also occur with congenital cytomegalovirus infection (CMV) and neuroblastoma. Heart disease is common and presents in 60% to 70% of affected neonates.[15,16] PDA and pulmonary arterial stenosis are characteristic pathological lesions though other heart disease may occur. Since widespread use of the MMR vaccine in the United States, the incidence of CRS has dropped dramatically and most cases occur in recent immigrants.[17] Universal vaccination is not the norm in developing countries and it is estimated that more than 100,000 cases of congenital rubella occur worldwide each year.

After discussion, the mother reports a lengthy febrile illness occurring when she was about 3 months pregnant. She reports significant joint pain as well as headaches and general malaise.

What is the risk of CRS with a primary infection at 12 -weeks' gestation?

A. 75%
B. 50%
C. 20%
D. 10%
E. 2%

Discussion

The correct answer is **B**. Fetal disease is common with primary maternal infection and unlike other infectious illnesses such as toxoplasmosis or herpes simplex virus, the risk decreases with advancing gestation. The highest risk is in the first 8 weeks of pregnancy (75%), and this decreases to 50% from weeks 9 to 12. Subsequently risk is increasingly low, and under 10% by the 20th week of pregnancy.[12,18]

Women should be tested routinely for immunity to rubella during pregnancy, and titers sent for exposure (IgG, IgM) if found to be nonimmune. The risk to the fetus may be high, depending on the timing of exposure. Routine childhood vaccination is recommended, as is postpartum vaccination of a nonimmunized woman. There is no disease-specific treatment for CRS, care is supportive. Growth and hearing should be monitored into childhood.

Objectives

1. Understand the timing and embryology of the development of the heart
2. Identify exposures, teratogens, and medications associated with an increased risk of congenital heart defects
3. Identify the clinical features associated with fetal alcohol exposure
4. Identify the clinical features associated with CRS

Genetics of Heart Disease

CASE 4

You are evaluating an infant in term nursery whose nurse reports hearing a loud murmur. The baby is 42-hour old and the mother reports the baby is eating well and has voided and stooled. He has a slight degree of visible jaundice. As you talk to the mother she reports that she had heart surgery when she was a child, but is unsure of her diagnosis or type of surgery.

Which of the following is NOT true about recurrence risk in CHD

A. Aortic stenosis (AS) is one of the most commonly recurring malformations seen in a parent and affected child
B. Having two affected siblings, but healthy parents, gives a recurrence risk of 8% to 10%
C. In recurrent familial CHD, concordance (same subtype of CHD) is expected in just over half of the cases
D. If the mother is the affected parent, the recurrence risk is higher
E. Asymptomatic lesions may be seen in up to 20% of first-degree relatives of patients with left-sided obstructive lesions

Discussion

The correct answer is **C**. Recurrence risk varies widely by the type of CHD and which relatives are affected. In the absence of specific genetic or single gene diagnosis, risk is estimated on the basis of epidemiologic data.[12,19,20] In general, an affected mother provides the highest degree of recurrence risk. If the parents are unaffected, recurrence risk from a single affected sibling is around 2%. These risk increase substantially if a second sibling is affected. Ventricular septal defect (VSD), aortic stenosis (AS) and atrioventricular septal defect (AVSD) are some of the most common recurring malformations seen in a mother or father and child; in part because these are usually associated with prolonged survival and the ability to bear children. Parental recurrence data for severe cyanotic heart disease is generally unavailable. There is substantial variability in concordance with the type of malformation between family members, both in terms of specific subtype and the general spectrum of CHD. Less than half (47%) of affected individuals will have recurrent CHD within the same spectrum. When asymptomatic first-degree relatives of those with significant CHD (e.g., HLHS) are evaluated routinely, up to 20% will have abnormal echocardiographic findings (e.g., bicuspid aortic valve).

With this history in mind, you perform a full evaluation. The baby is pink and well perfused. Lungs are clear to auscultation. A late peaking systolic murmur is heard at the left upper sternal border and the cardiac impulse is slightly leftward. Pulses are good in all extremities. You also note some minor facial dysmorphisms including a small ears and mouth and a sloped, bulbous nose.

Which of the following congenital cardiac anomalies would NOT be typical for the infant described above?
A. Double aortic arch with vascular ring
B. Transposition of the great arteries
C. Tetralogy of Fallot
D. Interrupted aortic arch
E. Truncus arteriosus

Discussion

The correct answer is **B**. The infant described above has clinical features consistent with 22q11.2 deletion syndrome, also known as DiGeorge syndrome. More than 80% of the affected infants will have congenital cardiac anomalies in addition to hearing loss, cleft lip and palate, and feeding difficulties.[21] Multiple genes have been identified from the deleted region of chromosome 22

and several (TBX1, CRKL, ERK2) are known to be involved in neural crest cell migration. Subsequent abnormalities in anterior heart field development result in conotruncal anomalies, the most typical of which are interrupted aortic arch, double aortic arch, and tetralogy of Fallot with or without pulmonary atresia.[22] Truncus arteriosus may also occur. Transposition of the great arteries has been described in infants diagnosed with 22q11.2 deletion but is atypical and diagnosed in <1% of cases.

Helpful Tip: The features of classic 22q11.2 deletion syndrome can be remembered with the mnemonic CATCH (Cardiac, Abnormal facies, Thymic aplasia, Cleft palate, Hypoparathyroidism/Hypocalcemia) but children can present with a variety of features. This is partially based on the size of the deletion but features can vary within a family. It may also be referred to as velocardiofacial syndrome.

Helpful Tip: Although 22q11.2 deletion syndrome can be inherited in an autosomal dominant fashion, this chromosome is highly prone to rearrangements. Therefore the majority (>90%) of cases are de novo mutations in a previously unaffected family.

Quick Quiz: Prenatal Diagnosis/Screening

Which of the following is FALSE regarding prenatal evaluation for congenital cardiac disease?
A. The majority of fetuses with CHD occur in a high-risk population
B. Prenatal diagnosis of HLHS has been shown to improve outcomes
C. The majority of fetuses with CHD do not show overt signs of cardiac failure during fetal life
D. Monochorionic pregnancy is an indication for fetal echocardiogram
E. The strongest evidence for a benefit of fetal intervention is in the treatment of fetal arrhythmias

Discussion

The correct answer is **A**. Although family history of CHD and certain maternal risk factors increase the risk of CHD and are an indication for fetal echocardiogram, the majority of cases occur in a low-risk population. Diagnosis is therefore dependent on routine prenatal US. Prenatal diagnosis of HLHS, coarctation, and TGA is associated with improved outcomes. Due to the differences in fetal circulation, most fetuses with CHD will not show signs of failure in utero. Monochorionic twins are at increased risk for anomalies and twin-twin transfusion syndrome (TTTS). Although a minority of infants with certain anatomy (e.g., HLHS with a restrictive atrial septum) may be considered candidates for fetal intervention, definitive data on outcomes is lacking. Treatment of a fetal arrhythmia is considered standard of care, and may result in improved cardiac function or resolution of hydrops.

CASE 5

A mother presents in labor with an estimated fetal weight of 800 g and is receiving magnesium for tocolysis. You obtain prenatal records which show her to be a 43-year-old G3P1 with one healthy daughter. Prenatal infectious laboratory work was unremarkable but the quad screen showed a low AFP and low estriol. The mother reports that prenatal US showed a cardiac abnormality. She has not yet had a fetal echo, cell-free fetal DNA testing, or an amniocentesis. The mother asks about possible chromosomal abnormalities and the risk of heart disease.

Which of the following has the highest risk of congenital heart malformation?
A. Trisomy 13 (Patau syndrome)
B. Trisomy 18 (Edward syndrome)
C. Monosomy X (Turner syndrome)
D. Tetrasomy 22p (Cat eye syndrome)
E. Trisomy 21 (Down syndrome)

Discussion

The correct answer is **B**. Known chromosomal disorders are associated with approximately 10% of cases of CHD and all of the above are commonly associated. Many chromosomal anomalies are associated with a high rate of spontaneous loss. Trisomy 21 occurs more frequently among live-born newborns and are therefore the most common chromosomal anomaly found in infants with CHD.[23,24] About half (40%–50%) of the patients with Down syndrome will have significant CHD. Almost all (90%–100%) infants with trisomy 18 will have CHD as will those with trisomy 13 (80%). About 50% of infants with Cat eye syndrome will have heart disease, most commonly abnormalities in pulmonary venous return (total anomalous pulmonary venous return [TAPVR], PAPVR). Girls with Turner syndrome are least likely to be affected, 25% to 35% and characteristically have systemic outflow abnormalities (coarctation, AS; http://ghr.nlm.nih.gov/condition/noonan-syndrome). Noonan syndrome is a disorder with autosomal domi-

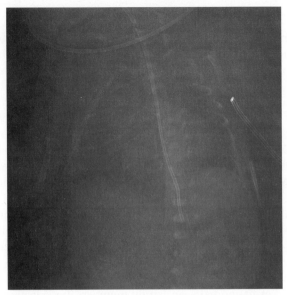

FIGURE 4-1. Portable Chest x-ray of the infant described in Case 5.

nant inheritance pattern that also frequently has associated cardiovascular anomalies (80%–85%). The most common finding is pulmonary valve stenosis, though other malformations can occur.[12] Most cases of Noonan syndrome result from mutations in one of the three genes, PTPN11, SOS1, or RAF1. The typical phenotype includes dysmorphic facial features, short neck, low hairline, broad chest, pectus excavatum or pectus carinatum, scoliosis, bleeding disorders, and cryptorchidism in affected males.

The infant delivers several days later and weighs 980 g. He is breathing spontaneously at delivery but with substantial respiratory effort and remains cyanotic and ultimately requires intubation. Saturations are in the low 90s on 40% oxygen after intubation and surfactant. He is well perfused. Several other abnormalities are noted including a large umbilical cord hernia and imperforate anus. He is notably dysmorphic with low set ears, heavy eyebrows, and microcephaly. Hands are held clenched but his general tone is fairly normal. A chest x-ray (CXR) is performed and findings are shown in Figure 4-1.

Which CHD is most consistent with this history and CXR?
A. VSD
B. HLHS
C. DORV
D. TOF
E. CoA

Discussion

The correct answer is **D**. This infant has clinical features compatible with trisomy 18.[23] The CXR reveals a boot-shaped heart which is consistent with the diagnosis of TOF. Tetralogy of Fallot consists of a grouping of four interrelated cardiac defects: (1) narrowing of the pulmonary outflow tract (pulmonary stenosis or atresia), (2) ventricular septal defect, (3) overriding aorta which is shifted to be more over the right ventricle, and (4) right ventricular hypertrophy. The degree of pulmonary obstruction varies widely leading to a range of presentation and of saturation on diagnosis. All the other listed malformations are seen in patients with trisomy 18, but this is the only one consistent with history and CXR.

Helpful Tip: Nuchal translucency (NT) thickness evaluation is now part of routine prenatal ultrasound evaluation in the first trimester, especially for high-risk mothers. Increased NT thickness is seen in infants with chromosomal anomalies and heart disease, but there is also an association between NT >99th percentile and CHD in the absence of a chromosomal disorder.[7]

Helpful Tip: Although congenital cardiac disease is more common in certain genetic syndromes, in the majority of cases CHD is isolated and infants have no associated anomalies. In most cases the cause is unknown.

CASE 6

An infant is seen in routine pediatric clinic for a 1-month checkup. He was born at term and pregnancy was complicated by mild maternal hypertension that did not necessitate early delivery. He has been gaining weight well and eating eagerly. The mother has no concerns. On examination you see a healthy and well-nourished infant in no distress. On cardiac examination you note a soft (2/6) high-pitched murmur heard throughout the chest and especially loud on the back and in the axilla. The remainder of the examination is benign. You reassure the mother, but refer the infant for an echocardiogram, which diagnoses mild peripheral pulmonic stenosis (PPS).

Which of the following genetic abnormalities is NOT associated with PPS?
A. 7q11.23 microdeletion
B. JAG1 deletion
C. PTPN11 mutation
D. TBX5 mutation
E. Chromosome 45 XO

Discussion

The correct answer is **D**. A degree of relative PPS is relatively common in infancy. The murmur results from turbulence which occurs at the peripheral branch points in the distal pulmonary arteries in response to the relatively increased pulmonary blood flow after birth. The murmur is characteristic but an echocardiogram should be considered to rule out true pulmonary stenosis and to follow the degree of obstruction. The PPS is often self-limited and improves as the child ages and the murmur should resolve by 6 months of age. However in rare cases, especially when seen in association with a genetic syndrome, PPS can become severe, causing right ventricular failure, and requiring treatment. Alagille syndrome is classically associated with PPS, but it can also be seen in Turner, Williams, and Noonan syndromes.[12]

JAG1 is a cell-signaling molecule which interacts with the notch receptor. Mutations or deletions in JAG1 are associated with Alagille syndrome which is characterized by cholestatic liver disease, vertebral anomalies, cardiovascular disease, and characteristic facial features. Tetralogy of Fallot and valvar pulmonary stenosis can be seen in addition to PPS.[25] Turner syndrome more commonly is associated with Coarctation of the Aorta, but PPS can also be seen. Williams syndrome is associated with a microdeletion of 7q11.23 which results in insufficient elastin production. Affected patients have characteristic facial features, mental retardation, hypercalcemia, as well as cardiovascular anomalies. Supravalvar Aortic Stenosis and pulmonary stenosis are seen in addition to Peripheral Pulmonic Stenosis.

An estimated 50% of patients diagnosed with Noonan syndrome will have a mutation in the PTPN11 gene which encodes another cell-signaling molecule, nonreceptor-type protein tyrosine phosphatase SHP2. Inheritance is autosomal dominant though the presentation is quite variable. Hypertrophic cardiomyopathy and pulmonary stenosis may result, which can be severe.

Transcription factors are implicated in a variety of types of CHD including those in the T-box family which cause velocardiofacial syndrome (TBX1 included in 22q11.2 deletion syndrome) and Holt–Oram syndrome (TBX5 mutation). Holt–Oram syndrome is characterized by abnormalities of the forearms and CHD, most commonly an Atrial Septal Defect but ventricular defects, conotruncal abnormalities, and single ventricle anatomy can also result. Peripheral pulmonary stenosis is not a typical finding. Arrhythmias, however, are frequently seen due to conduction system dysfunction.

Objectives

1. Identify the characteristics of known chromosomal abnormalities associated with CHD
2. Know the clinical features associated with 22q11.2 deletion
3. Know the recurrence risk associated with specific types of CHD
4. Know the risk of having an affected child in a parent with a personal history of CHD

Fetal Circulation and Imaging

CASE 7

A mother presents for prenatal counseling at 28 weeks' gestation. Her infant was diagnosed with CHD at 22 weeks. She asks about how the heart in utero is different from after birth.

Which of the following is TRUE regarding normal fetal circulation?
A. Because of preferential streaming, the left atrium contains the most well-saturated hemoglobin in the fetus
B. The right atrial pressure is typically higher than left atrial pressure
C. The right ventricle primarily ejects blood through the ductus arteriosus into the head and neck vessels
D. In the fetal heart, parallel circulation occurs so that the relative ventricular outputs can be different
E. Afterload is rarely a factor in ventricular output because in utero pressures are generally low

Discussion

The correct answer is **D**. As shown in Figure 4-2, multiple shunts operate in the fetal heart to divert the majority (up to 90%) of blood away from the lungs. Preferential streaming in the right atrium directs deoxygenated blood returning from the superior vena cava (SVC) out the ductus arteriosus and to the lower extremities and placenta for gas exchange. Blood returning from the inferior vena cava is mixed with that returning from the

placenta and is relatively more saturated as the ductus venosus contains the most well-oxygenated blood in the fetus. This blood is directed across the foramen ovale and into the left ventricle where it supplies the brain and upper extremities. These shunts create a parallel circulation with equal atrial pressures, so that an increase in afterload impacting just one of the ventricles will lead to decreased output volume and a compensatory increase by the other.[26] In contrast, the postnatal heart operates in series, with blood returning from the veins to the right heart, to the lungs, left heart, and then out to the body so that in the absence of residual shunts, the cardiac output (CO) from the ventricles must be equal.

The mother presents several weeks later and is now at 33-week gestation. The infant has developed ascites and a small pleural effusion. She states heart failure is common in the elder members of her family and wants to know how this situation is different. You explain that the fetal heart has a poor ability to increase contractility and handles increased pressures poorly.

Which of the following is NOT a reason the fetal heart has decreased ability to increase contractility compared to the adult?
A. Increased sympathetic stimulation and adrenoreceptor concentration resulting in tachycardia in response to increased afterload
B. Disorganized arrangement of the myofilaments in the immature heart
C. Use of glucose as the primary energy source instead of free fatty acids as in the adult heart
D. Lower active tension at similar muscle lengths
E. Decreased number of mitochondria and decreased size of the sarcoplasmic reticulum

Discussion

The correct answer is **A**. The immature heart is characterized by smaller cells with decreased energy supply, disorganization, and decreased sympathetic innervations. Myofibrils are less prevalent and less organized, resulting in lower active tension. Decreased numbers of mitochondria and amount of sarcoplasmic reticulum result in decreased energy supply and less calcium release for muscle contraction. Fetal heart cells have higher concentrations of DNA and unlike adult cells, respond to stress with hyperplasia (increase in number of cells) rather than hypertrophy. These factors result in a poor ability to increase contractility or stroke volume in response to increased end diastolic pressures and a flattened ventricular function curve. The fetal heart rate (HR) will increase in response to increased

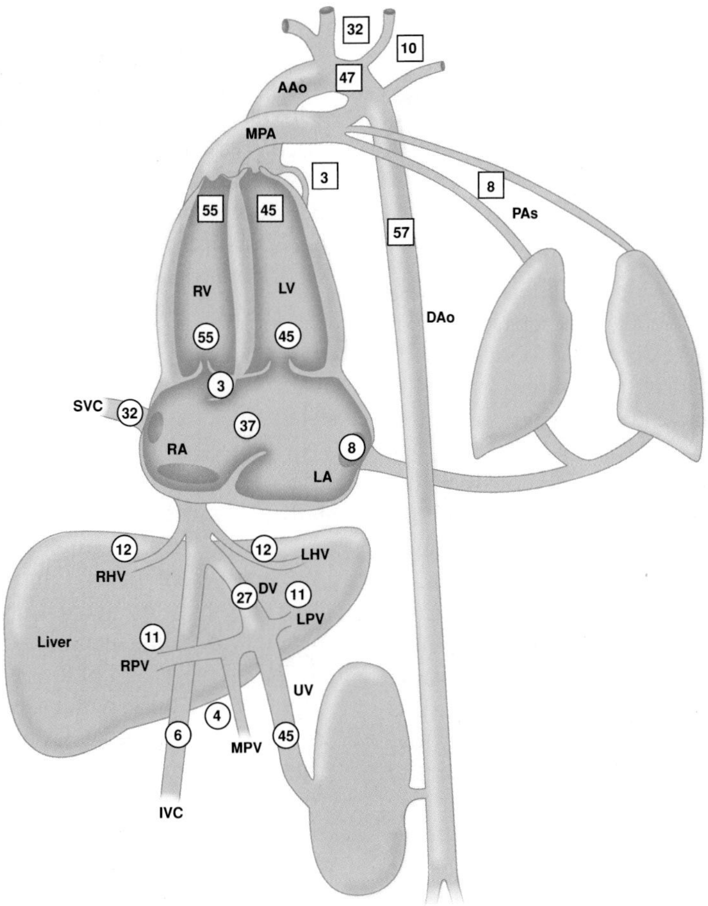

FIGURE 4-2. Normal fetal circulation with the typical percent of blood flow distribution shown in circles, and output shown in squares. Multiple shunts at the atrial and arterial level act to divert blood flow away from the pulmonary arteries and lungs, so that they receive only an estimated 8% of blood flow. (Reproduced with permission from Artman M, Mahony L, Teitel DF. *Neonatal Cardiology.* 2nd ed. New York: McGraw-Hill Professional; 2010.)

afterload; this is due to an inability to increase stroke volume rather than sympathetic innervation or adrenoreceptors, both of which are less in the developing heart.[27]

Helpful Tip: Even the normal fetal heart is already in a high contractile and low afterload state. This is combined with a relative inability to increase preload and low oxygen supply and thus a poor response to disease states.

In Table 4-1, which choice is correct regarding the direction of the forces leading to the development of hydrops fetalis?

TABLE 4-1.   **Quick Quiz: Hydrops Fetalis**

	PLASMA ONCOTIC PRESSURE	CAPILLARY FILTRATION COEFFICIENT	RIGHT ATRIAL PRESSURE	LYMPHATIC FLOW	INTERSTITIAL COMPLIANCE
A	+	+	–	+	+
B	–	+	+	–	+
C	–	+	–	+	+
D	+	–	+	–	–
E	–	–	+	–	+

Discussion

The correct answer is **B**. Hydrops fetalis is characterized by excess fluid accumulation in more than one compartment of the body: the chest, pericardial sac, abdomen, and usually last, the skin. Although often historically characterized as immune and nonimmune hydrops, with the introduction of Rho (D) immune globulin (RHOgam) the incidence of Rh disease and hydrops due to severe anemia is now responsible for less than 15% of cases of hydrops fetalis. Hydrops is the final common outcome of multiple disease processes including cardiac failure, compressive intrathoracic masses, severe anemia, infection, and a host of genetic and metabolic diseases.

Primary cardiac etiologies are responsible for approximately 20% of cases of hydrops and many other etiologies have a secondary component of heart failure. Abnormal cardiac anatomy, poor systolic or diastolic function, arrhythmias, severe anemia, and extrinsic compression due to a mass such as a congenital pulmonary airway malformation (CPAM) all lead to elevated right atrial pressure and impaired venous return. This is the most important factor in initiating the pathway that results in hydrops. Elevated pressures increase the hydrostatic pressure in the vessels and impair liver function leading to hypoalbuminemia and lower oncotic pressure. Lymph flow is several times higher in a healthy fetus than after birth and this is rapidly lost by elevated venous pressures leading to further interstitial fluid accumulation. The fetus also has a capillary filtration coefficient five times higher than that of the adult leading to leaking of fluid and even proteins from the capillaries. Infectious and inflammatory processes as well as genetic etiologies may worsen capillary leak. Interstitial compliance is increased, so that it takes a substantial volume for back pressure to build in the interstitium.[27,28]

Outcomes of neonates affected by hydrops fetalis are poor, especially when abnormalities are diagnosed in the first trimester or associated with pleural effusions.[29] Cases diagnosed during the first trimester are frequently due to aneuploidy. Overall mortality is above 50% but varies based on the underlying etiology. Potentially treatable causes such as anemia due to Parvovirus B19 and supraventricular tachycardia have the best chance for unimpaired survival.[30]

In the fetus with heart failure, which of the following prenatal imaging findings seen on echocardiogram and umbilical Doppler is most significantly associated with an increased risk of mortality?
A. Increased cardiac size/thoracic size ratio (C/T ratio >0.35)
B. Hepatic flow reversal in the ductus venosus
C. Umbilical venous atrial pulsations
D. Right atrial dilation
E. Tricuspid valve regurgitation

Discussion

The correct answer is **C**. The right heart is the harder working ventricle in the fetus and the right atrium is the site of venous return and mixing, so fetal heart failure is most apparent on the right side of the heart. All of the listed findings are associated with increasing degrees of heart failure either due to intrinsic heart disease or secondary to another pathologic problem causing secondary failure. Right atrial dilation is an early sign of altered fetal heart function and increased flow. Valvular disease may also result and worsen the degree of failure in the fetus. Eventually right heart dilation and poor contractility lead to impairment and reversal of venous return from the placenta, beginning as reversal in the inferior vena cava, then the ductus venosus, and finally atrial pulsations in the portal and umbilical vein. This is a strong predictor of fetal demise.[31]

Helpful Tip: Historically the vast majority of cases of hydrops fetalis were due to Rh isoimmunization and anemia; this has been markedly reduced with the introduction of Rhogam. Currently almost 90% of cases are due to other causes, referred to as "nonimmune" hydrops.

Helpful Tip: Edema can accumulate in a number of areas in hydrops, but peritoneal fluid is the most common. Placental edema can also occur.

Which of the choices below is CORRECT in listing the relative saturations in the fetal heart from highest to lowest for the listed structures? (see Fig. 4-3)
A. Ductus arteriosus > ascending aorta > descending aorta
B. Left ventricle > inferior vena cava > pulmonary arteries
C. Ductus venosus > right ventricle > ascending aorta
D. Ductus venosus > pulmonary veins > left ventricle
E. Ascending aorta > pulmonary artery > inferior vena cava

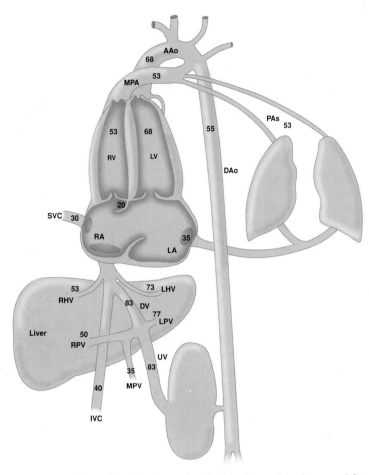

FIGURE 4-3. Hemoglobin saturations in the cardiac chamber and major blood vessels in the normal fetus. AAo, ascending aorta; DAo, descending aorta; DV, ductus venosus; LA, left atrium; LHV, left hepatic vein; LPV, left portal vein; LV, left ventricle; MPA, main pulmonary artery; MPV, main portal vein; PA's, branch pulmonary arteries; RA, right atrium; RHV, right hepatic vein; RPV, right portal vein; RV, right ventricle; SVC, superior vena cava; UV, umbilical vein; IVC, inferior vena cava. (Reproduced with permission from Artman M, Mahony L, Teitel DF. *Neonatal Cardiology*. 2nd ed. New York: McGraw-Hill Professional; 2010.)

Discussion

The correct answer is **E**. The ductus venosus contains newly oxygenated blood return from the placenta, with saturations in the 80s. This blood mixes to some degree in the right atrium but is primary directed into the left heart structures and ascending aorta. Lower saturations are found in the right ventricle and pulmonary arteries. In contrast to the postnatal environment, pulmonary venous return is quite desaturated as it returns to the left atrium.[26] Please refer to Figure 4-3 for detailed depiction of in utero hemoglobin saturation.

Helpful Tip: Normal fetal circulation directs relatively better oxygenated blood out the aorta and thus to the cerebral circulation, providing optimal oxygen delivery to the brain (though saturations are in the 60s). In infants with structural CHD this system is abnormal, and can result in relative cerebral immaturity and a higher risk for white matter injury.

Objectives

1. Understand patterns of blood flow in the fetal heart
2. Understand differences in function between the fetal heart and the neonatal heart
3. Describe saturations in each section of the fetal heart and major vessels
4. Understand the role of cardiac disease and function in the development of hydrops fetalis

Neonatal Transition/Pulmonary Hypertension

CASE 8

A 27-year-old woman presents in labor at 36 weeks. She reports a long history of chronic back pain that was aggravated by the pregnancy. She reports chronic opiate use that continued during the pregnancy, though she states she tried to take other medications instead. She also has a history of severe depression but stopped taking her medication during pregnancy. She did receive prenatal care and the baby had a normal 22-week ultrasound for anatomy.

The infant is delivered by cesarean section after a prolonged labor with rupture of membranes at delivery with meconium-stained fluid. She is vigorous and crying but noted to be cyanotic which continues into the 10th minute of life. A pulse oximetry probe is placed and reveals the saturation on the right hand at 65%, it is similar on the right foot. She is treated with supplemental oxygen with only partial improvement in saturations. The infant is eventually intubated due to continued hypoxemia. CXR is performed and reveals clear, dark lung fields and a normal cardiac silhouette.

What is the most likely finding on 2D echocardiogram?
A. Apical displacement of the septal and posteriolateral leaflets of the tricuspid valve with atrial enlargement and tricuspid stenosis
B. Bowing of the right ventricular septum with right-to-left shunting through a PDA
C. Atretic pulmonary valve with nonrestrictive atrial septum and VSD
D. L-looped transposition of the great vessels with VSD
E. Right ventricular hypertrophy with atrial right-to-left shunting and an absent-ductal shunt

Discussion

The correct answer is **E**. The clinical scenario is most consistent with primary pulmonary hypertension due to premature closure of the ductus arteriosus, which is described in (E). The typical findings of Ebstein anomaly are described in A, which may cause cyanosis depending on the degree of pulmonary outflow obstruction and right-to-left shunting. Tetraology of Fallot (A) can present with a murmur alone but severe cyanosis can result when accompanied by Pulmonary Atresia and a restrictive atrial septum; if the atrial shunt is not restrictive, desaturation is usually less pronounced than what is described in this scenario. Lung fields may be clear but the cardiac silhouette classically shows a boot-shaped

heart due to right ventricular hypertrophy. Transposition of the great arteries (TGA) may present with marked cyanosis and a normal appearing CXR in the dextro-looped heart (d-TGA), but this is not the typical presentation for the abnormally L(levo)-looped heart. In L-looped TGA, the right and left ventricle are transposed in addition to the great vessels, so that deoxygenated blood drains from the right atrium into the morphologic left ventricle (situated on the right), out to the pulmonary system, and back to the left heart and then to the systemic circulation (Fig. 4-4). Normal series circulation is maintained, so that figuration is commonly referred to as congenitally corrected TGA. However, other cardiac abnormalities are very frequent with L-TGA and so these infants may require cardiac surgery.

The echocardiographic findings as described in B more typically fit secondary pulmonary hypertension from a variety of causes including meconium aspiration syndrome and respiratory distress syndrome. CXR in these cases would typically show evidence of pulmonary disease rather than clear lung fields. Primary pulmonary hypertension can be caused by premature closure of the ductus arteriosus, but also may be idiopathic.[32]

Which medication is MOST likely to have caused the illness in this infant?
A. Acute opioid intoxication
B. Benzodiazepines
C. Selective serotonin reuptake inhibitors (SSRIs)
D. Ibuprofen
E. Valproic acid

Discussion

The correct answer is **D**. The clinical history is most compatible with premature closure of the ductus arteriosus and the most likely maternal exposure to cause this is nonsteroidal anti-inflammatory drugs (NSAIDs) such as ibuprofen. Many combination opioid-NSAID medications exist and may be taken inadvertently in cases of chronic opioid use. An association has also been documented between maternal intake of SSRIs and an increased risk of pulmonary hypertension in the neonate.[33,34] Population-based studies have shown at least a twofold increased risk of pulmonary hypertension associated with use late in the pregnancy, though the absolute risk remains low. Use of SSRIs early during pregnancy appears to have less of an impact. Opioid and benzodiazepine use just prior to delivery may cause acute apnea and cyanosis but they are not associated with an increased risk of cardiac anomalies or pulmonary hypertension. Valproic acid is an antimetabolite and maternal intake during pregnancy may result to a variety of facial anomalies, myelomeningocele, and a variety of complex congenital cardiac anomalies but its use is not specifically associated with pulmonary hypertension.

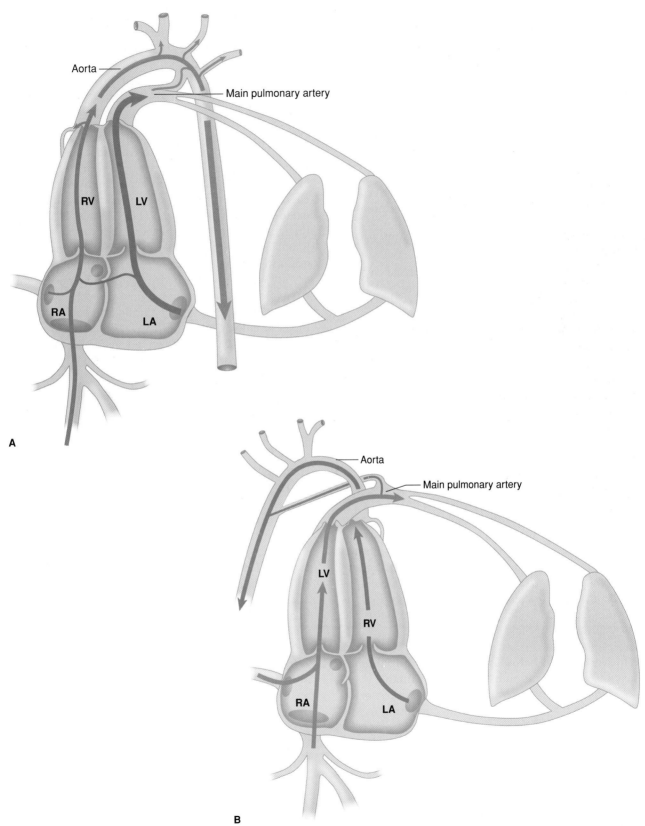

FIGURE 4-4. Classic d-Transposition of the Great Arteries (**A**) with parallel circulation and L-Transposition of the Great Arteries (**B**) with both atrial-ventricular and ventricular-arterial discordance, resulting in corrected circulatory pattern. (Reproduced with permission from Artman M, Mahony L, Teitel DF. *Neonatal Cardiology.* 2nd ed. New York: McGraw-Hill Professional; 2010.)

Helpful Tip: CXR findings help to categorize and eliminate causes of hypoxia. Abnormally clear lung fields are indicative of decreased pulmonary blood flow, whether from a structural abnormality such as PA or due to pulmonary hypertension. Opacified lung fields can indicate a primary pulmonary process, but also occur when there is impaired pulmonary venous return, such as in obstructed TAPVR.

Quick Quiz: Pulmonary Hypertension

Which of the findings below is NOT true about echocardiographic findings in an infant with pulmonary hypertension?
A. Pure right-to-left shunting through the PFO/atrial septum is rare
B. Ventricular septal bowing and decreased venous return may impact left ventricular output
C. Bidirectional flow through the PDA indicates the aortic and pulmonary pressures are roughly equal
D. Right atrial and right ventricular dilation may be seen along with pulmonary narrowing
E. Tricuspid regurgitation (TR) may not be present even in cases of significant pHTN

Discussion

The correct answer is **D**. Right atrial dilation and right ventricular dilation occur in pulmonary hypertension due to TR and back pressure from the pulmonary circulation, however the pulmonary artery is usually also dilated in cases of pulmonary hypertension, differing it from pulmonary valvular disease. Shunting through the PDA and PFO can aid in determining the diagnosis and degree of pulmonary hypertension but purely right-to-left shunting through the PFO is a late and severe finding often associated with RV failure. Left ventricule output can be affected in severe pulmonary hypertension. TR provides a potential estimate of RV pressure, but is not always present, especially in older infant.

Which statement below is TRUE regarding pulmonary vascular relaxation in the newborn infant?
A. The fetus has intrinsically low levels of nitric oxide synthase (NOS) and endothelin-1 resulting in low pulmonary vascular tone
B. Vaginal squeeze is essential in clearing fetal lung fluid and allowing normal transition to air breathing
C. Premature infants have immature relaxation mechanisms and thus elevated vascular tone when compared to term infants
D. Endothelial nitric oxide synthase (eNOS) is upregulated at the time of birth and acts via guanylate cyclase to produce cyclic GMP and allow smooth muscle relaxation

E. Without proper oxygenation, mechanical distention of the lungs has no significant effect on pulmonary vascular resistance (PVR) and pulmonary blood flow

Discussion

The correct answer is **D**. The system governing vascular tone is complex, allowing for a rapid transition from vasoconstriction to vasodilation in the first few minutes of life. In the term or late-preterm infant, high vascular tone is present due to low levels of oxygen and secretion of vasoconstrictors including endothelin and leukotriene. Production of vasodilatory substances such as nitric oxide (NO) and prostacyclin (PGI2) is low in the fetus though the ability to upregulate synthesis increases as the infant approaches delivery.[32] The hormonal changes that occur in the hours and days prior to spontaneous delivery are what begins clearance of lung fluid and pulmonary vascular dilatation, not vaginal squeeze.[35] At normal delivery, both oxygen content and mechanical stretch increase quickly after the first few breaths. In animal models both have been shown independently to result in pulmonary vessel relaxation; in the healthy term infant they work synergistically to rapidly lower pulmonary pressures. Although it is accurate that premature infants have impaired relaxation due to lower levels of intrinsic NO production, they actually have lower vascular tone and lower PVR compared to term infants.

Helpful Tip: Prostaglandins are involved in uterine contractions, so NSAIDs may also be used as tocolysis in women with preterm labor. However this poses a risk of ductal closure in the fetus, so use is limited to women at less than 32- weeks' gestation and only for 24 to 48 hours.

Helpful Tip: In utero PVR varies with gestational age with a nadir around 30 weeks and a subsequent increase. Therefore, despite significant lung disease, very-preterm infants are at lower risk for pulmonary hypertension than late-preterm and term infants.

Which is FALSE regarding the pathophysiology of idiopathic pulmonary hypertension (PPHN)?
A. Infants with idiopathic PPHN will have increased production and **high** levels of endogenous NO but this is ineffective against the thickened vessel walls of the pulmonary arteries
B. The presence of NSAIDs in newborn meconium is associated with increased risk and severity of pHTN
C. Smooth muscle cell hyperplasia is seen on autopsy specimens
D. Upregulation of phosphodiesterase 5 (PDE5) is seen in animal models of idiopathic PPHN
E. Endothelin levels are also increased, causing vasoconstriction and increased production of reactive oxygen species (ROS)

Discussion

The correct answer is **A**. Multiple abnormalities, both anatomic and at the enzyme level, are seen in neonates diagnosed with idiopathic pulmonary hypertension. Although the etiology is by definition unknown, it is clear that the process has begun in utero many days to weeks before birth.[32,36] Significant remodeling of the pulmonary arteries results in abnormal growth and extension of smooth muscle cells and altered endothelial cell function.[37] Vascular endothelial cells are responsible for production of nitric oxide synthase (eNOS) and thus NO. Production and activity are low in animal models of PPHN and metabolism of downstream messengers is increased. In addition, endothelin levels have been shown to be increased above normal levels. Both of these factors result in increased production of ROS such as peroxynitrite and superoxide. The presence of ROS will exacerbate vasoconstriction, cause inflammation and cell death, and worsen smooth muscle- cell hypertrophy.

The infant is placed on inhaled nitric oxide (iNO) with a minimal increase in saturations which remain in the high 60s and low 70s. Ventilation is appropriate with PCO_2 range between 35 toand 45 mm Hg. PaO_2 progressively declines and she becomes hypotensive and acidotic. Ultimately she is placed onto extracorporeal membrane oxygenation (ECMO).

Which of the following is ACCURATE about the use of iNO?
A. Use of iNO has resulted in decreased need for ECMO, decreased mortality, and shorter length of intubation in neonates with pulmonary hypertension
B. NO is not indicated until the oxygenation index (OI) is above 40
C. Infants with CHD are at increased risk for pulmonary hypertension and use of iNO may help optimize their physiology prior to surgery
D. Use of sildenafil, at phosphodiesterase 5 (PDE5) inhibitor will decrease the amount of available cyclic guanosine monophosphate (cGMP) thus overlapping with the role of nitric oxide
E. Use of iNO is contraindicated in CHD wherein systemic blood flow is dependent on right-to-left shunting across the ductus arteriosus

Discussion

The correct answer is **E**. The iNO presented the first available option for selective pulmonary vasodilation. Several other selective pulmonary vasodilators are now available and increasingly used in neonates and infants, but iNO remains the most well studied and most commonly used. Use has expanded beyond the population of neonates with acute hypoxic respiratory failure, failure of transition to postnatal circulation, and acute pulmonary hypertension. Use of nitric oxide in this population has shown about a 50% to 60% response rate, meta-analysis shows a decreased need for ECMO without a reduction in mortality. In addition, long-term outcomes including the incidence of hearing loss, cerebral palsy, and developmental delay (Mental Developmental Index or Motor Developmental Index on the Bayley Scales of Infant Development, 2nd Revision <2SD) were not improved in the patients treated with NO,[38] suggesting the illness may have already impacted the infant by the time he or she is ill enough to require iNO.

Oxygenation index is calculated from the amount of respiratory support and the resulting PaO_2 OI = [(mean airway pressure × FiO_2)/postductal PaO_2] × 100 and is commonly used as an indicator of disease severity. NO treatment should be started at an OI of 25 and ECMO considered at OI persistently above 40. Studies using NO in less ill infants (OI 15–25) have not shown a reduced need for ECMO but may potentially impact length of mechanical ventilation in certain infants. NO acts through guanylate cyclase to generate cGMP which decreases intracellular calcium concentrations and results in vasorelaxation. There are several other interacting parts of this complex pathway, including prostacyclin (PGI2) which acts through cyclic AMP to promote vasorelaxation. Effectiveness of NO is partially dependent on the amount of circulating phosphodiesterase 5 (PDE5) which degrades cGMP and thus stops relaxation. Sildenafil inhibits PDE5 and shows promise in the treatment of pulmonary hypertension in neonates, both alone and synergistically with iNO. It also may facilitate weaning from NO after recovery.[36]

Helpful Tip: Multiple processes can cause pulmonary hypertension and a subsequent need for ECMO, including RDS, pneumonia, aspiration syndromes, structural pulmonary anomalies, and pulmonary hypoplasia, in addition to idiopathic cases. Congenital diaphragmatic hernia (CDH) which results in pulmonary hypoplasia and structural vascular abnormalities, has poor response to therapies including nitric oxide and is now the single most common indication for neonatal ECMO.

Helpful Tip: NO can oxidize hemoglobin to methemoglobin (metHgb), impairing oxygenation. MetHgb level should be checked within 8 hours of initiation of iNO, but toxicity is rare at the current recommended maximum dose of 20 ppm.

Which factor does NOT help dilate the pulmonary vascular bed?
A. Decreased $PaCO_2$
B. Decreased thromboxane and endothelin-1
C. Hyperoxia (PaO_2 >100 mm Hg)
D. Increased prostaglandin (PGE1)
E. Increased prostacylin (PGI2)

Discussion

The correct answer is **C**. Many factors combine to cause rapid pulmonary vasorelaxation in the healthy term infant and provide potential therapeutic options. Arterial concentrations of CO_2 influence vascular tone and lower levels cause vasorelaxation though this may result in decreased cerebral perfusion. Normoxia is important in pulmonary vessel dilatation, but there is no evidence that hyperoxia has any benefit and may in fact be harmful. A natural reduction in endothelin and thromboxane should occur before delivery, as well as an increase in prostacyclin, all supporting the normal decline in PVR. Prostaglandin is commonly used in CHD to keep the ductus arteriosus patent, but also causes pulmonary vasorelaxation.

Congenital Heart Disease

Helpful Tip: Prenatal diagnosis of CHD allows for preparation of both the family and the medical team and may improve outcomes. However the likelihood of prenatal diagnosis varies based on the position of the infant, maternal habitus, skill of the examiner, and the type of lesion. Lesions causing abnormalities of one of the four main chambers are much easier to diagnose that outflow tract abnormalities. TGA and TAPVR specifically are often not diagnosed prenatally and can present with a dramatically ill infant.

Objectives

1. Identify known causes of pulmonary hypertension in the newborn
2. Describe the typical clinical presentation of newborns with pulmonary hypertension
3. Understand the pathophysiology of pulmonary hypertension
4. Know echocardiographic findings typically seen in newborn with pulmonary hypertension
5. Know the mechanism of action of inhaled NO and understand its use in the management of newborns with pulmonary hypertension

CASE 9

A newborn is born with oxygen saturations in the low 60s. An echocardiogram demonstrates Ebstein anomaly with severe tricuspid valve regurgitation.

Which of the following is the most likely cause of his cyanosis?
A. Right-to-left shunting at the ventricular level
B. Right-to-left shunting at the atrial level
C. Left-to-right shunting at the ventricular level
D. Left-to-right shunting at the atrial level
E. Aortopulmonary collaterals

Discussion

The correct answer is **B**. Ebstein anomaly is characterized by apical displacement of the septal tricuspid leaflet in the right ventricular cavity away from the tricuspid valve annulus and enlargement of the anterior tricuspid leaflet in a "sail-like" manner. The right ventricle is also abnormal, with the inlet portion thinned or atrialized, resulting in a smaller, functional right ventricular cavity. Associated defects in Ebstein anomaly include atrial and ventricular septal defects, pulmonary atresia or stenosis, and Wolff–Parkinson–White syndrome. At birth, while the pulmonary resistance is high, the degree of cyanosis in Ebstein anomaly will depend on the amount of right-to-left shunting at the atrial level. In neonates with mild tricuspid valve displacement and minimal pulmonary stenosis, the degree of shunting will decrease as the PVR falls and cyanosis will improve. If there is significant tricuspid valve displacement or right ventricular outflow tract obstruction (RVOTO), cyanosis will persist despite a fall in the PVR with progression to congestive heart failure. A VSD, if present, results in a left-to-right shunting and would not result in cyanosis. Aortopulmonary collaterals result in increased pulmonary blood flow and would also not result in cyanosis. The surgical management of Ebstein anomaly involves a systemic to pulmonary artery shunt alone for cyanosis or a shunt plus tricuspid valvuloplasty for cyanosis with significant tricuspid valve regurgitation and right ventricular dysfunction.[39]

CASE 10

A term newborn has cyanosis shortly after birth with oxygen saturations of 65%. Her chest radiograph shows decreased vascular markings.

Which of the following is the most likely congenital heart disease present?
A. Truncus arteriosus
B. Critical pulmonary stenosis
C. Tricuspid atresia with transposition of the great arteries
D. Hypoplastic left heart syndrome
E. Total anomalous pulmonary venous return

Discussion

The correct answer is **B**. The "five T's" of cyanotic congenital heart disease is a useful mnemonic describing transposition of the great arteries (TGA), tetralogy of Fallot, truncus arteriosus, total anomalous pulmonary venous return (TAPVR) and tricuspid valve abnormalities.[40] Tricuspid valve abnormalities include tricuspid atresia/stenosis, hypoplastic right ventricle syndrome, and tricuspid valve displacement or Ebstein anomaly. Critical pulmonary stenosis is also within the group of tricuspid valve abnormalities. Of the types of cyanotic congenital heart disease, only tetralogy of Fallot and tricuspid valve abnormalities are associated with decreased pulmonary blood flow. Both truncus arteriosus and hypoplastic left heart syndrome are at risk for excessive pulmonary blood flow once the pulmonary vascular resistance falls. Tricuspid atresia with transposition of the great arteries is functionally similar to hypoplastic left heart syndrome. Total anomalous pulmonary venous return is characterized by a left-to-right shunt resulting in increased pulmonary blood flow and potential pulmonary venous obstruction.

Helpful Tip: Prenatal diagnosis of TGA has been shown to improve survival. Certain echocardiographic features such as a restrictive foramen ovale or constriction of the ductus arteriosus are predictive of the need for emergent atrial septostomy.

CASE 11

A newborn is born at 40 weeks' gestation and has a prenatal diagnosis of TGA with intact ventricular septum. He is limp and cyanotic shortly after birth and requires tracheal intubation. A prostaglandin infusion is started. On examination, his HR is 150 beats/min, respiratory rate is 50 breaths/min, and blood pressure (BP) is 60/30 mm Hg. Simultaneous saturations in the right arm and left leg are 50% and 70%, respectively, on 50% FiO_2. His lungs are clear with no murmurs appreciated. An echocardiogram demonstrates a 5-mm patent foramen ovale with bidirectional flow, TGA, intact ventricular septum, a patent aortic arch, a PDA with flow from the pulmonary artery to the aorta, and normal pulmonary venous anatomy.

What is the most likely pathophysiology that is present in this patient?
A. Differential cyanosis from interrupted aortic arch
B. Differential cyanosis from pulmonary hypertension
C. Reverse differential cyanosis from a restrictive atrial septum
D. Reverse differential cyanosis from pulmonary hypertension
E. Reverse differential cyanosis from an interrupted aortic arch

Discussion

The correct answer is **D**. The patient in this scenario has reverse differential cyanosis with a lower oxygen saturation in the upper extremity compared to the lower extremity. This clinical finding is most often seen with TGA with CoA, interrupted aortic arch or persistent pulmonary hypertension.[41] The newborn in this vignette has TGA with persistent pulmonary hypertension. The echocardiogram describes a patent aortic arch and therefore interrupted aortic arch is excluded as an answer. A restrictive atrial septum would result in significant cyanosis, but not reverse differential cyanosis. A restrictive atrial septum may be the cause of persistent pulmonary hypertension, and a balloon atrial septostomy should be considered. Newborns with both TGA and persistent pulmonary hypertension are at risk for high morbidity and mortality. Therapies such as inhaled NO, pulmonary vasoactive drugs, restriction of ductal flow, and ECMO have helped to allow infants to proceed with an arterial switch operation once the persistent pulmonary hypertension resolves.[42]

CASE 12

An infant born at 27 weeks' gestation has a large PDA and has been unable to wean from ventilatory support. Three doses of indomethacin have been given without clinical change and surgical ligation being considered.

Which of the following statements is true regarding surgical ligation of a PDA?
A. Surgical ligation always results in increased left ventricular output
B. Surgical ligation is often associated with an improved neurodevelopmental outcome
C. Surgical ligation decreases the incidence of vocal cord paralysis
D. Surgical ligation decreases the incidence of necrotizing enterocolitis
E. Surgical ligation is often associated with ligation of the pulmonary artery

Discussion

The correct answer is **D**. A PDA can result in pulmonary overcirculation, left ventricular volume overload and systemic hypoperfusion. Surgical ligation is an option for a persistently PDA and one needs to understand both the benefits and risks of ligation.[43] The hemodynamic effects of ligation of a patent ductus ligation include decreased left ventricular output due to the decrease in left ventricular preload from removal of the shunt and possible increases in cerebral blood flow. Ligation of a ductus arteriosus has been shown to improve lung compliance. Neurodevelopmental outcome studies have not shown an association between surgical ligation and improved neurodevelopmental outcome. Ligation of a PDA has been shown to decrease the incidence of necrotizing enterocolitis in very low—birth-weight neonates.[44] Ligation of the pulmonary artery is a rare complication of ductal ligation.

PDA is an example of a left-to-right shunting that results in a volume load on the left ventricle. Preterm infants are more susceptible to left ventricular failure than term infants or older children.

Which of the following best characterizes the physiologic features that result in left ventricular failure?
A. Increased left ventricular diastolic volume and increased left ventricular end diastolic pressure
B. Decreased left ventricular diastolic volume and decreased left ventricular end diastolic pressure
C. Increased left ventricular diastolic volume and decreased left ventricular end diastolic pressure
D. Decreased left ventricular diastolic volume and increased left ventricular end diastolic pressure
E. Increased left ventricular diastolic volume and no change in left ventricular end diastolic pressure

Discussion

The correct answer is **A**. The left-to-right shunting that occurs with a PDA results in increased pulmonary venous return to the left atrium and left ventricle which results in increased left ventricular diastolic volume or preload.[45] The additional volume results in left ventricle dilation which increases left ventricular end diastolic pressures with a secondary increase in left atrial size and pressure. Overt left heart failure with pulmonary edema can ensue if compensatory mechanisms such as increased contractility and myocardial hypertrophy are not present to help ventricular performance. In newborn infants, and particularly premature infants, these compensatory mechanisms may not be well developed. The premature myocardium has fewer contractile elements, is less responsive to stretch and may not be able

to increase stroke volume in response to increased ventricular diastolic volume (Frank–Starling mechanism). The sympathetic nervous system may also be immature in a premature infant resulting in the inability to increase the force of contraction or HR. Premature infants have lower serum calcium concentrations which may further impair myocardial function.

Helpful Tip: Infants who have a surgical PDA ligation are at increased likelihood of neurodevelopmental impairment, chronic lung disease, and retinopathy of prematurity. However it is unknown whether this is due entirely to pre-existing factors such as higher illness severity in these patients, or is related to the procedure itself.

Objectives

1. Identify the common congenital heart defects associated with cyanosis in the newborn period
2. Understand the physiology associated with PDA resulting in heart failure
3. Describe complications associated with surgical closure of the PDA
4. Describe features associated with Ebstein anomaly

CASE 13

A 2-month-old female with trisomy 21 and a complete atrioventricular canal defect is transferred to the neonatal intensive care unit for the management of chronic respiratory failure, inability to wean ventilatory support and failure to thrive. She was born at 33 weeks' gestation and her birth weight was 1,500 g. Her current weight is 2,500 g and she is receiving continuous nasogastric feeds of a 27 kcal/oz formula. Her current medications include furosemide 1 mg/kg/dose twice daily and ranitidine 4 mg/kg/day. On examination, the infant is tachycardic, tachypneic, and the liver is palpable 4 cm below the right costal margin. Her chest radiograph shows increased pulmonary vascular markings and moderate cardiomegaly.

Which of the following is the best management for this patient?

A. Increase ventilator support to decrease respiratory distress
B. Increase caloric intake to optimize growth
C. Increase furosemide to improve diuresis
D. Start dopamine to augment CO
E. Refer for surgical repair of atrioventricular canal defect

Discussion

The correct answer is **E**. This infant is demonstrating signs of congestive heart failure from the atrioventricular canal defect. The left-to-right shunting in a complete atrioventricular canal defect occurs at both the atrial and ventricular levels and results in excessive pulmonary blood flow.[46] PVR is increased as a compensatory mechanism and due to the risk of permanent changes to the pulmonary vascular bed, surgery for a complete atrioventricular valve defect usually occurs before 6 months of age.[47] Early repair is indicated for the above patient due to her failure to thrive and trisomy 21. Patients with Down syndrome are at additional risk of fixed, elevated PVR possibly related to chronic nasopharyngeal obstruction and relative hypoventilation.[48] Increasing ventilator support, caloric intake, and diuretic therapy will help to alleviate the symptoms of congestive heart failure, but definitive repair is the best management strategy.

Helpful Tip: In a sick infant, a negative perinatal history (no maternal illness, no difficulties with labor or delivery) makes cardiac disease MORE likely.

Helpful Tip: Neonatal cardiac disease presents with one or more of three key signs: cyanosis, tachypnea, and decreased systemic perfusion. While other etiologies may be causative, infants with any of these three should be evaluated specifically for cardiac disease.

CASE 14

A 3-day-old infant is admitted for possible sepsis. He appears pale and is tachycardic and tachypneic. Physical examination reveals a systolic ejection murmur with a gallop, hepatomegaly, poor pulses, and decreased perfusion. A cardiology consultation is obtained and an echocardiogram reveals critical aortic stenosis (AS). Prostaglandin E1 is started immediately.

What additional echocardiographic findings will impact proceeding with an aortic valvotomy?

A. Amount of flow across the aortic valve
B. Amount of mitral valve regurgitation
C. Amount of mitral stenosis
D. Presence of a coarctation
E. Degree of right ventricular hypoplasia

Discussion

The correct answer is **C**. Neonatal critical aortic stenosis is part of a spectrum of CHD that ranges from an isolated stenotic aortic valve to HLHS. Therefore, it is important to know if the intracardiac structures are compatible with a two-ventricle repair in which the initial therapy would include aortic valvotomy.[49] The amount of flow across the aortic valve is usually negligible in critical AS as the majority of systemic flow is provided by the ductus arteriosus and has little impact on feasibility of a biventricular repair. Mitral valve regurgitation is often present in critical AS, and therefore, is also of limited use in surgical planning. Aortic valve and mitral valve dimensions have been shown to have predictive value for biventricular repair. Additional variables include left ventricular dimensions and mass as well as endocardial fibroelastosis (EFE). A coarctation should increase the suspicion of additional left-sided obstructions, but in the absence of the variables mentioned above, critical AS with a coarctation does not preclude a two-ventricle repair.

CASE 15

A 3-day-old infant with critical coarctation undergoes resection with end-to-end anastomosis via a left thoracotomy. He has significant hypertension immediately after surgery requiring initiation of a nitroprusside infusion. On examination, the infant appears to be in no distress with HRs in the 140s. The BPs in all four extremities are equal. There are no murmurs auscultated. His abdomen is soft and nontender.

Which of the following is the best explanation for the infant's hypertension?

A. Residual coarctation
B. Increased sympathetic stimulation resulting in vasoconstriction
C. Decreased parasympathetic stimulation resulting in vasoconstriction
D. Increased levels of angiotensin I
E. Mesenteric arteritis

Discussion

The correct answer is **B**. Postoperative hypertension after coarctation repair can be puzzling in the absence of a residual coarctation, hence the term paradoxical hypertension. Though the exact etiology is unknown, there appears to be a biphasic effect to the rise in BP.[50,51] Surgical stimulation of the sympathetic nerve fibers located between the media and adventitia of the aortic isthmus results in release of norepinephrine with subsequent vasoconstriction and BP elevation. This is thought to be responsible for the hypertension in the first 24 hours after coarctation repair. Sympathetic nerve stimulation also causes the juxtaglomerular cells to release renin with activation of the renin–angiotensin system and this is postulated as the mechanism for the hypertension seen 2 to 3 days after surgery. Residual coarctation and mesenteric arteritis are both potential postoperative complications, but unlikely in an infant with no BP differential and a reassuring abdominal examination. Angiotensin I levels are increased, but angiotensin I is inactive and it is angiotensin II that is a potent vasoconstrictor.

CASE 16

A 2-month-old, ex–28-week premature infant with Tetralogy of Fallot is working on weight gain prior to surgical repair. He has respiratory failure and remains on mechanical ventilation. His baseline saturations are in the mid-80s. You are called to the bedside because his saturations dropped to the 50s during a feed and the saturations are not improving with increased FiO_2. A stat CXR reveals appropriate endotracheal tube position and clear lung fields.

What is the rationale for using phenylephrine in this situation?
A. Phenylephrine decreases pulmonary vascular resistance and will increase pulmonary blood flow
B. Phenylephrine increases pulmonary vascular resistance and will increase systemic blood flow
C. Phenylephrine decreases systemic vascular resistance and will increase pulmonary blood flow
D. Phenylephrine decreases systemic vascular resistance and will increase systemic blood flow
E. Phenylephrine increases systemic vascular resistance and will increase pulmonary blood flow

Discussion

The correct answer is **E**. Hypercyanotic spells can be a life-threatening event in an infant with TOF if not properly

recognized and treated. Dynamic subpulmonary obstruction, from possible catecholamine surge, is thought to play a role in the fall in pulmonary blood flow with resultant cyanosis and hyperpnea. Another potential mechanism involves a fall in pulmonary blood flow due to a decrease in the ratio of systemic vascular resistance to PVR. Treatment for a hypercyanotic spell is therefore directed at both explanations.[52] Sedation or neuromuscular blockade in an intubated patient, increased inspired oxygen, and knee-to-chest maneuvers can work to terminate the spell. Right ventricular preload can also be augmented with a crystalloid or colloid bolus. Phenylephrine can be effective by increasing systemic vascular resistance and allowing for increased pulmonary blood flow. Persistent hypercyanosis unresponsive to medical management may require mechanical circulatory support or emergent surgical intervention.

Helpful Tip: Infants with tetralogy of Fallot and pulmonary stenosis (TOF/PS) typically have a systolic murmur from the pulmonary outflow tract which may change or disappear during hypercyanotic episodes or "tet spells."

Helpful Tip: Although patients with tetralogy of Fallot and pulmonary atresia or severe pulmonary stenosis often require prostaglandin therapy and neonatal surgery, they are at less risk from hypercyanotic episodes than their less affected counterparts. Even patients with mild stenosis and good oxygenation, referred to as "pink tets," are at risk and families should be counseled accordingly.

CASE 17

A neonate has profound cyanosis and respiratory acidosis shortly after birth requiring endotracheal intubation and mechanical ventilation. An echocardiogram reveals TOF with absent pulmonary valve syndrome. On conventional settings with a set peak inspiratory pressure of 35 mm Hg, the neonate continues to have severe respiratory compromise with a $PaCO_2$ of 98 mm Hg.

Which of the following strategies have been shown to be most effective in this scenario?
A. Switch to volume ventilation
B. Switch to pressure regulated volume control ventilation
C. Place patient in a prone position
D. Initiate rescue ECMO
E. Initiate high-frequency ventilation

Discussion

The correct answer is **C**. In TOF with absent pulmonary valve syndrome, there is massive enlargement of the main and branch pulmonary arteries, resulting in compression of the trachea and bronchial tree. Neonates present with severe respiratory distress, cyanosis, and air trapping. The hypoxemia is a result from a combination of right-to-left shunting at the VSD as well as ventilation–perfusion mismatch. Endotracheal intubation and mechanical ventilation are necessary as well as high-positive end-expiratory pressures to help stent open the airways. Prone positioning can help relieve tracheal compression.[53] Other modes of ventilation have not been shown to be effective. ECMO may be considered a rescue therapy, but these neonates are better served with early surgical repair which includes plication of the pulmonary arteries.

Helpful Tip: Infants with cyanosis due to impaired pulmonary blood flow (atresia, stenosis, severe TR) will usually have the majority of shunting at the atrial level as the obstruction is typically prior to the ductus arteriosus. Unlike infants with pulmonary hypertension or transposition, saturations in the upper and lower parts of the body are usually equal.

CASE 18

A newborn is delivered with a prenatal diagnosis of PA and intact ventricular septum. He is placed on a prostaglandin infusion and an echocardiogram demonstrates a small right ventricle, PA with intact ventricular septum, and confluent pulmonary arteries supplied by a ductus arteriosus. His oxygen saturation is 80% on room air.

What is the most appropriate next step in management?
A. Surgical repair with relief of outflow tract obstruction
B. Palliation with placement of a Blalock–Taussig shunt
C. Cardiac catheterization
D. Emergent balloon atrial septostomy
E. Emergent intubation

Discussion

The correct answer is **C**. In patients with PA and intact ventricular septum, it is important to confirm the coronary circulation as this will impact the type of surgical

palliation.[54] This is best performed with coronary artery angiography by cardiac catheterization. If there is right ventricular dependent coronary circulation, where large areas of the myocardium receive coronary blood flow from the right ventricle, relief of the RVOTO would result in lowering of the right ventricular pressure with subsequent myocardial hypoperfusion, infarct, and dysfunction. A restrictive atrial septum is rare due to the obligatory right-to-left shunting at the atrial level, and atrial septostomy is not indicated. Oxygen saturations of 80% are appropriate for this type of mixing lesion.

CASE 19

A newborn is transferred from the nursery with a pulse oximetry of 85% and a murmur. You perform a hyperoxia test to assess for cyanotic heart disease. On room air, the PaO_2 in the right radial artery is 55 mm Hg. In 100% inspired oxygen, the PaO_2 is 100 mm Hg. What is the most likely diagnosis?
A. D-transposition of the great arteries
B. Pulmonary atresia with intact ventricular septum
C. Truncus arteriosus
D. Tetralogy of Fallot
E. No cyanotic heart disease

Discussion

The correct answer is **C**. In cyanotic infants with suspected CHD, the hyperoxia test is a sensitive and specific tool in the initial evaluation. The hyperoxia test can help distinguish between pulmonary and cardiac causes of cyanosis.[55] Proper technique of the hyperoxia test is important for accurate interpretation. Measurement of the PaO_2 should be obtained in a preductal vessel such as the right radial artery and 100% inspired oxygen should be given for a minimum of 10 minutes before obtaining a repeat arterial blood gas. The normal response to 100% inspired oxygen is a PaO_2 of >200 mm Hg. In pulmonary disease, the PaO_2 is low in room air and will increase to greater than 150 mm Hg with 100% inspired oxygen. In cardiac disease, the PaO_2 is less than 150 mm Hg with 100% inspired oxygen and can be less than 50 mm Hg depending on the type of CHD. In cardiac lesions with a parallel circulation, such as TGA, or cardiac lesions with restricted pulmonary blood flow, such as TOF with severe pulmonary stenosis or PA with intact ventricular septum, the PaO_2 is less than 40 mm Hg in room air and less than 50 mm Hg in 100% inspired oxygen. Cardiac lesions with complete mixing and unrestricted pulmonary blood flow, such as truncus arteriosus, HLHS, or other single ventricle variants will have a PaO_2 in the 50 to 60 mm Hg range in room air and PaO_2 will be less than 150 mm Hg in 100% inspired oxygen.

Helpful Tip: A hyperoxia test helps to evaluate for heart disease. A PaO_2 of greater than 150 mm Hg will virtually exclude cyanotic heart disease, though an echocardiogram may still be indicated to evaluate for acyanotic heart disease or pulmonary hypertension.

CASE 20

A 1-week-old infant, born at 38 weeks' gestation, has known CHD and is awaiting surgical palliation. He has had difficulty with oral intake and is receiving nasogastric feeds. Today, he develops grossly bloody stools and an abdominal radiograph reveals dilated loops of bowel with pneumatosis.

Which of the following cardiac lesions is most likely to be present in this infant?
A. PA with intact ventricular septum
B. Aortopulmonary window
C. Ebstein malformation
D. TOF
E. Complete atrioventricular canal defect

Discussion

The correct answer is **B**. CHD is one of the risk factors associated with necrotizing enterocolitis in term infants. The incidence of necrotizing enterocolitis in infants with CHD has been reported as high as 3.5%, which is 10- to 100-fold higher than reported population-wide rates.[56] The principle underlying mechanism of necrotizing enterocolitis in infants with CHD is thought to be related to mesenteric ischemia. Specifically, cardiac lesions with the potential for significant runoff from the systemic to pulmonary circulation appear to be associated with a higher risk. Of the possible answer choices, only an aortopulmonary window has the potential for a significant left-to-right shunting that would result in impaired mesenteric perfusion. Other high-risk lesions include HLHS, univentricular heart disease with aortic arch obstruction, and truncus arteriosus.

Helpful Tip: Increased risk for necrotizing enterocolitis persists in infants with cardiac disease even after surgical repair. It is unknown whether this is related to continued relative hypoxia, abnormal vasculature, or other factors.

CASE 21

A 4-day-old term male presents to the intensive care unit in profound shock. His postnatal course was benign and he was discharged at 2 days of life. His parents report that he has been fussy and not feeding well for the last 24 hours. You are unable to palpate any femoral pulses on your examination and order an emergent echocardiogram. The echocardiogram reveals HLHS.

Which of the following statements is accurate regarding detection of critical CHD in newborns?
A. An echocardiogram should be performed prior to discharge
B. Pulse oximetry is highly sensitive and should be performed immediately after delivery
C. Pulse oximetry is highly sensitive and should be performed after 24 hours of birth
D. Pulse oximetry is highly specific and should be performed immediately after delivery
E. Pulse oximetry is highly specific and should be performed after 24 hours of birth

Discussion

The correct answer is **E**. Early detection of critical CHD can significantly improve morbidity and mortality. Physical examination findings, such as heart murmurs or overt cyanosis, may not be evident for the first 48 hours due to ductal patency and newborns may be discharged from the hospital prior to diagnosis. Pulse oximetry has been studied as a potential screening tool and has been shown to be highly specific for detection of critical CHD.[57,58] False-positive rates were affected by the timing of the test with significantly lower false-positive rates when the test was performed after 24 hours of life compared to before 24 hours of life. An echocardiogram is only indicated if there are clinical signs or symptoms concerning for CHD.

Quick Quiz: Pulse Oximetry Screening

Which of the following would NOT be detected by pulse oximetry screening?
A. Tetralogy of Fallot with Pulmonary Atresia
B. Interrupted Aortic Arch
C. Large Ventriculoseptal Defect
D. Hypoplastic Left Ventricle

Discussion

The correct answer is **C**. Pulse oximetry screening, either using the foot or right hand and foot together, has been shown to be effective in detection of critical CHD. It is now recommended by the AAP and AHA. Cyanotic heart disease and defects resulting in complete mixing or decreased systemic outflow will be detected. However, clinically important, but non-critical heart disease, such as a ventricular septal defect, atrioventricular canal, or Tetralogy of Fallot with mild pulmonary stenosis will not be detected.

CASE 22

A term infant has HLHS and is awaiting surgical palliation. He remains on a prostaglandin E1 infusion. He had persistent apnea requiring endotracheal intubation. He is noted to have decreased perfusion with decreased urine output and an arterial blood gas reveals a pH of 7.5, $PaCO_2$ 30, PaO_2 28, HCO_3 22, and BE –3. His ventilator settings are as follows: tidal volume 8 mL/kg, rate 12, PEEP 5, pressure support 8 and FiO_2 0.21, and his oxygen saturations are 88%.

Which of the following is the best respiratory strategy for this infant?
A. Decrease minute ventilation
B. Increase minute ventilation
C. Increase FiO_2
D. Increase $FiCO_2$
E. Elective extubation

Discussion

The correct answer is **D**. In HLHS, a balance between pulmonary and systemic blood flow is critically important in the preoperative period. The tendency is toward increased pulmonary blood flow as PVR falls with the potential for systemic compromise, as described in the above vignette. Limitation of pulmonary blood flow includes avoidance of excessive oxygen administration and respiratory alkalosis. Methods to increase PVR include hypoxia and hypercarbia.[59] Hypercarbia can be achieved by hypoventilation or delivery of additional carbon dioxide. Hypoventilation often leads to atelectasis and alveolar hypoxemia and is not the preferred method. Addition of carbon dioxide to the inspired gas mixture is relatively simple and allows for quick adjustments to the $PaCO_2$. Increasing minute ventilation and FiO_2 are both incorrect as these maneuvers will further exacerbate respiratory alkalosis and increase pulmonary blood flow. Elective extubation is not indicated due to the history of persistent apnea and changes to the inspired gas mixture must be used with caution in patients who are spontaneously breathing.

CASE 23

You are examining a newborn male who is a couple of hours old and note prominent carotid pulses, but absent femoral pulses. Auscultation of the chest reveals a systolic murmur as well as a gallop. The liver is palpable 3 cm below the right costal margin. You are concerned about coarctation of the aorta and order an echocardiogram. The echocardiogram reveals a widely patent aortic arch with hyperdynamic ventricular function. There are no structural abnormalities, but the SVC has a diameter that is greater than the aortic arch and all the heart chambers are dilated.

Which of the following is the next best course of action?
A. Request a cardiac catheterization for better delineation of the aortic arch
B. Order a brain MRI/MRA
C. Start dopamine
D. Start PGE1
E. Start milrinone

Discussion

The correct answer is **B**. The neonate in this scenario has signs of high output cardiac failure. The vein of Galen malformation, though rare, is the most common hemodynamically significant extracardiac arteriovenous malformation in neonates.[60] The discrepancy between the carotid and femoral pulses may mimic aortic coarctation. Auscultation of the fontanelle may reveal a cranial bruit. Intractable congestive heart failure in a neonate with a vein of Galen malformation is associated with high morbidity and mortality rates. Early diagnosis with neuroimaging is necessary to optimize medical and surgical management.

Helpful Tip: Cranial vascular malformations may present with symptoms of heart failure. Increased SVC flow and flow reversal in the descending aorta with otherwise normal anatomy may be indicators of vascular steal phenomena from a large lesion.

Objectives

1. Identify commonly encountered preoperative and postoperative complications in patients with specific types of CHD
2. Identify common clinical presentation in the newborn period for specific congenital heart defects
3. Understand benefits of predischarge pulse oximetry screening in all newborns to detect serious CHD
4. Generate list of differential diagnoses of congenital heart defects based on clinical presentation

Cardiomyopathy

CASE 24

A mother presents for induced delivery due to excessive fetal growth with an estimated fetal weight of 4,300 g at 38 weeks. Maternal labs are negative but she does have a history of diabetes diagnosed 5 years ago which was treated with diet alone prior to pregnancy. She states her blood sugars have been difficult to control and she has required insulin for the last 3 months. Her most recent HgbA1C was 9.6%.

Induction is unsuccessful though the infant tolerates labor well. After 16 hours and lack of progress, a cesarean section is performed. The infant is crying and vigorous and weighs 4.45 kg. He is hypoglycemic and admitted to the NICU for closer observation. At 6 hours of life you notice a systolic crescendo–decrescendo murmur at the left sternal border. Femoral pulses are palpable but the infant has hypotension as well as worsening acidosis and elevated lactate.

Which of the following is FALSE regarding hypertrophic cardiomyopathy (HCM)?
A. The most common causes of hypertrophic cardiomyopathy (HCM) presenting in the fetal and newborn period are maternal diabetes (IDM) and twin-twin transfusion syndrome (TTTS)
B. The diagnosis of hypertrophic cardiomyopathy requires that thickening (hypertrophy) of the ventricle is seen in the absence of primary outflow tract obstruction
C. Systolic dysfunction occurs first, followed by impaired diastolic filling
D. Monophasic filling of the ventricle is abnormal and a negative prognostic sign
E. The larger, recipient twin is at risk for hypertrophic cardiomyopathy due to fluid overload

Discussion

The correct answer is **C**. The most frequently diagnosed etiologies of hypertrophic cardiomyopathy are secondary in the infant of a diabetic mother and TTTS.[61] However, there is a growing awareness of genetic and metabolic causes including storage disorders, fatty acid oxidation disorders, and carnitine deficiency, so that many cases once termed idiopathic may now be diagnosed. Noonan syndrome and Beckwith–Wiedemann syndrome are also causes. Hypertrophic cardiomyopathy is characterized by abnormal thickening of one or both ventricles, greater than two standard deviations from the mean, or greater than 4 mm at the posterior wall in the term infant. Hypertrophy is a normal response to the increased resistance seen in diseases such pulmonic or aortic stenosis, so

evaluation must also be completed for anatomical abnormalities. When heart failure occurs it is usually associated with diastolic dysfunction with impairment of the normal triphasic filling from atria to ventricle. Systolic dysfunction and secondary outflow tract obstruction may also occur. All three are negative prognostic factors.

The incidence of both primary structural CHD and acquired cardiac disease is increased several fold in twins affected by TTTS. The recipient twin is at risk for progressive cardiac dysfunction and failure due to hypervolemia and excessive hormone production by both twins. Increased levels of atrial natriuretic peptide (ANP), endothelin-1, and VEGF are seen in the recipient twin. Hypovolemia activates the renin–angiotensin system in the donor twin but a portion of this is passed through the placenta.[62] Cardiac compromise is more common in the recipient twin and presents with right atrial dilatation and hypertension which can progress to biventricular hypertrophy and RVOTO. The mechanism by which hypertrophy occurs has not been fully elucidated, but is thought to be produced in response to increase afterload resulting from a combination of fluid overload and endocrine factors.

Which of the following is a potential cause of primary cardiomyopathy?
A. Anomalous left coronary artery from the pulmonary artery (ALCAPA)
B. Hemochromatosis
C. EFE
D. Myotubular myopathy
E. Respiratory chain defects

Discussion

The correct answer is **C**. All of the above are potential causes of cardiomyopathy. A myriad of diseases can lead to cardiomyopathy due to chronic ischemia, energy failure, infiltrative disease, and primary structural muscle abnormalities. EFE may occur as a primary disorder or secondary to congenital heart defects or mitochondrial myopathies. Histopathology shows collagen and elastic fiber deposits in the endocardium. Abnormal echogenicity may be seen on echocardiogram.

CASE 25

A 7-day-old, ex–35-week infant is recovering nicely in the neonatal intensive care unit. She was born after spontaneous labor and a maternal fever was noted prior to delivery, but cultures were negative and antibiotics discontinued. She has been breathing comfortably and working on oral feeding when she begins to decline. Tachypnea and desaturation are noted and worsen until she requires intubation and subsequently inotropic support. CXR reveals a massively enlarged cardiac silhouette.

Which of the following is NOT a possible cause of dilated cardiomyopathy (DCM)?
A. Undiagnosed coarctation of the aorta
B. Human immunodeficiency virus (HIV) infection
C. Coxsackie B virus infection
D. Eagle–Barrett syndrome (Prune Belly)
E. Mitochondrial cytopathy

Discussion

The correct answer is **D**. This history is classic for a perinatally acquired viral infection with subsequent decompensation. With severe DCM the most frequently encountered infectious agent is enterovirus, with Coxsackie B the most frequent serotype. However many other infectious agents have been shown to cause an acute myocarditis in the neonate including parvovirus, influenza, adenovirus, and HIV.[63] Genetic and metabolic causes of DCM are also seen, though Eagle–Barrett syndrome is associated with hypertrophic disease. Undiagnosed structural heart disease and arrhythmias may also eventually result in secondary dilation and systolic failure.

The prognosis for DCM and enterovirus infection specifically is poor, with supportive care being the primary therapy and a potential need for heart transplant.[64,65] The role of intravenous immune globulin (IVIG) and steroids are unclear. Infants diagnosed with DCM during fetal life frequently have hydrops fetalis and the mortality may exceed 80%. Perinatal infection caries a substantial risk of both mortality (31%–75%) and permanent cardiac damage. Treatable causes (e.g., arrhythmia) have a better prognosis.

Objectives

1. Identify potential causes of cardiomyopathy in the neonate
2. Describe the common clinical presentation of neonatal cardiomyopathy
3. Understand therapeutic options in newborns with a cardiomyopathy
4. Describe clinical features associated with hypertrophic cardiomyopathy in pregnancies affected by maternal diabetes

Hypotension and Hypertension in the Fetus/Newborn

CASE 26

An infant is born after spontaneous preterm labor at 28 weeks; two doses of betamethasone were given. The infant is intubated and receives surfactant, then extubated to CPAP. An umbilical arterial line is placed to monitor blood gases. The infant is well perfused and has voided once. At 12 hours of life, the arterial pressure is 34/20 (mean arterial pressure 25).

Which of the following is NOT true about BP in the premature infant?
A. Treatment of hypotension is associated with an increase in cerebral and renal blood flow but not an improvement in long-term outcome
B. Hypotension, when defined as a pressure two standard deviations below the mean for age, is associated with normal systemic blood flow in the majority of infants
C. Intra-arterial systolic BP directly correlates with left ventricular output
D. Associations have been demonstrated between low systemic BP and cerebral injury
E. The BP at which cerebral autoregulation is lost is poorly defined

Discussion

The correct answer is **C**. The relationship between BP and perfusion is complex, especially in the newborn and premature infant. BP in the normal range may be due to an adequate amount of blood flow, but may also be due to vasoconstriction with abnormally decreased flow. In a similar way, statistically low BP for age is not an indicator of decreased flow in most infants.[66,67] In addition, the presence of intracardiac and extracardiac shunts (e.g., patent foramen ovale, PDA) which are especially impactful in preterm infants, cause left ventricular output to correlate poorly with both BP and blood flow.[68]

Clinical shock and lactic acidosis are associated with negative outcomes in premature and term infants. Studies have also shown that infants with BP that statistically falls below the documented normal range for age are at increased risk for intraventricular hemorrhage and ischemia. However, this is complicated by the facts that the normal range is poorly defined for many infants and not all infants with low BP have low blood flow. Some experts recommend more direct measurement of perfusion via functional echocardiogram and measurement of SVC flow but its use is not currently widespread.[69] Treatment of hypotension, whether by fluid bolus, inotropy, or steroids, has been shown to increase BP but there is no compelling evidence that treatment changes long-term outcomes.

Which of the following is NOT a potential benefit of delayed cord clamping?
A. Increased hemoglobin
B. Increased SVC flow
C. Decreased IVH
D. Decreased jaundice
E. Increased mean arterial pressure

Discussion

The correct answer is **D**. Delayed (30–180 seconds) umbilical cord clamping and umbilical cord milking have several potential benefits on hemodynamic stability and iron stores in infants <32 weeks. Studies have shown decreased rates of IVH and transfusion, but there is little long-term data available. Infants who received delayed cord clamping are more likely to have elevated bilirubin requiring phototherapy.[70,71]

Helpful Tip: BP is a product of flow (CO) and resistance (systemic vascular resistance). Patients may therefore have low BP but adequate flow, if SVR is low.

Which of the following is NOT typically associated with a lower BP in late-preterm and term infants?
A. Severe RDS
B. Fetomaternal hemorrhage
C. Maternal spinal anesthesia
D. Hypercarbia
E. Maternal tobacco use

Discussion

The correct answer is **E**. Observational studies have shown that larger, more mature infants have a higher mean BP due in part to maturity of the cardiac muscle and adrenoreceptors. Even in cases of hemorrhage, hypotension is a later finding due to release of catecholamines and vasopressin in response to low BPs. Severe lung disease, such as RDS is associated with lower BPs, as are pneumonia and sepsis. Hypercarbia may cause local vasodilation in the cerebral circulation but compensatory mechanisms limit the systemic impact and pulmonary vasoconstriction occurs. Maternal tobacco use has been shown to cause increased BPs and increased reactivity in neonates which may persist postnatally.[72]

Which of following is FALSE concerning BP in the newborn?
A. Low–birth-weight infants have a lower normal BP until they reach term-corrected gestational age
B. Oscillometric BP measurement is best for mean BP, worst for diastolic pressure
C. The appropriate size BP cuff is 40% to 70% of the arm circumference
D. Intra-arterial pressures average 5 mm Hg lower than oscillometric pressures
E. BPs can increase significantly during feeding or sucking on a pacifier

Discussion

The correct answer is **A**. Low–birth-weight infants initially have a lower BP followed by a rapid rise over the next 1 to 2 weeks. By 1 month of age, BP norms are the similar for all infants, regardless of gestational age. For example by 2 weeks of age, the 50th percentile for mean BP in a 26-week infant is almost 40.[73] Noninvasive BP measurement is used commonly due to ease and low risk of complications. On average, cuff BPs read slightly higher than intra-arterial pressures, this may be more significant in the smallest infants. Appropriate cuff size is important and should be one of the first things evaluated when an infant has high or low BP.[74] Although clinically difficult, the most accurate BPs are obtained when the infant is lying undisturbed, sleeping or resting, and distant from feeds.

Helpful Tip: Although frequently used for premature infants, the guideline of a mean arterial pressure equal to the gestational age has essentially no scientific basis. Outcomes data show an MAP < GA does not necessarily increase risk for mortality, especially if perfusion is good. Conversely, using this adage in an older-preterm infant can lead to under treatment of significant hypotension.

Helpful Tip: As a general guideline, a persistent systolic BP >90 mm Hg or a diastolic BP of >60 mm Hg are cause for concern and evaluation in full-term infants. Age-specific nomograms are available for preterm infants.

Which of the following is TRUE concerning hypertension in the neonate?
A. Risk of thrombosis from an appropriately placed umbilical arterial catheter (UAC) is low
B. The most common causes of hypertension in the term neonate are volume overload, CoA, and hyperthyroidism
C. Due to capillary leak, infants undergoing ECMO are rarely hypertensive
D. Most infants with even significant hypertension are asymptomatic
E. Formerly preterm infants are a low risk for hypertension, unless born small for gestational age

Discussion

The correct answer is **D**. Symptomatic hypertension is rare though irritability and poor feeding are sometimes seen in addition to serious complications such as heart failure and intracranial hemorrhage. The most common presentation remains the asymptomatic infant. The two most frequently documented causes of hypertension in the neonatal intensive care unit are umbilical catheter thrombus and renal or renovascular disease. Infants with renal disease or urologic obstruction have an estimated 20% incidence of hypertension, compared to 10% for infants on ECMO and 1% in the overall population.[73,75] coarctation of the aorta is the most common cardiac cause of hypertension. Hypervolemia is rare unless iatrogenic and usually causes only transiently increased BP, if at all. Due to impairment of renal development and use of umbilical catheters and nephrotoxic medications, ex-preterm infants are a higher than normal risk for hypertension. An association between hypertension and chronic lung disease is also seen. Studies are conflicting regarding infants born small for gestational age with some showing lower BPs initially, but higher into childhood.

Objectives

1. Know common causes of hypotension in the preterm infant
2. Know common causes of hypertension in the newborn
3. Understand the relationship between BP and perfusion

Cardiovascular Effects of Hypoxic Ischemic Encephalopathy/Asphyxia

CASE 27

A healthy, 26-year-old G1P0 mother at 39 weeks presents in Labor and Delivery triage with complaint of rupture of membranes and pain. On examination the umbilical cord is present in the vagina and fetal heart tones are in the 80s. An emergency C-section is performed. At delivery the infant is limp, cyanotic, and apneic with a barely palpable HR in the 30s. Resuscitation is begun and the infant is given bag-mask ventilation, then intubated as chest compressions are begun. Epinephrine is administered via the ETT, then again after an umbilical venous line is placed. Subsequently there is improvement in HR and some gasping is noted at 18 minutes of age. Apgars are 1, 1, 2, 4, and 6. Initial blood gas done at 45 minutes of life shows a mixed

acidosis: 6.9/78/120/-16. The infant remains intubated and neurologic examination reveals a hypotonic infant responsive only to painful stimulation.

The infant above has severe hypoxic ischemic encephalopathy (HIE).

Which of the following echocardiographic signs is NOT typical in a neonate with severe HIE?
A. Regional wall or septal motion abnormalities
B. Decreased left ventricular shortening fraction
C. Tricuspid valve incompetence
D. Increased right ventricular pressure with premature closure of the ductus arteriosus
E. Mitral valve incompetence

Discussion

The correct answer is **D**. HIE frequently involves other organ systems in addition to the nervous system. Over 80% of cases will include involvement of the kidneys, liver, or cardiovascular system. Systemic hypotension is very frequent, while cardiac-specific involvement is less so, but still occurs in approximately 30% of patients with moderate or severe HIE.[76,77] Electrocardiography (ECG) can show specific T-wave abnormalities as well as Q-waves and even segmental infarction. These have prognostic implications but clinically ECG is used infrequently. Echocardiography in cases of severe HIE shows characteristic anomalies including decreased left ventricular (LV) function and lower shortening fraction, focal wall motion abnormalities, septal dyskinesia, papillary muscle hyperechogenicity and valvular incompetence. Tricuspid valve incompetence, regurgitation, and pulmonary hypertension are also more common in infants with HIE, but this is typically associated with a persistently PDA, not premature closure.

Cardiac biomarkers show consistent association with HIE and severity of illness.

Which of the following biomarkers are sensitive to myocardial injury AND can be used to predict cardiovascular compromise in infants with HIE?
1. Creatine kinase-muscle brain isoenzyme (CK-MB)
2. Troponin-T
3. Troponin-I
4. B-type natriuretic peptide (BNP)

A. 1, 2, 3
B. 2, 3
C. 4
D. 2, 3, 4
E. All of the above

Discussion

The correct answer is **B**. Multiple small studies have evaluated known markers of cardiac dysfunction in cases of severe HIE. Troponin-I and troponin-T are structural proteins in cardiac myocytes and well-established markers of cardiac ischemia in children as well as adults. Both have been shown to be significantly elevated in neonates with severe HIE compared to mild HIE and term controls. Elevated troponin-T levels are associated with decreased stroke volume (SV) and LV output. Significantly elevated troponin-I and troponin-T levels are risk factors for early mortality. CK-MB is a cardiac isoenzyme expressed in myocardial muscle. Although it is elevated in infants with HIE compared to controls, it is not specific for those with cardiovascular compromise.[78] BNP is a peptide hormone secreted by the walls of the ventricles in response to volume overload and ventricular stress. It is increasingly used in the management of heart failure in adults and children and may play a role in the evaluation of PDA. It is sensitive to myocardial dysfunction and pulmonary hypertension. N-terminal-pro-BNP (NTpBNP) is an inactive by product with a longer half-life and may also be useful. Elevated BNP has shown an association with intraventricular hemorrhage and death in preterm infants with a PDA, but has not currently been shown to be predictive of outcomes in infants with HIE.

Helpful Tip: BNP levels may be useful in guiding diagnosis and management of PDA. Several small studies have shown a correlation between an elevated BNP level and hemodynamically significant PDA.[79,80]

Helpful Tip: A low HR is commonly seen in infants undergoing whole body cooling. An HR of 80 to 100 is typical but it may also be slightly lower. The infant should be evaluated to determine if any treatment is required.

The infant is treated with standard-of-care, whole-body cooling, and cooled to an esophageal temperature of 33.5°C. The HR decreases with cooling as expected.

Which of the following is the expected decrease in CO for an infant undergoing total-body hypothermia?
A. None
B. 5%
C. 10%
D. 25%
E. 33%

Discussion

The correct answer is **E**. Mild therapeutic hypothermia, either selective-head cooling or whole-body cooling, is now standard of care for moderate and severe HIE. Hypothermia results in a decreased metabolic rate and energy utilization overall, but has several specific cardiovascular implications. Sinus bradycardia is a common and expected side effect of the lower temperature. However, stroke volume does not increase in compensation, and in fact is decreased in infants undergoing therapeutic hypothermia. This leads to a significant reduction in CO to approximately 67% before cooling level.[76] This is in addition to any cardiac-specific sequelae of the hypoxic ischemic event. Inotropic use is a common, but mostly temporary, need during therapeutic hypothermia.[81]

Helpful Tip: Infants with HIE and high oxygen requirement (>50%) should be monitored for pulmonary hypertension. This can be done continuously with preductal (on the right hand) and postductal (on either foot) pulse oximetry monitoring. A difference of 10% indicates significant pulmonary hypertension with shunting at the ductal level.

The infant has an increasing oxygen requirement and eventually requires 100% oxygen to maintain saturations above 80%. A pre- and postductal saturation difference is noted. Echocardiogram reveals findings consistent with pulmonary hypertension. The infant is started on dopamine at 10 µg/kg/min to raise systemic BP in hopes of improving the degree of shunt through the PDA.

Which of the following is NOT true?
A. Approximately one-third of infants with HIE will have specific cardiac dysfunction
B. Infants with HIE have increased rates of pulmonary hypertension
C. Whole-body cooling increases the incidence and severity of pulmonary hypertension in infants with HIE
D. More than 60% of neonates with HIE will receive inotropic support
E. There is insufficient evidence to show whether inotropic support improves mortality or neurodevelopmental outcomes in neonates with HIE

Discussion

The correct answer is **C**. Cardiovascular effects of moderate–severe HIE are common with the majority of patients experiencing systemic hypotension (>60%) and the need for inotropy, which as discussed previously, is increased by therapeutic hypothermia. Cardiac-specific effects, such a focal ventricular wall infarction or valve incompetence, are seen in approximately one-third of patients in whom echocardiograms are performed. Although the majority of affected infants receive volume resuscitation and inotropic support, there is not adequate data to demonstrate a beneficial effect on outcome.[76,81]

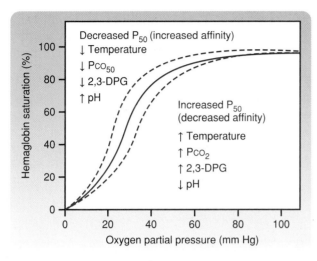

FIGURE 4-5. Factors that shift the oxyhemoglobin dissociation curve. Changes in blood pH shift the oxyhemoglobin dissociation curve. An increase in CO_2 production by tissue and release into blood results in the generation of hydrogen ions (H+) and a decrease in pH. This shifts the dissociation curve to the right, which has a beneficial effect by aiding in the release of O_2 from Hgb for diffusion into tissues. The shift to the right in the dissociation curve is due to the decrease in pH and to a direct effect of CO_2 on Hgb. This effect of CO_2 on the affinity of Hgb for O_2 is known as the Bohr effect, and it serves to enhance O_2 uptake in the lungs and delivery of O_2 to tissues. Conversely, as blood passes through the lungs, CO_2 is exhaled, thereby resulting in an increase in pH, which causes a shift to the left in the oxyhemoglobin dissociation curve. Increased body temperature, such as during exercise, shifts the oxyhemoglobin dissociation curve to the right and enables more O_2 to be released to tissues where it is needed because the demand increases. During cold weather, a decrease in body temperature, especially in the extremities (lips, fingers, toes, and ears), shifts the O_2 dissociation curve to the left (higher Hgb affinity). (Reproduced with permission from Koeppen BM, Stanton BA. *Berne and Levy Physiology.* 6th ed. Philadelphia, PA: Mosby/Elsevier; 2009.)

The process of pulmonary artery relaxation that normally occurs after birth is complex and requires oxygenation and perfusion to occur as expected. The hypoxia and acidosis that occur in neonates with HIE impair this process and lead to an increased frequency of pulmonary hypertension, which is seen in 20% to 25% of infants.[82] Despite concerns, analysis of available studies of mild therapeutic hypothermia has not shown this to increase the frequency of pulmonary hypertension or the need for extra corporeal membrane oxygenation (ECMO) (Fig. 4-5).

Objectives

1. Understand the impact of ischemia on CO and function
2. Identify typical finding on the EKG in infants with HIE
3. Identify biomarkers of cardiac dysfunction in neonates with HIE

Electrocardiography, Electrophysiology, and Dysrhythmias

Which of the following is a normal electrocardiographic finding in a premature infant in comparison to a term infant?
A. Relative bradycardia
B. Longer QRS interval
C. Longer QT interval
D. LV predominance
E. RV predominance

Discussion

The correct answer is **D**. The initial electrocardiogram in infants <35 weeks' gestation differs from that of a term infant.[83] The premature infant usually has relative tachycardia with HRs less than 200 beats/min. The QRS duration, as well as the PR interval and the QT interval, is usually shorter than term infants. The electrocardiogram of a premature infant is also characterized by left ventricular dominance, compared to the right ventricular dominance that can be seen up to 6 months in term infants.

Helpful Tip: Adenosine should be administered rapidly over 1 to 2 seconds, followed immediately by a saline flush. If central access is available, the dose should be administered as close to the heart as possible. Multiple side effects are possible, including significant bradycardia.

CASE 28

A newborn presents with a narrow complex tachycardia with HRs in the 200s. He is irritable with moderate tachypnea. You think he may be in supraventricular tachycardia and give a dose of adenosine. His rhythm changes to the rhythm strip are shown in Figure. 4-6.

What is the most effective method for terminating this tachycardia?
A. IV amiodarone
B. IV lidocaine
C. IV digoxin
D. Oral propranolol
E. Direct current cardioversion

Discussion

The correct answer is **E**. In patients with narrow complex tachycardia, adenosine can be therapeutic or diagnostic. Adenosine slows the conduction through the

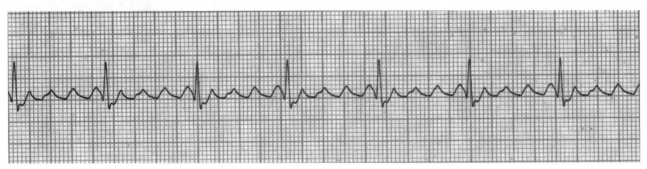

FIGURE 4-6. Rhythm strip for the infant described in Case 28.

atrioventricular node and atrial flutter waves can be better visualized. The rhythm strip demonstrates atrial flutter with 4:1 atrioventricular block. Amiodarone, digoxin, and β blockers have all been used to treat atrial flutter, but cardioversion is the most effective therapy. Neonatal atrial flutter can have significant morbidity with heart failure or hydrops and therefore sinus rhythm should be established as quickly as possible.[84] The recurrence rate of atrial flutter is low.

Which of the following is the most common cause of complete heart block in a newborn without structural heart disease?
A. Maternal anti-Ro and anti-La autoantibodies
B. Maternal ANA autoantibodies
C. Maternal antithyroid antibodies
D. Maternal methadone use
E. Fetal hypoxemia

Discussion

The correct answer is **A**. Congenital complete heart block is commonly seen with l-TGA and polysplenia. In the majority of patients without structural heart disease, the most common cause of congenital heart block (CHB) is transmission of maternal anti-Ro and anti-La autoantibodies.[85] Although the precise mechanism is unknown, it is thought to be an immune-mediated tissue injury of the atrioventricular node or His bundle. ANA autoantibodies have not been shown to be associated with neonatal lupus and complete heart block. Maternal antithyroid antibodies, methadone use and fetal hypoxemia can cause sinus bradycardia, but have not been shown to cause complete heart block.

Quick Quiz: Heart Block

What is the risk of congenital heart block in an infant born to a mother with known anti-Ro antibodies?
A. <1%
B. 3%
C. 10%
D. 45%

Discussion

The correct answer is **B**. CHB is rare event, occurring in <1/20,000 infants. Women with lupus and anti-Ro antibody have a 3% risk of a child with neonatal lupus syndrome and CHB, though recurrence risk is higher (18%–20%).[86]

Helpful Tip: CHB has a high mortality rate, especially when associated with structural heart disease or hydrops fetalis. Outcome is dependent on the ventricular rate. A slightly low rate in the 70s or 80s is often fairly well tolerated, while lower rates, especially under 55 bpm often result in fetal death.

CASE 29

A 2-week-old infant has a resting HR of 260 beats/min. There is no heart murmur and a chest radiograph reveals normal heart size. The infant is breathing comfortably with normal BPs and perfusion. An electrocardiogram reveals tachycardia with narrow QRS complexes. You apply ice to the face for 30 seconds without any change to the cardiac rhythm.

What is the most appropriate next step in management?
A. IV verapamil
B. DC cardioversion
C. Oral propranolol
D. IV adenosine
E. IV digoxin

Discussion

The correct answer is **D**. Supraventricular tachycardia is the most common arrhythmia seen in neonates and infants and is a type of re-entrant tachycardia propagated by the presence of an accessory pathway.[87] The electro-cardiogram typically demonstrates a narrow QRS with an HR that is not variable. Supraventricular tachycardia can result in congestive heart failure if prolonged, and therefore, termination of the tachycardia is recommended. Eliciting a dive reflex with facial submersion in cold water or placing ice to the face for 30 seconds is a method to terminate supraventricular tachycardia. Adenosine, which blocks the atrioventricular node, is also quite effective in the disruption of the re-entry mechanism. DC cardioversion should be reserved for an infant who is hemodynamically unstable. Verapamil has been shown to have deleterious effects in children less than 1 year of age and should be avoided. Propranolol and digoxin are medications used to prevent recurrence of supraventricular tachycardia, but have limited roles in the acute termination of supraventricular tachycardia.

CASE 30

A newborn baby is noted to have complete heart block shortly after delivery with an HR of 50 beats/min.

Which of the following medications would be most useful to increase the HR?
A. Atropine infusion
B. Digoxin infusion
C. Dobutamine infusion
D. Isoproterenol infusion
E. Milrinone infusion

Discussion

The correct answer is **D**. The most common fetal arrhythmia requiring intervention in the delivery room is congenital complete heart block. Rapid assessment and intervention can prevent poor cardiac output, ventricular failure, and pericardial effusion.[88] Isoproterenol is a nonspecific β agonist with no α-adrenergic activity resulting in inotropy and chronotropy.[89] It can increase the ventricular escape rate in cases of complete heart block. Atropine acts by blocking the action of acetylcholine and is only effective in reversing atrioventricular block from excessive vagal stimuli, but would not be indicated in this scenario. Digoxin may slow the ventricular rate and should be avoided. Dobutamine and milrinone are both effective for inotropy, but have little effect on chronotropy.

Objectives

1. Identify common EKG patterns in the preterm infant
2. Know common causes of congenital heart block
3. Know common causes of supraventricular tachycardia in the newborn
4. Understand appropriate evaluation and management for newborns with supraventricular tachycardia
5. Understand the physiologic implications for newborns with congenital heart block

Pharmacology

CASE 31

A 3-day-old male with pulmonary atresia and intact ventricular septum is maintained on a prostaglandin E1 infusion (PGE1). His surgical repair has been delayed due to Group B streptococcus bacteremia.

The parents inquire about the side effects of PGE1.

Which of the following is an accurate statement?
A. Prostaglandin E1 can result in cutaneous vasodilation
B. Prostaglandin E1 can cause primary hypoxia and tracheal intubation may be warranted
C. Prostaglandin E1 can cause hypothermia
D. Prostaglandin E1 can cause significant hypertension
E. Neurologic sequelae, such as seizures, are uncommon with prostaglandin E1 administration

Discussion

The correct answer is **A**. Prostaglandin E1 has allowed for the stabilization of infants with critical CHD who are dependent on a PDA for pulmonary or systemic blood flow or intracardiac mixing prior to palliation or repair. The main side effects of prostaglandin E1 include apnea, cutaneous vasodilation, hypotension, hyperthermia, and seizures.[90] Hypoxia can occur with prolonged apnea, but prostaglandin E1 does not cause primary hypoxia. The incidence of side effects correlates with the dose and duration of prostaglandin E1 with higher doses and longer duration resulting in more adverse effects.

Helpful Tip: Prostaglandin infusion is typically dosed from 0.01 to 0.1 µg/kg/min. In infants with that already have ductal patency (e.g., prenatally diagnosed CHD) a lower dose (0.02 µg/kg/min) is often adequate and will decrease the incidence of side effects such as apnea and fever.

Helpful Tip: Long-term prostaglandin treatment may be necessary in neonates who are premature or have significant comorbidities. Usage >14 days is associated with specific side effects including gastric outlet obstruction, cortical hyperostosis, and renal tubular impairment.[91]

CASE 32

A 1-month-old infant has a large atrioventricular canal defect and has signs of congestive heart failure. Her medications include digoxin and furosemide. Her electrolytes are as follows: sodium 130, potassium 3, chloride 88, carbon dioxide 32, BUN 17, and creatinine 0.3.

Which of the following would be the best medical management?
A. Add acetazolamide
B. Add chlorothiazide
C. Add calcium
D. Decrease digoxin
E. Decrease furosemide

Discussion

The correct answer is **E**. This infant has hypokalemic, hypochloremic metabolic alkalosis produced by furosemide, a loop diuretic.[92] The appropriate intervention would be to decrease the furosemide dosage as well as add potassium chloride supplementation. A thiazide diuretic may worsen the excessive potassium and chloride urine loss. Acetazolamide is a weak diuretic which results in renal loss of HCO_3 ions and while it can aid in the treatment of hypochloremic alkalosis, it is usually ineffective unless the diuretic dosage is decreased and potassium chloride is added.

Table 4-2 profiles various inotropes with sites of action and hemodynamic effects. Which of the following is correct?

TABLE 4-2.

DRUG	α	β₁	β₂	CARDIAC OUTPUT
A. Epinephrine	+++	+++	+++	↑↑
B. Norepinephrine	+++	+++		↑ or ↓
C. Dopamine		++	+	↑↑
D. Dobutamine	+		+	↑↑
E. Isoproterenol		+++	+++	↑↑

Discussion

The correct answer is **A**. Commonly used catecholamines include dopamine, epinephrine, and norepinephrine that are endogenous, and dobutamine and isoproterenol, which are synthetic.[93] Epinephrine is a potent direct agonist of both α and β receptors. A low-dose infusion results in predominant β-adrenoreceptor activation while higher doses stimulate α receptors. Epinephrine increases heart rate and contractility and therefore increases cardiac output. Norepinephrine primarily acts on α receptors resulting in increased systemic vascular resistance and arterial BP with little change in contractility or cardiac output. Dopamine, at low doses, stimulates dopaminergic receptors and increases renal, mesenteric, and coronary blood flow. At moderate doses, dopamine activates β-adrenergic receptors and increases contractility and HR. At high doses, dopamine has predominant α-adrenergic effects resulting in peripheral vasoconstriction and increases in heart rate and blood pressure. Dobutamine is primarily a β1 agonist with additional β2 and α activity. Dobutamine is useful for increasing inotropy without increasing HR. Isoproterenol is a pure β1 and β2 agonist without α effects. Isoproterenol is useful for maintaining the heart rate in children with bradycardia and atrioventricular heart block.

CASE 33

A 2-week-old infant born at 28 weeks' gestation has been successfully extubated and weaned onto CPAP support. On physical examination, the infant has moderate to severe work of breathing and a murmur is heard at the left sternal border between the second and third intercostal spaces. There are palpable palmar pulses. You are concerned that the ductus arteriosus has reopened and would like to start medical therapy with a nonselective cyclooxygenase inhibitor.

Which of the following is a true statement regarding indomethacin and ibuprofen?
A. Indomethacin has less renal toxicity than ibuprofen
B. Indomethacin has less risk of necrotizing enterocolitis than ibuprofen
C. Ibuprofen is less effective for ductal closure than indomethacin
D. Ibuprofen has less deleterious effect on cerebral blood flow than indomethacin
E. Ibuprofen has a higher risk of intraventricular hemorrhage than indomethacin

Discussion

The correct answer is **D**. Indomethacin and ibuprofen are medications that have been used as alternatives to surgical ligation for a PDA.[94] Ibuprofen has been shown to have equal efficacy to indomethacin with possibly less vascular compromise. Unlike indomethacin, ibuprofen does not decrease mesenteric or cerebral blood flow. Ibuprofen also has less effect on renal perfusion than indomethacin. Controlled, randomized trials have shown no difference in the incidence of necrotizing enterocolitis or intraventricular hemorrhage between ibuprofen and indomethacin.[95]

Helpful Tip: Indomethacin prophylaxis can be given to infants <1,000 g for the first 3 days of life, this practice has been shown to result in a decrease in the rates of PDA and PDA requiring surgery, but not to have a definitive impact on the incidence of chronic lung disease.

Which of the following is NOT a known side effect of indomethacin?
A. Oliguria
B. Decreased platelet aggregation
C. Decreased mesenteric perfusion
D. Hypernatremia
E. Decreased cerebral perfusion

Discussion

The correct answer is **D**. Indomethacin administration has a number of known side effects due to decreased renal perfusion including decreased urine output, fluid retention, creatinine elevation, and electrolyte abnormalities including hyponatremia. Decreased mesenteric and cerebral perfusion also occurs and is likely one of the factors leading to a lower rate of intraventricular hemorrhage. Platelet dysfunction is seen, and can result in clinically significant bleeding.

CASE 34

A newborn female born at 30 weeks' gestation has hypotension and signs of compromised systemic perfusion. You have given volume replacement without significant clinical improvement and are considering inotropic therapy.

Which of the following statements is most accurate regarding dopamine and dobutamine use in preterm infants?
A. Dopamine primarily increases mean blood pressure by increasing stroke volume
B. Dobutamine primarily increases mean BPs by increasing stroke volume
C. Dobutamine primarily increases mean BPs by increasing systemic vascular resistance
D. Dopamine is preferred for hypotension and shock caused by myocardial dysfunction
E. Dobutamine is preferred for hypotension and shock caused by sepsis

Discussion

The correct answer is **B**. Both dopamine and dobutamine are inotropic agents used for systemic hypotension. Dopamine is a sympathomimetic amine that directly stimulates α1- and β1-adrenergic receptors. At low concentrations, dopamine causes vasodilation by the activation of dopaminergic receptors in the renal, mesenteric, and coronary vascular beds. At moderate concentrations, dopamine is a direct β1-adrenergic agonist and increases cardiac output. At high doses, dopamine is a direct α1-adrenergic agonist and results in increased systemic vascular resistance. Dobutamine is a synthetic catecholamine that acts primarily on β1 receptors with additional β2- and α1-adrenergic effects. Randomized, controlled trials investigating the use of dopamine and/or dobutamine in preterm infants have demonstrated that dobutamine mainly increases mean blood pressure by an increase in stroke volume while dopamine increases mean blood pressure by an increase in systemic vascular resistance.[96,97] Therefore, for hypotension and shock related to vasodilation from sepsis, dopamine, and epinephrine may be more effective than dobutamine. For hypotension and shock related to myocardial dysfunction, such as in perinatal asphyxia, dobutamine may be more effective in restoring myocardial contractility without a significant increase in systemic vascular resistance.

Helpful Tip: Although volume replacement is often first-line therapy for hypotension due to its ease and rapidity, newborn infants are rarely volume depleted unless an event such as a placental abruption, has occurred. Thus inotropy should be considered early. However, infants with significant third spacing may have substantial volume requirements.

Objectives

1. Know side effects associated with the use of prostaglandin E
2. Know side effects associated with the use of indomethacin and ibuprofen for the treatment of a PDA

3. Understand the indications to use dopamine and dobutamine in the newborn
4. Identify side effects associated with the use of diuretics

Neurodevelopmental Outcome

Children with CHD are at increased risk for neurodevelopmental disorders or disabilities.

Which of the following is a correct statement regarding risk stratification for the development of neurodevelopmental disorders or disabilities?
A. An infant with acyanotic heart disease requiring open heart surgery in the neonatal period is in a low-risk category
B. An infant with cyanotic heart disease not requiring open heart surgery in the neonatal period is in a low-risk category
C. A newborn with CHD and trisomy 21 is in a low-risk category
D. A newborn with CHD and macrocephaly is in a high-risk category
E. A newborn with CHD born at 34 weeks is in a high-risk category

Discussion

The correct answer is **E**. Risk factors for neurodevelopmental disorders or disabilities in children with CHD have been identified.[98] The high-risk category includes: patients requiring open heart surgery for cyanotic or acyanotic CHD in the neonatal or infancy period, patients with cyanotic heart disease who do not require open heart surgery in the neonatal or infancy period but have sequelae of chronic hypoxemia, and CHD associated with comorbidities such as prematurity <37 weeks, suspected genetic syndromes, history of mechanical support or cardiopulmonary resuscitation, perioperative seizures, or microcephaly.

Helpful Tip: Children with CHD, especially those in certain high-risk categories, are at substantial risk for neurodevelopmental delay. Risks should be discussed with family during initial hospitalization and developmental follow-up is indicated, especially for high-risk infants.

Objective

1. Understand the risk for developmental delay among children with a history of CHD.

REFERENCES

1. Jenkins KJ, Correa A, Feinstein JA, et al. Noninherited risk factors and congenital cardiovascular defects: Current knowledge: A scientific statement from the American Heart Association Council on Cardiovascular Disease in the Young: Endorsed by the American Academy of Pediatrics., *Circulation.* 2007;115(23):2995–3014.
2. Matok I, Gorodischer R, Koren G, et al. Exposure to folic acid antagonists during the first trimester of pregnancy and the risk of major malformations. *Br J Clin Pharmacol.* 2009;68(6):956–962.
3. Ionescu-Ittu R, Marelli AJ, Mackie AS, et al. Prevalence of severe congenital heart disease after folic acid fortification of grain products: Time trend analysis in Quebec, Canada. *BMJ.* 2009;338:b1673.
4. Hoffman JI, Kaplan S. The incidence of congenital heart disease. *J Am Coll Cardiol.* 20021;39(12):1890–1900.
5. Sardor GG, Smith DF, MacLeod PM. Cardiac malformations in the fetal alcohol syndrome. *J Pediatr.* 1981;98(5):771–773.
6. Serrano M, Han M, Brinez P, et al. Fetal alcohol syndrome: Cardiac birth defects in mice and prevention with folate. *Am J Obstet Gynecol.* 2010;203(1):75e7–75.e15
7. Hunter LE, Simpson JM. Prenatal screening for structural congenital heart disease. *Nat Rev Cardiol.* 2014;11(6):323–334.
8. Srivastava, D. Molecular and morphogenetic cardiac embryology: Implications for congenital heart disease. In: Artman M, Mahony L, Teitel DF, eds. *Neonatal Cardiology.* New York NY: McGraw-Hill, Medical Pub. Division; 2002:2.
9. Maschhoff KL, Baldwin HS. Molecular determinants of neural crest migration. *Am J Med Genet.* 2000;97(4):280–288.
10. Lin CJ, Lin CY, Chen CH, et al. Partitioning the heart: Mechanisms of cardiac septation and valve development. *Development.* 2012;139(18):3277–3299.
11. Mahler GJ, Butcher JT. Cardiac developmental toxicity. *Birth Defects Res C Embryo Today.* 2011;93(4):291–297.
12. Blue GM, Kirk EP, Sholler GF, et al. Congenital heart disease: Current knowledge about causes and inheritance. *Med J Aust.* 2012;197(3):155–159.
13. Jones KL, Smith DW. *Environmental Agents, in Smith's Recognizable Patterns of Human Malformation.* 6th ed. Philadelphia, PA: Elsevier Saunders; 2006:646.
14. Todorova K, Mazneĭkova V, Ivanov S, et al. The frequency of mild and severe fetal malformations in diabetic women with high values of glycosilated hemoglobin in early pregnancy (abstract only). *Akush Ginekol (Sofiia).* 2005;44(3):3–10.
15. Peckham CS. Clinical and laboratory study of children exposed in utero to maternal rubella. *Arch Dis Child.* 1972;47(254):571–577.
16. Taeusch HW, Ballard RA, Gleason CA. *Avery's Diseases of the Newborn.* 8th ed. Philadelphia, PA: Elsevier Saunders; 2005.
17. Reef SE, Redd SB, Abernathy E, et al. The epidemiological profile of rubella and congenital rubella syndrome in the United States, 1998–2004: The evidence for absence of endemic transmission. *Clin Infect dis.* 2006;43 (suppl 3):S126–S132.
18. Dewan P, Gupta P. Burden of Congenital Rubella Syndrome (CRS) in India: A systematic review. *Indian pediatr.* 2012;49(5):377–399.
19. Goldmuntz E. The genetic contribution to congenital heart disease. *Pediatr Clin North Am.* 2004;51(6):1721–1737.
20. Benson DW The genetics of congenital heart disease: A point in the revolution. *Cardiol Clin.* 2002;20(3):385–394, vi.

21. Goldmuntz E, Emanuel BS. Genetic disorders of cardiac morphogenesis. The DiGeorge and velocardiofacial syndromes. *Circ Res.* 1997;80(4):437–443.

22. Momma K. Cardiovascular anomalies associated with chromosome 22q11.2 deletion syndrome. *Am J Cardiol.* 2010; 105(11):1617–1624.

23. Jones KL, Smith DW. *Chromosomal Abnormality Syndromes, in Smith's Recognizable Patterns of Human Malformation.* 6th ed. Philadelphia, PA: Elsevier Saunders; 2006:7.

24. Pierpont ME, Basson CT, Benson DW, Jr., et al. Genetic basis for congenital heart defects: Current knowledge: A scientific statement from the American Heart Association Congenital Cardiac Defects Committee, Council on Cardiovascular Disease in the Young: Endorsed by the American Academy of Pediatrics. *Circulation.* 2007;115(23):3015–3038.

25. Marín-García J. Advances in molecular genetics of congenital heart disease. *Rev Esp Cardiol.* 2009;62(3):242–245.

26. Artman M, Mahony L, Teitel DF. Perinatal cardiovascular physiology. In: Artman M, Mahony L, Teitel DF, eds. *Neonatal Cardiology.* New York, NY: McGraw-Hill, Medical Pub. Division; 2002:39.

27. Huhta JC. Fetal congestive heart failure. *Semin Fetal Neonatal Med.* 2005;10(6):542–552.

28. Bellini C, Hennekam RC, Fulcheri E, et al. Etiology of nonimmune hydrops fetalis: A systematic review. *Am J Med Genet A.* 2009;149A(5):844–851.

29. Iskaros J, Jauniaux E, Rodeck C. Outcome of nonimmune hydrops fetalis diagnosed during the first half of pregnancy. *Obstet Gynecol.* 1997;90(3):321–325.

30. Santo S, Mansour S, Thilaganathan B, et al. Prenatal diagnosis of non-immune hydrops fetalis: What do we tell the parents? *Prenat Diagn.* 2011;31(2):186–195.

31. Tulzer G, Gudmundsson S, Wood DC, et al. Doppler in nonimmune hydrops fetalis. *Ultrasound Obstet Gynecol.* 1994; 4(4):279–283.

32. Steinhorn RH. Neonatal pulmonary hypertension. *Pediatr Crit Care Med.* 2010;11(2 suppl):S79–S84.

33. Kieler H, Artama M, Engeland A, et al. Selective serotonin reuptake inhibitors during pregnancy and risk of persistent pulmonary hypertension in the newborn: Population based cohort study from the five Nordic countries. *BMJ.* 2012; 344:d8012.

34. Chambers CD, Hernandez-Diaz S, Van Marter LJ, et al. Selective serotonin-reuptake inhibitors and risk of persistent pulmonary hypertension of the newborn. *N Engl J Med.* 2006; 354(6):579–587.

35. Derbent A, Tatli MM, Duran M, et al. Transient tachypnea of the newborn: Effects of labor and delivery type in term and preterm pregnancies. *Arch Gynecol Obstet.* 2011;283(5):947–951.

36. Steinhorn RH. Pharmacotherapy for pulmonary hypertension. *Pediatr Clin North Am.* 2012;59(5):1129–1146.

37. Wojciak-Stothard B, Haworth SG. Perinatal changes in pulmonary vascular endothelial function. *Pharmacol Ther.* 2006; 109(1–2):78–91.

38. Finer N, Barrington K. Nitric Oxide for respiratory failure in infants born at or near term. *Cochrane Database Syst Rev.* 2006;(4):CD000399.

39. Bove EL, Hirsch JC, Ohye RG, et al. How I manage neonatal Ebstein's anomaly. *Semin Thorac Cardiovasc Surg Pediatr Card Surg Annu.* 2009;:63–65.

40. Waldman JD, Wernly JA. Cyanotic congenital heart disease with decreased pulmonary blood flow in children. *Pediatr Clin North Am.* 1999;46(2):385–404.

41. Wernovsky G. Transposition of the great arteries. In: Allen HD, Driscoll DJ, Shaddy RE, et al., eds. *Moss and Adams' Heart Disease in Infants, Children and Adolescents.* Philadelphia, PA: Lippincott Williams & Wilkins; 2008:1038.

42. Roofthooft MT, Bergman KA, Waterbolk TW, et al. Persistent pulmonary hypertension of the newborn with transposition of the great arteries. *Ann Thorac Surg.* 2007;83(4):1446–1450.

43. Noori S. Pros and cons of patent ductus arteriosus ligation: Hemodynamic changes and other morbidities after patent ductus arteriosus ligation. *Semin Perinatol.* 2012;36(2):139–145.

44. Cassady G, Crouse DT, Kirklin JW et al. A randomized, controlled trial of very early prophylactic ligation of the ductus arteriosus in babies who weighed 1000 g or less at birth. *N Engl J Med.* 1989;320(23):1511–1516.

45. Schneider DJ. The patent ductus arteriosus in term infants, children, and adults. *Semin Perinatol.* 2012;36(2):146–153.

46. Cetta F, Minich LL, Edwards WD, et al. Atrioventricular septal defects. In: Allen HD, Driscoll DJ, Shaddy RE, et al., eds. *Moss and Adams' Heart Disease in Infants, Children and Adolescents.* Philadelphia, PA: Lippincott Williams & Wilkins; 2008:646.

47. Yamaki S, Yasui H, Kado H, et al. Pulmonary vascular disease and operative indications in complete atrioventricular canal defect in early infancy. *J Thorac Cardiovasc Surg.* 1993;106(3):398–405.

48. Clapp S, Perry BL, Farooki ZQ, et al. Down's syndrome, complete atrioventricular canal and pulmonary vascular obstructive disease. *J Thorac Cardiovasc Surg.* 1990;100(1):115–121.

49. Rhodes LA, Colan SD, Perry SB et al. Predictors of survival in neonates with critical aortic stenosis. *Circulation.* 1991;84(6): 2325–2335.

50. Fox S, Pierce WS, Waldhausen JA. Pathogenesis of paradoxical hypertension after coarctation repair. *Ann Thorac Surg.* 1980;29(2):135–141.

51. Sealy WC. Paradoxical hypertension after repair of coarctation of the aorta: A review of its causes. *Ann Thorac Surg.* 1990;50(2):323–329.

52. Rajagopal SK, Thiagarajan, RR. Perioperative care of children with tetralogy of Fallot. *Curr Treat Options in Cardiovasc Med.* 2011;13:464–474.

53. Heinemann MK, Hanley FL. Preoperative management of neonatal tetralogy of Fallot with absent pulmonary valve syndrome. *Ann Thorac Surg.* 1993;55(1):172–174.

54. Giglia TM, Mandell VS, Connor AR et al. Diagnosis and management of right ventricle dependent coronary circulation in pulmonary atresia with intact ventricular septum. *Circulation.* 1992;86(5):1516–1528.

55. Lennox EG. Cardiology. In: Tschudy MM, Arcara KM, eds. *The Harriet Lane Handbook.* Philadelphia, PA: Elsevier Mosby; 2012.

56. McElhinney DP, Hedrick HL, Bush DM, et al. Necrotizing enterocolitis in neonates with congenital heart disease: Risk factors and outcomes. *Pediatrics.* 2000;106(5):1080–1087.

57. Mahle WT, Newburger JW, Matherne GP et al. Role of pulse oximetry in examining newborns for congenital heart disease: A scientific statement from the American Heart Association and American Academy of Pediatrics. *Circulation.* 2009;120(5): 447–458.

58. Thangaratinam S, Brown K, Zamora J et al. Pulse oximetry screening for critical congenital heart defects in asymptomatic newborn babies: A systematic review and meta-analysis. *Lancet*. 2012;379(9835):2459–2464.

59. Theilen U, Shekerdemian L. The intensive care of infants with hypoplastic left heart syndrome. *Arch Dis Child Fetal Neonatal Ed*. 2005;90(2):F97–F102.

60. Diebler C, Dulac O, Renier D et al. Aneurysms of the vein of Galen in infants aged 2 to 15 months. Diagnosis and natural evolution. *Neuroradiology*. 1981;21(4):185–197.

61. Pedra SR, Smallhorn JF, Ryan G, et al. Fetal cardiomyopathies: Pathogenic mechanisms, hemodynamic findings, and clinical outcome. *Circulation*. 2002;106(5):585–591.

62. Martins Y, Silva S, Matias A, Blickstein I. Cardiac morbidity in twin-twin transfusion syndrome? *J Perinat Med*. 2012;40(2):107–114.

63. Sivasankaran S, Sharland GK, Simpson JM. Dilated cardiomyopathy presenting during fetal life. *Cardiol Young*. 2005;15(4):409–416.

64. Freund MW, Kleinveld G, Krediet TG, et al. Prognosis for neonates with enterovirus myocarditis. *Arch Dis Childhood Fetal Neonatal Ed*. 2010;95(3):F206–F212.

65. Nathan M, Walsh R, Hardin JT, et al. Enteroviral sepsis and ischemic cardiomyopathy in a neonate: Case report and review of literature. *ASAIO J*. 2008;54(5):554–555.

66. Cayabyab R, McLean CW, Seri I. Definition of hypotension and assessment of hemodynamics in the preterm neonate. *J Perinatol*. 2009;29 (suppl 2):S58–S62.

67. Barrington KJ. Hypotension and shock in the preterm infant. *Semin Fetal Neonatal Med*. 2008;13(1):16–23.

68. Kluckow M, Evans N. Low systemic blood flow in the preterm infant. *Semin Neonatol*. 2001;6(1):75–84.

69. Evans N. Assessment and support of the preterm circulation. *Early Hum Dev*. 2006;82(12):803–810.

70. Sommers R, Stonestreet BS, Oh W, et al. Hemodynamic effects of delayed cord clamping in premature infants. *Pediatrics*. 2012;129(3):e667–e672.

71. Rabe H, Diaz-Rossello JL, Duley L, et al. Effect of timing of umbilical cord clamping and other strategies to influence placental transfusion at preterm birth on maternal and infant outcomes. *Cochrane Database Syst Rev*. 2012;8: CD003248.

72. Cohen G, Vella S, Jeffery H, et al. Cardiovascular stress hyperreactivity in babies of smokers and in babies born preterm. *Circulation*. 2008;118(18):1848–1853.

73. Flynn JT. Hypertension in the neonatal period. *Curr Opin Pediatr*. 2012;24(2):197–204.

74. Stebor AD. Basic principles of noninvasive blood pressure measurement in infants. *Adv Neonatal Care*. 2005;5(5):252–261.

75. Blowey DL, Duda PJ, Stokes P, et al. Incidence and treatment of hypertension in the neonatal intensive care unit. *J Am Soc Hypertens*. 2011;5(6):478–483.

76. Armstrong K, Franklin O, Sweetman D, et al. Cardiovascular dysfunction in infants with neonatal encephalopathy. *Arch Dis Child*. 2012;97(4):372–375.

77. Shah P, Riphagen S, Beyene J, Perlman M. Multiorgan dysfunction in infants with post-asphyxial hypoxic-ischaemic encephalopathy. *Arch Dis Child Fetal Neonatal Ed*. 2004;89(2):F152–F155.

78. Sweetman D, Armstrong K, Murphy JF, et al. Cardiac biomarkers in neonatal hypoxic ischaemia. *Acta Paediatr*. 2012; 101(4):338–343.

79. Chen S, Tacy T, Clyman R. How useful are B-type natriuretic peptide measurements for monitoring changes in patent ductus arteriosus shunt magnitude? *J Perinatol*. 2010;30(12):780–785.

80. Mine K, Ohashi A, Tsuji S, et al. B-type natriuretic peptide for assessment of haemodynamically significant patent ductus arteriosus in premature infants. *Acta Paediatr*. 2013;102(8):e347–e5352.

81. Shankaran S, Laptook AR, Ehrenkranz RA, et al. Whole-body hypothermia for neonates with hypoxic-ischemic encephalopathy. *N Engl J Med*. 2005;353(15):1574–1584.

82. Lapointe A, Barrington KJ. Pulmonary hypertension and the asphyxiated newborn. *J Pediatr*. 2011;158(2 suppl):e19–e24.

83. Tipple M. Interpretation of electrocardiograms in infants and children. *Images Paediatr Cardiol*. 1999;1(1):3–13.

84. Casey FA, McCrindle BW, Hamilton RM et al. Neonatal atrial flutter: Significant early morbidity and excellent long-term prognosis. *Am Heart J*. 1997;133(3):302–306.

85. Olah KS, Gee H. Antibody mediated complete congenital heart block in the fetus. *Pacing Clin Electrophysiol*. 1993;16(9): 1872–1879.

86. Friedman D, Duncanson LJ, Glickstein J, Buyon J. A review of congenital heart block. *Images Paediatr Cardiol*. 2003;5(3):36–48.

87. Dubin AM. Arrhythmias in the newborn. *Neoreviews*. 2000; 1(8):e146–e151.

88. Johnson B, Ades A. Delivery room and early postnatal management of neonates who have prenatally diagnosed congenital heart disease. *Clin Perinatol*. 2005;32(4):921–946, ix.

89. Tabbutt S, Helfaer MA, Nichols DG. Pharmacology of cardiovascular drugs. In: Nichols DG, Ungerleider RM, Spevak PJ, et al., eds. *Critical Heart Disease in Infants and Children*. Philadelphia, PA: Mosby Elsevier; 2006:173.

90. Lewis AB, Freed MD, Heymann MA, et al. Side effects of therapy with prostaglandin E1 in infants with critical congenital heart disease. *Circulation*. 1981;64(5):893–898.

91. Tálosi G, Katona M, Túri S. Side-effects of long-term prostaglandin E(1) treatment in neonates. *Pediatr Int*. 2007;49(3):335–40.

92. Segar JL. Neonatal diuretic therapy: Furosemide, thiazides, and spironolactone. *Clin Perinatol*. 2012;39(1):209–220.

93. Shekerdemian LS, Reddington A. Cardiovascular pharmacology. In: Chang AC, Hanley FL, Wernovsky G, et al., eds. *Pediatric Cardiac Intensive Care*. Baltimore, MD: Williams & Wilkins; 1998:45.

94. Narayanan-Sankar M, Clyman RI. Pharmacology review: Pharmacologic closure of patent ductus arteriosus in the neonate. *Neoreviews*. 2003;4(8):e215–e221.

95. Ohlsson A, Walia R, Shah S. Ibuprofen for the treatment of patent ductus arteriosus in preterm and/or low birth weight infants. *Cochrane Database Syst Rev*. 2008;(1):CD003481.

96. Osborn D, Evans N, Kluckow M, et al. Randomized trial of dobutamine versus dopamine in preterm infants with low systemic blood flow. *J Pediatr*. 2002;140(2):183–191.

97. Zhang J, Penny DJ, Kim NS, et al. Mechanisms of blood pressure increase induced by dopamine in hypotensive preterm neonates. *Arch Dis Child Fetal Neonatal Ed*. 1999;81(2):F99–F104.

98. Marino BS, Lipkin PH, Newburger JW et al. Neurodevelopmental outcomes in children with congenital heart disease: Evaluation and management: A scientific statement from the American Heart Association. *Circulation*. 2012;126(9):1143–1172.

Chapter 5
RESPIRATORY FUNCTION
Ravi Mangal Patel, MD, MSc

CASE 1

A male infant is delivered at 25 weeks of gestation by cesarean section for worsening maternal preeclampsia. He develops respiratory distress within minutes after birth, including grunting and subcostal retractions. He is placed on continuous positive airway pressure (CPAP) with a positive end-expiratory pressure (PEEP) of 6 cm H_2O. However, he subsequently requires endotracheal intubation and initiation of mechanical ventilation. A chest radiograph is obtained (Fig. 5-1).

Of the following, which is the most likely cause for this infant's respiratory distress?
A. Pneumonia
B. Surfactant deficiency
C. Transient tachypnea of the newborn
D. Apnea of prematurity
E. Persistent pulmonary hypertension of the newborn (PPHN)

Discussion

The correct answer is **B**. The most likely cause of respiratory distress in this preterm infant is RDS, which is secondary to surfactant deficiency. The risks of RDS decrease as gestational age increases, although term infants remain at risk for the disease. The chest radiograph in Figure 5-1 demonstrates lung fields with the classic "ground glass" appearance seen in surfactant deficiency due to air-distended bronchioles and ducts within a background of alveolar atelectasis as well as low lung volumes. Pneumonia, particularly those due to Group B Strep (GBS) infection, can have a similar radiographic appearance as RDS. However, this infant was delivered for a maternal indication (preeclampsia), making an

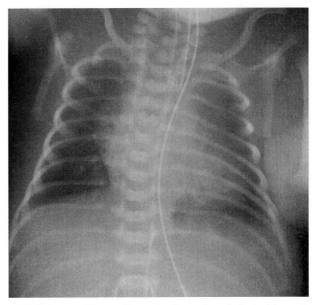

FIGURE 5-1. Chest radiograph of a newborn infant with respiratory distress.

infectious process unlikely. Although infants with apnea of prematurity can require mechanical ventilation secondary to apneic episodes, the presentation of apnea of prematurity typically occurs several days after birth and should not be associated with grunting and retractions. Patients with transient tachypnea of the newborn can present with respiratory distress in the delivery room. However, the clinical course of transient tachypnea of the newborn is typically not as severe as the presentation of this infant and rarely requires the support of mechanical ventilation. Finally, infants with RDS can develop persistent PPHN. However, this would not be the most likely underlying cause of respiratory distress.

Which of the following medications administered to the mother before delivery would have decreased the risk of respiratory distress in this patient?
A. Magnesium sulfate
B. Terbutaline
C. Penicillin
D. Betamethasone
E. Hydrocortisone

Discussion

The correct answer is **D**. The American College of Obstetricians and Gynecologists (ACOG) recommends that a single course of corticosteroids, either dexamethasone or betamethasone, be administered to pregnant women between 24 and 34 weeks of gestation who are at risk of preterm delivery within 7 days.[1] The administration of corticosteroids reduces the risks of RDS, perinatal mortality, and other morbidities before 32 weeks of gestation. The efficacy of use at 32 to 33 weeks of gestation is unclear, but treatment may be beneficial.

You decide to administer surfactant through the endotracheal tube (ETT) for this patient.

In randomized trials, preterm infants with RDS who receive surfactant, compared to placebo, were found to have a HIGHER risk of which of the following?
A. Mortality
B. Pulmonary hemorrhage
C. Pulmonary interstitial emphysema
D. Pneumothorax
E. A and D

Discussion

The correct answer is **B**. Treatment with surfactant is associated with a small, but increased risk of pulmonary hemorrhage.[2] The pathophysiology of pulmonary hemorrhage is thought to be related to rapid changes in pulmonary capillary blood flow leading to vessel rupture. Initial treatment of a pulmonary hemorrhage should focus on attempting to tamponade pulmonary bleeding by increasing PEEP to increase alveolar distention and decrease pulmonary blood flow. The use of surfactant for the treatment of RDS decreases the risk of mortality, pulmonary interstitial emphysema, and pneumothorax in preterm infants.[3,4]

Which of the following components of surfactant is responsible for improving lung mechanics?
A. Surfactant protein A
B. Surfactant protein D
C. Phosphatidylcholine
D. Phosphatidylglycerol (PG)
E. Sphingomyelin

Discussion

The correct answer is **C**. Phosphatidylcholine (also known as lecithin) is the primary phospholipid in surfactant involved in lowering alveolar surface tension. The majority of surfactant is dipalmitoylphosphatidylcholine, which accounts for almost half of surfactant by weight and is the component with the greatest physiologic activity. In contrast, surfactant proteins contribute to approximately 10% of surfactant mass.[5]

Despite intensive care, the patient expires on the first postnatal day. The family consents to autopsy.

Upon autopsy examination of this infant, which of the following pathologic findings is most likely to be identified?
A. Gram-positive cocci in the alveolar spaces
B. Absence of pulmonary capillaries
C. Dense material lining the respiratory ducts and bronchioles
D. Interstitial thickening and fibrosis
E. C and D

Discussion

The correct answer is **C**. The classic histologic feature of RDS is the hyaline membrane. This membrane is a dense hyaline material that lines the distal airway structures, primarily the alveolar ducts, and stains acidophilic with hematoxylin and eosin.[6] The membrane was first described in Hochheim in 1903 and is formed from cellular debris from injured epithelium. In contrast, interstitial thickening and fibrosis is seen in infants with bronchopulmonary dysplasia (BPD) and is not a histologic finding of RDS. Infections with gram-positive cocci, such as GBS, may complicate or contribute to the death of infants with RDS. However, in this infant who was delivered secondary to maternal indication, a primary infectious process contributing to early mortality would be unlikely.

Helpful Tip: Surfactant improves lung compliance by decreasing alveolar surface tension.

Helpful Tip: Pneumonia secondary to GBS can have a similar radiographic appearance as RDS.

Alveolar collapse resulting in decreased alveolar ventilation in infants with RDS can be explained by which of the following laws or principles?
A. Dalton law
B. LaPlace law
C. Fick law
D. Bernoulli principle
E. Poiseuille law

Discussion

The correct answer is **B**. LaPlace law states that the pressure (*P*) within a sphere (or alveolus) is directly related to the surface tension (*T*) of the liquid and inversely related to the radius (*r*) of the sphere by the following equation: $P = 2\ T/r$. Surfactant, by directly lowering the surface tension in direct proportion to surface area, allows establishment and maintenance of a functional residual capacity (FRC) by preventing alveolar collapse at the end of expiration. In the absence of surfactant, alveolar pressure will vary inversely with alveolar radius (by LaPlace law), and smaller alveoli will tend to collapse, with resultant overexpansion of larger units.[7]

Objectives

1. Know the pathophysiology and risk factors for respiratory distress syndrome (RDS)
2. Recognize the clinical and imaging features of RDS
3. Recognize the pathologic features of RDS
4. Know the clinical strategies and therapies used to decrease the risk and severity of RDS
5. Know the management of RDS, including surfactant replacement
6. Know the effects of surface tension on alveolar and airway stability and lung mechanics

CASE 2

A 7-day-old 30 weeks of gestation female infant who is not receiving any respiratory support is noted to have three episodes of desaturation and bradycardia over the prior 24 hours. A recording of one of these episodes is shown (Fig. 5-2). Her vital signs are otherwise normal. She is tolerating advancement of enteral feeding. A complete blood count (CBC) and chest radiograph are both unremarkable.

What is the most likely cause of this infant's desaturation and bradycardia?
A. Sepsis
B. Obstructive apnea
C. Central apnea
D. Congenital heart disease
E. B and C

Discussion

The correct answer is **C**. Apnea, defined as pauses in respiration of 20 seconds or more, is seen in at least 85% of

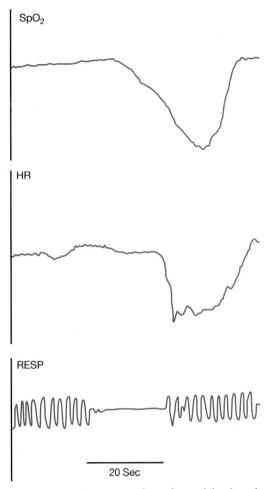

FIGURE 5-2. Monitor tracing of an infant with bradycardia and desaturation. The pulse oximetry tracing (SpO_2), heart rate waveform (HR), and respiratory rate waveform (RESP) are depicted.

infants <34 weeks of gestation at birth.[8] Episodes of apnea of prematurity are most commonly seen between 5 and 10 days of postnatal age, although can be seen within 1 day after birth.[9] Other causes of apnea, such as sepsis, should be excluded. However, sepsis is unlikely in this infant who has otherwise normal vital signs and a normal CBC and chest radiograph. While obstructive and mixed apnea is seen in older preterm infants, the timing of apnea and the monitor recording (Fig. 5-2) suggest that the episodes are triggered by primary central apnea (followed by bradycardia and desaturation) that is characteristic of apnea of prematurity.

The patient is subsequently started on caffeine therapy and she demonstrates a decrease in the frequency of apnea episodes. However, the patient's mother is concerned about the risks of caffeine therapy.

In a large, multicenter clinical trial evaluating the efficacy and safety of caffeine therapy, which of the following was more common in infants randomized to caffeine treatment compared to placebo?
A. Necrotizing enterocolitis
B. Decreased weight gain
C. BPD
D. Patent ductus arteriosus (PDA)
E. C and D

Discussion

The correct answer is **B**. Caffeine is widely used for the treatment of apnea of prematurity and is thought to decrease apneic episodes by increasing chemoreceptor responsiveness and enhancing respiratory mechanics. In the Caffeine for Apnea of Prematurity (CAP) trial, infants randomized to caffeine treatment had a greater weight loss in the first 3 weeks after initiation of treatment, although these differences were no longer present by 4 weeks of age.[10] In contrast, infants randomized to caffeine, compared to placebo, had a *lower* incidence of both BPD and PDA. In addition, no significant difference in the incidence of necrotizing enterocolitis was seen between groups.

Quick Quiz: Control of Breathing

Of the following statements regarding control of neonatal breathing, which statement is TRUE?
A. Inhalation of CO_2 decreases ventilation
B. Hyperoxia results in an immediate increase in ventilation, followed by a later decrease in ventilation
C. Hypoxia results in an immediate decrease in ventilation, followed by a later increase in ventilation
D. Acidosis results in a decrease in ventilation
E. Overdistention of the lungs decreases ventilation

Discussion

The correct answer is **E**. The newborn infant has a number of pulmonary reflexes in response to acidosis, CO_2, and oxygen.[11] Overdistention of the lungs results in a decrease in ventilation and this effect is mediated by the Hering–Breuer reflex. Inhalation of CO_2 results in an increase in the partial pressure of carbon dioxide ($PaCO_2$) that, similar to acidosis, increases the hydrogen ion concentration at the ventrolateral surface of the medulla, and results in increases in respiratory drive. In contrast, hypoxia results in a brief increase in ventilation followed by a decrease in ventilation, while hyperoxia does the opposite.

Helpful Tip: Apnea of prematurity is one of the most common problems encountered in very low–birth-weight infants.

Objectives

1. Know the pathophysiology of apnea of prematurity
2. Know the management of apnea of prematurity
3. Know the effects of pulmonary reflexes and oxygen, carbon dioxide, and hydrogen ion concentrations on control of neonatal breathing

CASE 3

A male infant is delivered by elective repeat cesarean section at 38 weeks of gestation because of maternal request secondary to a history of prior cesarean delivery. Upon admission to the nursery, the infant is found to have a pulse rate of 160 bpm and a respiratory rate of 90 breaths per minute. Pulse oximetry shows an oxygen saturation (O_2Sat) of 92% in room air. Over the next 24 hours, the infant remains in room air and the respiratory rate decreases to 40 to 50 breaths per minute and O_2Sat increases to 99%.

Of the following, which is the most likely cause for this infant's presentation?
A. Blood aspiration
B. RDS
C. Transient tachypnea of the newborn
D. Physiologic tachypnea
E. Sepsis

Discussion

The correct answer is **C**. The most likely cause of respiratory distress in this term infant is transient tachypnea of the newborn. The characteristic feature is the presence of respiratory distress, primarily the presence of tachypnea, soon after birth. Tachypnea usually persists for hours or up to several days with subsequent complete resolution.[12] A more severe clinical course than the one described is typically seen with blood aspiration. RDS is unlikely, given the short duration of respiratory distress and the lack of a need for respiratory support. Sepsis is also unlikely in this infant who underwent an elective cesarean delivery.

Which of the following risk factors is likely to have contributed to the infant's respiratory distress?
A. Male sex
B. Maternal history of prior cesarean section
C. Cesarean delivery before 39 weeks of gestation
D. Absence of labor
E. C and D

Discussion

The correct answer is **E**. Among term infants delivered by elective cesarean, delivery before 39 weeks of gestation has been associated with an increased risk of neonatal respiratory morbidity.[13] In addition, the absence of labor may lead to a delay in clearance of fetal lung fluid, which is one of the hallmarks of transient tachypnea of the newborn.[14] Currently, ACOG recommends that elective cesarean delivery should not be performed before 39 weeks of gestation unless fetal lung maturity can be confirmed.[15]

Helpful Tip: Elective delivery should not occur before 39 weeks of gestation.

Had the mother in the previous scenario decided to undergo amniocentesis to test for fetal lung maturity prior to delivery, which of the following results would be consistent with fetal lung maturity?
A. Lecithin to sphingomyelin ratio (L/S ratio) of 1.5
B. L/S ratio of 3.5
C. Phosphatidylcholine less than 2% of total phospholipids
D. PG less than 2% of total phospholipids
E. B and D

Discussion

The correct answer is **B**. Both the L/S ratio and the presence of PG in amniotic fluid are clinically used to determine fetal lung maturity.[15] Lecithin, also known as phosphatidylcholine, is a major component of surfactant and the relative abundance of lecithin in amniotic fluid is standardized to sphingomyelin, a general membrane lipid in amniotic fluid. PG is a minor component of surfactant that typically appears in sufficient quantities several weeks after the increase in lecithin. Assessment of PG is less impacted by contamination from blood or meconium, compared to lecithin, although it appears later in pregnancy than lecithin. Commonly used criteria to determine fetal lung maturity include an L/S ratio greater than 2 and the presence of PG (PG greater than 2–3% of total phospholipids).

The clearance of fetal lung fluid at birth is primarily mediated by
A. Nitric oxide
B. Closure of the PDA
C. Oxygen
D. Epithelial sodium channels
E. Surfactant

Discussion

The correct answer is **D**. The rapid clearance of fetal lung fluid is mediated by transepithelial sodium reabsorption through amiloride-sensitive sodium channels (ENaC) within the alveolar epithelial cells.[14] Infants delivered by elective cesarean section are less likely to clear fetal lung fluid, as labor is an important mediator of the active clearance of fetal lung fluid.

Objectives

1. Know the pathogenesis, pathophysiology, and risk factors for transient tachypnea of the newborn infant
2. Know the clinical features of transient tachypnea of the newborn infant
3. Know the prevention and management of transient tachypnea of the newborn infant
4. Know the timing of the biochemical maturation of the lung and the physiological and biochemical factors affecting this maturation

CASE 4

You are called to the delivery room for a term infant who develops unexpected, severe respiratory distress at birth. Labor and delivery were uncomplicated. You administer 100% oxygen by bag-mask ventilation. However, you are unable to increase O_2Sat above 40% by 5 minutes of age and subsequently perform endotracheal intubation and initiate mechanical ventilation. The mother received no prenatal care. The infant requires escalation in both peak inspiratory pressure (PIP) and PEEP to maintain pulse oximetry above 70%. At 2 hours of age, he develops sudden severe bradycardia and cardiopulmonary resuscitation is started. A chest radiograph is obtained (Fig. 5-3).

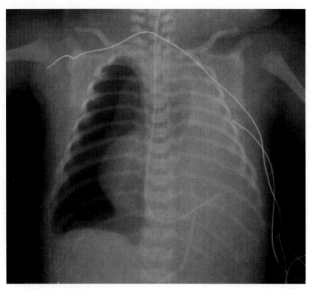

FIGURE 5-3.   Chest radiograph of a newborn infant with severe respiratory distress at birth with sudden deterioration.

What is the most likely UNDERLYING cause of respiratory distress in this infant?
A. Meconium aspiration
B. Chorioamnionitis
C. Pneumothorax
D. Congenital diaphragmatic hernia (CDH)
E. Congenital pulmonary airway malformation (CPAM)

Discussion

The correct answer is **D**. This patient has clinical and radiographic features of CDH. The presence of severe, unexpected respiratory distress at birth should lead to the immediate consideration of a possible CDH. Clinical features include asymmetric chest rise, a scaphoid abdomen, and auscultation of bowel sounds in the affected hemithorax. The diagnosis of CDH is confirmed by chest radiograph (Fig. 5-3), which demonstrates a nasogastric tube terminating in the left hemithorax. Patients with CDH are at risk of pneumothorax, including tension pneumothorax, as seen in this infant. However, this is not the underlying cause of respiratory distress in this infant and the pneumothorax is likely related to a combination of poor lung compliance and high ventilatory pressures.

The infant receives cardiopulmonary resuscitation including positive pressure ventilation, chest compressions in a 3:1 ratio, and two doses of intravenous epinephrine 4 minutes apart. However, he remains bradycardic with a heart rate <40 bpm.

Which of the following is the most appropriate next step in management of this patient?
A. Administer intravenous atropine
B. Administer intravenous epinephrine at 0.1 mg/kg
C. Perform synchronized cardioversion
D. Perform needle decompression at the second midclavicular intercostal space
E. Perform needle decompression at the fourth midclavicular intercostal space

Discussion

The correct answer is **D**. This patient has cardiopulmonary arrest in the setting of a large right tension pneumothorax. Immediate evacuation is required to allow restoration of spontaneous circulation and continued cardiopulmonary resuscitation is unlikely to be successful without evacuation of extrapleural air. Evacuation can be performed by either needle decompression (preferred in emergent situations) or chest tube thoracostomy. The appropriate location for needle decompression is the second intercostal space in the midclavicular line.[16] The fourth intercostal space should be avoided to minimize injury to breast and nipple structures.

Helpful Tip: Immediate evacuation of a tension pneumothorax is needed to prevent obstructive shock and cardiovascular collapse.

After successful cardiopulmonary resuscitation, the infant is transitioned from a conventional ventilator to a high-frequency oscillatory ventilator (HFOV) with a mean airway pressure (MAP) of 18 cm H_2O and inspired oxygen concentration of 100%. An arterial blood gas obtained from the umbilical arterial catheter demonstrates a pH of 7.3, $PaCO_2$ of 50 mm Hg, and a partial pressure of oxygen (PaO_2) of 40 mm Hg. Your center typically initiates extracorporeal membrane oxygenation (ECMO) based on a patient's oxygenation index (OI).

Using the information provided, what is this patient's OI?
A. 20
B. 30
C. 36
D. 40
E. 45

Discussion

The correct answer is **E**. OI is a measure of a patient's oxygenation status and is calculated by the following formula: OI = ([MAP] × [percent of inspired oxygen])/ PaO_2 in mm Hg. For this patient, the calculated OI = ([18] × [100])/40 = 45. If the fraction of inspired oxygen (FiO_2) is provided, multiply the value by 100.

You decide your patient requires ECMO and discuss the risks of ECMO with the patient's family, including the risks of bleeding complications. You also discuss survival rates for infants requiring ECMO.

Survival on ECMO is highest for which of the following neonatal diseases?
A. CDH
B. Neonatal sepsis
C. Meconium aspiration syndrome
D. RDS
E. PPHN

Discussion

The correct answer is **C**. Based on data from the ECMO Life Support Organization (ELSO), survival for neonatal ECMO is highest for infants with meconium aspiration syndrome with survival rates exceeding 90%.[17] In contrast, CDH has the lowest survival for infants requiring ECMO.

Objectives

1. Plan appropriate therapy for an infant with extrapulmonary causes of respiratory distress
2. Recognize the clinical and imaging features of extrapulmonary causes of respiratory distress
3. Know the risks of positive pressure ventilation and CPAP
4. Know the pathophysiology of air leaks and how to manage air leaks
5. Recognize clinical and imaging features of air leaks
6. Know the indications and risks of extracorporeal membrane oxygenation (ECMO)

CASE 5

A term infant delivered by elective repeat cesarean at 39 weeks of gestation is diagnosed with a pulmonary abnormality at a referring hospital and transferred to you for further evaluation and treatment. A sepsis evaluation, including CBC and blood culture, at the referring hospital is unremarkable. The infant has mild tachypnea but does not require supplemental oxygen. A chest radiograph and computerized tomography of the chest are shown in Figures 5-4 and 5-5, respectively.

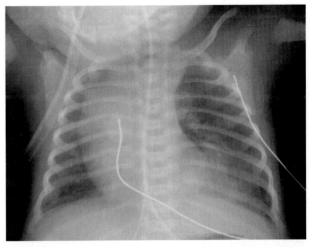

FIGURE 5-4. Chest radiograph of an infant with an undiagnosed pulmonary abnormality.

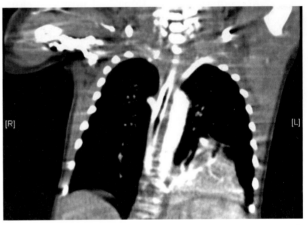

FIGURE 5-5. Computerized tomography of the chest with intravenous contrast in an infant with an undiagnosed pulmonary abnormality.

Of the following, which is the most likely diagnosis?
A. CPAM
B. Bronchopulmonary sequestration
C. CDH
D. Congenital lobar emphysema
E. Bronchogenic cyst

Discussion

The correct answer is **B**. Bronchopulmonary sequestrations are masses of pulmonary tissue that receive blood supply from the aorta (Fig. 5-5) and are not directly connected to the tracheobronchial tree. In contrast, CPAMs are connected to the tracheobronchial tree and do not demonstrate vascularity. CPAMs are typically diagnosed by antenatal ultrasound or after diagnostic evaluation following recurrent pneumonias affecting a single part of the lung. Both bronchogenic cysts and congenital lobar emphysemas would have radiolucent, cystic appearances on a chest radiograph, instead of the radiopaque lesion seen in the lower left lung field in Figure 5-4.

Quick Quiz: Congenital Pulmonary Airway Malformation

Of the following types of CPAMs, which is the most common CPAM subtype diagnosed after birth?
A. Type 0
B. Type 1
C. Type 2
D. Type 3
E. Type 4

Discussion

The correct answer is **B**. Type 1 is the predominant type of CPAM, comprising 50% to 65% of postnatal cases. Type 1 CPAMs typically present within the first week to month of life, if not diagnosed antenatally. However, Type 1 CPAMs can also be seen in older children and young adults. This type consists of single or multiple large cysts (3–10 cm in diameter) surrounded by smaller cysts and compressed normal lung parenchyma.[18] The next most common subtype is Type 2 lesions, which account for 10% to 40% of postnatal CPAMs and consist of smaller cysts (0.5–2.0 cm in diameter) and are associated with a higher incidence of cardiac, renal, and chromosomal anomalies.

Quick Quiz: Congenital Pulmonary Lyymphangiectasia

Patients with congenital pulmonary lymphagiectasia can present with severe respiratory distress after birth and develop pleural effusions.

Analysis of pleural fluid obtained from these patients would likely reveal which of the following?
A. Elevated triglyceride level and low lymphocyte percentage
B. Elevated triglyceride level and high lymphocyte percentage
C. Elevated triglyceride level and absent lymphocytes
D. Normal triglyceride level and low lymphocyte percentage
E. Normal triglyceride level and high lymphocyte percentage

Discussion

The correct answer is **B**. The pleural effusions in patients with congenital pulmonary lymphangiectasia are

secondary to accumulation of chylous fluid, which is diagnosed by the presence of a high triglyceride level and elevated cell count with predominance of lymphocytes.[19] However, this test may not be reliable in infants who are malnourished or are not receiving enteral nutrition or receiving feedings with fat intake limited to only medium-chain triglycerides. Treatment for this disorder is generally supportive and both antiplasmin and somatostatin treatment may be beneficial in some infants.[20]

Helpful Tip: Limiting enteral fat intake to only medium-chain triglycerides may decrease chylous effusions.

Objectives

1. Recognize the clinical and imaging features of congenital malformations of the lung
2. Recognize the appropriate management for an infant with congenital malformations of the lung
3. Recognize the clinical and laboratory manifestations of hydrothorax/chylothorax
4. Plan the therapeutic management of hydrothorax/chylothorax

CASE 6

Induction of labor is initiated for a woman at 42 weeks and 2 days of gestation. This is her first pregnancy. Labor is complicated by nonreassuring fetal heart tracings and her infant is subsequently delivered by emergent cesarean delivery. Meconium-stained amniotic fluid is noted at delivery. The infant is depressed at birth, with a heart rate less than 100 bpm and he undergoes tracheal suctioning with return of thick meconium. He requires subsequent intubation, mechanical ventilation, and admission to the neonatal intensive care unit.

Of the following chest radiographs (Fig. 5-6), which is the most consistent with the clinical scenario presented?
A. Image A
B. Image B
C. Image C
D. Image D
E. Images A and D

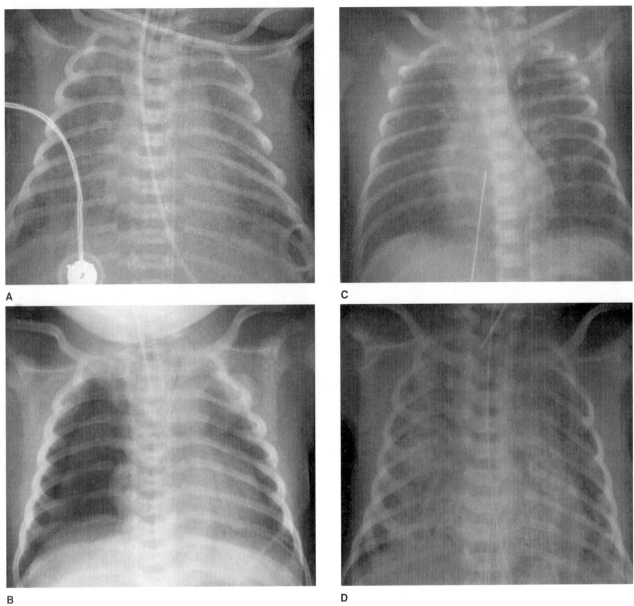

FIGURE 5-6.   Chest radiographs of neonates with various etiologies of respiratory failure.

Discussion

The correct answer is **E**. Both images A and D (Fig. 5-6) show the characteristic radiographic features of meconium aspiration syndrome, with normal to high lung volumes and bilateral *heterogeneous* pulmonary infiltrates. Postterm infants, such as the one in this scenario, are at higher risk than other term infants for meconium aspiration. Importantly, radiographic features of meconium aspiration syndrome can be difficult to distinguish from neonatal pneumonia. In contrast, image C is from an infant with RDS and shows *homogenous* bilateral hazy lung fields. Image B is from an infant with pulmonary hypoplasia and decreased lung volumes with a right pneumothorax.

Helpful Tip: Meconium aspiration syndrome can be difficult to distinguish from a neonatal pneumonia on a chest radiograph.

After admission to the neonatal intensive care unit, you decide to administer surfactant.

In randomized trials, surfactant administration, when compared to placebo, in infants with meconium aspiration has led to:
A. Decreased need for ECMO
B. Decreased length of hospital stay
C. Decreased mortality
D. A and B
E. A, B, and C

Discussion

The correct answer is **D**. In full- and near-term infants with meconium aspiration syndrome, surfactant treatment in clinical trials resulted in a decreased need for subsequent ECMO and a reduction in the length of hospital stay.[21] However, there was no significant reduction in mortality with surfactant treatment, compared to placebo, in infants with meconium aspiration syndrome.

After administration of surfactant, the infant continues to have poor oxygenation with an OI above 25. You decide to initiate therapy with inhaled nitric oxide (iNO).

Of the following, which mechanism is primarily responsible for pulmonary vasodilatation that results from iNO therapy?
A. Decrease in cyclic adenosine monophosphate
B. Increase in cyclic adenosine monophosphate
C. Decrease in cyclic guanosine monophosphate (cGMP)
D. Increase in cGMP
E. A and C

Discussion

The correct answer is **D**. Nitric oxide stimulates guanylate cyclase, which results in an increase in cGMP and activates cGMP-dependent protein kinases.[22] As a result, iNO decreases intracellular calcium in vascular smooth muscles which results in pulmonary vascular relaxation and increases in pulmonary blood flow.

Of the following, treatment with iNO results in an increase in which of the following compounds?
A. Cyanohemoglobin
B. Methemoglobin
C. NO_2
D. B and C
E. A, B, and C

Discussion

The correct answer is **D**. Elevations of methemoglobin and NO_2 are two important potential side effects of treatment with iNO. In clinical trials of iNO, treatment was associated with increased levels of methemoglobin and

NO_2 when compared to placebo. However, clinically significant elevations of these levels are uncommon. In addition, increases are dose dependent and usually seen at iNO doses above 20 to 80 parts-per-million.[23,24]

Which of the following statements about treatment with iNO in near-term and term infants with hypoxic respiratory failure and/or PPHN of the newborn is TRUE?
A. Treatment with iNO decreases mortality
B. Treatment with iNO increases mortality
C. Treatment with iNO decreases the need for ECMO
D. Treatment with iNO decreases mortality and the need for ECMO
E. Treatment with iNO decreases mortality but does not decrease the need for ECMO

Discussion

The correct answer is **C**. In two clinical trials of near-term and term infants, treatment with iNO, when compared to placebo, resulted in a decreased need for ECMO.[25,26] However, both trials did not demonstrate any significant difference in mortality between groups.

Quick Quiz: Persistent Pulmonary Hypertension of the Newborn

Which of the following is not a risk factor for the development of PPHN?
A. RDS
B. Meconium aspiration syndrome
C. PDA
D. Asphyxia
E. Pneumonia

Discussion

The correct answer is **C**. Of the following, only PDA is not a risk factor for PPHN. Patients with a PDA typically have a left-to-right shunt leading to pulmonary overcirculation, pulmonary edema, and congestive heart failure.[27] If left untreated for a prolonged period of time, a long-standing left-to-right shunt in patients with a PDA can result in morphologic changes in the pulmonary vasculature and reversal of the ductal shunt resulting in a right-to-left shunt (Eisenmenger syndrome) from late-onset pulmonary hypertension. However, this is a different clinical entity than PPHN.[28] Meconium aspiration syndrome is the most common cause of PPHN.[29] Other causes of PPHN include RDS, sepsis, pneumonia, maternal nonsteroidal anti-inflammatory medication use, and CDH.[30] Finally, idiopathic PPHN is seen in a small number of infants without an identifiable cause. Typically, infants with idiopathic PPHN have no evidence of parenchymal lung disease on chest radiographs and demonstrate decreased pulmonary vascular markings or "black lungs."

Of the following congenital heart lesions, which can have a similar clinical presentation as PPHN?
A. Coarctation of the aorta
B. Total anomalous pulmonary venous return (TAPVR)
C. Hypoplastic left heart syndrome
D. A and B
E. A, B, and C

Discussion

The correct answer is **E.** Congenital heart disease should always be considered in the differential diagnosis of PPHN.[31] Infants with TAPVR can be difficult to differentiate from PPHN. Both obstructed TAPVR and PPHN can result in severe hypoxemia with right-to-left atrial level shunts. In patients with PPHN, identifying the pulmonary venous anatomy by echocardiography can be challenging, but determining the pulmonary venous anatomy is critical in differentiating between these two diagnoses in patients with severe hypoxemia. Infants with critical coarctation of the aorta (or interrupted aortic arch) can have a pre- and postductal O_2Sat differential that is similar to patients with PPHN. Finally, infants with hypoplastic left heart syndrome, particularly those with a restrictive atrial septum, can present with severe cyanosis and hypoxemia.[32] Importantly, these patients may worsen with the administration of high amounts of oxygen, as this can lead to steal of pulmonary blood flow from the systemic circulation.

Which of the following changes is likely to have the largest effect on decreasing pulmonary vascular resistance (PVR)?
A. Increase in pH from 7.1 to 7.2
B. Increase in pH from 7.2 to 7.3
C. Increase in pH from 7.3 to 7.4
D. Increase in PaO_2 from 25 to 50 mm Hg
E. Increase in PaO_2 from 50 to 100 mm Hg

Discussion

The correct answer is **D.** The pulmonary vasculature can demonstrate significant vasoreactivity to changes in pH and PaO_2.[33] Each of the changes listed will result in a decrease in PVR, although the most substantial decrease occurs with an increase in PaO_2 from 25 to 50 mm Hg. Increases in PaO_2 beyond 75 mm Hg result in marginal decreases in PVR. Similarly, a 0.1 unit increase in pH from 7.1 to 7.2 has the largest effect on decreasing PVR, while additional 0.1 unit increases in pH have lesser

effects. The relationship between pH, PaO_2, and PVR is shown in Figure 5-7.

Objectives

1. Know the pathogenesis, pathophysiology, pathologic features, and risk factors of meconium aspiration syndrome
2. Recognize the clinical features and differential diagnosis of persistent pulmonary hypertension
3. Know how to manage meconium aspiration syndrome
4. Know the clinical and imaging features of meconium aspiration syndrome
5. Know the mechanisms of action, indications and techniques of administration, and effects and risks of inhaled pulmonary vasodilators such as nitric oxide

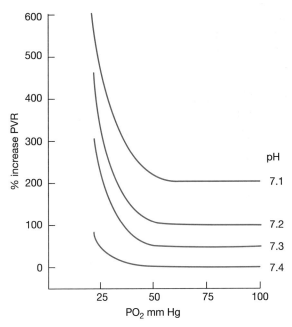

FIGURE 5-7. Pulmonary vascular resistance (PVR) responses to changes in pH and PO_2. (Reproduced with permission from Rudolph AM, Yuan S. Response of the pulmonary vasculature to hypoxia and H+ ion concentration changes. *J Clin Invest.* 1966; 45(3):399–411.)

CASE 7

You are called to assess a term infant at 45 minutes of life. Pregnancy was complicated by gestational diabetes, polyhydramnios, and maternal opioid abuse. At birth, the infant is active and vigorous and requires routine resuscitation along with frequent oropharyngeal suctioning. The 5-minute Apgar score is 9. The infant then develops two episodes of coughing and gagging with cyanosis. A nasogastric tube is inserted and a chest and abdominal radiograph is obtained (Fig. 5-8).

Of the following, which is the most likely diagnosis?
A. Tracheal atresia
B. Isolated esophageal atresia (EA)
C. EA with proximal tracheoesophageal fistula (TEF)
D. EA with distal TEF
E. Cyanotic congenital heart disease

Discussion

The correct answer is **D**. The clinical scenario of coughing and gagging with cyanosis in a newborn infant should lead to consideration of possible EA and/or TEF. Clues to the diagnosis include the presence of polyhydramnios and the need for frequent oropharyngeal suctioning after birth. The diagnosis is confirmed by chest radiograph with coiling of the nasogastric tube in the proximal esophagus as seen in Figure 5-8. The presence of bowel gas suggests that

there is a distal TEF in addition to an EA. In contrast, absent bowel gas would be expected in an isolated EA or an EA with proximal TEF. The presence of a TEF should prompt investigation of associated anomalies, including cardiac, renal, vertebral, and anorectal malformations.

Of the following types of tracheoesophageal malformations in Figure 5-9, which is the most common?
A. Image A
B. Image B
C. Image C
D. Image D
E. Image E

Discussion

The correct answer is **A**. A proximal EA with distal TEF is the most common type of tracheoesophageal malformation, comprising approximately 87% of all lesions (Fig. 5-9, Image A). Less common types of malformations include an isolated esophageal malformation (Image B), an isolated TEF (Image C), an EA with double TEF (Image D), and an EA with proximal TEF (Image E). Initial treatment is focused on stabilization of the patient and ligation of the TEF. Approach to repair of the EA depends largely on the distance between the proximal and distal portions of the esophagus and repair can be challenging. The presence of an imperforate anus in a

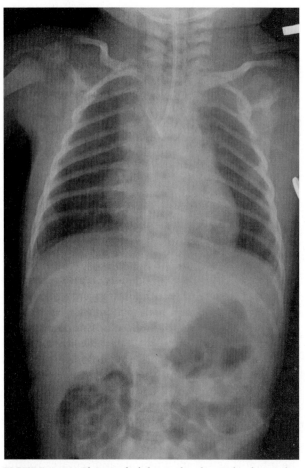

FIGURE 5-8. Chest and abdominal radiograph of an infant with choking and cyanosis.

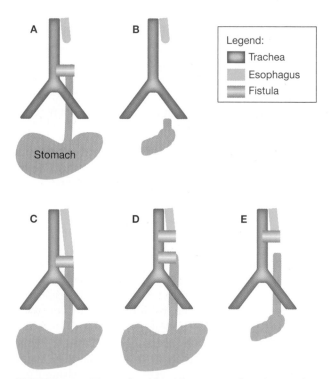

FIGURE 5-9. Types of esophageal atresias and tracheoesophageal fistulae. The size of the stomach correlates with the presence (large) or absence (small) of gastrointestinal gas.

patient with a TEF-EA should alert you to the risk of rapid pulmonary decompensation. Patients on respiratory support can develop rapid abdominal distention due to a lack of ability to decompress the bowel gas, which can lead to progressive respiratory compromise.

During which phase of lung development did this tracheoesophageal anomaly likely occur?

A. Embryonic
B. Saccular
C. Canalicular
D. Pseudoglandular
E. Alveolar

Discussion

The correct answer is **A**. Both TEF and airway atresias (laryngeal, tracheal) commonly arise during the embryonic phase of lung development in the first 7 weeks of gestation. The embryonic phase is characterized by the development of the conducting airways (trachea and bronchi).

Helpful Tip: The presence of polyhydramnios and need for frequent suctioning or gagging with feeding should alert you to the possibility of a tracheoesophageal malformation.

Quick Quiz: Morphologic Development of the Lung

The lungs of an infant born at 32 weeks of gestation would be in which of the following phases of development?

A. Embryonic
B. Saccular
C. Canalicular
D. Pseudoglandular
E. Alveolar

Discussion

The correct answer is **B**. The morphologic development of the lungs passes through five phases from initial development to the presence of definitive alveoli at 36 weeks of gestation. The characteristic structures of each phase of lung development and corresponding gestational ages as defined by Warren and Anderson are shown in Table 5-1.[34]

Of the following factors, which is not involved in lung development?

A. Fibroblast growth factor
B. Vitamin A
C. GATA-6
D. NOX
E. GLI

Discussion

The correct answer is **D**. A number of molecular factors are involved in early lung development, which is regulated in part by the interactions of the lung and surrounding mesenchyme.[35] Patients with mutations in the fibroblast growth factor receptor 2 (FGFR2), such as infants with Pfeiffer, Apert, and Crouzon syndrome, demonstrate a variety of defects including laryngomalacia, tracheomalacia, lobar atresia, and pulmonary aplasia. In knockout mice without the GLI gene, a variety of airway and lung defects are seen. Similarly, vitamin A deprivation results in tracheal stenosis and pulmonary agenesis. Finally, GATA-5 and GATA-6 are members of the zinc-finger family of transcription factors and play a role in lung cell differentiation. Of the factors listed, only NOX is not known to be involved in lung development.

TABLE 5-1. **Morphologic Development of the Lung**

PHASE	MORPHOLOGIC CHARACTERISTICS AND STRUCTURES	APPROXIMATE WEEKS OF GESTATION
Embryonic	Trachea and bronchi; absent type II pneumocytes	0–7
Pseudoglandular	Conducting airways and terminal bronchioles; immature and undifferentiated type II pneumocytes	7–17
Canalicular	Respiratory bronchioles, alveolar ducts, and primitive alveoli; immature and differentiated type II pneumocytes	17–27
Saccular	Enlarged peripheral airways and thinned alveolar walls; developing laminar bodies	28–36
Alveolar	Definitive alveoli; mature type II pneumocytes	36 and greater

Objectives

1. Plan appropriate therapy for an infant with extrapulmonary causes of respiratory distress
2. Recognize the clinical features of extrapulmonary causes of respiratory distress
3. Recognize the imaging features of extrapulmonary causes of respiratory distress
4. Know the stages and mediators of normal and abnormal cellular and structural development of all components of the lung

CASE 8

You are asked to consult with an African-American woman who is at 23 and 6/7 weeks of gestation and is expecting twins, one a male and the other a female. She presented at 22 weeks of gestation with preterm labor and premature rupture of membranes and is now suspected to have chorioamnionitis. She has not received antenatal steroids. She asks you about the risks of her infants developing BPD.

Of the following, which is the strongest risk factor for BPD?
A. Chorioamnionitis
B. Gestational age
C. Male sex
D. Failure to receive antenatal steroids
E. Twin gestation

Discussion

The correct answer is **B**. The risk of BPD is inversely related to gestational age and gestational age is the strongest predictor of BPD risk.[36] Almost two-thirds of infants with BPD are born before 28 weeks of gestation.[37] Additional antenatal risk factors for BPD include the presence of chorioamnionitis, male sex, and failure to receive antenatal steroids. Furthermore, the risk of BPD varies by race and ethnicity.

The following day, at 24 weeks of gestation, the mother delivers both twins. They receive mechanical ventilation in the delivery room and are admitted to the neonatal intensive care unit. You discuss potential treatments that may reduce the risk of BPD with the mother.

Treatment with which of the following medications has NOT been shown to reduce the risk of BPD?
A. Surfactant
B. Caffeine
C. Vitamin A
D. Dexamethasone
E. None of the above

Discussion

The correct answer is **A**. Limited pharmacologic therapies are available to decrease the incidence of BPD in high-risk preterm infants.[38] Of the therapies listed, treatment with surfactant has not been shown to decrease the incidence of BPD.[4,39] Vitamin A is a retinoid that is important in lung development, growth, and repair after injury.[40] In a meta-analysis, vitamin A therapy in clinical trials resulted in a decrease in the incidence of BPD (defined as oxygen at 36 weeks' postmenstrual age).[41] Caffeine is a common treatment of apnea of prematurity and in a large clinical trial, treatment with caffeine compared to placebo, resulted in a reduction in BPD.[10] However, this was not the primary outcome of the trial. Both early and late treatment with dexamethasone significantly reduces the incidence of BPD in preterm infants.[42,43] However the routine clinical use of dexamethasone is no longer recommended by the American Academy of Pediatrics due to the increased risk of cerebral palsy resulting from treatment.[44]

On postnatal day 4, both twins remain on mechanical ventilation and are receiving an FiO_2 of 0.5 to 0.6, a PIP of 22 cm H_2O, a PEEP of 4 cm H_2O, and a ventilator rate of 45 breaths per minute. You attempt to adjust ventilator settings to improve oxygenation in both of these patients.

Compared to baseline (solid black line) (Fig. 5-10), which of the following changes (dotted lines) is the most likely to improve oxygenation?
A. A
B. B
C. C
D. D
E. E

Discussion

The correct answer is **D**. In infants receiving mechanical ventilation, oxygenation is most likely to be improved by increasing the MAP, assuming the FiO_2 is held constant. The MAP is the area under the solid line and changes in PEEP have the most influence on MAP and, therefore, oxygenation. Decreasing PEEP (answer E) is likely to worsen the oxygenation status for this infant. Increasing the PIP (answer A) and

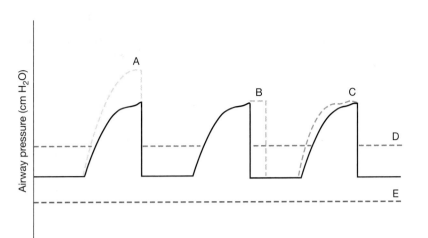

FIGURE 5-10. Airway pressure waveform from an infant with respiratory distress syndrome receiving pressure-targeted synchronized intermittent mandatory ventilation.

inspiratory time (answer B) will improve oxygenation, but not as significantly as changes in PEEP. Increasing the flow (answer C) is likely to have minimal impact on oxygenation.

Over the next 12 hours, Twin A requires an increase in ventilator rate from 45 to 60 breaths per minute to maintain $PaCO_2$ within target ranges.

Considering the change in ventilator rate, which of the following *additional* changes in Figure 5-10 would have increased the risk of pneumothorax in this patient?
A. A
B. B
C. C
D. D
E. E

Discussion

The correct answer is **B**. As the ventilator rate increases, simultaneously increasing the inspiratory time will result in significant decrease in the expiratory time. Short expiratory times can lead to incomplete expiration resulting in air trapping. This can place the patient at increased risk for pneumothorax.

Helpful Tip: Oxygenation is dependent on MAP.

Helpful Tip: Insufficient expiratory time can lead to air trapping and increase the risk of pneumothorax.
You review the pressure–volume curve for Twin A to determine the current lung compliance and guide additional ventilator adjustments.

Compared to baseline (solid line), which of the following changes is likely to result in the shift in the pressure–volume curve (dotted line) depicted in Figure 5-11?
A. Increase in PIP
B. Increase in inspiratory time
C. Decrease in expiratory time
D. Increase in flow
E. Increase in PEEP

Discussion

The correct answer is **E**. The major change noted in the compliance curve in Figure 5-11 is a decrease in the opening pressure, which is the point at which an increase in airway pressure begins to result in a change in lung volume. Increasing the PEEP will increase alveolar recruitment and shift the inflection point for opening pressure to the left.

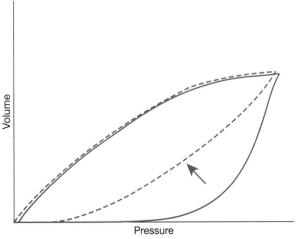

FIGURE 5-11. Pressure–volume curve of an infant with respiratory distress syndrome.

You return to the unit 12 weeks later and both twins remain hospitalized and continue to receive respiratory support. Twin A is currently on a nasal cannula with 1 L per minute of flow and receiving an FiO_2 of 0.28. Twin B is currently on CPAP at a pressure of 5 cm H_2O and receiving an FiO_2 of 0.30.

Which of the following statements is TRUE?
A. Twin A has mild BPD and Twin B has moderate BPD
B. Twin A has moderate BPD and Twin B has severe BPD
C. Twin A has mild BPD and Twin B has severe BPD
D. Both twins have moderate BPD
E. Both twins have severe BPD

Discussion

The correct answer is **B**. The diagnosis of BPD is primarily based on the amount of supplemental oxygen an infant requires at 36 weeks' postmenstrual age. Based on the NIH consensus definition of BPD (Table 5-2),[45] both infants in the scenario have met clinical criteria for the diagnosis of BPD. However, as noted in Table 5-2, the severity of BPD is based on the level of oxygen and need for positive pressure.

To aid in your diagnosis of BPD, you obtain a chest radiograph for Twin A.

Of the following radiographs in Figure 5-12, which is most likely to be seen in an infant with severe BPD?
A. Image A
B. Image B
C. Image C
D. Image D

Discussion

The correct answer is **C**. The image shown in answer C is consistent with cystic BPD, which is a severe form of BPD.

First described by Northway et al.[46] in 1967, BPD remains one of the most common serious morbidities affecting extremely preterm infants.[47] The radiograph in Figure 5-12 demonstrates the "small, rounded areas of lucency alternating with areas of irregular density in both lungs" that was first described by Northway et al. Over time, this severe form of "Old" BPD, characterized by intense inflammation and disruption of normal pulmonary structures, has been replaced with "New" BPD, which is characterized by diffusely reduced alveolar development and is typically milder in severity than "Old" BPD.[37]

Helpful Tip: Preterm infants who are receiving no respiratory support at 36 weeks' postmenstrual age can be diagnosed with mild BPD if they were treated with supplemental oxygen for 28 or more days.

Helpful Tip: The threshold of supplemental oxygen requirement that differentiates moderate and severe BPD is 30%.

Quick Quiz: Bronchopulmonary Dysplasia

Which of the following statements regarding BPD is FALSE?
A. BPD is an independent risk factor for adverse neurodevelopmental outcomes
B. Infants with BPD are at higher risk of readmission following hospital discharge
C. Infants with BPD are at higher risk of complications from respiratory syncytial virus (RSV)
D. Symptomatic PDA is more common in infants with BPD
E. Prophylactic indomethacin treatment decreases BPD

TABLE 5-2.   NIH Definition of Bronchopulmonary Dysplasia

GESTATIONAL AGE AT BIRTH	LESS THAN 32 WEEKS	32 WEEKS OR GREATER
Time of assessment	36 weeks' postmenstrual age (PMA) or discharge home, whichever comes first	Greater than 28 days but less than 56 days postnatal age or discharge to home, whichever comes first
	Treatment with oxygen >21% for at least 28 days *PLUS*	
Mild BPD	Breathing room air at 36 weeks' PMA or discharge, whichever comes first	Breathing room air by 56 days postnatal age or discharge, whichever comes first
Moderate BPD	Need for <30% oxygen at 36 weeks' PMA or discharge, whichever comes first	Need for <30% oxygen at 56 days postnatal age or discharge, whichever comes first
Severe BPD	Need for >30% oxygen and/or positive pressure (ventilator or CPAP) at 36 weeks' PMA or discharge, whichever comes first	Need for >30% oxygen and/or positive pressure (ventilator or CPAP) at 56 days postnatal age or discharge, whichever comes first

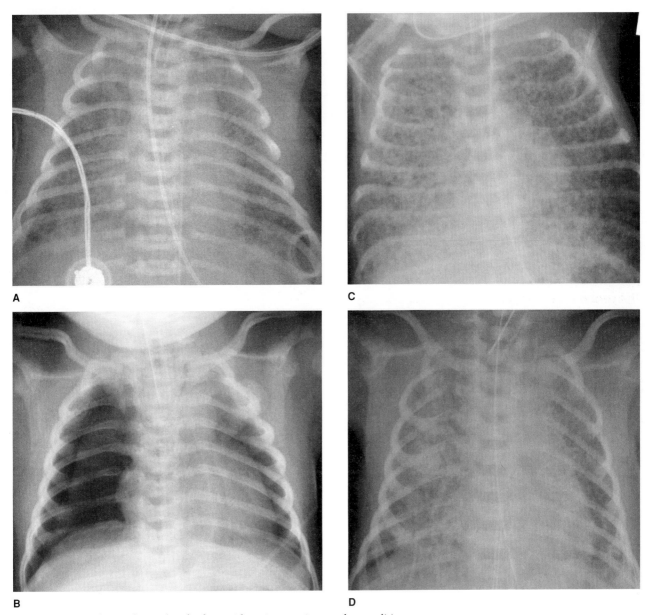

FIGURE 5-12. Chest radiographs of infants with various respiratory abnormalities.

Discussion

The correct answer is **E**. Infants with a symptomatic PDA are more likely to develop BPD although this association has not been demonstrated to be causal. In the Trial of Indomethacin Prophylaxis in Preterms (TIPP), treatment with indomethacin prophylaxis resulted in a reduction in symptomatic PDA but did not decrease BPD.[48,49] Currently, there is not a clinical consensus among neonatologists regarding the optimal circumstances and clinical criteria for the treatment of a PDA in preterm infants.

Helpful Tip: Although a symptomatic PDA is associated with BPD, closure of a PDA has not been shown to decrease the risk of BPD in randomized, controlled trials.

Quick Quiz: Bronchopulmonary Dysplasia

Which of the following hospitalized infants has severe BPD?

A. A 12-week-old infant born at 24 weeks of gestation receiving 25% oxygen by nasal cannula

B. A 28-day-old infant born at 24 weeks of gestation receiving 40% oxygen by CPAP

C. A 60-day-old infant born at 32 weeks of gestation receiving 40% oxygen by mechanical ventilation

D. A 5-week-old infant born at 33 weeks of gestation receiving 30% oxygen by CPAP

E. None of the above

Discussion

The correct answer is **C**. Based on Table 5-2, only the patient in answer C would meet the guidelines for severe BPD. Answer A is consistent with moderate, not severe, BPD. Both answers B and D describe patients who may go on to develop severe BPD, but have not met criteria based on either postmenstrual age (36 weeks) or postnatal age.

Which of the following candidate mechanisms is NOT involved in the pathophysiology of BPD?

A. Arrest of lung development
B. Cytokine-mediated lung inflammation and pulmonary edema
C. Volutrauma from mechanical ventilation
D. Barotrauma from high PEEP
E. Pulmonary interstitial thickening

Discussion

The correct answer is **D**. Lung injury from excessive tidal volumes and excessive inspiratory pressures are thought to contribute to the development of BPD.[45] Low, not high PEEP, has been linked to BPD. In addition, arrest of lung development, cytokine-mediated lung inflammation and edema, and pulmonary interstitial thickening are all candidate mechanisms of BPD.

At 28 days of postnatal age, which of the following is the strongest predictor of moderate-to-severe BPD?

A. Gestational age
B. Birth weight
C. Race
D. Need for positive pressure ventilation
E. FiO$_2$

Discussion

The correct answer is **D**. The risk of BPD varies inversely with gestational age and birth weight. For infants at birth and in the first few postnatal days (postnatal days 1 and 3), both gestational age and birth weight are the strongest predictors of BPD risk.[36] However, over time these baseline factors become less important and the predicted risk of BPD is primarily determined by the level of respiratory support and FiO$_2$. Not surprisingly, these are the two strongest predictors of BPD risk at 21 and 28 days of postnatal age, with level of respiratory support being the major predictor.

Objectives

1. Know the pathogenesis, pathophysiology, and pathologic features of BPD/chronic lung disease
2. Know the prenatal and postnatal risk factors for BPD/chronic lung disease and be aware of various preventative strategies
3. Recognize the clinical features of BPD/chronic lung disease
4. Know the management of BPD/chronic lung disease
5. Recognize the radiographic features of BPD/chronic lung disease
6. Know the prognosis, long-term complications, and permanent sequelae of BPD
7. Know the indications and techniques of positive pressure ventilation, including volume- and pressure-targeted ventilator modes
8. Recognize the factors (including pressure–volume and flow–volume relationships) that alter lung compliance

CASE 9

You are asked to evaluate a term infant who was born at 40 weeks of gestation. The mother recently emigrated from Mexico. She had reported fever and malaise 1 week prior to delivery. The infant is born by vaginal delivery and the amniotic fluid is noted to be "chocolate" colored. The patient receives CPAP in the delivery room due to respiratory distress. However, the patient has severe retractions and cyanosis and endotracheal intubation is performed. Upon admission to the neonatal intensive care unit, the infant is placed on a conventional ventilator and a chest radiograph is obtained (Fig. 5-13).

Of the following, which is the most likely diagnosis?

A. Meconium aspiration
B. Bacterial pneumonia
C. Viral pneumonia
D. Transient tachypnea of the newborn
E. RDS

Discussion

The correct answer is B. The clinical scenario and chest radiograph are consistent with a neonatal bacterial pneumonia. Although the chest radiographic could be seen in a patient with meconium aspiration syndrome, the lack of meconium-stained amniotic fluid makes this diagnosis unlikely.

Of the following, what additional finding would be likely in this case?

A. Maternal herpes simplex genital lesions at delivery
B. Maternal history of untreated syphilis
C. Maternal history of GBS colonization
D. Placental microabscesses
E. Placental abruption

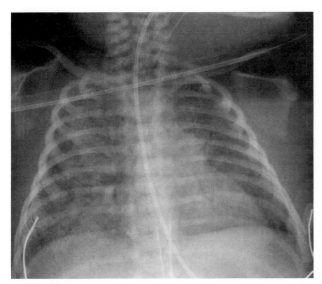

FIGURE 5-13.   Chest radiograph of an infant with respiratory distress.

Discussion

The correct answer is **D**. The history of "flu-like" symptoms in the mother and "chocolate"-colored amniotic fluid is classically associated with infection with *Listeria monocytogenes*. Upon examination of the placenta, microabscesses containing *L. monocytogenes* are likely to be found. GBS infection is a common pathogen in neonatal pneumonia although colonization is unlikely to lead to "flu-like" symptoms in the mother. Infections caused by herpes simplex virus and *Treponema pallidum* can lead to respiratory distress. However, the "chocolate"-colored amniotic fluid and radiographic appearance of lung fields seen in Figure 5-13 make these diagnoses unlikely.

Over the next 2 hours the patient requires escalation of ventilator support with increases in PIP, ventilator rate, and FiO$_2$. You are concerned about further clinical deterioration and consider broadening antimicrobial coverage.

Of the following antibiotics, which is the most effective for the likely causative organism in this infant?
A. Ampicillin
B. Gentamicin
C. Cefotaxime
D. Ceftazidime
E. Cefepime

Discussion

The correct answer is **A**. Ampicillin is the preferred treatment for infections caused by *L. monocytogenes*. Synergistic therapy with an aminoglycoside such as gentamicin should be considered, although gentamicin as monotherapy should not be used. Antimicrobials such as cefotaxime, ceftazidime, and cefepime are effective against gram-negative

organisms but are unlikely to be effective against *L. monocytogenes*, which is a gram-positive rod.

After updating the mother on her infant's condition, you obtain additional history including a detailed assessment of risk factors for infection.

Of the following, which is the most likely to be reported by the mother of this infant?
A. Exposure to cat feces
B. Consumption of unpasteurized cheeses
C. Recurrent skin infections
D. Painful genital lesions
E. A child with upper respiratory symptoms

Discussion

The correct answer is **B**. Of the answers listed, only consumption of unpasteurized cheeses is associated with Listeria infection in pregnant women. Exposure to cat feces is a risk factor for Toxoplasmosis infection. Recurrent skin infections would be likely in a mother colonized with methicillin-resistant *Staphylococcus aureus*. Painful genital lesions should raise immediate suspicion for herpes simplex infection. A household contact with upper respiratory symptoms would be likely in a viral, not bacterial, infection.

Despite escalation in conventional ventilator settings, you are unable to effectively ventilate the infant. You decide to place the infant on an HFOV. After 1 hour on HFOV, you obtain an arterial blood gas with the following values: pH = 7.45, PaCO$_2$ = 28 mm Hg, and PaO$_2$ = 35 mm Hg. You are currently on the following HFOV settings: MAP = 16 cm H$_2$O, amplitude = 33, frequency = 10 Hz, and FiO$_2$ = 1.

Of the following, which is the most appropriate adjustment in HFOV settings?
A. Decrease in MAP
B. Decrease in amplitude
C. Increase in amplitude
D. Decrease in frequency
E. Decrease in FiO$_2$

Discussion

The correct answer is **B**. After transitioning to an HFOV, this patient is being overventilated as evidenced by a PaCO$_2$ of 28 mm Hg. Ventilation in HFOV is influenced by both amplitude and frequency and decreasing amplitude will decrease ventilation and allow for the PaCO$_2$ to rise. In contrast, increasing the amplitude or decreasing the frequency would further increase ventilation and lead to further decreases in PaCO$_2$. Changes in MAP and FiO$_2$ influence oxygenation, but not ventilation, in patients receiving HFOV.

Despite providing an FiO_2 of 1, you are unable to adequately oxygenate your patient. You recall that MAP can improve oxygenation and decide to increase the MAP on the HFOV from 16 to 20 cm H_2O.

Of the following, which change in your patient's cardiovascular physiology would you anticipate?
A. Increase in preload
B. Decrease in preload
C. Increase in contractility
D. Decrease in afterload
E. None of the above

Discussion

The correct answer is **B**. The use of a high MAP can lead to a high intrapleural pressure and compromise venous return to the heart resulting in a decrease in preload. Consequently, this can lead to a decrease in cardiac output. Therefore, attention to hemodynamic parameters is important when adjusting ventilator parameters on a HFOV to ensure that improving pulmonary function does not result in cardiovascular compromise.

Helpful Tip: Expiration in a patient receiving HFOV is an active process.

Helpful Tip: High MAP can compromise cardiac output.

Objectives

1. Know the pathogenesis and causative agents in an infant in whom neonatal pneumonia is suspected
2. Know the clinical, imaging, and laboratory features and plan the management of an infant in whom neonatal pneumonia is suspected
3. Know the indications for and techniques of high-frequency ventilation
4. Know the effects and risks of high-frequency ventilation
5. Know how intrapleural pressure affects cardiovascular function

CASE 10

A term male is transferred to your center for further care. Oligohydramnios was present upon review of the antenatal history. Upon assessment after admission to your unit, the patient is noted to be receiving an FiO_2 of 0.8 by CPAP at a pressure of 6 cm H_2O. He has poor chest rise

and bilateral palpable abdominal masses. After placement of a urinary catheter, a large volume of urine is obtained. A chest radiograph demonstrates radiolucent lung fields with lung inflation to the seventh vertebral body.

Of the following, which is the most likely UNDERLYING cause of the clinical presentation in this infant?
A. PPHN
B. Pulmonary hypoplasia
C. Oligohydramnios
D. Posterior urethral valves
E. Infantile polycystic kidney disease

Discussion

The correct answer is **D**. The underlying clinical presentation is due to Potter sequence, which is typically caused by oligohydramnios due to severe *bilateral* renal disease. In this male infant, the presence of bilateral palpable abdominal masses and a large volume of urine output obtained following urinary catheter placement suggest urethral obstruction. In addition, the presence of radiolucent lung fields and low lung volumes indicate likely pulmonary hypertension and pulmonary hypoplasia. Posterior urethral valves are the most common bilateral renal disease affecting male infants. Patients with severe oligohydramnios can have compression of the chest wall resulting in restricted chest wall movement, pulmonary hypoplasia, and associated pulmonary hypertension. Although answers A, B, and C are all in the sequence leading to the clinical presentation seen in this infant, the underlying cause is posterior urethral valves.

The patient requires endotracheal intubation and mechanical ventilation. The FiO_2 is increased to 1. Arterial blood gas PaO_2 measurements are obtained from the right radial and left posterior tibial arteries.

Of the following PaO_2 measurements (in mm Hg), which is NOT likely to be found in this patient?
A. Right radial PaO_2: 50; left posterior tibial PaO_2: 50
B. Right radial PaO_2: 30; left posterior tibial PaO_2: 30
C. Right radial PaO_2: 50; left posterior tibial PaO_2: 30
D. Right radial PaO_2: 30; left posterior tibial PaO_2: 50
E. All are compatible with a primary diagnosis of PPHN

Discussion

The correct answer is **D**. Patients with PPHN can demonstrate severe hypoxemia, as is noted in the blood gas measurements in this patient receiving 100% oxygen. In the presence of an open PDA, patients with PPHN can have a significant difference (5–10% or greater) between their preductal (higher value) and postductal (lower value) oxygen levels (obtained from the right radial and left posterior tibial blood gas measurements, respectively). If the PDA is closed or systemic blood pressure is elevated, a ductal shunt may not be apparent (answers A and B). Importantly, these patients can be difficult to distinguish from cyanotic congenital heart disease and frequently require assessment of cardiac anatomy by echocardiogram. The PaO_2 relationship in answer D is compatible with reversal of pre- and postductal saturation differential and can be found in patients with a primary diagnosis of transposition of the great vessels.

Based on an arterial PaO_2 measurement of 30 mm Hg, $PaCO_2$ measurement of 40 mm Hg, and assuming you are at sea level, what would be the alveolar–arterial (A-a) oxygenation gradient for this patient?
A. 400
B. 521
C. 608
D. 633
E. 713

Discussion

The correct answer is **D**. The A-a gradient can be calculated by obtaining the PAO_2 (alveolar oxygen tension) and subtracting this value from the arterial oxygen tension (PaO_2), which is typically provided. The PAO_2 for this patient can be calculated using the following equation: $PAO_2 = FiO_2 \times$ (barometric pressure – pH_2O) – $PaCO_2/R$. The R (respiratory quotient) is 0.8, barometric pressure at sea level is 760 mm Hg and the pH_2O is 47 mm Hg. Using the values provided, we obtain the following: $PAO_2 = 1.0 \times (760 - 47) - 40/0.8 = 663$ mm Hg. Subtracting PaO_2 from this value (663 – 30) provides you with an A-a gradient of 633 mm Hg. The A-a gradient can be helpful when evaluating infants with hypoxemia. The presence of a large A-a gradient, as seen in this infant, can indicate problems with ventilation–perfusion mismatch, a right-to-left shunt as seen in pulmonary hypertension, or a problem with oxygen diffusion from the alveoli into the arterial circulation.

Of the following oxygen saturations determined by pulse oximetry, which would be most compatible with an arterial pH measurement of 7.4, $PaCO_2$ measurement of 40 mm Hg, and PaO_2 measurement of 30 mm Hg in a newborn infant whose temperature is 36.7°C?
A. 30%
B. 50%
C. 70%
D. 90%
E. 95%

Discussion

The correct answer is **C**. The relationship between the arterial PaO_2 and the O_2Sat is determined by the oxygen–hemoglobin dissociation curve. At an arterial oxygen tension of 30 mm Hg, the typical O_2Sat in a newborn with predominance of fetal hemoglobin will be around 70% assuming normal values for pH, $PaCO_2$, and temperature.[50]

A decrease in the patient's pH from 7.4 to 7.25 would have which of the following effects on oxygenation, assuming the PaO_2 and all other factors remain unchanged?
A. Oxygen saturation would decrease
B. Oxygen saturation would increase
C. Oxygen saturation would remain unchanged
D. Oxygen index would increase
E. Oxygen index would decrease

Discussion

The correct answer is **A**. A number of factors can shift the oxygen dissociation curve to the left or right including pH, pCO_2, temperature, and 2,3-diphosphoglycerate (DPG). These are further described in Table 5-3. A decrease in the patient's pH would shift the oxygen–hemoglobin dissociation curve to the left, allowing hemoglobin to release more oxygen to the tissues and result in lower arterial Oxygen saturation. The Oxygen index is based on a patient's PaO_2, not hemoglobin saturation, and would remain unchanged in this scenario.

Quick Quiz: Oxygen Uptake, Transport and Delivery

Which of the following principles explains the relationship between pH, pCO_2, and hemoglobin's affinity for oxygen?
A. Haldane effect
B. Bohr effect
C. Niels effect
D. LaPlace law
E. Henry law

TABLE 5-3. **Factors Influencing a Shift in the Oxygen Dissociation Curve of Hemoglobin**

SHIFT OF CURVE TO THE LEFT (INCREASED O_2 AFFINITY)	SHIFT OF CURVE TO THE RIGHT (DECREASED O_2 AFFINITY)
Alkalosis (increase in pH)	Acidosis (decrease in pH)
Decrease in pCO_2	Increase in pCO_2
Decrease in temperature (hypothermia)	Increase in temperature (hyperthermia)
Decrease in 2,3-DPG	Increase in 2,3-DPG
Fetal hemoglobin (HbF)	Adult hemoglobin (HbA)

Discussion

The correct answer is **B**. The Bohr effect explains the relationship between acid and base status determined by the effect of pH and pCO_2 on hemoglobin's affinity for oxygen (Table 5-3). The Haldane effect explains the property of hemoglobin in which deoxygenation of hemoglobin increases its ability to carry carbon dioxide.

Objectives

1. Recognize the laboratory, imaging, and other diagnostic features of persistent pulmonary hypertension
2. Know the causes of and how to evaluate arterial hypoxemia in an infant with a structurally normal heart
3. Know how to calculate an alveolar–arterial oxygen gradient
4. Know the various factors affecting oxygen uptake, transport, and delivery
5. Know how to interpret arterial blood gas measurements

CASE 11

A 3-week-old infant is referred to your center after failing attempts at extubation. After birth, she developed respiratory distress and stridor that progressively worsened and did not respond to oxygen by nasal cannula. She was subsequently intubated and placed on a ventilator with immediate improvement in respiratory distress. An evaluation of infectious causes was unremarkable. Extubation was attempted several times. However, within hours of extubation, she developed stridor and respiratory distress and required reintubation. A flow–volume curve is provided in Figure 5-14.

Of the following, which is the most likely cause of this infant's UNDERLYING respiratory problem?
A. Congenital central hypoventilation syndrome
B. Laryngomalacia
C. Pierre Robin sequence
D. Vascular ring
E. Vocal cord paralysis

Discussion

The correct answer is **D**. The presence of stridor should alert you to the possibility of airway obstruction. The flow–volume curve in Figure 5-14 demonstrates obstruction to expiratory flow that is consistent with an

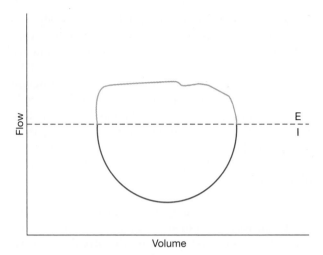

FIGURE 5-14. Flow–volume loop of an infant with respiratory distress. The expiratory (E) and inspiratory (I) phases are indicated above and below the dotted line, respectively.

intrathoracic airway obstruction. Of the choices listed, only a vascular ring is a cause of intrathoracic airway obstruction. Vascular rings can be difficult to diagnose and require a high index of suspicion. Dynamic compression of the trachea is typically seen during bronchoscopy and imaging studies, including magnetic resonance imaging, computerized tomography with contrast or echocardiography, can be useful in delineating the vascular anatomy. The two most common types of vascular rings are double aortic arch and right aortic arch with ligamentum arteriosum.[51] Congenital central hypoventilation syndrome is a rare respiratory disorder caused by dysfunction of the autonomic nervous system.[52] Infants are typically unresponsive to abnormal elevations in CO_2 and can have potentially lethal periods of apnea during sleep. The disease is caused by mutations in the paired-like homeobox 2B (PHOX2B) gene. Laryngomalacia, Pierre Robin sequence, and vocal cord paralysis are all causes of *extrathoracic* upper airway obstruction.

Which of the following clinical findings would you expect to find in this infant?
A. Apnea
B. Inspiratory stridor
C. Biphasic stridor
D. Expiratory stridor
E. Grunting

Discussion

The correct answer is **D**. Infants with intrathoracic airway obstruction, such as those with vascular rings, present with expiratory stridor. In contrast, infants with upper airway obstruction above the level of the vocal cords present with inspiratory stridor. Both inspiratory

TABLE 5-4. **Causes of Airway Obstruction in Infants and Associated Clinical Symptoms**

LEVEL OF AIRWAY OBSTRUCTION	CAUSES	CLINICAL SYMPTOMS
Supraglottic	Pierre Robin sequence Choanal atresia	Stridor with inspiration
Laryngeal	Laryngomalacia Paralysis of vocal cords Subglottic stenosis	Stridor with both inspiration and expiration (biphasic)
Intrathoracic	Tracheal stenosis Tracheomalacia Vascular rings Mediastinal lesions	Stridor with expiration

and expiratory stridor (biphasic) is seen in infants with obstruction at the level of the vocal cords. Laryngomalacia is the most common congenital anomaly of the larynx, accounting for over half of cases.[53] Patients with laryngomalacia typically have biphasic stridor, although the inspiratory component can worsen with agitation or in the supine position. Most cases of laryngomalacia improve over time without surgical intervention. Common causes of airway obstruction in infants and their associated clinical findings are listed in Table 5-4.

Quick Quiz: Airway Obstruction

Of the following, which finding is NOT commonly seen in patients with Pierre Robin sequence?
A. Micrognathia
B. Glossoptosis
C. Cleft palate
D. Retrognathia
E. Macroglossia

Discussion

The correct answer is **E**. Clinical findings in Pierre Robin sequence include micrognathia (small mouth), glossoptosis (downward displacement of the tongue), retrognathia (posterior positioning of the maxilla), and cleft palate.[54] The sequence is thought to be caused primarily by hypoplasia of the mandible which leads to displacement of the tongue and disruption in closure of the palate. Patients can have a varying spectrum of airway obstruction ranging from no obstruction to severe obstruction with respiratory failure. Treatment is typically individualized and surgical interventions to relieve the airway obstruction include tongue–lip adhesion, mandibular distraction, and tracheostomy. Macroglossia is seen in patients with Beckwith–Wiedemann syndrome and Down syndrome, but not Pierre Robin sequence.

You are called to the delivery room for a term infant with unexpected respiratory distress. The infant is cyanotic despite the administration of supplemental oxygen. However, his cyanosis improves with crying. You are unable to pass a catheter through both nares. His heart rate is 140 bpm and respiratory rate is 50 breaths per minute.

Of the following, which is the most appropriate immediate next step in management of this patient?
A. Perform endotracheal intubation
B. Place an oral airway
C. Place a laryngeal mask airway
D. Place a nasal airway
E. Obtain ENT consultation

Discussion

The correct answer is **B**. This patient has choanal atresia, which is caused by a bony or membranous obstruction across the posterior choanae.[55] As neonates are obligate nasal breathers, complete nasal obstruction can lead to significant respiratory distress. Immediate management is directed toward ensuring airway patency by placement of an oral airway to compensate for the nasal obstruction. A nasal airway would be ineffective in a patient with nasal obstruction. A laryngeal mask airway can be useful in patients with oral or oropharyngeal airway obstructions. However, this would be poorly tolerated without sedation or anesthesia. Patients with choanal atresia and severe respiratory distress may require endotracheal intubation. However, in a patient with a normal heart rate and respiratory rate, an oral airway should be attempted first. Evaluation of associated anomalies, including the CHARGE association (**C**oloboma, **H**eart disease, **A**tresia choanae, **R**etarded growth and retarded development and/or CNS anomalies, **G**enital hypoplasia, and **E**ar anomalies and/or deafness), should be considered in patients with choanal atresia.[56]

Of the following statements regarding nasal flaring and grunting, which is TRUE?
A. Nasal flaring helps maintain FRC
B. Grunting helps decrease airway resistance
C. Nasal flaring helps decrease airway resistance
D. Grunting helps increase airway diameter
E. Grunting results from expiration against abducted vocal cords

Discussion

The correct answer is **C**. Nasal flaring and grunting are common signs of respiratory distress in the newborn. Nasal flaring results from contraction of the alae nasi muscles, which leads to a marked reduction in nasal resistance.[57] Importantly, nasal resistance in a newborn accounts for a large component of total airway resistance. Grunting results from expiration against partially adducted (closed) vocal cords. This results in increased airway pressure that helps maintain FRC by providing effective PEEP.

You have replaced a dislodged ETT in a patient with a larger ETT. The new ETT diameter is twice as large. However, having forgotten to cut the length of the tube after reintubation, the new ETT is twice as long.

Quick Quiz: Airway Resistance

What is the effective change in the airway resistance of your patient?
A. Increase by eightfold
B. Increase by fourfold
C. No change
D. Decrease by fourfold
E. Decrease by eightfold

Discussion

The correct answer is **E**. According to Poiseuille law, resistance to flow (R) is directly proportional to the length of a tube (L) and inversely proportional to the radius of a tube (r) raised to the fourth power according to the following relationship: $R \approx L/r^4$. Therefore, changes in the radius of an ETT have a much larger effect on airway resistance than changes in the length of an ETT. In this scenario, a twofold increase in the radius of the ETT will lead to a 16-fold reduction in the airway resistance. Accounting for the twofold increase in airway resistance by the doubling of the ETT length, the effective change in resistance is a net decrease in resistance by eightfold.

You are discussing how airway resistance can vary with different pulmonary disorders in infants. An infant with which of the following pulmonary disorders would be expected to have the lowest airway resistance?
A. Meconium aspiration syndrome
B. Severe BPD
C. Treacher Collins syndrome
D. RDS
E. Pierre Robin sequence

Discussion

The correct answer is **D**. Of the following disorders, only RDS is characterized by low airway resistance. Patients with meconium aspiration syndrome and severe BPD have high airway resistance caused by abnormal conduction airways. In contrast, patients with Treacher Collins syndrome and Pierre Robin sequence have high airway resistance caused by abnormalities of their upper airway.

Which of the following statements about airway resistance is FALSE?
A. Decreasing the density of inspired gas will affect turbulent flow
B. Airways have increased resistance during inspiration compared to expiration
C. Increasing the density of inspired gas will not affect laminar flow
D. Airway resistance accounts for the majority of respiratory system resistance
E. Nasal resistance accounts for the majority of airway resistance

Discussion

The correct answer is **B**. Airways dilate during inspiration and therefore have less resistance compared to expiration. The density of a gas can affect turbulent flow, which primarily affects the large airways. In contrast, laminar flow that involves the smaller airways is unaffected by the density of gas. A combination of helium and oxygen, which has a lower density than room air, can be used therapeutically to decrease airway resistance in patients with upper airway obstruction. Over half of the total respiratory system resistance is accounted by airway resistance, with the remaining resistance comprising lung and chest wall resistance. Similarly, nasal resistance is the primary determinant of airway resistance in newborn infants.

Quick Quiz: Time Constant

Which of the following statements is TRUE?
A. Expiratory time on a ventilator should be set in direct proportion to a patient's time constant
B. Administration of surfactant to an infant with RDS will not impact the time constant
C. Increasing the airway resistance will decrease the time constant
D. Decreasing the compliance will decrease the time constant
E. Bronchodilation in an infant with BPD will increase the time constant

Discussion

The correct answer is **D**. The time constant is a function of compliance and resistance and is a measure of the amount of time for a given volume of air to exit the lung. Infants with RDS have a low lung compliance and low airway resistance and, therefore, have a relatively low time constant. However, administration of surfactant increases lung compliance and, as a result, will also increase the time constant assuming no change in airway resistance. In infants with BPD and airway hypertrophy, bronchodilation will decrease airway resistance and decrease the time constant. A patient's inspiratory time, not expiratory time, should be proportional to the time constant.

Helpful Tip: The presence of expiratory stridor should alert you to the possibility of a serious airway problem, vascular anomaly, or mediastinal mass.

Helpful Tip: Nasal, oral, and laryngeal mask airways can be helpful in the management of patients with upper airway obstruction.

Objectives

1. Know the clinical features of an infant with airway obstruction
2. Know the appropriate diagnostic evaluation and management of an infant with airway obstruction
3. Know the factors that affect airway resistance and how resistance changes with various lung disorders
4. Know the factors that influence upper airway patency
5. Know the principles governing gas flow, including airway diameter, turbulence, and time constants

CASE 12

You are caring for a 5-month-old former 24 weeks of gestation infant whose mother is planning to move from Atlanta, GA to Denver, CO over the summer. The mother requests that her infant be air transported to Denver to be closer to family. Your patient is currently receiving an FiO_2 of 0.40 by OxyHood. Atlanta is at sea level and the atmospheric pressure in Denver is 631 mm Hg.

What would be the expected oxygen requirement for your patient in Denver, assuming all other respiratory parameters remain unchanged?
A. 0.40
B. 0.45
C. 0.49
D. 0.52
E. 0.55

Discussion

The correct answer is **C**. The atmospheric pressure is inversely proportional to altitude and, at higher altitudes, a lower atmospheric pressure results in a proportionally lower PaO_2. The relationship between the inspired oxygen level in Atlanta ($FiO_{2|Atlanta}$) and Denver ($FiO_{2|Denver}$) can be determined using the alveolar gas equation. As the patient's pCO_2 is unchanged, this component can be removed and you are left with the following relationship: $(P_{ATM|Atlanta} - P_{H2O}) \times FiO_{2|Atlanta} = (P_{ATM|Denver} - P_{H2O}) \times FiO_{2|Denver}$. As Atlanta is at sea level, the $P_{ATM|Atlanta}$ is 760 mm Hg. The $P_{ATM|Denver}$ and $FiO_{2|Atlanta}$ are provided and the P_{H2O} is 47 mm Hg. Therefore, you are able to solve for $FiO_{2|Denver}$ after entering the known variables. $(760 - 47) \times 0.4 = (631 - 47) \times FiO_{2|Denver}$. $FiO_{2|Denver} = ([760 - 47] \times 0.4)/(631 - 47) = 0.49$.

During air transport, your patient requires intubation and mechanical ventilation secondary to poor oxygenation. Upon arrival to Denver, he is placed on a mechanical ventilator at a rate of 40 breaths per minute and an FiO_2 of 0.8. His pulse rate is 150 bpm, respiratory rate is 50 breaths per minute, and mean arterial pressure is 60 mm Hg. The PaO_2 on an arterial blood gas is 60 mm Hg, the $PaCO_2$ is 45 mm Hg, and hemoglobin concentration is 9.5 mg/dL. You discuss ways to improve oxygen delivery with the accepting physician in Denver.

Of the following, which change would lead to the greatest increase in oxygen delivery in this patient?
A. Increase in the PaO_2 from 60 to 100 mm Hg
B. Increase in ventilator rate from 40 to 50 breaths per minute
C. Increase in O_2Sat from 95% to 100%
D. Increase in hemoglobin from 9 to 12 mg/dL
E. Decrease in heart rate from 160 to 120 bpm

Discussion

The correct answer is **D**. Oxygen delivery (DO_2) is dependent on both cardiac output and the oxygen content of arterial blood. The two primary determinants of cardiac output are heart rate (HR) and stroke volume (SV). In this patient, decreasing the heart rate would result in a decrease in cardiac output and therefore decrease in DO_2. Increasing ventilation is unlikely to improve DO_2 in this patient, particularly in the setting of a normal $PaCO_2$. While increases in O_2Sat, PaO_2, and hemoglobin (Hb) will all result in an increase in DO_2, the change in hemoglobin is likely to have the greatest impact. Changes in PaO_2, beyond any associated improvement in O_2Sat, is likely to have minimal impact on DO_2. The relationship between the cardiac, respiratory, and hematologic factors influencing DO_2 is as follows: $DO_2 = (HR \times SV) \times (1.34 \times O_2Sat \times Hb + PaO_2 \times 0.003)$.

Over the next 2 weeks, your patient continues to deteriorate with refractory oxygenation despite broad-spectrum antimicrobial therapy and increases in ventilator support with escalation of FiO_2 to 1. You discuss the potential complicating factors in this patient with the accepting physician in Denver.

Of the following, which is the most likely complicating factor in this patient?
A. PDA
B. Pulmonary hypertension
C. Surfactant protein B deficiency
D. Infection with RSV
E. Alveolar–capillary dysplasia

Discussion

The correct answer is **B**. Patients with severe BPD, as the one described in this scenario, are at risk of developing pulmonary hypertension. One study estimated that one in six extremely low–birth-weight infants (<1,000 g at birth) develop pulmonary hypertension that persists to hospital discharge.[58] In contrast to extremely low–birth-weight infants without pulmonary hypertension, infants with pulmonary hypertension are lower in gestation age, more likely to have severe BPD, and have a fivefold greater risk of mortality. Respiratory decompensation due to PDA, surfactant

protein B deficiency, and alveolar–capillary dysplasia are likely to present early in the neonatal course and the latter two diagnoses are frequently lethal with survival to 5 months of age highly unlikely. Infection with RSV can lead to severe respiratory problems in infants with severe BPD. However, RSV infection is unlikely during the summer months.

You discuss potential pharmacologic therapies for this patient with the physician in Denver.

Of the following, which is NOT a treatment for pulmonary hypertension?
A. Epoprostenol
B. Isoproterenol
C. Sildenafil
D. Bosentan
E. iNO

Discussion

The correct answer is **B**. The pharmacologic approaches to late pulmonary hypertension, as seen in this infant, are varied.[58] Common therapies include the use of iNO and sildenafil, which both increase cGMP and result in pulmonary vascular relaxation. Additional treatments in patients with refractory pulmonary hypertension include epoprostenol, a naturally occurring prostaglandin with potent vasodilatory activity that is administered by continuous infusion, and bosentan, an endothelin receptor antagonist that is orally administered. Importantly, the risk profile and off-label use of these medications in neonates and infants needs to be weighed against the benefits of therapy. Isoproterenol is a beta-agonist used in infants with congenital heart block, but is not used clinically for the treatment of pulmonary hypertension.

Objectives

1. Know the effects of changes in altitude on oxygenation
2. Know how acute and chronic lung disease affects cardiovascular function
3. Know the various factors affecting oxygen uptake, transport, and delivery, including the blood and circulation
4. Know the prognosis, long-term complications, and permanent sequelae of BPD

CASE 13

You are rounding in the neonatal intensive care unit and decide to intubate and administer surfactant to a 1-day-old 26 weeks of gestation infant who is receiving

CPAP and has an escalating oxygen requirement. After completing rounds, you walk by the bedside and realize the patient's ETT has not been shortened. You are concerned about the dead space that this is contributing to the infant. The patient's $PaCO_2$ is 60 mm Hg and the expired CO_2 detected by end-tidal CO_2 monitoring is 40 mm Hg.

Of the following, what is the physiologic dead space volume as a percent of the infant's total tidal volume?
A. 10%
B. 20%
C. 33%
D. 50%
E. 66%

Discussion

The correct answer is **C**. The ratio of dead space volume to tidal volume is determined by the following equation: $(PaCO_2 - PeCO_2)/PaCO_2$. You are provided with the patient's $PaCO_2$ (60 mm Hg) and the $PeCO_2$ (40 mm Hg) is the expired CO_2 detected by capnography. Therefore, the ratio of dead space volume to tidal volume = (60 − 40 mm Hg)/60 mm Hg = 0.33 or 33%.

You decide to allow permissive hypercapnea for your patient and ventilate your patient using a volume-targeted mode.

Which of the following statements about permissive hypercapnea is TRUE?
A. CO_2 elimination is inversely proportional to alveolar ventilation (V_A)
B. CO_2 elimination is proportional to alveolar CO_2
C. An increase in alveolar CO_2 and similar decrease in V_A would result in unchanged CO_2 elimination
D. B and C
E. A, B, and C

Discussion

The correct answer is **D**. CO_2 elimination (VCO_2) is proportional to both V_A and alveolar CO_2 (P_ACO_2) by the following equation: $K \times VCO_2 = P_ACO_2 \times V_A$, where K is a constant. The use of permissive hypercapnea involves accepting higher values of $PaCO_2$ by using lower tidal volumes to minimize ventilator-associated lung injury.[59]

Which of the following statements regarding gas exchange is TRUE?
A. The movement of gas between the alveoli and pulmonary capillary bed is an active process
B. The rate of gas exchange across a membrane is proportional to the thickness of the membrane
C. The rate of gas exchange across a membrane is inversely proportional to the diffusion coefficient
D. The rate of gas exchange across a membrane is inversely proportional to the concentration difference of gas across the membrane
E. The rate of gas exchange across a membrane is directly proportional to the area of the membrane

Discussion

The correct answer is **E**. Fick law governs gas exchange and states that the rate of diffusion of a gas across a membrane is proportional to the diffusion coefficient of the gas(es) involved, the area of the membrane and the concentration difference of the gases across the membrane, and inversely proportional to the length or thickness of the membrane. The movement of gas between the pulmonary capillary bed and alveoli is a passive, not active, process.

The use of CPAP in the delivery room in infants with RDS is directed at maintaining which of the following lung volumes?
A. Vital capacity (VC)
B. Residual volume (RV)
C. Expiratory reserve volume (ERV)
D. Inspiratory reserve volume (IRV)
E. Functional residual capacity (FRC)

Discussion

The correct answer is **E**. Maintaining FRC is an important goal of therapy in infants with RDS to recruit alveoli and allow for alveolar gas exchange. Frequently, the retention of airway liquid after birth complicates respiratory failure secondary to RDS.[60] The recruitment of an adequate FRC allows for gas exchange throughout the respiratory cycle, instead of only during the period of inspiration. Another consideration for ventilation in the delivery room is the use of a long inflation time to overcome the long time constant associated with moving liquid through the airways. Definitions of key lung volume measures are provided in Table 5-5.[61]

Quick Quiz: Lung Volume

You are attempting to determine the FRC in a newborn infant who is mechanically ventilated. You decide to use the helium dilution technique. You begin with a 50-mL

TABLE 5-5. Definition and Clinical Determination of Key Lung Volumes

LUNG VOLUME MEASUREMENT	DEFINITION	CLINICAL METHOD(S) FOR DETERMINATION
Functional residual capacity (FRC)	The volume of gas in the lung that is in communication with the airways at the *end* of expiration	Helium dilution or nitrogen washout
Tidal volume (TV)	The volume of gas exchanged in and out of the lung in a single respiratory cycle	Pneumotachometer or plethysmograph
Vital capacity (VC)	The total gas exchange capacity of the lung	Difficult to measure, but can be approximated by measuring tidal volume during crying
Thoracic gas volume (TGV)	Volume of gas in the thorax at the end of expiration (FRC plus gas that is not in communication with the airways)	Body plethysmograph while an infant is breathing against an occluded airway

gas mixture in a balloon that contains 15% helium in oxygen. You connect the balloon to the ETT of the infant for a total of eight respiratory cycles and then remove the balloon and clamp it shut and place the infant back on the ventilator. The concentration of helium in the balloon is now 10%.

What is this patient's FRC?
A. 5 mL
B. 10 mL
C. 25 mL
D. 50 mL
E. 75 mL

Discussion

The correct answer is **C**. Techniques to determine FRC include the helium dilution method[62] and the nitrogen washout method.[63] Measurements of FRC can be useful in determining lung growth, although are not commonly performed in routine clinical practice. The nitrogen washout technique uses the amount of nitrogen displaced by another gas, typically oxygen, to measure the effective FRC. The helium dilution technique used the relative dilution of helium based on the initial (C_i) and final (C_f) concentration of helium and volume of gas (V_g) inspired to determine the FRC. The FRC can be calculated by the following: $FRC = V_g \times (C_i/C_f) - V_g$. Using the values provided in this case, the FRC = 50 mL × (0.15/0.10) − 50 mL = 25 mL.

Of the following statements comparing normal newborn respiratory mechanics to an adult, which answer is TRUE?
A. The healthy newborn lung has a higher compliance than an adult lung
B. The chest wall of a newborn infant is less compliant than an adult
C. Neonates have a longer time constant than adults
D. Airway resistance is lower in newborn infants compared to adults
E. All of the above statements are false

Discussion

The correct answer is **E**. There are several important differences between the newborn and adult lung.[64] The newborn lung is less compliant than an adult lung although the chest wall is more compliant. The compliant chest wall is one reason that newborn infants, and not adults, demonstrate chest wall retractions during respiratory distress. In addition, neonates have shorter time constants and higher airway resistance than adults. The largest contribution of airway resistance in newborn infants is upper airway resistance, which is primarily determined by nasal resistance.

Of the following statements regarding respiratory muscle function and development, which answer is TRUE?
A. The diaphragm muscle is a secondary muscle involved in respiration
B. The neonatal diaphragm muscle generates a larger tetanic force than the adult muscle
C. The diaphragm is innervated by the vagus nerve
D. Birth trauma typically affects the right hemidiaphragm
E. All of the above statements are false

Discussion

The correct answer is D. Unilateral paralysis of the diaphragm can be seen in infants with injury to the phrenic nerve during birth, with or without associated brachial plexus injury.[65] Breech position is an important risk factor and the right side of the diaphragm is more commonly affected than the left. Infants typically present with respiratory distress after birth and the chest radiograph demonstrates elevation of the hemidiaphragm. Confirmation of diaphragm paralysis can be made with ultrasound or fluoroscopy, although high PEEP may lead to false-negative studies. Some infants spontaneously recover from the injury, while others require plication of the diaphragm. The diaphragm is innervated by the phrenic nerve, not the vagus nerve, which comes of the C3, C4, and C5 cervical spinal cord roots. Phrenic nerve injury can be seen in infants who have undergone a chest tube thoracostomy or thoracotomy for closure of a PDA, repair of a TEF, or placement of a Blalock–Taussig shunt. The diaphragm is the major muscle involved in human respiration. In comparison to an adult, the neonatal diaphragm muscle has a lower tetanic force and a much larger fraction of power output is needed to establish adequate ventilation.[66]

Objectives

1. Know the concepts of anatomic and physiologic dead space
2. Know the determinants of gas exchange
3. Know the basic gas laws and their clinical applications
4. Know the factors that determine residual lung volume, FRC, and tidal volume, and how they change with various pulmonary disorders
5. Know the indications for and techniques of CPAP
6. Plan the ventilatory therapy for infants with respiratory failure of different etiologies
7. Distinguish the differences in pulmonary mechanics between the neonate and adult
8. Know the interpretation and limitations of methods for measuring pulmonary function
9. Know the developmental characteristics of respiratory muscle function

CASE 14

You are mechanically ventilating a 3-kg term infant who has returned from surgery for the placement of a ventriculoperitoneal shunt secondary to congenital hydrocephalus.

The current ventilator settings are ventilator rate of 35 breaths per minute, PIP of 24 cm H_2O, PEEP of 4 cm H_2O, and inspiratory time of 0.3 seconds. Upon examination, the infant's chest rise is excessive. The expiratory tidal volume measurement by the ventilator is 40 mL.

What is this patient's lung compliance?
A. 0.5 mL/cm H_2O
B. 0.6 mL/cm H_2O
C. 0.67 mL/cm H_2O
D. 1.67 mL/cm H_2O
E. 2 mL/cm H_2O

Discussion

The correct answer is **E**. Lung compliance is determined by measuring a change in volume by a given change in pressure (compliance = Δ Volume/Δ Pressure). In this patient, the Δ Pressure is 20 cm H_2O (PIP – PEEP), and the Δ Volume is the expiratory tidal volume of 40 mL. Therefore the compliance is 40 mL/20 cm H_2O = 2 mL/cm H_2O. Infants such as the patient in this scenario, who are undergoing ventilation due to postoperative respiratory failure secondary to anesthesia or sedation without an underlying primary pulmonary process, are likely to have high respiratory system compliance due to both high lung compliance and high chest wall compliance.

Helpful Tip: An individual patient's lung compliance should be considered when deciding the appropriate type and level of respiratory support.

Helpful Tip: In patients who are receiving pressure-targeted ventilation, tidal volumes can change rapidly due to dynamic changes in lung compliance and need to be monitored carefully.

Due to a medical error, the patient receives three times the desired volume of intravenous fluids and gains 20% of birth weight on postoperative day 1.

Of the following, which change in respiratory mechanics would you expect for this patient on postoperative day 1 compared to the prior day?
A. Increase in airway resistance
B. Decrease in airway resistance
C. Increase in lung compliance
D. Decrease in lung compliance
E. Increase in function residual capacity

Discussion

The correct answer is **D**. An excessive amount of fluid administration places this infant at risk of pulmonary edema, which is the excessive accumulation of fluid in the airspaces of the lung. The mechanism for pulmonary edema in this patient would be an increase in intravascular pressure related to the intravascular fluid load which would result in an increase in transvascular fluid flow.[67] Additional causes of edema include decreases in interstitial pressure, decreases in microvascular oncotic pressure, and increases in membrane permeability due to capillary leak from sepsis or other inflammatory conditions. Treatments for pulmonary edema include fluid restriction, optimization of cardiac function, diuretics, and the use of PEEP. Pulmonary edema is a common problem in infants with PDA and the use of adequate PEEP is a key part of conservative management.[68,69]

Helpful Tip: The use of PEEP can be helpful to treat or prevent pulmonary edema from a hemodynamically significant PDA.

Objectives

1. Plan the ventilatory therapy for infants with respiratory failure of different etiologies
2. Recognize the factors that alter lung compliance and chest wall compliance and how they change with various pulmonary disorders and gestational age
3. Know the interpretation and limitations of methods for measuring pulmonary function
4. Know the causes of pulmonary edema and its effect on lung function

CASE 15

A 2-day-old term female born at 40 weeks of gestation is referred to your center for ECMO. She presented at the referring hospital with respiratory distress after birth and was initially treated with CPAP. Her chest radiograph was consistent with RDS, although she did not have any risk factors. A full sepsis evaluation was negative. On postnatal day 1, she was intubated and given surfactant, which resulted in transient clinical improvement. However, the following day she deteriorated and was referred to your center. Upon admission to your center, the OI is 60 and an echocardiogram demonstrates normal cardiac anatomy. You decided to initiate ECMO. Over the next 2 weeks, you are unable to wean your patient off ECMO despite multiple attempts.

Upon further testing, which of the following abnormalities is likely to be discovered?
A. Surfactant protein A deficiency
B. Surfactant protein B deficiency
C. Surfactant protein C deficiency
D. Surfactant protein D deficiency
E. ADCB-2 deficiency

Discussion

The correct answer is **B**. Surfactant deficiencies are rare disorders that are frequently lethal and can initially present as severe neonatal respiratory failure with a radiographic appearance similar to RDS.[70] Of the surfactant proteins, deficiencies of surfactant protein B (SP-B) and C (SP-C) are the two deficiencies with recognized clinical phenotypes. SP-B deficiency presents in the neonatal period and is typically fatal. In contrast, SP-C deficiency has a variable onset from infancy to adulthood and more commonly presents beyond the neonatal period as idiopathic lung disease. ABCA-3, not ADCB-2, deficiency is another inherited surfactant disorder that presents in the neonatal period and is thought to be related to a defective ability to transport lipids essential for surfactant function into lamellar bodies. Gene testing is the preferred method to test for surfactant disorders and both SP-B and ABCA-3 demonstrate autosomal recessive inheritance, while SP-C can have sporadic or autosomal dominant inheritance.

You send gene testing and the results show a loss-of-function mutation in the gene encoding SP-B. The mother of your patient asks about any potential treatments for her daughter.

Of the following treatments, which has been shown to increase long-term survival in infants with SP-B deficiency who survive beyond the neonatal period?
A. Corticosteroids
B. Exogenous surfactant
C. iNO
D. HFOV
E. Lung transplantation

Discussion

The correct answer is **E**. Most infants with SP-B deficiency die in the neonatal period. However, in 1994 the first infant with SP-B deficiency underwent lung transplantation.[71] In a single-center experience with lung transplantation, infants with SP-B and ABCA-3 deficiency typically underwent transplant at a median of 100 and 140 postnatal days, respectively. Currently, there are no mechanism-specific interventions for infants with surfactant disorders. Therefore, lung transplantation is one of the few options to allow for long-term survival in

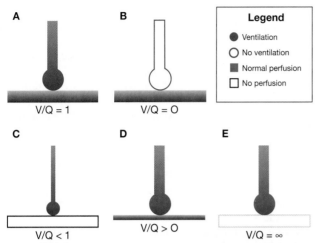

FIGURE 5-15. Various ventilation (V) and perfusion (Q) relationships. The width of the respective alveolar unit (*blue*) or capillary unit (*red*) is proportional to the relative amount of ventilation or perfusion, respectively, for a given alveolar unit.

infants who are able to survive beyond the neonatal period.

Of the following ventilation and perfusion relationships depicted in Figure 5-15, which is the most likely to be seen in a patient similar to the one described in the previous scenario with severe parenchymal lung disease but no evidence of pulmonary hypertension?

A. Image A
B. Image B
C. Image C
D. Image D
E. Image E

Discussion

The correct answer is **C**. Mismatching of ventilation (V) and perfusion (Q) is seen in infants with severe cardiopulmonary illnesses. In a patient with severe parenchymal lung disease, the V/Q is likely to be less than one as the V_A will be reduced while the alveolar perfusion will remain unchanged, as is shown in answer C.

Of the following ventilation and perfusion relationships depicted in Figure 5-15, which is consistent with dead space ventilation?

A. Image A
B. Image B
C. Image C
D. Image D
E. Image E

Discussion

The correct answer is **E**. Dead space ventilation is seen where there is V_A without alveolar perfusion. In this situation, the V/Q approaches infinity and results in wasted respiratory work. Gas that remains in the conducting airways or that reaches nonperfused alveoli are both examples of dead space ventilation.

Objectives

1. Know the inherited surfactant disorders
2. Know the causes and the effects of ventilation/perfusion mismatching
3. Know the concepts of anatomic and physiologic dead space

ACKNOWLEDGMENT

Supported by the National Center for Advancing Translational Sciences of the National Institutes of Health under Award Number UL1TR000454.

REFERENCES

1. ACOG Committee on Obstetric Practice. ACOG Committee Opinion No. 475: antenatal corticosteroid therapy for fetal maturation. *Obstet Gynecol*. 2011;117(2 Pt 1):422–424.
2. Raju TN, Langenberg P. Pulmonary hemorrhage and exogenous surfactant therapy: a metaanalysis. *J Pediatr*. 1993;123(4):603–610.
3. Seger N, Soll R. Animal derived surfactant extract for treatment of respiratory distress syndrome. *Cochrane Database Syst Rev*. 2009;(2):CD007836.
4. Soll RF. Prophylactic synthetic surfactant for preventing morbidity and mortality in preterm infants. *Cochrane Database Syst Rev*. 2000;(2):CD001079.
5. Possmayer F, Yu SH, Weber, JM, et al. Pulmonary surfactant. *Can J Biochem Cell Biol*. 1984;62:1121–1133.
6. Claireaux AE. Hyaline membrane in the neonatal lung. *Lancet*. 1953;265(6789):749–753.
7. Smith BT. The pulmonary surfactant: quantity and quality. *N Engl J Med*. 1979;300(3):136–137.
8. Barrington K, Finer N. The natural history of the appearance of apnea of prematurity. *Pediatr Res*. 1991;29(4 Pt 1):372–375.
9. Krauss AN. Apnea in infancy: pathophysiology, diagnosis, and treatment. *N Y State J Med*. 1986;86(2):89–96.
10. Schmidt B, Roberts RS, Davis P, et al. Caffeine therapy for apnea of prematurity. *N Engl J Med*. 2006;354(20):2112–2121.
11. Carlo WA, Martin RJ, Fanaroff AA. The respiratory system. In: Fanaroff AA, Martin RJ, Walsh MC, eds. *Fanaroff and Martin's*

Neonatal-Perinatal Medicine: Diseases Of The Fetus And Infant. Philadelphia, PA: Mosby Elsevier; 2006:1110–1111.

12. Avery ME, Gatewood OB, Brumley G. Transient tachypnea of newborn. Possible delayed resorption of fluid at birth. *Am J Dis Child*. 1966;111(4):380–385.

13. Tita AT, Landon MB, Spong CY, et al. Timing of elective repeat cesarean delivery at term and neonatal outcomes. *N Engl J Med*. 2009;360(2):111–120.

14. Jain L, Eaton DC. Physiology of fetal lung fluid clearance and the effect of labor. *Semin Perinatol*. 2006;30(1):34–43.

15. American College of Obstetricians and Gynecologists. ACOG Committee Opinion No. 394, December 2007. Cesarean delivery on maternal request. *Obstet Gynecol*. 2007;110(6):1501.

16. Yu VY, Liew SW, Robertson NR. Pneumothorax in the newborn. Changing pattern. *Arch Dis Child*. 1975;50(6):449–453.

17. Conrad SA, Rycus PT, Dalton H. Extracorporeal life support registry report 2004. *ASAIO J*. 2005;51(1):4–10.

18. Azizkhan RG, Crombleholme TM. Congenital cystic lung disease: contemporary antenatal and postnatal management. *Pediatr Surg Int*. 2008;24(6):643–657.

19. Bellini C, Boccardo F, Campisi C, et al. Congenital pulmonary lymphangiectasia. *Orphanet J Rare Dis*. 2006;1:43.

20. Esther CR Jr, Barker PM. Pulmonary lymphangiectasia: diagnosis and clinical course. *Pediatr Pulmonol*. 2004;38(4):308–313.

21. El Shahed AI, Dargaville P, Ohlsson A, et al. Surfactant for meconium aspiration syndrome in full term/near term infants. *Cochrane Database Syst Rev*. 2007;(3):CD002054.

22. Abman SH. Recent advances in the pathogenesis and treatment of persistent pulmonary hypertension of the newborn. *Neonatology*. 2007;91(4):283–290.

23. Miller OI, Celermajer DS, Deanfield JE, et al. Guidelines for the safe administration of inhaled nitric oxide. *Arch Dis Child Fetal Neonatal Ed*. 1994;70(1):F47–F49.

24. Taylor MB, Christian KG, Patel N, et al. Methemoglobinemia: toxicity of inhaled nitric oxide therapy. *Pediatr Crit Care Med*. 2001;2(1):99–101.

25. Neonatal Inhaled Nitric Oxide Study Group. Inhaled nitric oxide in full-term and nearly full-term infants with hypoxic respiratory failure. *N Engl J Med*. 1997;336(9):597–604.

26. Clark RH, Kueser TJ, Walker MW, et al. Low-dose nitric oxide therapy for persistent pulmonary hypertension of the newborn. Clinical inhaled nitric oxide research group. *N Engl J Med*. 2000;342(7):469–474.

27. Hamrick SE, Hansmann G. Patent ductus arteriosus of the preterm infant. *Pediatrics*. 2010;125(5):1020–1030.

28. Schneider DJ, Moore JW. Patent ductus arteriosus. *Circulation*. 2006;114(17):1873–1882.

29. Singh BS, Clark RH, Powers RJ, et al. Meconium aspiration syndrome remains a significant problem in the NICU: outcomes and treatment patterns in term neonates admitted for intensive care during a ten-year period. *J Perinatol*. 2009;29(7):497–503.

30. Dhillon R. The management of neonatal pulmonary hypertension. *Arch Dis Child Fetal Neonatal Ed*. 2012;97(3):F223–F228.

31. Konduri GG, Kim UO. Advances in the diagnosis and management of persistent pulmonary hypertension of the newborn. *Pediatr Clin North Am*. 2009;56(3):579–600.

32. Barron DJ, Kilby MD, Davies B, et al. Hypoplastic left heart syndrome. *Lancet*. 2009;374(9689):551–564.

33. Rudolph AM, Yuan S. Response of the pulmonary vasculature to hypoxia and H+ ion concentration changes. *J Clin Invest*. 1966;45(3):399–411.

34. Warren JB, Anderson JM. Core concepts: respiratory distress syndrome. *Neoreviews*. 2009;10(7):351–361.

35. Perl AK, Whitsett JA. Molecular mechanisms controlling lung morphogenesis. *Clin Genet*. 1999;56(1):14–27.

36. Laughon MM, Langer JC, Bose CL, et al. Prediction of bronchopulmonary dysplasia by postnatal age in extremely premature infants. *Am J Respir Crit Care Med*. 2011;183(12):1715–1722.

37. Baraldi E, Filippone M. Chronic lung disease after premature birth. *N Engl J Med*. 2007;357(19):1715–1722.

38. Laughon MM, Smith PB, Bose C. Prevention of bronchopulmonary dysplasia. *Semin Fetal Neonatal Med*. 2009;14(6):374–382.

39. Soll RF. Prophylactic natural surfactant extract for preventing morbidity and mortality in preterm infants. *Cochrane Database Syst Rev*. 2000;(2):CD000511.

40. Veness-Meehan KA. Effects of retinol deficiency and hyperoxia on collagen gene expression in rat lung. *Exp Lung Res*. 1997;23(6):569–581.

41. Darlow BA, Graham PJ. Vitamin A supplementation to prevent mortality and short- and long-term morbidity in very low birthweight infants. *Cochrane Database Syst Rev*. 2011;(10):CD000501.

42. Halliday HL, Ehrenkranz RA, Doyle LW. Early (<8 days) postnatal corticosteroids for preventing chronic lung disease in preterm infants. *Cochrane Database Syst Rev*. 2010;(1):CD001146.

43. Halliday HL, Ehrenkranz RA, Doyle LW. Late (>7 days) postnatal corticosteroids for chronic lung disease in preterm infants. *Cochrane Database Syst Rev*. 2009;(1):CD001145.

44. Watterberg KL; American Academy of Pediatrics. Committee on Fetus and Newborn. Policy statement–postnatal corticosteroids to prevent or treat bronchopulmonary dysplasia. *Pediatrics*. 2010;126(4):800–808.

45. Jobe AH, Bancalari E. Bronchopulmonary dysplasia. *Am J Respir Crit Care Med*. 2001;163(7):1723–1729.

46. Northway WH Jr, Rosan RC, Porter DY. Pulmonary disease following respirator therapy of hyaline-membrane disease. Bronchopulmonary dysplasia. *N Engl J Med*. 1967;276(7):357–368.

47. Stoll BJ, Hansen NI, Bell EF, et al. Eunice Kennedy Shriver National Institute of Child Health and Human Development Neonatal Research Network. Neonatal outcomes of extremely preterm infants from the NICHD Neonatal Research Network. *Pediatrics*. 2010;126(3):443–456.

48. Schmidt B, Davis P, Moddemann D, et al. Long-term effects of indomethacin prophylaxis in extremely-low-birth-weight infants. *N Engl J Med*. 2001;344(26):1966–1972.

49. Schmidt B, Roberts RS, Fanaroff A, et al. TIPP Investigators. Indomethacin prophylaxis, patent ductus arteriosus, and the risk of bronchopulmonary dysplasia: further analyses from the Trial of Indomethacin Prophylaxis in Preterms (TIPP). *J Pediatr*. 2006;148(6):730–734.

50. Nelson NM, Prodhom LS, Cherry RB, et al. A further extension of the in vivo oxygen-dissociation curve for the blood of the newborn infant. *J Clin Invest.* 1964;43:606–610.

51. Humphrey C, Duncan K, Fletcher S. Decade of experience with vascular rings at a single institution. *Pediatrics.* 2006;117(5):e903–e908.

52. Marion TL, Bradshaw WT. Congenital central hypoventilation syndrome and the PHOX2B gene mutation. *Neonatal Netw.* 2011;30(6):397–401.

53. Masters IB. Congenital airway lesions and lung disease. *Pediatr Clin North Am.* 2009;56(1):227–242.

54. Scott AR, Tibesar RJ, Sidman JD. Pierre Robin sequence: evaluation, management, indications for surgery, and pitfalls. *Otolaryngol Clin North Am.* 2012;45(3):695–710.

55. Ramsden JD, Campisi P, Forte V. Choanal atresia and choanal stenosis. *Otolaryngol Clin North Am.* 2009;42(2):339–352.

56. Pagon RA, Graham JM Jr, Zonana J, et al. Coloboma, congenital heart disease, and choanal atresia with multiple anomalies: CHARGE association. *J Pediatr.* 1981;99(2):223–227.

57. Carlo WA, Martin RJ, Fanaroff AA. The respiratory system. In: Fanaroff AA, Martin RJ, Walsh MC, eds. *Fanaroff and Martin's Neonatal-Perinatal Medicine: Diseases of the Fetus and Infant.* Philadelphia, PA: Mosby Elsevier; 2006:1088.

58. Bhat R, Salas AA, Foster C, et al. Prospective analysis of pulmonary hypertension in extremely low birth weight infants. *Pediatrics.* 2012;129(3):e682–e689.

59. Miller JD, Carlo WA. Permissive hypercapnia in neonates. *Neoreviews.* 2007;8(8):e345–e352.

60. Hooper SB, Te Pas AB, Lewis, RA, et al. Establishing functional residual capacity at birth. *Neoreviews.* 2010;11(9):474–483.

61. Carlo WA, Martin RJ, Fanaroff AA. The respiratory system. In: Fanaroff AA, Martin RJ, Walsh MC, eds. *Fanaroff and Martin's Neonatal-Perinatal Medicine: Diseases of the Fetus and Infant.* Philadelphia, PA: Mosby Elsevier; 2006:1092–1093.

62. Gaultier C. Lung volumes in neonates and infants. *Eur Respir J Suppl.* 1989;4:130S–134S.

63. Gerhardt T, Hehre D, Bancalari E, et al. A simple method for measuring functional residual capacity by N2 washout in small animals and newborn infants. *Pediatr Res.* 1985;19(11):1165–1169.

64. Nelson NM. Neonatal pulmonary function. *Pediatr Clin North Am.* 1966;13(3):769–799.

65. Schifrin N. Unilateral paralysis of the diaphragm in the newborn infant due to phrenic nerve injury, with and without associated brachial palsy. *Pediatrics.* 1952;9(1):69–76.

66. Sieck GC, Mantilla CB, Fahim MA. Functional development of respiratory muscles. In: Polin RA, Fox WW, Abman SH, eds. *Fetal and Neonatal Physiology.* Philadelphia, PA: W.B. Saunders Co.; 2004:848–863.

67. Carlton DP. Pathophysiology of edema. In: Polin RA, Fox WW, Abman SH, eds. *Fetal and Neonatal Physiology.* Philadelphia, PA: W.B. Saunders Co.; 2004:1357–1361.

68. Robertson NR. Prolonged continuous positive airways pressure for pulmonary oedema due to persistent ductus arteriosus in the newborn. *Arch Dis Child.* 1974;49(7):585–587.

69. Vanhaesebrouck S, Zonnenberg I, Vandervoort P, et al. Conservative treatment for patent ductus arteriosus in the preterm. *Arch Dis Child Fetal Neonatal Ed.* 2007;92(4):F244–F247.

70. Gower WA, Wert SE, Nogee LM. Inherited surfactant disorders. *NeoReviews.* 2008;9(10):e458–e467.

71. Faro A, Hamvas A. Lung transplantation for inherited disorders of surfactant metabolism. *NeoReviews.* 2008;9(10):e468–e476.

Chapter 6

GENETICS AND DYSMORPHOLOGY
Margaret P. Adam, MD and Angela Sun, MD

CASE 1

You are asked to evaluate a 1-day-old term male with an absent left hand. On physical examination, he has normal growth parameters and is not noted to have any dysmorphic facial features. His right arm appears completely normal with a normal hand and normal palmar flexion creases. He is noted to have a normal appearing upper and lower left arm, which ends transversely just before the location of where the left hand would be. Radiographs of the upper left arm demonstrate an intact and normal appearing humerus, radius, and ulna. You explain to the medical student that this infant has an isolated congenital anomaly.

You explain that a congenital anomaly
A. By definition is genetic in nature
B. Occurs in 5% to 7% of the general population
C. Is a structural defect that deviates from the normal standard
D. Can be subdivided into major anomalies, minor anomalies, and disruptive anomalies
E. Is typically associated with a 25% recurrence risk

Discussion

The correct answer is **C**. Congenital is a term that refers to a feature that is present at birth. As such, congenital does not imply etiology and does not mean that a feature is due to a genetic cause. An anomaly is considered a structural defect that deviates from the normal standard. Anomalies can be subdivided into major anomalies (those that are of cosmetic importance or require surgical and/or medical management) and minor anomalies (those that have no major surgical or cosmetic importance). Examples of major anomalies are bladder exstrophy, cleft lip with or without

cleft palate, and microtia/anotia. Examples of minor anomalies are syndactyly between the 2nd and 3rd toe, ear pits, and/or tags, and single transverse palmar crease.

In the case above, the infant could have a limb reduction defect due to an in utero vascular disruption to the developing hand or due to amniotic bands sequence (Fig. 6-1). To distinguish between these possibilities, placental pathology could be undertaken to determine if there were amniotic bands present. However, the absence of pathology in the placenta does not absolutely exclude the possibility of amniotic bands sequence. An evaluation for constriction bands on the extremities would also be evidence of possible amniotic bands sequence. Both vascular disruptive defects and amniotic bands sequence are typically sporadic events with a low recurrence risk for future pregnancies.

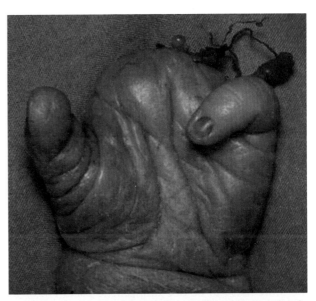

FIGURE 6-1. Terminal limb deficiency due to amniotic bands. Note the strands of amnion in which the fingers were entwined and the nubbin of tissue in the area of where the index finger would be. (Used with permission of H. Eugene Hoyme.)

Most isolated congenital anomalies are due to a combination of genetic and environmental factors. Therefore, most isolated defects have a recurrence risk that is less than the recurrence risk for an autosomal recessive condition (25%). Empiric recurrence risks for many anomalies (based on the type of anomaly, the severity of the anomaly, and the family history) are published[1]; however, most empiric recurrence risks fall within the range of 3% to 5%, particularly if there is no known family history of a similarly affected individual or a family history of a similarly affected individual who is not a first-degree relative.

You further explain to the medical student that most birth defects can be divided into mechanistic categories.

The transverse limb reduction defect described above most likely falls into which mechanistic category?
A. Deformation
B. Disruption
C. Malformation
D. Subformation
E. Ciliopathy

Discussion

The correct answer is **B**. Birth defects can be divided into probable mechanistic categories that help the clinician decide if there is likely to be a strong genetic contribution.[2] Each mechanism is associated with different diagnostic and recurrence risk implications. The mechanistic categories include deformations, disruptions, and malformations. Deformations are an abnormality of structure that arises from prenatal mechanical forces that are exerted on an otherwise normally formed structure or tissue. For example, unusual head shape or clubbed feet due to in utero constraint from oligohydramnios or twinning. Disruptions are structural defects that result from the destruction or interruption of intrinsically normally developing tissues. This mechanism tends to lead to birth defects that do not follow the typical patterns seen during embryologic development, but instead affect a group of tissues that may not be embryologically related. Examples of disruptions include terminal transverse limb reduction defects due to amniotic bands or segmental intestinal atresias caused by vascular disruptions. Malformations are structural defects that arise from an intrinsically abnormal developmental process. Examples of malformations include congenital heart defects and structural brain malformations, such as holoprosencephaly or polymicrogyria. Malformations are more likely to be due to a genetic condition or to result from genetic susceptibilities. Deformations and disruptions are in general less likely to be due to a genetic condition or genetic susceptibility.

CASE 2

You next evaluate a 3-day-old term African-American male born to a 41-year-old G2P2 mother. He is noted to have bilateral postaxial polydactyly of the hands.

The next evaluation for this infant should be a(n)
A. Full skeletal survey to evaluate for a skeletal dysplasia
B. Chromosomal microarray to evaluate for a chromosome abnormality
C. Ophthalmologic evaluation to evaluate for retinal pigmentation anomalies
D. Complete blood count to evaluate for thrombocytopenia
E. Pedigree to evaluate for a family history of polydactyly

Discussion

The correct answer is **E**. In babies who have anomalies, it is helpful to collect a complete family history, including whether other family members have similar anomalies. For example, a newborn who is found to have bilateral postaxial (ulnar) polydactyly of the hands may have a parent who had unilateral or bilateral postaxial polydactyly that was removed as an infant. Isolated postaxial polydactyly can be inherited as an autosomal dominant condition with reduced penetrance, particularly in individuals who are of African descent.[3] The number of limbs affected can vary from individual to individual, even within the same family. Because of reduced penetrance, a first-degree relative (parent) may not be affected, while a second-degree relative (grandparent, aunt, uncle) may be affected. Therefore, it is important to ask about second- and third-degree relatives when taking a family history.

A full skeletal survey in this situation would not be necessary unless there was evidence of decreased length, of disproportion (limbs appearing too short compared to the trunk or trunk appearing too short compared to the limbs), or of underlying bony abnormalities, such as pectus anomaly or congenital scoliosis, on physical examination.

Chromosomal microarray is likely not necessary unless there is evidence of dysmorphic features, growth retardation, family history of multiple anomalies and/or intellectual disability, or the finding of other anomalies in this infant.

Postaxial polydactyly can be seen in individuals with Bardet–Biedl syndrome, a disorder of cilia that is typically associated with the development of obesity in those older than 1 year of age, the development of cone-rod retinal dystrophy (typically presenting as night blindness in early childhood), hypogonadism in males, renal abnormalities, and intellectual disability. While this diagnosis could remain in the differential diagnosis, if a family history of nonsyndromic postaxial polydactyly is ellicited, this diagnosis would be unlikely.

Thrombocytopenia can be seen with bilateral absence of the radius but presence of the thumbs in thrombocytopenia-absent radius (TAR) syndrome; however, these individuals do not have postaxial polydactyly.

The mother states that her maternal grandfather and her sister both have a history of postaxial polydactyly. However, you also note that the infant has bilateral transverse palmar creases. He otherwise appears normal with normal growth parameters.

You explain to the medical student that the palmar creases found in this infant likely signifies
A. Trisomy 21
B. Trisomy 18
C. A single-gene disorder
D. A minor anomaly
E. A normal phenotypic variant

Discussion

The correct answer is **D**. It is important to note that the prevalence of a given feature varies based on sex, race, and ethnic background of the individual. A feature that is present in less than 4% of the general population being studied is considered a minor anomaly.[4] Those rare features that occur in greater than 4% of the population being studied are considered a normal phenotypic variant. Therefore, minor anomalies may overlap with normal phenotypic variants depending on the demographics of the population. An example of this is that single transverse palmar crease is considered a minor anomaly in those of Caucasian ancestry, in which it is found unilaterally in 4% and bilaterally in 1% of the general Caucasian population. However, it is considered a normal phenotypic variant in individuals of Chinese descent, in which it is found unilaterally in 16.8% and bilaterally in 6.6% of healthy Chinese newborns.[5] Given that this infant has no other dysmorphic features, it is unlikely that he has Down syndrome or trisomy 18, despite the fact that his mother was 41 years at the time of delivery. Similarly, without any other known congenital anomalies or dysmorphic features, a single-gene disorder is unlikely.

Helpful Tip: A careful physical examination for minor anomalies may lead to the finding of unsuspected associated major malformations or to the recognition of a genetic syndrome.

CASE 3

You are called to attend the cesarean section delivery of 35-week twins. The pregnancy was otherwise uncomplicated. Upon delivery, twin A is noted to have a unilateral clubbed foot. The family history is significant for an older sibling who had a ventricular septal defect (VSD). The parents are wondering if the finding of clubbed foot could be genetic.

You answer that
A. Because there is a family history of a previous child with a birth defect, it is more likely that the clubbed foot is genetic
B. Clubbed foot is a minor anomaly, making it less likely to be genetic
C. Clubbed foot in this instance is most likely a deformation, meaning it is not likely to be genetic
D. Unilateral clubbed foot is rarely genetic, while bilateral clubbed foot is usually genetic
E. Clubbed foot in this instance is likely a disruption, meaning it is not likely to be genetic

Discussion

The correct answer is **C**. The overall clinical scenario helps to determine the likelihood that a birth defect is associated with a genetic predisposition. For example, the finding of isolated unilateral clubbed foot in a twin gestation is likely to have a very low recurrence risk (<1%), while the recurrence risk for isolated (nonsyndromic) bilateral clubbed feet in a baby with no evidence of in utero constraint may be as high as 5%.[1] Clubbed foot is considered a major anomaly, as it typically requires some type of medical or surgical correction. The finding of a family history of a sibling with an isolated malformation that is unrelated to the birth defect seen in the proband does not increase the likelihood that the birth defect in the proband is genetic. Likewise, clubbed foot (whether unilateral or bilateral) can be due to a genetic cause in some instances and due to nongenetic causes in other instances.

Both twins are admitted to the neonatal intensive care unit for mild prematurity. Twin B has done well clinically. She is breathing comfortably on room air and has been nippling all of her feeds. She has stooled once and has normal urine output. You note that she has cupped ears, long palpebral fissures, and a deep sacral dimple, the base of which you are not able to visualize. Her physical features do not resemble that of Twin A. The parents report that Twin B does not resemble either of them or her 2-year-old sibling.

The next most appropriate evaluation for Twin B is
A. Ultrasound of the sacral spine to evaluate for spinal dysraphism
B. Ophthalmologic evaluation for retinal or optic colobomas
C. Renal ultrasound to evaluate for a structural renal anomaly
D. CT scan of the temporal bones to evaluate for Mondini dysplasia
E. CMA to evaluate for a chromosome abnormality

Discussion

The correct answer is **A**. Minor anomalies may be the key to the diagnosis of an occult malformation or of a genetic syndrome, which is typically described based on the constellation and pattern of minor anomalies. Approximately 15% to 20% of normal newborns have one minor anomaly, which is associated with an approximately 3% risk of an associated major malformation. Approximately 0.8% of newborns will have two minor anomalies, with an associated 10% risk of an accompanying major malformation. Only 0.5% of newborns will have three or more minor anomalies, with an overall risk of a coexistent major malformation being 20%.[6] For example, cutaneous markers over the vertex of the scalp or in the lumbosacral area are associated with an increased risk of a dysraphic state of the spine and would warrant consideration of further head/spine imaging. While the search for other malformations, such as renal anomalies, certainly could be undertaken, it is likely low yield in the absence of a firm genetic diagnosis in an otherwise asymptomatic individual (i.e., absence of electrolyte abnormalities or evidence of renal insufficiency). While cupped ears could signify an internal ear malformation, a hearing evaluation in this instance would be most useful. In the absence of hearing loss, a CT scan of the temporal bones is unlikely to be abnormal. Chromosomal microarray certainly could be pursued as a next step, but the constellation of features seen in this infant could also represent a single-gene disorder and a genetics consultation would help to determine the most appropriate type of genetic testing for this infant.

CASE 4

You are asked to evaluate a 2-day-old female because of facial asymmetry. The history is significant for a difficult vaginal vertex delivery that required forceps assistance. While quiet, the infant appears completely normal with no dysmorphic features. However, when the infant cries, there is asymmetry noted in the oral area, with drooping of the left corner of the mouth unaccompanied by drooping of the right corner of the mouth. The infant has preserved an equal nasolabial fold depth bilaterally and is able to close both eyes equally well.

The most likely explanation for this finding is
A. The infant sustained an injury to the right facial nerve during forceps delivery
B. The infant sustained an injury to the left facial nerve during forceps delivery
C. The infant has unilateral congenital absence of the right depressor anguli oris muscle
D. The infant has unilateral congenital absence of the left depressor anguli oris muscle
E. The infant sustained a brainstem injury involving the facial nerve nucleus

Discussion

The correct answer is **C**. The infant described has asymmetric crying facies due to congenital absence of the right depressor anguli oris muscle. This can be distinguished from a facial nerve palsy by the presence of equal nasolabial fold depth bilaterally and the bilateral ability to firmly close both eyes and wrinkle the forehead equally on both sides.

Asymmetric crying facies can be an isolated finding or part of a genetic syndrome.

Which genetic syndrome is most commonly associated with asymmetric crying facies?
A. Williams syndrome
B. Down syndrome
C. Oculoauriculovertebral syndrome (Goldenhar syndrome)
D. Velocardiofacial syndrome (22q11 deletion syndrome)
E. Prader–Willi syndrome (PWS)

Discussion

The correct answer is **D**. The most common syndrome associated with asymmetric crying facies is velocardiofacial syndrome caused by a deletion on 22q11.

Individuals with nonsyndromic asymmetric crying facies are at increased risk above the general population risk for congenital anomalies, including congenital heart defects, skeletal anomalies, genitourinary malformations, gastrointestinal malformations, and central nervous system anomalies.[7] Therefore, in an infant with asymmetric crying facies, a careful physical examination should be undertaken with a low threshold to perform further imaging studies of the heart, abdomen, skeletal system, and central nervous system. In addition, evaluation for features of the 22q11 deletion syndrome and consideration of genetic testing for this condition is appropriate.[8]

Objectives

1. Describe the difference between a major malformation and a minor anomaly
2. Differentiate between a malformation, a deformation, and a disruption
3. Determine the recurrence risk for multifactorial disorders
4. Distinguish between a facial nerve palsy and asymmetric crying facies

CASE 5

You are called to attend the cesarean section delivery of a term footling breech infant born to a 24-year-old G2P1 mother. You are told that there were no known pregnancy complications. A first-trimester screen apparently demonstrated a normal nuchal translucency measurement of 1.8 mm at 12 weeks 0 days gestation. Adjusted risks for this pregnancy calculated through sequential screening included a risk of trisomy 21 of 1:5092 and a risk of trisomy 18 of 1:7732. Prenatal ultrasounds were normal. No amniocentesis was performed. At birth the infant is noted to have dysmorphic features, including upslanting palpebral fissures, small ears with overfolded helices, and a protruding tongue. Hands reveal a transverse crease on the left hand but normal flexion creases on the right hand. There is an increased space between the 1st[t] and 2nd toes. You suspect Down syndrome.

Which of the following genetic tests would be most appropriate to confirm the diagnosis?
A. Fluorescence in situ hybridization (FISH) for chromosome 21
B. Routine karyotype
C. High-resolution karyotype
D. Chromosomal microarray
E. No confirmatory genetics studies are needed, as the diagnosis of Down syndrome can be made on clinical grounds alone

Discussion

The correct answer is **B**. While it is true that a diagnosis of Down syndrome can be made on clinical grounds, confirmatory karyotype is typically performed for recurrence risk counseling. In addition, routine karyotype may detect the 1% to 2% of Down syndrome cases that occur due to a mosaic chromosome complement, such as 46,XY/47,XY,+21. Individuals with mosaic Down syndrome typically have a better cognitive prognosis than do individuals with Down syndrome who do not have mosaicism. Some individuals with mosaic Down syndrome can have intelligence quotient (IQ) levels that approach the low normal range, although this is not universally true.

The FISH testing, as opposed to karyotype, can be used on a STAT basis to return a result typically within 24 to 48 hours after the blood is drawn. However, FISH testing alone will not determine which individuals have Down syndrome due to a chromosomal translocation (approximately 3–4% of cases) and which individuals have the more typical three free standing copies of chromosome

21. It is this distinction that is important for recurrence risk counseling.[9]

High-resolution karyotype in the above scenario also is not indicated, as the cytogenetics laboratory need only assess for gross chromosomal number and not for smaller and more subtle chromosome deletions and/or duplications. High-resolution karyotype may be used to detect suspected balanced or unbalanced chromosomal translocations (in which small pieces of two chromosomes have switched places with one another). It should be noted, however, that even at its highest resolution, a karyotype can detect deletions and duplications that are about 3 to 5 megabases (Mb; million base pairs) and larger.[10] This means that most microdeletion and microduplication conditions, such as the 22q11 deletion syndrome (velo-cardiofacial syndrome; DiGeorge syndrome), cannot be detected by high-resolution karyotype alone.

A chromosomal microarray, also known as array comparative genomic hybridization, is a newer technology used to evaluate chromosomes at very high resolution, on the order of kilobases (thousands of base pairs) as opposed to megabases. There are several different array platforms. Oligonucleotide array platforms compare a control genome to the patient's genome using oligonucleotide probes (similar to FISH technology but using probes that are much smaller and spread throughout the genome at standard intervals with increased density in gene-rich regions). Single nucleotide polymorphism (SNP) array platforms compare the alleles at millions of polymorphic base pair sites distributed primarily throughout coding regions, where SNPs are better characterized. Some platforms combine oligonucleotides and SNPs. While both platforms can give information about small duplications or deletions of genetic material (at a resolution higher than traditional FISH technology), SNP arrays have the advantage of evaluating parent of origin, and therefore may be able to give information about isodisomic uniparental disomy (when two homologous chromosomal segments are inherited from the same parent instead of one segment from one parent and the other segment from the other parent). This can be important for genetic segments that are imprinted (a gene that is expressed only from the maternally or paternally derived chromosome, with the other homologue silenced). Furthermore, SNP arrays can give information about consanguinity, as there may be multiple contiguous areas of allele homozygosity detected in individuals whose parents are closely related.

Chromosomal microarrays cannot determine the position of any particular genetic segment within the genome, meaning that it cannot detect Robertsonian translocations or balanced translocations. Therefore, in an individual with suspected Down syndrome, CMA can certainly detect the addition of an extra copy of chromosome 21

but cannot answer the question of whether the extra copy is translocated onto another chromosome or whether there are three free standing copies of chromosome 21.

Helpful Tip: Chromosomal microarray is a first-line test for individuals without a recognizable genetic syndrome who have multiple congenital anomalies, intellectual disability, and/or autism.

The family is surprised that their child has Down syndrome. They state that they were told that their risk of having a baby with Down syndrome was low because the mother's age is younger than 35 years. They ask you to explain how their prenatal testing could have been normal if their baby has Down syndrome.

You explain that
A. There could have been a blood sample error that lead to the normal maternal screening results
B. The baby could have mosaic Down syndrome, which might lead to normal prenatal testing
C. The blood and ultrasound testing they had prenatally were screening and not diagnostic tests
D. The family must carry a translocation which lead to Down syndrome, and therefore prenatal testing was falsely normal
E. The ultrasound was probably interpreted falsely as being normal

Discussion

The correct answer is **B**. Approximately 70% of babies with Down syndrome are born to women who are under age 35 years at delivery.[11] Ultrasound examination followed by maternal blood testing evaluates for markers that suggest there is a problem with the fetus and/or placenta. None of this testing is diagnostic for a chromosome abnormality; it is only suggestive. Therefore, first-trimester screening (nuchal translucency combined with maternal serum levels of free beta-human chorionic gonadotropin hCG [β-hCG] and pregnancy-associated plasma protein A [PAPP-A]) and second-trimester screening (measurement of maternal serum alpha-fetoprotein [MSAFP], hCG, estriol [uE3], and dimeric inhibin A [DIA]) can generate a risk for trisomy 21, trisomy 18, and in some laboratories trisomy 13. The risk estimated by these ultrasound and analyte markers is then compared to a woman's age-related risk for having a child with one of these conditions. Sometimes the risks generated through first-trimester screening and second-trimester screening are combined and called integrated screening (when results are not disclosed to the patient until all test results are returned) or sequential screening (when the results of the first-trimester screen are disclosed to the mother if they are abnormal). The first-trimester screen alone can detect about 90% of fetuses with Down syndrome and trisomy 18 with an approximately 5% false-positive rate. Sequential or integrated screening can detect approximately 95% of fetuses with Down syndrome but retains the 5% false-positive rate. Ultrasounds may be read as normal in up to 20% of fetuses with Down syndrome.[11,12]

The only way to truly determine if the fetus has a chromosome abnormality is through specific diagnostic testing, which traditionally includes either a chorionic villus sampling between 10 and 12 weeks of pregnancy or an amniocentesis, typically performed after 15 weeks of pregnancy. Newer technology using fetal DNA isolated from maternal blood (the so-called cell-free fetal DNA testing) is just entering the clinical arena and is currently validated to detect Down syndrome (and other trisomies) by assessing if extra fetal genetic material derived from chromosome 21 (or the chromosome in question) is present in maternal blood. However, since it is a DNA-based test and not a fetal karyotype, it also cannot determine if Down syndrome in the fetus is due to a translocation. The false-positive rate for this type of testing is still being investigated in large cohorts of pregnant women, but may be as low as 0.1%.[13] Therefore, a confirmatory traditional prenatal diagnostic test, such as amniocentesis, is currently recommended in those who undergo cell-free fetal DNA diagnostic testing.

The baby has been noted to have low tone and difficulty breastfeeding, but is able to feed well using a preemie nipple. His glucose levels have been normal. He appears to be breathing comfortably on room air with an oxygen saturation of 97% pre- and postductally. His four extremity blood pressures have been normal and femoral pulses are strong and equal bilaterally. His lungs are clear to auscultation and he does not have a cardiac murmur. He has had normal urine output. You request a lactation consultation. The parents are wondering what further medical evaluations need to be performed.

Which of the following medical evaluations is NOT indicated within the first month of life?
A. Echocardiogram to assess for a congenital heart defect
B. Complete blood count
C. Hearing screen
D. Thyroid function tests
E. Renal ultrasound to assess for renal anomalies

Discussion

The correct answer is **E**. Structural renal and urinary tract anomalies are not common in Down syndrome and a renal ultrasound is not indicated routinely for an indi-

vidual with Down syndrome who is asymptomatic.[9] The other evaluations are considered standard screening that should be completed in the neonatal period. Individuals who have a normal cardiac examination should still undergo an echocardiogram to detect minor cardiac problems, even if they had a previous normal fetal echocardiogram. Approximately 50% of individuals with Down syndrome will have a congenital heart defect. Complete blood count is used to assess for polycythemia and for leukemoid reaction (increased white blood cell count or transient myeloproliferative disorder), which can be a risk factor for the future development of leukemia. Hearing screening is routinely performed in all newborns born in the United States. Congenital hypothyroidism is more common in individuals with Down syndrome and can be assessed initially through newborn screening in those states that use thyroid-stimulating hormone (TSH) as a screen for hypothyroidism. In those states in which only a free thyroxine (T4) level is assessed through newborn screening, a TSH level should be sent.

Helpful Tip: Congenital hypothyroidism can be missed in the newborn period if only a free T4 is obtained.

The family states that they are definitely planning on having more children in the future but are concerned about their recurrence risk.

Which of the following is true about this family's recurrence risk for having another child with Down syndrome?
A. If their baby has Down syndrome due to three free standing copies of chromosome 21, then their recurrence risk depends on whether the extra copy of chromosome 21 was maternally or paternally inherited
B. If their baby has Down syndrome due to three free standing copies of chromosome 21, then their recurrence risk will remain very low, likely less than 1%
C. If their baby has Down syndrome due to three free standing copies of chromosome 21, then the family is not at an increased risk of having a child with a different trisomy, such as trisomy 18 or trisomy 13
D. If their baby has Down syndrome due to a translocation between chromosomes 14 and 21, then their recurrence risk depends on whether the translocation was maternally or paternally inherited
E. If their baby has Down syndrome due to a translocation between chromosomes 14 and 21, then their recurrence risk is closest to 50%

Discussion

The correct answer is **D**. Younger women who have a child with trisomy 21 due to three free standing copies of chromosome 21 are more likely to have a genetic susceptibility to nondisjunction. For a woman younger than age 35, the recurrence risk for having another child affected with trisomy 21 is approximately 1% above the baseline age-related risk. In addition, women who have had one child with a trisomy are at a slightly increased risk of having a child with a different trisomy, again due to the likely genetic susceptibility to nondisjunction. Regardless of family history, as women age their risk of having a child with a trisomy, such as trisomy 21, increases. After age 35, the recurrence risk for this woman to have another child with Down syndrome will return to her age-related risk.

For women who have a child with Down syndrome due to a translocation, it is important to determine if one of the parents carries a balanced chromosomal rearrangement that could be inherited. In this situation, the recurrence risk depends upon the sex of the parent who carries the translocation and which chromosome is involved in the translocation with chromosome 21.[14] Whereas most cases of trisomy 21 due to three free standing copies of chromosome 21 are due to a nondisjunction event in the generation of the oocyte, a small subset is due to a nondysjunction event during spermatogenesis. However, in general practice determining parent of origin for the extra chromosome 21 in those with three free standing copies of chromosome 21 is not performed clinically and recurrence risks are not adjusted based on parent of origin of the extra chromosome 21.

Helpful Tip: When evaluating for a balanced chromosomal translocation or rearrangement, karyotype must be used as opposed to chromosomal microarray.

CASE 6

Next you are asked to evaluate a term female born to a 33-year-old G4P4 mother with no prenatal care. The mother is obese but did not have screening for diabetes during the pregnancy. She denies any polyuria or polydypsia during the pregnancy but does estimate that she gained 60 lb during the pregnancy. She denies any recreational drug, prescription drug, alcohol, or tobacco use during the pregnancy. On examination, the infant has cutis aplasia at the vertex of the scalp, microcephaly, bilateral cleft lip and palate, and a heart murmur. An echocardiogram detects tetralogy of Fallot. The preliminary head magnetic resonance imaging (MRI) study suggests holoprosencephaly.

Based on the clinical features of this infant, what is the most likely diagnosis?
A. Trisomy 13
B. Trisomy 18
C. Trisomy 21
D. The 22q11 deletion syndrome
E. Diabetic embryopathy

Discussion

The correct answer is **A**. Salient features of trisomy 13 include the following: holoprosencephaly, microcephaly with sloping forehead; cleft lip and palate; cutis aplasia congenita; and congenital heart defects. Median survival for those with trisomy 13 is 2–3 days. Approximately 80% of affected individuals die in the first month of life, with only 5% surviving the first 6 months of life. While long-term survivors have been described, it is quite rare, despite correction of congenital anomalies, such as cleft palate or congenital heart defects.[2]

Cutis aplasia congenita is characterized by the localized or widespread absence of skin at birth. It most commonly appears as an ulcerated or membranous defect of the skin, typically positioned near the midline of the scalp vertex, at or in proximity to the posterior parietal hair whorl. However, cutis aplasia congenita can be found anywhere on the body and more than one lesion can be present. While most defects are superficial and do not require specific treatment aside from infection precautions, some can extend deep, even to the surface of the scalp (Fig. 6-2). Deep lesions may require plastic surgery. Once the lesion has healed, no hair will grow in that area. Cutis aplasia congenita can be found in a number of genetic syndromes, including trisomy 13, or may be an isolated finding.

Salient features of trisomy 18 include the following: prominent occiput; clenched hands with overlapping of the index finger over the third finger and the fifth finger over the fourth; nail hypoplasia; short sternum; and rockerbottom feet with dorsiflexion of the great toe. A variety of congenital heart defects can be detected but do not correlate with outcome. 50% of affected individuals die within the first week of life; 5% to 10% of affected individuals will survive the first year of life. Therefore, long-term survival is possible but rare, even with interventions for such anomalies as congenital heart defects. Those who survive have severe cognitive impairment.

While tetralogy of Fallot is a common congenital heart defect in those with the 22q11 deletion syndrome, the other features described above would be unusual for this condition. Cleft palate can also be seen in the 22q11 deletion syndrome, but cleft lip with or without cleft palate is unusual.

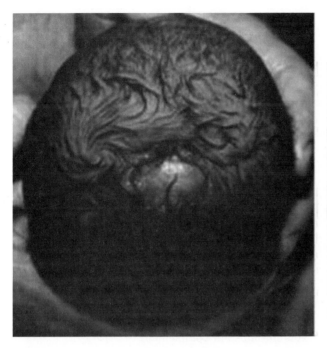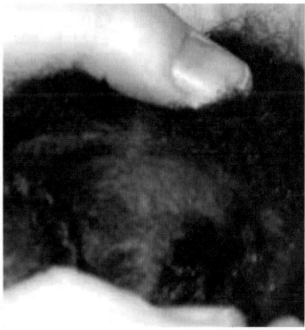

FIGURE 6-2.   Cutis aplasia. The left panel demonstrates a severe area of cutis aplasia that extends to the skull (Used with permission of H. Eugene Hoyme). Note that this is a typical location for cutis aplasia. The right panel demonstrates an area of healed cutis aplasia in which no hair grows.

Individuals with diabetic embryopathy can have many types of congenital anomalies, although cleft lip and palate and cutis aplasia congenita would be unusual, making trisomy 13 the most likely diagnosis in this case.

CASE 7

You are asked to evaluate a 4-day-old phenotypic female who was found to have coarctation of the aorta. The prenatal history is significant for a large cystic hygroma detected on a 12-week ultrasound. Serial prenatal ultrasounds were performed, which documented slow resolution of the cystic hygroma. A fetal echocardiogram was also performed and was normal. The mother declined amniocentesis. After birth the infant was noted to have weak and delayed femoral pulses compared to the right radial pulse, which prompted echocardiogram. On further physical examination you note that the neck appears webbed with a broad chest and widely spaced nipples. The ears are low set and posteriorly rotated. The remainder of the physical examination is normal, including normal female external genitalia.

In order to confirm the diagnosis, what is the most appropriate next test?
A. Routine karyotype
B. High-resolution karyotype
C. FISH for the 22q11 deletion syndrome
D. Chromosomal microarray
E. Molecular genetic testing for Noonan syndrome

Discussion

The correct answer is **A**. The most likely diagnosis for this infant is Turner syndrome. Turner syndrome represents a genetic continuum in which there is presence of one entire X chromosome with the absence of all or part of the second sex chromosome (X or Y), either in all cells examined or in a mosaic fashion.[15] The most common karyotype is 45,X, followed by 45,X/46,XY and 45,X/46,XX. Short stature is common in those with Turner syndrome, typically due to absence of the *SHOX* gene, which is on the short arm of the X chromosome.

In normal early female embryonic development, each cell will inactivate one X chromosome. The choice of which X chromosome to inactivate is random. However, all daughter cells derived from the ancestral cell will retain the same inactive X chromosome. It should be noted that certain genes on the X chromosome escape X inactivation, which accounts for the fact that women who only have one X chromosome do not have a normal phenotype. Individuals with Turner syndrome can have the following features: short stature; webbed neck; broad chest with widely spaced nipples; congenital heart defects (typically left-sided congenital heart defects, such as bicuspid aortic valve or coarctation of the aorta); renal anomalies; ovarian dysgenesis; and lymphedema of the dorsum of the hands and feet. The findings of webbed neck and broad chest with widely spaced nipples is not specific to Turner syndrome and can be seen in any individual (male or female) who had a cystic hygroma in utero.

Performing a high-resolution karyotype in this case would offer little more information than a routine karyotype, although subtle rearrangements of one of the X chromosomes can sometimes lead to features of Turner syndrome. While the 22q11 deletion syndrome is associated with congenital heart defects and dysmorphic features, the features described here are more consistent with Turner syndrome.[16] Chromosomal microarray testing could detect this chromosome difference, but at present is not as sensitive at detecting chromosomal mosaicism as routine karyotype. Some of the phenotypic features of Turner syndrome overlap with that of Noonan syndrome, including prenatal detection of cystic hygroma, postnatal webbed neck with broad chest and widely spaced nipples, and lowest and posteriorly rotated ears. However, coarctation of the aorta is not a common congenital heart defect in those with Noonan syndrome. Therefore, Noonan syndrome would remain in the differential diagnosis but molecular genetic testing for Noonan syndrome would be indicated only after Turner syndrome has been excluded.

You order a peripheral blood karyotype on this infant and the results are returned as 45,X[15]/46,XY[5].

What is the next most important evaluation for this infant?
A. Obtaining follicle-stimulating hormone (FSH) and leutenizing hormone (LH) levels to evaluate for evidence of hypogonadism
B. Obtaining a testosterone level to evaluate for testes
C. Obtaining an antimullerian hormone (AMH) level to evaluate for Sertoli cell function
D. Obtaining a renal ultrasound to evaluate for structural renal anomalies
E. Obtaining a pelvic and inguinal ultrasound to evaluate for a uterus and gonads

Discussion

The correct answer is **E**. It is imperative to determine if there are gonads present and where they may be located. While renal ultrasound is also an important evaluation in an individual with Turner syndrome, in the absence of electrolyte abnormalities or renal insufficiency, this

evaluation can wait. Measurement of FSH and LH levels may also establish if functional gonads are present, but will not provide information on gonadal location or distinguish between nonfunctioning dysgenetic gonads and absent gonads. In addition, interpretation of these hormone levels in a newborn can be difficult. It would be unlikely that this infant has significant production of testosterone (produced by the Leydig cells of the testes) because there is no evidence of virilization of the external genitalia. Similarly, AMH (which is produced by the Sertoli cells of the testes) may be a marker of gonadal composition and function but will not determine the location of the gonads or distinguish between dysgenetic gonads or absent gonads.

You discuss with the parents of this infant the chromosome difference and the need for surgical repair of the coarctation of the aorta. The parents are curious about long-term medical management for an individual with this chromosome complement.

All of the following evaluations/treatments are recommended EXCEPT
A. Growth hormone therapy if short stature becomes apparent
B. Periodic echocardiogram to evaluate for aortic root dilation
C. Spinal radiographs to evaluate for vertebral anomalies
D. Removal of any gonadal remnants
E. Hormone replacement therapy in adolescence and adulthood

Discussion

The correct answer is **C**. While the development of scoliosis in individuals with Turner syndrome is increased above the general population risk, frank vertebral anomalies are uncommon. Clinical screening for the development of scoliosis is recommended in this patient population during childhood and adolescence, but spine radiographs are only indicated for those with clinical signs of scoliosis.[15]

The external genitalia of individuals with a 45,X/46,XY chromosome complement can appear as normal male, as normal female, or as ambiguous. However, if genetic material derived from the Y chromosome is present in a subset of cells, it is possible that the affected individual has a dysgenetic gonad. In this case there is an approximately 7% to 10% risk of the development of gonadoblastoma or dysgerminoma in the dysgenetic gonad.[17] In those individuals who are assigned a female sex of rearing (as in this case), the gonads must be removed due to the increased risk of gonadoblastoma. In individuals with a 45,X/46,XY chromosome complement who have been assigned a male sex of rearing, the decision to retain the gonads is complex. If the gonads are retained in the scrotum, the individual must undergo surveillance for the development of gonadoblastoma. Tumor screening protocols vary and no consensus guidelines have been developed. Tumor screening protocols typically involve at least annual physical examination with palpation of the gonads by a healthcare professional and at least annual testicular ultrasound beginning in late childhood or at the initiation of puberty.

Currently, growth hormone is offered to individuals with a 45,X cell line as early as 2 years of age, if growth velocity is subnormal.

Approximately 3% to 8% of individuals with Turner syndrome, regardless of karyotype, have aortic root dilation, which can lead to aortic aneurysm, dissection, rupture, and death.[15] This is even true for those who have no other known congenital heart defect. Therefore, screening for aortic root dilation and aortic disease in individuals with Turner syndrome has been suggested. Individuals with Turner syndrome are also predisposed to the development of hypertension, which is often idiopathic in nature.

Since the vast majority of individuals with Turner syndrome have either streak gonads or dysgenetic gonads that have been removed, lifelong hormone replacement therapy is typically indicated starting in adolescence. Rarely individuals with Turner syndrome due to a structural X chromosome anomaly or a 45,X/46,XX chromosome complement will undergo spontaneous puberty due to the presence of functional ovarian tissue. These individuals, however, are at increased risk for the development of premature ovarian failure (POF).

CASE 8

A 35-year-old G1P0 mother undergoes amniocentesis for maternal age. The result is 47,XXX. The obstetrician asks you to meet with this family prenatally to discuss appropriate postnatal management of their daughter.

Which of the following evaluations are recommended after birth?
A. Echocardiogram
B. Renal ultrasound
C. Pelvic ultrasound
D. Echocardiogram, renal ultrasound, and pelvic ultrasound
E. No specialty evaluations are needed after birth

Discussion

The correct answer is **E**. Individuals with 47,XXX typically have no abnormal clinical features at birth. These individuals appear as completely normal females with normal internal and external anatomy. They typically have normal fertility. Occasionally babies with 47,XXX have mild hypotonia. As they grow, individuals with 47,XXX tend to have tall stature for their family background. They typically have normal intelligence, although their measured IQ levels may be less than expected for their family background. They may have mild speech delay, learning disabilities, and poor motor coordination, although these are variable features.[18]

You are discussing sex chromosome anomalies with the medical student on rotation in the neonatal intensive care unit.

Which of the following is true regarding the diagnosis of Klinefelter syndrome (47,XXY)?
A. Approximately 50% of individuals with Klinefelter syndrome require supplemental testosterone therapy in adulthood
B. All individuals with Klinefelter syndrome have infertility
C. Individuals with Klinefelter syndrome typically have mental retardation
D. Individuals with Klinefelter syndrome typically have short stature
E. Individuals with Klinefelter syndrome frequently have hypogonadism, which usually manifests as cryptorchidism and small phallus at birth

Discussion

The correct answer is **B**. Individuals with 47,XXY (Klinefelter syndrome) may have no phenotypic features at birth. Due to hypogonadism, individuals with Klinefelter syndrome may have small, hard testes and small phallus, although this is typically not noted until adolescence. In adolescence and adulthood, affected individuals tend to have tall stature with long limbs and may develop truncal obesity. They may also develop gynecomastia. Most men with Klinefelter syndrome require supplemental testosterone therapy; infertility in men with 47,XXY is universal, with some men coming to medical attention due to this problem.

Individuals with Klinefelter syndrome may have speech and language delays and they may have a shy and reserved personality. While most have an IQ that falls within the normal range, it is often at the lower level of normal (mean IQ 85–90).[2]

Objectives

1. The basic features of the common trisomies
2. The basic features of the most common sex chromosome abnormalities
3. The most useful medical evaluations after the diagnosis of a numerical chromosome abnormality
4. When to order a karyotype versus a chromosomal microarray
5. The advantages and limitations of chromosomal microarray compared to karyotype

CASE 9

You are asked to meet with a family prenatally because the fetus was detected as having a likely truncus arteriosus on a 20-week ultrasound. Fetal growth has been normal and no other anomalies have been detected on a level II ultrasound done by a maternal–fetal medicine group. The family history is negative for other individuals with congenital heart defects, other birth defects, or learning problems. The family has been offered the possibility of prenatal diagnostic testing in this pregnancy but is undecided as to whether they wish to pursue this.

Which genetic test(s) is(are) most appropriate to order in a prenatal setting?
A. Karyotype alone
B. Karyotype with FISH for 22q11 deletion
C. Karyotype with FISH for 15q11 deletion
D. Karyotype with sequencing for *TBX1*
E. Karyotype with sequencing for *NKX2.5*

Discussion

The correct answer is **B**. In an infant with a congenital heart defect, the most common genetic causes are large chromosomal abnormalities and the 22q11 deletion syndrome. Karyotype alone will detect large chromosomal anomalies but cannot detect the 22q11 deletion or other microdeletion syndromes (see Table 6-1 for a list of common deletion syndromes and their associated features). In any fetus or infant with a known or suspected conotruncal heart defect, testing for the 22q11 deletion syndrome (via FISH testing or CMA) is indicated. The most common congenital heart defect in those with the 22q11 deletion syndrome is tetralogy of Fallot; however, the most specific cardiac lesion is interrupted aortic arch type B.[16,19] See Table 6-2 for a list of congenital heart defects and the most specific associated genetic syndrome.

Deletion of 15q11 can lead to either PWS or Angelman syndrome, depending on whether the deletion occurred on the paternally derived chromosome or on the maternally derived chromosome, respectfully. Neither of these microdeletion syndromes is typically associated with congenital heart defects. Mutations in both *TBX1* and *NKX2.5* have been associated with isolated conotruncal congenital heart defects, but in the absence of a family history of similarly affected individuals, sequencing of these genes would not be indicated in a prenatal setting.

The family decides to undergo prenatal testing and it is determined that the fetus has the 22q11 deletion syndrome. The family is interested in knowing what postnatal studies will be needed after the child is born.

All of the following evaluations are recommended in the neonatal period EXCEPT
A. Echocardiogram
B. Renal ultrasound
C. Ionized calcium level
D. Urine calcium to creatinine ratio
E. Complete blood count with differential

Discussion

The correct answer is **D**. One of the most common microdeletion syndromes is the 22q11 deletion syndrome (also called DiGeorge syndrome or velocardiofacial syndrome). These conditions are all one and the same, caused by a common 3-Mb deletion on chromosome 22q11. There have been over 80 features described in association with this condition, although most individuals with this condition have only a handful of these features. Common features may include: congenital heart defects (conotruncal anomalies such as tetralogy of Fallot and truncus arteriosus); palatal anomalies (cleft palate, submucous cleft palate, velopharyngeal insufficiency); maldevelopment of the thymus (although severe clinical immunodeficiency is uncommon); typical facial features (short and narrow palpebral fissures, laterally builtup nose, bulbous nasal tip, small ears with overfolded helices); normal intelligence with learning disabilities (mean IQ 75); hypocalcemia; and psychiatric problems (depression, bipolar disorder, and schizophrenia).[16]

Neonates with a known diagnosis of the 22q11 deletion syndrome should undergo an echocardiogram (even if a prenatal echocardiogram was normal); renal ultrasound to detect structural renal anomalies; an ionized calcium level to assess for hypoparathyroidism (with referral to an endocrinologist if low); measurement of thyroid function (TSH at a minimum); and assessment of humoral immune response and measurement of absolute

TABLE 6-1.   Common Chromosomal Deletion Syndromes and Their Associated Features

DELETION SYNDROME	PERCENTAGE DETECTABLE BY KARYOTYPE	DYSMORPHIC FEATURES	CONGENITAL ANOMALIES	FUNCTIONAL DEFICITS
1p36 deletion	25%	• Straight eyebrows • Deep-set eyes • Large and late-closing anterior fontanel • Brachydactyly and/or camptodactyly • Short feet	• Brain anomalies • Congenital heart defects • Renal anomalies • Skeletal anomalies (rib anomalies; scoliosis)	• Hypotonia • Seizures • Intellectual disability (typically severe to profound)

4p- (Wolf–Hirschhorn syndrome)	50–60%	• "Greek warrior helmet" facial appearance
		  • Broad, flat nasal bridge
		  • High forehead
		  • Widely spaced eyes
		• Poorly formed ears
		• Microcephaly
			• Cleft lip and/or palate
			• Congenital heart defects
			• Urinary tract malformations
			• Scoliosis
			• Structural brain anomalies
				• Hypotonia
				• Seizures
				• Failure to thrive/growth retardation
				• Intellectual disability (moderate to severe)

5p- (Cri du Chat syndrome)	>90%	• Microcephaly • Micrognathia • Widely spaced eyes • Downslanting palpebral fissures • Round face • Abnormal shape to ears/ear tags	• Partial webbing of fingers and/or toes • Inguinal hernia • Congenital heart defects	• High pitched cat-like cry • Hypotonia • Intellectual disability (moderate to severe)
7q11.2 (Williams syndrome)	<1%	• Bitemporal narrowing of the forehead • Periorbital fullness • Small jaw • Stellate/lacy pattern of irides • Full lips/wide mouth	• Supravalvar aortic stenosis and/or peripheral pulmonic stenosis • Arteriopathy can affect any artery (can result in renovascular hypertension) • Strabismus	• Hypercalcemia/hypercalciuria • Failure to thrive in infancy • Overfriendly personality • Mild cognitive impairment
15q11–q13 (Prader–Willi syndrome)	<70%	• Short stature • Bitemporal narrowing of the forehead • Almond-shaped eyes • Small hands and feet	• Cryptorchidism (hypogonadism in both males and females) • Strabismus • Scoliosis	• Hypotonia in infancy • Failure to thrive (often requiring feeding tube) in infancy • Hyperphagia develops around 5 years of age • Mild cognitive impairment
15q11–q13 (Angelman syndrome)	<1	• Microcephaly develops with time • Dysmorphic features may be absent • Prognathia • Wide mouth, widely spaced teeth	• Strabismus • Scoliosis	• Hypotonia in infancy • Ataxic gait • Seizures • Frequent laughter • Excitability/hand flapping • Absent to minimal speech
16p11	Unlikely	• No consistent dysmorphic features	• No consistent anomalies	• Autism • Cognitive impairment • Variable phenotype, with some individuals who have no symptoms

(continued)

TABLE 6-1. **Continued**

DELETION SYNDROME	PERCENTAGE DETECTABLE BY KARYOTYPE	DYSMORPHIC FEATURES	CONGENITAL ANOMALIES	FUNCTIONAL DEFICITS
17p11.2 (Smith–Magenis syndrome)	Variable	• Short stature • Brachydactyly • Upslanting palpebral fissures • Tented appearance to upper lip	• Middle ear and laryngeal anomalies with coarse, deep voice • Cardiac defects • Iris anomalies/microcornea	• Mild to moderate infantile hypotonia • Failure to thrive in infancy • Chronic sleep disturbance • Mild to moderate cognitive impairment
22q11	Unlikely	• Short palpebral fissures • Bulbous nasal tip • Small ears with overfolded helices	• Conotruncal heart defects • Palatal anomalies (cleft palate; VPI) • Structural renal anomalies	• Hypocalcemia • Immune dysfunction • Learning disabilities

lymphocyte count (with followup T and B cell subsets and referral to an immunologist if low). The immunologic studies may be abnormal in those who are clinically ill as a neonate, so repeat studies should be considered prior to administration of live viral vaccines.[20]

Since infants with the 22q11 deletion syndrome are predisposed to low calcium levels as opposed to high calcium levels (which may be seen in Williams syndrome due to deletion of 7q11), there is no need to assess the urinary excretion of calcium.

The family mentions that they are interested in having more children at some point in the future.

What is the recurrence risk for this family to have another affected child?

A. Since the 22q11 deletion syndrome is inherited in an autosomal dominant fashion, the recurrence risk will be 50% with each future pregnancy
B. Since neither parent has features of the 22q11 deletion, their recurrence risk is close to 1%
C. Their recurrence risk is the same as the incidence of this condition in the general population (about 1/4,000)
D. Since the 22q11 deletion syndrome is inherited in an autosomal recessive fashion, the recurrence risk will be 25% with each future pregnancy
E. The recurrence risk cannot be determined until parental testing for the 22q11 deletion has been performed

Discussion

The correct answer is **E**. There can be extensive clinical variability in the features of the 22q11 deletion

syndrome, even among members of the same family. This does not appear to be due to the size of the deletion itself, as 90% of individuals have the exact same deletion, which is mediated by long terminal repeat elements present in the DNA architecture itself. The reason for such clinical variability is unknown. However, due to this variability, it may not always be possible to detect this condition in a mildly affected parent without a full medical evaluation and parental testing. Approximately 10% of the 22q11 deletion syndrome is inherited from a parent, some of whom will not be diagnosed until the birth of a more severely affected child. FISH testing should be offered to both parents of an affected child to help refine their recurrence risk. If FISH testing is normal for both parents, then the recurrence risk is approximately 1%, based on the risk of gonadal mosaicism for the deletion in one of the parents. Because this family has an affected child, their risk will be above the general population incidence of the condition. The 22q11 deletion syndrome is inherited in an autosomal dominant fashion, so in the event that one of the parents is found to have the 22q11 deletion, the recurrence risk will be 50% with each future pregnancy.

Objectives

1. The most common features of the 22q11 deletion syndrome
2. The appropriate medical evaluations for those affected with the 22q11 deletion syndrome
3. Appropriate genetic counseling for the family of an affected child

TABLE 6-2.   **Congenital Heart Defects and Their Most Specific Associated Syndrome**

CARDIAC MALFORMATION	GENETIC SYNDROME	SYNDROMIC ETIOLOGY
Atrioventricular canal	Down syndrome	47,XX,+21 or 47,XY,+21
Coarctation of the aorta	Turner syndrome	45,X
Conotruncal heart defects	22q11 deletion syndrome	Deletion of 22q11
Peripheral pulmonary artery stenosis	Noonan syndrome	>10 genes; mutations in *PTPN11* account for ~50% of cases
Supravalvular aortic stenosis	Williams syndrome	Deletion 7q11

CASE 10

A 33-week male is admitted to the NICU for prematurity. On physical examination, he is noted to have a grade II hypospadias, but no other external anomalies. His growth parameters are all appropriate for his gestational age. In discussing his care with the family, the mother mentions that at the time of conception, she took several doses of valproic acid (VPA) that was prescribed to her for bipolar disorder. She also drank approximately two glasses of wine per week until she discovered she was pregnant at about 5 weeks of gestation. She denies any other prescription medication use, recreational drug use, or smoking during the pregnancy. She is wondering if the in utero VPA and/or alcohol exposure caused her son's hypospadias.

You answer that

A. These early exposures during pregnancy are unlikely to be related to his hypospadias
B. Since the formation of the external genitalia occurs during the first trimester, it is possible that VPA lead to his birth defect
C. The combination of VPA use and alcohol consumption early in the first trimester could have caused his birth defect
D. Since VPA use during pregnancy is associated with neural tube defects and this infant has a birth defect in the pelvic area, a spine MRI would be indicated to evaluate for an occult neural tube defect
E. Alcohol typically causes birth defects when used heavily in the second and third trimesters of pregnancy

Discussion

The correct answer is **A**. Approximately 80% of pregnant women are exposed to at least one medication or chemical during pregnancy, with the average number of exposures being four.[21] A teratogen is defined as an exposure during pregnancy that has a harmful effect on the fetus. Teratogens can be medications, chemicals, a maternal condition (e.g., insulin-dependent diabetes), or a fetal condition that leads to a harmful effect, most commonly a miscarriage, a birth defect, growth retardation, or neurocognitive abnormalities.

The timing of the exposure is a main factor in determining fetal outcome. In general, the first 15 days after fertilization (which corresponds to weeks 2–4 of gestation based on last menstrual period) are considered the "all or none" period, in which an exposure will either cause a miscarriage (due to severe, unrecoverable damage to the embryo) or there will be no phenotypic affect at all (complete loss of a few cells for which the embryo can compensate). The VPA exposure in this case was likely during this time period and therefore would not be postulated to have caused a fetal affect. The most sensitive time for causing structural birth defects in pregnancy is during the middle to late first trimester (15–60 days postfertilization). It is during this time period that organogenesis occurs and that structural birth defects can result from disruption of the normal developmental processes.[22] VPA exposure during the middle to late first trimester has been associated with neural tube defects; however, in the absence of a gross neural tube defect or an abnormal neurologic examination, spinal MRI would not be indicated for this infant. Hypospadias would not be a typical birth defect seen in either VPA exposure or in fetal alcohol syndrome.

Exposures during the second and third trimester of pregnancy are not likely to result in structural birth defects, with the exception of vascular disruptive defects. Exposures in the second and third trimesters, however, can lead to impaired or abnormal fetal growth and to impaired IQ, as brain development occurs throughout gestation and well into postnatal life.

You are explaining to a pediatric resident that a teratogen is defined as an exposure during pregnancy that produces a pattern of anomalies in exposed individuals at greater than the background risk for birth defects.

What is the background risk of birth defects?
A. 0.5% to 1%
B. 1% to 2%
C. 3% to 4%
D. 5% to 7%
E. 6% to 8%

Discussion

The correct answer is **C**. The background risk of birth defects in the general population is 3% to 4%. An exposure is considered teratogenic if it results in a consistent pattern of anomalies (major malformations and/or minor anomalies) in exposed individuals at greater than the background risk of birth defects.

Helpful Tip: Women who sustain a potential teratogenic exposure prior to 15 days postfertilization (up to 4 weeks' gestation as estimated by last menstrual period) are unlikely to deliver an infant with a phenotype related to that exposure.

CASE 11

A 28-year-old G2P1 mother delivers a term infant with lower limb anomalies, including sacral agenesis, shortened and bowed femurs, shortened and bowed fibula with hypoplastic tibia, bilateral talipes equinovarus, and preaxial polydactyly of the feet (Fig. 6-3). He has a heart murmur, and an echocardiogram has been ordered but is pending. The remainder of the physical examination is normal with no upper limb anomalies and no facial dysmorphic features. The maternal history is significant for alcoholism prior to pregnancy. The mother reports that she stopped drinking as soon as she found out she was

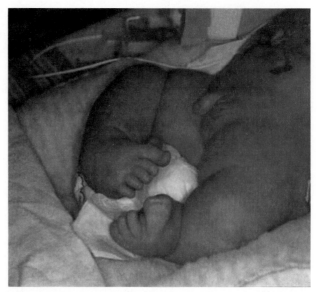

FIGURE 6-3.   Lower limb anomalies seen in the infant in Case 11.

pregnant. She also has a history of insulin-dependent diabetes diagnosed at age 16 years. She states that her glucose control during the pregnancy was good, but the medical records suggest that she had limited prenatal care in the first trimester with several documented blood glucose levels in the 250 to 300 mg/dL range. Her blood glucose control significantly improved starting in the mid-second trimester and was well controlled in the third trimester. The mother also reports that she has an uncle with Down syndrome, but no medical records are available to confirm this diagnosis.

What is the most likely etiology for this infant's features?
A. Diabetic embryopathy
B. Fetal alcohol syndrome
C. Translocation Down syndrome
D. Holt–Oram syndrome
E. Achondroplasia

Discussion

The correct answer is **A**. Diabetes is one of the most common maternal medical complications during pregnancy, and can be either overt (present and diagnosed prior to pregnancy) or gestational (diagnosed during pregnancy, regardless of whether insulin is required for treatment). Women who have insulin-dependent diabetes prior to pregnancy have a 6% to 8% chance of having a child with a birth defect and a 7- to 10-fold increased risk of having a child with a major structural anomaly that is fatal or requires surgery, even if their diabetes is well controlled during pregnancy.[23,24] Women with gestational diabetes likely have a risk that is above the general population risk of having a child with a birth defect, but their risk may be lower than women with insulin-dependent diabetes diagnosed prior to pregnancy.

Women who have poorly controlled diabetes during the first trimester of pregnancy are at risk of having an infant with diabetic embryopathy, including cardiac malformations, central nervous system malformations, renal and urinary tract anomalies, and skeletal anomalies.[25] Caudal regression syndrome, which is characterized by maldevelopment of the sacrum and lower limbs, vertebral anomalies, renal anomalies, imperforate anus, neural tube defects, and genitourinary malformations, is a commonly known association with maternal diabetes, although genetic causes for this type of birth defect have also been discovered. The finding of sacral hypoplasia/aplasia, hypoplasia of the tibia, and preaxial polydactyly of the feet is highly suggestive of diabetic embryopathy.[24] The underlying mechanism that leads to diabetic embryopathy is poorly understood, although it has been postulated that increased oxidative stress caused by hyperglycemia and other metabolic derangements in the mother leads to excessive embryonic cell apoptosis.[26]

The types of limb anomalies seen in this infant would be very unusual for fetal alcohol syndrome, in which individuals typically have prenatal growth retardation, microcephaly, and facial dysmorphic features, including short palpebral fissures, a long and smooth philtrum, and a thin vermillion of the upper lip. Individuals with Down syndrome likewise typically have facial dysmorphic features and do not have the types of limb anomalies described in this infant.

Holt–Oram syndrome is typically characterized by congenital heart defects (often ASD or VSD) and asymmetric upper limb anomalies, such as thumb hypoplasia or duplication, radial–ulnar anomalies, and phocomelia (severe hypoplasia or aplasia of the upper portion of a limb so that the hand/fingers attach directly to the trunk). Lower limb involvement is typically not seen in Holt–Oram syndrome.

While this infant has reduced length of the lower extremities, he does not have other features of achondroplasia, the most common form of short limb dwarfism. Individuals with this condition typically do not have polydactyly or sacral agenesis; in addition, the upper extremities would be expected to be shortened. The child would also be anticipated to have macrocephaly with frontal bossing, a depressed nasal bridge, and midfacial hypoplasia.

Helpful Tip: Pregnant women with pre-existing diabetes should undergo a high-level ultrasound and a fetal echocardiogram to screen for fetal birth defects.

You note that unlike many infants born to women with gestational diabetes, this infant is not macrosomic and does not have several other complications common to infants of diabetic mothers, such as hypoglycemia, polycythemia, hyperbilirubinemia, or electrolyte abnormalities.

What is the most likely explanation for why this infant does not display some of the most common features seen in infants born to women with gestational diabetes?
A. The mother had pre-existing diabetes and not gestational diabetes
B. The above complications are more likely to occur when diabetes is poorly controlled during the second and third trimesters
C. The infant likely has a genetic syndrome and not issues related to maternal diabetes
D. The above complications are more likely to occur if oral hypoglycemic medications are used to control maternal diabetes during pregnancy and not if insulin is used
E. The above findings are seen only when the infant possesses genetic susceptibilities to them and are unrelated to maternal glucose control during pregnancy

Discussion

The correct answer is **B**. Women who have poorly controlled diabetes after the first trimester, regardless of whether diabetes was diagnosed prior to or during the pregnancy, have an increased risk for diabetic fetopathy. Diabetic fetopathy is characterized by fetal macrosomia, hypoglycemia, polycythemia, hyperbilirubinemia, electrolyte abnormalities (i.e., hypocalcemia, hypomagnesemia), and cardiomyopathy, leading to increased obstetrical and neonatal complications but not to birth defects. The level of maternal glucose control inversely correlates with the degree of diabetic fetopathy. The means by which maternal diabetes is controlled does not play a role in whether an infant develops diabetic fetopathy. The absence of evidence of diabetic fetopathy in an infant with birth defects consistent with diabetes does not preclude diabetic embryopathy as the cause.

CASE 12

A woman with a known seizure disorder that is refractory to antiepileptic medications other than phenytoin was maintained on phenytoin throughout her pregnancy. She delivers a term female infant. On examination, the infant appears nondysmorphic and has normal growth parameters. The infant has appropriate tone and appears to be feeding well. The pediatric resident is surprised that the infant does not have any birth defects or other anomalies despite the fact that a known teratogenic medication was used throughout pregnancy.

What is the most likely reason why this infant does not display any birth defects or other anomalies?
A. The mother of the infant was likely noncompliant with the medication, so the infant likely did not have a significant exposure
B. The use of supplemental folic acid during the pregnancy can reverse all of the teratogenic effects of this medication
C. Genetic susceptibilities play a role in whether an exposed fetus sustains affects from a teratogenic exposure
D. Phenytoin is not known to be teratogenic during pregnancy
E. The teratogenic effects of this medication are only present when a woman also consumes alcohol during the pregnancy

Discussion

The correct answer is **C**. It is important to realize that teratogenic affects have been clearly demonstrated for only about 30 drug treatments in humans.[27] Table 6-3 lists several known teratogens and the features they may produce in exposed pregnancies. Avoiding all drugs during pregnancy can be dangerous to both maternal and fetal health, as untreated maternal conditions, such as diabetes and hypertension, can lead to serious birth defects and/or fetal demise. Even those substances that are clearly teratogenic, such as isotretinoin, methotrexate, VPA, carbamazepine, and thalidomide, cause birth defects in only a subset of exposed individuals. While both the timing of the exposure during pregnancy and the dose of the exposure are important factors in determining if a fetus will be affected, genetic susceptibilities (most of which have not yet been identified) likely also play a role in whether an exposed fetus sustains affects. Supplemental folic acid during pregnancy may decrease the risk of having a child with a neural tube defect and therefore is used in those who are taking VPA during pregnancy; however, folic acid supplementation will not

TABLE 6-3.   List of Teratogens and their Common Affects

TERATOGEN	COMMON AFFECTS
Isotretinoin (Accutane)	• Aural atresia (hypoplastic or absent ears) • Conotruncal heart malformations • Hydrocephalus and brain malformations • Cognitive deficits
Maternal alcohol use (fetal alcohol syndrome)	• Prenatal growth retardation, affecting length and/or weight, that persists postnatally • Structural central nervous system anomaly (brain malformation and/or microcephaly) • Characteristic facial features (short palpebral fissures; long and smooth philtrum; thin upper lip) • Cognitive and/or neurobehavioral deficits
Maternal diabetes	• Caudal regression syndrome • Congenital heart defects • Central nervous system anomalies • Renal anomalies
Methotrexate	• Craniosynostosis • Hypertelorism (widely spaced eyes) • Limb defects (ulnar digit deficiency; syndactyly) • Congenital heart defects
Phenytoin	• Mild to moderate growth retardation • Wide anterior fontanel • Widely spaced eyes • Hypoplasia of distal phalanges with small nails • Borderline to mild cognitive impairment
Thalidomide	• Skeletal anomalies, including phocomelia (absence of the middle portion of the limb), particularly of the upper extremity
Valproic acid	• Neural tube defects • Congenital heart defects • Hyperconvex nails • Cleft lip

eliminate the risk of having a child with a neural tube defect.

Objectives

1. The definition of a teratogen
2. That the dose and timing of an exposure determines the likelihood that it will cause a fetal affect
3. That medication use during pregnancy may be necessary to avoid adverse fetal outcomes
4. That only a subset of individuals who sustain an adverse exposure during pregnancy will demonstrate an affect

CASE 13

An infant girl is born with hypotonia. She has no other congenital anomalies. An oligonucleotide Chromosomal microarray is sent and returns with a deletion of 15q11–q13.

Based on this finding, what condition does this infant have?
A. PWS
B. Angelman syndrome
C. Williams syndrome
D. Down syndrome
E. It is not possible to tell which condition she has without further molecular characterization

Discussion

The correct answer is **E**. Deletion of 15q11–q13 can lead to either PWS or Angelman syndrome, depending on whether the deletion arose on the maternally derived (Angelman syndrome) or on the paternally derived (PWS) chromosome. PWS and Angelman syndrome are caused by deletion or abnormal expression of genes from the same chromosomal region (15q11–q13) but result in very different phenotypes in older individuals; in early infancy, it may not be possible to distinguish between these two conditions on clinical grounds alone, particularly in a female who may not have discernible hypogonadism on external examination of the genitalia.

Genomic imprinting is the cause of the different phenotypes that result from deletion of 15q11–q13. Some cases are due to abnormal methylation of the 15q11–q13 region without a frank deletion. Neither FISH nor oligonucleotide CMA testing can determine if the deletion arose on the maternally or paternally derived chromosome. Therefore, parent-specific methylation testing of this region is the most informative and most sensitive way of detecting and differentiating between these two disorders.

Further methylation testing is done and determines that this infant has Angelman syndrome. You are discussing the case with your resident and mention that Angelman syndrome is an example of a condition that can be caused by epigenetic changes.

What is meant by the term epigenetics?
A. Modification in gene expression that is not caused by changes in the DNA sequence itself
B. Modification in gene expression caused by sequence alterations in noncoding areas of the DNA
C. Modification in gene expression caused by differential splicing of a gene
D. Modification in gene expression caused by sequence alterations in the promoter region of the gene
E. Modification in gene expression caused by pathogenic mutations in the coding region of the gene

Discussion

The correct answer is **A**. Epigenetics refers to regulation of gene expression without changing the DNA sequence itself. Examples of epigenetic modification that can affect whether a gene is expressed or silenced include DNA methylation and histone modification.

CASE 14

An infant is born at 34 weeks with an omphalocele, macrosomia, and macroglossia. You suspect Beckwith–Wiedemann syndrome (BWS).

This condition can be associated with all of the following medical complications EXCEPT
A. Transient hypoglycemia
B. Body asymmetry which typically improves over time
C. Macroglossia that could require feeding therapy
D. Continued growth leading to gigantism in adulthood
E. A predisposition to the development of embryonal tumors

Discussion

The correct answer is **D**. Beckwith-Wiedemann syndrome is characterized by macrosomia, typically present from birth. The macrosomia may persist into childhood and early adolescence, but adults with this condition typically have growth parameters that are within the normal range (although they may be within the upper limits of normal). Individuals with this condition may have umbilical abnormalities, such as omphalocele or umbilical hernia. They are often born mildly premature (typically after 30 weeks' gestation). They may present with macroglossia, which may result in feeding difficulties and/or the need for speech therapy. Tongue reduction surgery may be indicated in severe cases leading to breathing difficulties.[28]

After birth, individuals with Beckwith-Wiedemann syndrome may have transient hypoglycemia, which often resolves spontaneously. They may be noted to have asymmetry as a result of segmental overgrowth (termed hemihyperplasia), which typically improves over time in most affected individuals.

On abdominal ultrasound they tend to have renomegaly and can also be noted to have adrenomegaly. They have an increased risk of the development of embryonal tumors, particularly Wilms tumor and hepatoblastoma, although neuroblastoma is observed rarely. Because of these issues, individuals with a clinical diagnosis of Beckwith-Wiedemann syndrome undergo tumor screening, which consists most commonly of serum AFP levels every 6 weeks to 3 months until approximately 2 to 3 years of age (to screen for hepatoblastoma) and abdominal ultrasound to include views of the liver and both kidneys every 3 months until 8 years of age (to screen for Wilms tumor).

The family is concerned about whether BWS is an inherited condition.

Beckwith-Wiedemann syndrome is inherited in what manner?
A. An autosomal recessive fashion
B. An autosomal dominant fashion
C. An X-linked fashion
D. Due to an imprinting defect in most cases
E. Due to a mitochondrial disorder in most cases

Discussion

The correct answer is **D**. Beckwith-Wiedemann syndrome can result from a variety of genetic mechanisms, although abnormalities of imprinting (gain of methylation of certain genes, loss of methylation of other genes, or a combination of these) are the most common. A subset of individuals have uniparental disomy of all or part of chromosome 11p15, which leads to an abnormal methylation pattern typically affecting more than one gene. Because imprinting problems are the most common etiology for this condition, recurrence risks for an affected individual and for an affected individual's parents are typically very low.

Objectives

1. What the term epigenetics means
2. How different genetic conditions can be due to abnormalities of the same genetic locus

CASE 15

A 31-year-old G1P0 female delivers a term male with normal growth parameters. The mother reports that she and her husband have infertility and used in vitro fertilization (IVF) with intracytoplasmic sperm injection (ICSI) to conceive this pregnancy. Both parents report that they are healthy. The mother of the infant reports that her brother has mental retardation and her father has a movement disorder.

This couple's infertility could have been due to all of the following conditions EXCEPT
A. One of the individuals in this couple could carry a balanced chromosomal translocation
B. One of the individuals in this couple could carry an unbalanced chromosomal translocation
C. The father has a Y chromosome microdeletion that includes the AZF loci, which leads to azoospermia
D. The father has Klinefelter syndrome (47,XXY)
E. The mother carries a premutation for Fragile X on one of her X-chromosomes

Discussion

The correct answer is **B**. If one of the individuals in this couple carried an unbalanced chromosomal translocation, that individual would be expected to have some type of symptom, such as cognitive impairment, dysmorphic features, or congenital anomalies. Individuals who carry balanced chromosomal translocations (in which there is no net gain or loss of genetic material) are expected to have no overt symptoms, but they are at risk for having multiple miscarriages and/or children with an unbalanced chromosome complement.

One of the causes of male factor infertility is deletion of the AZF loci on the long arm of the Y chromosome (Y-chromosome microdeletion). Individuals who have these deletions typically do not have overt physical features. As long as the *SRY* gene is present on the short arm of the Y-chromosome, typical male genital development will occur, with or without the AZF loci. Other genetic causes of male factor infertility include Klinefelter syndrome (47,XXY), in which males may have unrecognized symptoms prior to their diagnosis of infertility.

Fragile X syndrome is due to expansion of a triplet repeat at the beginning (or 5′ end) of the *FMR1* gene. Women who carry between 54 and 200 CGG repeats (so-called premutation) typically do not have Fragile X syndrome itself, but they are at increased risk for the development of POF (cessation of menses prior to age 40 years) and Fragile X tremor/ataxia syndrome

(FXTAS). A family history of mental retardation (particularly in males) and the presence of older individuals with movement disorders (a male who has FXTAS due to a premutation) could be consistent with a family history of Fragile X syndrome.[29]

Helpful Tip: In couples who have experienced three or more miscarriages, a chromosome analysis should be performed on each member of the couple to evaluate for a balanced chromosomal translocation. This cannot be performed using CMA, as CMA will only detect a net gain or loss of genetic material and does not evaluate for the arrangement of the genetic material.

The mother reports that she was diagnosed with POF as the cause of her infertility. She also reports that as part of her evaluation for POF, she was tested for Fragile X syndrome and found to have a premutation (CGG expansion in the range of 150 repeats). The family decided not to pursue prenatal testing for Fragile X syndrome in their son but would like to have him tested now. You note that their son has no dysmorphic features, no congenital anomalies, and normal growth parameters.

Which of the following is true?
A. Testing is not indicated, as their son has no features of the condition
B. Their son has a 50% chance of being affected
C. Their son has a 100% chance of being affected
D. Their son has a 25% chance of being affected
E. CGG expansions occur only through the paternal lineage, so their son is only at risk of being a premutation carrier

Discussion

The correct answer is **B**. Throughout the genome there are many repeated sequences. Short repeat sequences of three nucleotides (such as CGG-CGG-CGG) can be unstable during human meiosis, the process by which haploid germ cells are created from diploid precursor cells. The expansion of such sequences can occur outside of the coding region of a gene or within the coding sequence of the gene. When they occur within the coding sequence of the gene, they can result in the formation of an abnormal protein, as each trinucleotide (or three nucleotides together) codes for a specific amino acid that will be added to the protein product. An example of a trinucleotide repeat that occurs within a gene and that alters protein function, leading to disease, is Huntington disease. In other situations, expansion of repeats directly outside of the gene (i.e., at the 5′ or beginning portion of the coding sequence of the gene) can become methylated (methyl groups are added to the

repeating elements once they reach a certain length). When this happens, the gene next to the methylated repeat element can be turned off (an example of epigenetic regulation), resulting in no transcription of the gene, which means that no protein product is made. An example of this phenomenon is Fragile X syndrome.

In the question, the mother has 2 X chromosomes; therefore her son either inherited the X chromosome without the Fragile X premutation (50% chance) or the X chromosome with the Fragile X premutation (50% chance). However, as triplet repeat expansions in Fragile X syndrome are unstable during female meiosis, there is virtually a 100% chance that the mother's premutation expanded to a full mutation (>200 CGG repeats) in the egg. Therefore, a male who inherited the X chromosome with the expanded repeats would be expected to be affected by Fragile X.

You ask the mother of this baby to provide more information about her brother with mental retardation. She states that he is unable to live independently although he is able to participate in activities of daily living with support. He is toilet trained. She provides a picture of him, which demonstrates the appearance of macrocephaly and a long, thin face. You suspect that he is affected by Fragile X syndrome.

Which of the following statements about Fragile X syndrome is true?
A. Males with Fragile X syndrome have macroorchidism at birth
B. Females who carry Fragile X syndrome are not at risk for learning problems
C. Fragile X syndrome is one of the most common inherited forms of cognitive impairment
D. Only males with a head circumference two standard deviations above the mean or greater should be tested for Fragile X syndrome
E. The average IQ in males with Fragile X syndrome is 80

Discussion

The correct answer is **C**. Fragile X syndrome is one of the most common inherited forms of cognitive impairment, previously denoted as mental retardation. Mental retardation is defined as an IQ level of less than 70. The term "mental retardation," however, has come to be regarded as derogatory within the general population, such that other terms, such as "cognitive impairment" or "intellectual disability" have largely replaced it. However, neither cognitive impairment nor intellectual disability (both of which denote an IQ level of less than 70) should be confused with learning disabilities, in which individuals can have a normal IQ level but may have functional learning deficits that require special help in school. Developmental disability denotes a situation in which an infant or young child is noted to be behind his/her age-matched peers with regard to developmental progress. This term implies that an individual has the ability to "catch up" to his/her same-aged peers. In those who are adolescents or older and are still behind their peers developmentally, the term developmental delay is less appropriate, as it is unlikely that the affected individual will be able to catch up to his/her same-aged peers.

Males with Fragile X syndrome typically have a head circumference that is >50th percentile for age. At birth and in early infancy individuals with this condition may have hypotonia, gastroesophageal reflux disease, and frequent otitis media, but the other features of Fragile X syndrome typically develop over time. Macroorchidism is not present at birth but may develop after puberty. Therefore, Fragile X syndrome is difficult to diagnose through clinical features alone in young children, and molecular genetic testing to determine the number of CGG repeats is required for diagnosis. Chromosome analysis or karyotype will not detect Fragile X syndrome. In the above case, testing for Fragile X syndrome can be pursued to determine whether this baby is affected. The earlier that the diagnosis is made, the earlier interventional therapies can be instituted, which help to optimize developmental outcome.

Although Fragile X syndrome was originally thought to be inherited in an X-linked recessive fashion (in which males are affected and carrier females are unaffected) it has now been realized that the features of Fragile X syndrome can affect both males and females. The degree of intellectual impairment in females depends primarily upon X-inactivation. If the X chromosome which has the expanded repeat is the X chromosome that is expressed in most cells, then the female will be affected, sometimes to the same degree that is seen in affected males. However, affected females are typically less severely impaired than males, who often have IQ levels in the 30 to 50 range.[30]

Helpful Tip: Any male with developmental delay or intellectual impairment who does not have a known diagnosis should be tested for Fragile X syndrome.

As you are explaining more about Fragile X syndrome to the medical student, she asks you about other conditions that are due to triplet repeat expansion.

Which of the following disorders is also due to a triplet repeat expansion?
A. Trisomy 18
B. Marfan syndrome
C. Triploidy
D. Duchenne muscular dystrophy
E. Myotonic dystrophy type 1

Discussion

The correct answer is **E**. Myotonic dystrophy type 1 is caused by a CTG trinucleotide repeat in the noncoding region of *DMPK*. Individuals with myotonic dystrophy can have mild features, classic features, or congenital myotonic dystrophy. Congenital myotonic dystrophy is characterized by hypotonia with severe muscle weakness at birth, which may be accompanied by respiratory insufficiency and shortened lifespan. Individuals with congenital myotonic dystrophy typically have less severely affected parents, and occasionally a parent may not have noticeable features of the condition.[31]

Marfan syndrome is an autosomal dominant connective tissue disorder that is characterized by involvement primarily of the cardiovascular, ocular, and skeletal systems. Early onset of features in the neonatal period, so-called Neonatal Marfan syndrome, is present in less than 15% of affected individuals.[32] Affected infants may have typical features of the condition, including dolichostenomelia (extremities that are disproportionately long for the size of the trunk), thin body build, arachnodactyly (long fingers), hyperextensible joints, scoliosis, chest wall deformity (pectus carinatum or excavatum), joint contractures (more common when the condition presents in the neonatal period), loose and redundant skin, and high-arched palate. Cardiovascular manifestations can include mitral valve prolapse and aortic root dilatation (typically at the level of the sinuses of Valsalva). Ophthalmologic anomalies may include myopia and ectopia lentis (dislocation of the lens).

Triploidy is due to the presence of an entire extra monosomic set of chromosomes (e.g., 69,XXX or 69,XXY), such that the affected individual has three copies of each chromosome instead of two copies. The extra set of chromosomes can either be paternally derived, in which case the placenta is typically large with cystic changes (partial molar placenta), or maternally derived, in which case the placenta may be small without molar changes. Most triploid pregnancies result in either a miscarriage or stillbirth, but live born infants have been reported. Physical features typically include small for gestational age growth parameters, widely spaced eyes, congenital heart defects, and syndactyly of fingers three and four. Triploidy is typically sporadic with a resultant low recurrence risk.[2]

Duchenne muscular dystrophy is one of the most common forms of muscular dystrophy. It is inherited in an X-linked fashion, with males having severe features of the condition with shortened life span.

In many triplet repeat expansion disorders, the age of onset of symptoms is earlier and the severity of symptoms worsens with each generation.

What is the term used to describe this phenomenon?
A. Anticipation
B. Variable expressivity
C. Codominance
D. Digenic inheritance
E. Mosaicism

Discussion

The correct answer is **A**. Conditions that are caused by triplet repeat expansions may be subject to anticipation, where the age of onset is earlier and the severity of symptoms worsens with each generation. Anticipation should not be confused with variable expressivity, in which individuals with the same mutation in the same family may have differing features, with some who seem to have earlier onset and more severe features compared to other family members. Variable expressivity can be seen in many genetic conditions, including Marfan syndrome and the 22q11 deletion syndrome. However, with variable expressivity the features are sometimes milder in successive generations, which do not occur with anticipation. The cause for variable expressivity is frequently unknown, although modifier genes and environmental differences may play a role in the expression of the condition in the affected individual.

Codominance refers to the situation in which both alleles are equally expressed and both exert a phenotypic affect. Digenic inheritance refers to a disease which results from the inheritance of mutations in two different genes cooccurring to cause the phenotype in an individual. Mosaicism is the occurrence of two or more cell lines with different genetic constitutions in the same individual. The term mosaicism implies that all cell lines can be derived from the same ancestral cell line.

The medical student reminds you that this family used IVF with ICSI to conceive this pregnancy. She asks you whether this could confer additional risks to their son.

Which of the following is true of IVF and/or ICSI?
A. IVF alone does not increase the risk of birth defects
B. The risk of birth defects in those who undergo IVF with ICSI is twice that of those who undergo IVF without ICSI
C. Neither IVF nor IVF with ICSI increases the risk of birth defects
D. There is no difference between the rate of birth defects in those who undergo IVF alone versus those who undergo IVF with ICSI
E. IVF does not impact epigenetic modification or imprinting

Discussion

The correct answer is **D**. There is an increased risk of birth defects in those who undergo IVF, but this risk appears to be the same for IVF alone and for IVF with ICSI.[33] The absolute risk of birth defects and the types of birth defects seen varies from study to study. Whether IVF with or without other embryo manipulation increases the risk of having a child with an epigenetic or imprinting defect has been the subject of much research. Current evidence suggests that IVF does impact epigenetic modification, but whether this truly leads to an increase in genetic diseases caused by epigenetic mechanisms (e.g., Angelman syndrome or BWS) in the offspring is still unclear.[34]

Objectives

1. The clinical features of Fragile X syndrome
2. What is meant by a triplet repeat expansion disorder
3. The difference between anticipation and variable expressivity
4. The risks if IVF

CASE 16

An infant is born with multiple congenital anomalies, including vertebral anomalies, a congenital heart defect, and a unilateral multicystic dysplastic kidney.

All of the following conditions are in the differential diagnosis for this constellation of findings EXCEPT
A. CHARGE syndrome
B. The 22q11 deletion syndrome
C. Osteogenesis imperfecta (OI)
D. Fanconi anemia
E. VACTERL association

Discussion

The correct answer is **C**. When an infant is born with multiple congenital anomalies, the most likely etiology is a chromosome abnormality. However, there are a number of single-gene disorders and nonchromosomal conditions that can lead to multiple congenital anomalies in specific patterns.

Helpful Tip: Not every individual with a genetic condition will have all of the features that have been described to be associated with that particular condition.

The combination of vertebral anomalies, congenital heart defect, and renal anomalies occurring together is common. The differential diagnosis for this group of anomalies depends on the evaluation of other organ systems combined with a thorough physical examination to evaluate for dysmorphic features. Conditions that may commonly present with this constellation of features includes CHARGE (**C**oloboma, **H**eart defects, Choanal **A**tresia, **R**etarded growth and development, **G**enital anomalies, **E**ar anomalies/hearing loss) syndrome, Fanconi anemia, the 22q11 deletion syndrome, and VAC-TERL (**V**ertebral anomalies, **A**nal atresia, **C**ardiac defects, **T**racheoesophageal fistula with esophageal atresia, **R**enal anomalies/dysplasia, **L**imb defects) association. Each of these conditions, however, has distinguishing features (see Table 6-4). In CHARGE syndrome, individuals frequently have colobomas of the iris, retina, and/or optic nerve, which are unusual in the other conditions listed. Because colobomas of the retina and/or optic nerve can occur without coloboma of the iris, an ophthalmology evaluation is indicated for those with the combination of congenital heart defect, vertebral anomalies and renal anomalies.[35] Likewise, in those who present with choanal atresia or choanal stenosis, CHARGE syndrome should be within the differential diagnosis and a search for other features of this condition should be undertaken. The typical appearance of the ear in an individual with CHARGE syndrome is shown in Figure 6-4.

Fanconi anemia most frequently is accompanied by radial ray/thumb anomalies, which are not common in CHARGE syndrome or the 22q11 deletion syndrome. The bone marrow features of Fanconi anemia may not be present at birth or even in early childhood.[36]

OI includes a group of conditions associated with increased fracture of bones with or without bony deformities. Individuals with OI can have a variety of different findings depending on the type of OI present. Type I is the mildest type, in which individuals typically appear normal at birth without bony deformities or fractures. They may have blue slcerae at birth, although this can be seen in normal infants under 1 year of age. Type II OI is the perinatal lethal form in which individuals have multiple fractures at birth and have undermineralization of the calvarium. Types III and IV can be associated with

TABLE 6-4. Distinguishing Features of CHARGE Syndrome, Fanconi Anemia, the 22q11 Deletion Syndrome, and VACTERL Association

SYNDROME	INHERITANCE PATTERN	ANOMALIES	ETIOLOGY
CHARGE	Autosomal dominant (many cases *de novo*)	• Coloboma (iris, retina, and/or optic nerve) • Heart defects • Choanal atresia (unilateral or bilateral) • Retarded growth and development • Genital anomalies • Ear anomalies/hearing loss	• Mutations in *CHD7* account for ~65% of cases • Remainder of cases, etiology unknown
Fanconi anemia	Primarily autosomal recessive	• Congenital heart defects • Bone marrow failure (typically in the first decade) • Ear anomalies/hearing loss • Increased risk of malignancy • Pigmentation anomalies (i.e., café au lait spots) • Thumb anomalies (absent, hypoplastic, triphalangeal) • Skeletal anomalies	• Multiple single genes (at least 15 known genes)
22q11 deletion (aka DiGeorge syndrome, velocardiofacial syndrome)	Autosomal dominant	• Conotruncal heart defects • Palatal anomalies (cleft palate; VPI) • Scoliosis (rare vertebral/spine anomalies) • Structural renal anomalies	• 22q11 deletion
VACTERL association (NOT a syndrome)	Not typically inherited	• Vertebral anomalies • Anal atresia| • Cardiac defects • Tracheoesophageal fistula with esophageal atresia • Renal anomalies/dysplasia • Limb defects (often radial ray anomalies)	• Unknown in most cases • May see this constellation of features as part of diabetic embryopathy • May not be genetic

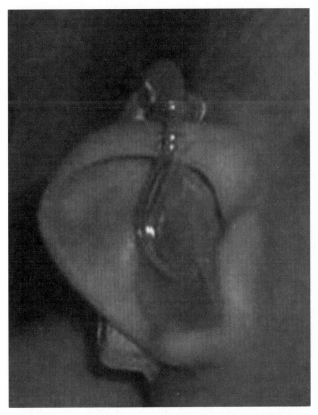

FIGURE 6-4. Typical ear configuration in an infant with CHARGE syndrome. Note the hearing aid, which denotes that the infant has hearing loss.

bony deformities at birth, in utero fractures or fractures with routine care. Blue sclera may or may not be present. Dentinogenesis imperfecta (translucent gray or brown teeth that break and wear easily) is also a variable feature, found more commonly in OI types II and III. Individuals with OI typically develop short stature and they may develop hearing loss in later childhood/adulthood, but they typically to not have other congenital anomalies that affect the heart or kidney.[37]

CASE 17

You are called 3 minutes after the vaginal delivery of a 39-week infant male born to a 35-year-old G4P0012 mother. The pregnancy was uncomplicated. His mother is group B strep (GBS) negative with no recent illnesses and no fever during delivery. The infant had a nuchal cord noted at the time of delivery. Immediately after

birth the baby was noted to be flaccid, apneic, and cyanotic. He does not respond to stimulation and suctioning. The 1-minute Apgar score is 4 and at 5 minutes you assign another Apgar score of 4. You give several minutes of positive pressure ventilation and then start continuous positive airway pressure (CPAP). He has slow improvement in his color but he remains flaccid and appears to be responsive only to painful stimuli with eye opening. On physical examination he is noted to have all growth parameters at the 10th percentile for gestational age. He has a tall forehead with a large anterior fontanelle that extends into the metopic suture. He has a depressed nasal bridge with anteverted nares. Genitourinary examination is normal male. He has no other anomalies on examination except extreme hypotonia with difficulty to elicit reflexes.

All of the following conditions are within your differential diagnosis EXCEPT
A. Spinal muscular atrophy
B. PWS
C. A peroxisomal disorder
D. Congenital myotonic dystrophy
E. 22q11 deletion syndrome

Discussion

The correct answer is **E**. While this infant is noted to have some dysmorphic features, it would be unusual for a child with the 22q11 deletion syndrome (DiGeorge syndrome; velocardiofacial syndrome) to present with this degree of hypotonia and unresponsiveness after a normal delivery at term. The other conditions listed can all result in significant hypotonia that is typically noted immediately after birth.

Which of the following clinical evaluations would be appropriate to pursue to help direct further genetic testing?
A. Head MRI
B. Ophthalmology evaluation
C. Skeletal survey
D. Echocardiogram
E. All of the above

Discussion

The correct answer is **E**. At this early juncture, the differential diagnosis for this degree of hypotonia is large and further clinical evaluations can be helpful in determining an appropriate course of action to direct further testing. While infection is a primary cause of acute illness in the neonate, once an infectious etiology has been appropriately excluded, further clinical evaluations to determine a possible etiology for hypotonia are warranted. Hypotonia can be caused by a problem in the central nervous system, the peripheral nervous system, and/or the muscular system. Furthermore, both chromosomal abnormalities and inborn errors of metabolism can affect one or more of these systems.

Head MRI is most useful in determining if there is an underlying brain malformation which can explain hypotonia. In addition, certain biochemical genetic conditions (i.e., aminoacidopathies like maple syrup urine disease; peroxisomal disorders like Zellweger syndrome) will result in white matter changes which can alert the physician to an inborn error of metabolism.

Ophthalmologic evaluation is also helpful in determining if cataracts or other eye anomalies are present, which can be seen in chromosome abnormalities, inborn errors of metabolism and some myopathies, such as congenital myotonic dystrophy.

A skeletal survey is helpful in the evaluation of peroxisomal disorders and other genetic syndromes which may be associated with multiple congenital anomalies. In peroxisomal disorders, chondrodysplasia punctata (stippling of the epiphyses) of the patella(e) and long bones may be seen. The finding of chondrodysplasia punctata is not specific for peroxisomal disorders, however, and can be seen as a finding in individuals with congenital disorders of bones and cartilage (i.e., X-linked chondrodysplasias types 1 and 2) or as a result of a teratogenic exposure (warfarin embryopathy; vitamin K deficiency in the fetus due to maternal gastrointestinal malabsorption, including previous maternal bariatric surgery).[38,39]

In a neonate with hypotonia and respiratory distress, a genetic syndrome involving a congenital heart defect must also be considered, for which an echocardiogram would be indicated.

While taking the family history, it is determined that the patient's parents are both healthy and well. The patient's father has a brother (the patient's paternal uncle) with a clinical diagnosis of Duchenne muscular dystrophy. The paternal uncle is currently 19 years of age and became wheelchair bound at age 11 years. The paternal uncle currently has significant respiratory compromise and cardiomyopathy. He was diagnosed with Duchenne muscular dystrophy on the basis of muscle biopsy, which was not confirmed through molecular genetic testing.

In light of this further information, which of the following is true?

A. A serum creatine phosphokinase (CK) level would not be a useful test at this age, as individuals with Duchenne muscular dystrophy typically do not have elevations of their CK level until later childhood
B. It is extremely unlikely that the hypotonia in this patient is related to the family history, as Duchenne muscular dystrophy is an X-linked condition
C. A muscle biopsy would be indicated to evaluate for the presence of dystrophin protein through immunohistochemistry
D. Genetic testing for Duchenne muscular dystrophy is now available and is indicated for this patient, despite the fact that the patient's uncle has a clinical diagnosis of Duchenne muscular dystrophy that was not confirmed through genetic testing
E. It is most likely that the reason this patient has severe hypotonia is that he also has Duchenne muscular dystrophy, which is an autosomal dominant condition with reduced penetrance

Discussion

The correct answer is **B**. DMD is an X-linked condition which primarily affects males. Females who carry a mutation in the *DMD* gene are typically asymptomatic in childhood but they have an increased risk of developing dilated cardiomyopathy in adulthood. Since the patient is male, he inherited the Y chromosome from his father and the X chromosome from his mother. DMD is a severe condition in males and is not known to have reduced penetrance; therefore, it would be expected that if the patient's father had inherited DMD he would be symptomatic, which he is not. In addition, severe hypotonia at birth is not a feature of DMD and therefore the likelihood that the patient has DMD as a cause of his hypotonia is extremely low and molecular genetic testing of *DMD* would not be warranted.[40]

Males affected with DMD typically have significantly elevated serum CK levels (>10 times the normal range) from early infancy. Therefore, measurement of serum CK level in a known at-risk male would be an appropriate screening test prior to pursuing molecular genetic testing. Of note, CK levels may gradually decrease with advancing age in affected males due to muscle loss over time, but will never be in the normal range.

While muscle biopsy with Western blot analysis and immunohistochemical staining for the dystrophin protein was the gold standard for diagnosis in the past, molecular genetic testing is now considered a first-line test for suspected DMD. It is most useful to perform molecular genetic testing on a known affected relative first; however, if it is difficult or impossible to obtain molecular genetic testing on a previously diagnosed family member (i.e., no

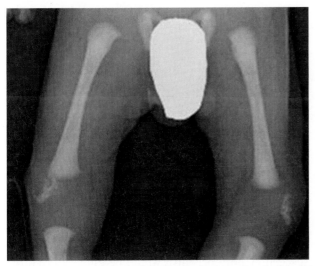

FIGURE 6-5.   Radiograph of the femurs for the patient in Case 17.

living relative to test), molecular genetic testing can be pursued on a symptomatic at-risk individual.

Helpful Tip: The presence of male-to-male transmission of a condition excludes the possibility of X-linked inheritance.

Further evaluations for this infant include an echocardiogram that is normal and an abdominal ultrasound that demonstrates liver and renal cysts. A head MRI shows delayed myelination and bifrontal cortical thickening consistent with pachygyria. A radiograph of the femurs is represented in Figure 6-5.

Laboratory values are as follows:

Sodium	144 mEq/L
Potassium	3.4 mEq/L
Chloride	109 mEq/L
Bicarbonate	30 mEq/L
BUN	4 mEq/L
Creatinine	0.7 mEq/L
Glucose	85 mg/dl
AST	120 IU/L
ASL	59 IU/L
Creatine kinase	91 IU/L
Capillary blood gas:	pH 7.32; pCO$_2$ 64 mmHg; pO$_2$ 51 mmHg; bicarbonate 32 mEq/L

Which of the following laboratory tests would be indicated next?

A. Plasma very long chain fatty acids
B. Plasma amino acids
C. Urine organic acids
D. Plasma ammonia level
E. Plasma acylcarnitine profile

Discussion

The correct answer is **A**. The clinical features, which include severe hypotonia, large anterior fontanelle, liver dysfunction, and chondrodysplasia punctata (Fig. 6-5) is very suggestive of a peroxisomal disorder, such as Zellweger syndrome. Plasma very long chain fatty acid analysis is the most informative initial screening test for this group of disorders. While plasma ammonia level would be indicated in this situation, the clinical findings of abnormal gyral pattern and chondrodysplasia punctata would argue against an inborn error of metabolism such as ornithine transcarbamylase (OTC) deficiency. In the absence of acidosis and other significant electrolyte abnormalities, an organic acidemia or aminoacidopathy would be less likely. A fatty acid oxidation disorder, for which an acylcarnitine profile would screen, would be unlikely in the absence of hypoglycemia.

Objectives

1. The distinguishing features between CHARGE syndrome, the 22q11 deletion syndrome, Fanconi anemia, and VACTERL association
2. How to assess when the family history is relevant to a patient's condition
3. What evaluations are most useful in the initial investigation of a hypotonic neonate

CASE 18

A 5-day-old infant is admitted for suspected sepsis. He has been breastfeeding inconsistently and developed vomiting and decreased urine output over the past few days. The prenatal history was unremarkable. The mother was GBS positive, and the infant was delivered at 36 weeks' gestational age via cesarean section due to preterm labor. On admission, his weight is 10% below birth weight. He is noted to be jaundiced, and the liver extends 4 cm below the costal margin. He has bilateral cataracts. His laboratory studies demonstrate the following: elevated WBC count, AST 375 IU/L, ALT 298 IU/L, total bilirubin 17 mg/dL, conjugated bilirubin 7 mg/dL, prothrombin time 19, INR 1.9, PTT 42. An infectious workup and antibiotics are initiated. His blood culture grows *Escherichia coli*. Once stable, enteral feeds are started with breast milk. His jaundice worsens and he develops bloody stools.

Which study can help establish the underlying diagnosis?
A. Abdominal x-ray
B. Rubella serology
C. Urine-reducing substances
D. Cytomegalovirus DNA polymerase chain reaction (PCR)
E. Liver biopsy

Discussion

The correct answer is **C**. This infant presents with classic features of galactosemia including failure to thrive, cataracts, hepatomegaly, jaundice, liver dysfunction, bleeding diathesis, and *E. coli* sepsis. Galactosemia is caused by deficiency of the enzyme galactose-1-phosphate uridylyltransferase (GALT), which is required to break down galactose. Decreased or absent enzyme activity results in accumulation of toxic substrates and impairment of other biochemical pathways, leading to complications in the neonatal period and later in life. Galactosemia is usually diagnosed through newborn screening programs. The test consists of measuring GALT activity from a blood spot. Molecular genetic testing is also available. However, in an acutely ill newborn, urine-reducing substances can be performed rapidly and can help guide appropriate intervention. The presence of reducing substances in the absence of glucosuria, along with the clinical presentation above, strongly suggests a diagnosis of galactosemia. Other causes of direct hyperbilirubinemia, such as biliary atresia or Alagille syndrome, would not be expected to cause the constellation of features above. Liver biopsy would not be indicated at this early stage of evaluation. Congenital infections cause various complications but not the presentation above.

Helpful Tip: Galactosemia should be within the differential diagnosis of a neonate or young infant who develops *E. coli* sepsis.

What is the most appropriate treatment for this condition?
A. Continue breastfeeding
B. Switch to an elemental formula with supplemental breastfeeding
C. Switch to an elemental formula and add carnitine supplementation
D. Switch to a soy-based formula
E. Switch to a low protein formula

Discussion

The correct answer is **D**. Treatment consists of eliminating galactose and its sources from the diet, including lactose, which is a disaccharide of galactose and glucose. Breastfeeding must be discontinued, and soy-based formulas are used. Neither low protein formula

nor carnitine supplementation is needed in patients with galactosemia.

What is the most likely cause for the bloody stools seen in this case?
A. Necrotizing enterocolitis
B. Sepsis
C. Milk protein allergy
D. Intussusception
E. Coagulopathy from liver dysfunction

Discussion

The correct answer is **E**. The bloody stools in this case are due to coagulopathy resulting from liver dysfunction rather than from necrotizing enterocolitis or from intussusception, both of which would be unlikely given the patient's age. Milk protein allergy is unlikely given the other features seen in this patient. Sepsis alone would not be expected to lead to bloody stools.

Objective

1. The clinical features of galactosemia

CASE 19

A 30-year-old G2P1 female presents at 35 weeks' gestational age with icteric sclerae. Her previous pregnancy was uncomplicated, and the current pregnancy has been unremarkable thus far. She notes normal fetal movements, and ultrasounds and laboratory studies have been normal. Starting 2 days ago, her family members noted that her eyes appeared yellow, so she presented for further evaluation. Her vital signs are stable. She complains of mild abdominal pain. Her liver enzymes and bilirubin level are elevated. Upon further diagnostic evaluation, she is diagnosed with acute fatty liver of pregnancy (AFLP). The biophysical profile is normal.

After delivery, the baby should be monitored for which of the following?
A. Hyperammonemia
B. Lactic acidosis
C. Hypoglycemia
D. Hypernatremia
E. Hypocalcemia

Discussion

The correct answer is **C**. AFLP is a rare complication that arises in the third trimester. Sometimes pregnant women also have features of maternal HELLP (**H**emolysis,

Elevated Liver enzymes, and Low Platelets) syndrome. There is a well-described association between mothers with AFLP and fetuses affected with LCHAD (long chain 3-hydroxyacyl-CoA dehydrogenase) deficiency. These mothers are obligate carriers of the condition. Other fatty acid oxidation disorders have been reported to cause AFLP or maternal HELLP syndrome including medium-chain acyl-CoA dehydrogenase (MCAD) deficiency, carnitine palmitoyltransferase I (CPT-I) deficiency, and trifunctional protein deficiency. The characteristic feature of fatty acid oxidation disorders is hypo- or nonketotic hypoglycemia. Indeed, some infants die of an apparent SIDS event once they begin to sleep through the night. During an acute crisis, patients may develop a Reye-like syndrome with severe hepatic dysfunction. During these episodes, hyperammonemia can occur, but otherwise it is not a concern. Electrolyte disturbances are not associated with defects in fatty acid oxidation.

What is the best screening test to evaluate for a fatty acid oxidation disorder?
A. Plasma amino acids
B. Plasma acylcarnitine profile
C. Urine organic acids
D. Very long chain fatty acids
E. Lipid profile

Discussion

The correct answer is **B**. A plasma acylcarnitine profile is the best screening test for an underlying fatty acid oxidation disorder. However, the acylcarnitine profile may be normal during periods of wellness, so a single normal test drawn in an asymptomatic individual cannot rule out the diagnosis. If the index of suspicion is high, a plasma acylcarnitine profile should be obtained after a fast or during a hypoglycemic episode. Molecular genetic testing can also be pursued if a specific fatty acid oxidation disorder is suspected; however, this is not routinely done in the absence of either an abnormal acylcarnitine profile which suggests a specific fatty acid oxidation disorder or in the absence of a family history of a specific disorder. An acylcarnitine profile is now a routine part of the newborn screen in most states. Plasma amino acids are used to screen for aminoacidopathies, such as phenylketonuria, and urea cycle disorders. Urine organic acids are helpful in the diagnosis of many inborn errors of metabolism including fatty acid oxidation disorders, but an acylcarnitine profile is the first-line test in diagnosing a fatty acid oxidation disorder. Very long chain fatty acids are indicated for the work-up of peroxisomal disorders. A lipid profile will likely be normal and would not be helpful in this case.

Objective

1. Which common biochemical assays are used to screen for which types of inborn errors of metabolism

CASE 20

You are seeing a 3-month-old female for new onset of seizures. She does not have a history of fever or other symptoms of illness. Her history is remarkable for poor growth despite regular breastfeeding. On examination, she is nondysmorphic. You note that her extremities are thin but her abdomen is somewhat protuberant. The liver edge is palpable 5 cm below the costal margin. She has mild hypotonia.

All of the following evaluations are indicated initially EXCEPT
A. Chromosomal microarray
B. Glucose level
C. Calcium level
D. Liver function tests
E. Head CT scan

Discussion

The correct answer is **A**. Initial evaluation for an infant with seizures would include an infectious work-up and measurement of electrolytes and glucose. Head imaging should also be considered to evaluate for a mass-occupying lesion (including an infectious abscess) or intracranial hemorrhage. In an infant with hepatomegaly, liver function tests would also be indicated. As part of the liver function tests, an ammonia level should be obtained, although hyperammonemia is more typically associated with encephalopathy as opposed to frank seizures. At this early stage, Chromosomal microarray would be less useful, particularly in an infant who is nondysmorphic. If the remainder of the evaluation is normal, Chromosomal microarray could be considered, as seizures with growth retardation even in the absence of dysmorphic features can be seen with small chromosome abnormalities. Therefore, a chromosome abnormality would remain within the differential diagnosis. Her laboratory studies reveal the following:

Sodium	139 mEq/L
Potassium	5.0 mEq/L
Chloride	103 mEq/L
Bicarbonate	15 mEq/L
Glucose	39 mg/dl
AST	111 IU/L
ALT	106 IU/L
Ammonia	20 mcmol/L

Both lactic acid and uric acid levels are elevated

Based on these findings, what is the most likely diagnosis?
A. MCAD deficiency
B. A mitochondrial disorder
C. Propionic acidemia
D. A glycogen storage disease
E. OTC deficiency

Discussion

The correct answer is **D**. This child has glycogen storage disease, likely type I. Glycogen storage diseases are caused by defects in the synthesis or breakdown of glycogen. There are more than 10 types which are classified based on involvement of the liver, muscle, or both. Type I is the most common and typically presents between 3 and 6 months of age with poor growth and hepatomegaly. Secondary complications include lactic acidosis, hyperuricemia, and hypertriglyceridemia. Older children can develop gout, pancreatitis, renal disease, and hepatic adenomas. The fatty acid oxidation disorders, such as MCAD deficiency, are characterized by hypo- or nonketotic hypoglycemia but typically do not have the other features seen in this infant, such as hepatomegaly or elevated lactic acid or uric acid. Mitochondrial disorders can present with seizures, growth deficiency, and elevated lactic acid, and but the finding of hyperuricemia in the setting of the clinical features above strongly suggest glycogen storage disease type I. While this child does have mild acidosis, propionic acidemia is not typically associated with hepatomegaly or seizures unless the patient is suffering from an acute crisis. OTC deficiency is an X-linked condition which can affect females as severely as males. These patients would have hyperammonemia due to impaired function of the urea cycle.

The long-term management of this condition involves which of the following?
A. Carnitine supplementation
B. Protein-restricted diet
C. Fat-restricted diet
D. Medium chain triglycerides (MCTs) oil
E. Cornstarch

Discussion

The correct answer is **E**. In individuals with glycogen storage disease, hypoglycemia may be asymptomatic as patients develop tolerance to chronically low blood sugar, although hypoglycemic seizures can occur. The goal of treatment is maintaining glucose homeostasis. Cornstarch acts as a slow-release form of glucose and helps maintain normal blood sugar levels between meals. A low fat diet and MCT oil is prescribed for defects in long chain fatty acid oxidation. Secondary carnitine

deficiency is a feature of many inborn errors of metabolism but not the glycogen storage diseases. Protein restriction is not necessary in glycogen storage diseases.

Objective

1. Which dietary treatments are used for several common inborn errors of metabolism

CASE 21

A 5-day-old male is admitted for poor feeding and dehydration. The pregnancy and delivery were unremarkable. His mother has tried breastfeeding and formula, but he does not seem to tolerate either. He spits up after most feeds, and sometimes his emesis is projectile. He does not seem interested in feeding and his parents have to wake him for most feeds. The child has a maternal uncle who is cognitively impaired. The parents are not sure what the maternal uncle's diagnosis is other than he was told to follow a "vegetarian" diet. On examination, the infant's heart rate is 140, blood pressure 85/60 mm Hg, and respiratory rate 70. He is somnolent and does not cry when examined. His initial laboratory studies reveal the following:

Venous blood gas pH	7.47, pCO_2 22 mm Hg, pO_2 51 mm Hg
Bicarbonate	16 mEq/L
AST	179 IU/L
ALT	201 IU/L
Ammonia	683 mcmol/L

What disorder do you suspect?
A. VLCAD deficiency
B. Methylmalonic acidemia
C. OTC deficiency
D. Citrullinemia
E. Hyperornithinemia-hyperammonemia-homocitrullinuria syndrome

Discussion

The correct answer is **C**. The differential diagnosis of hyperammonemia includes all of the above disorders, but the most common causes are urea cycle disorders and organic acidemias (in particular methylmalonic and propionic acidemia). Fatty acid oxidation disorders such as VLCAD deficiency can present with a Reye-like syndrome, and liver failure of any etiology will result in elevated ammonia levels. One of the keys to distinguishing between these disorders is the acid–base status. This patient's blood gas reveals a respiratory alkalosis, which is only seen in the urea cycle disorders. The organic acidemias and fatty acid oxidation disorders give rise to a metabolic acidosis. In addition, the history of an affected male related through the maternal side of the family indicates an X-linked pattern of inheritance. Of the urea cycle disorders, only OTC deficiency is X-linked. Citrullinemia and all others are autosomal recessive in their mode of inheritance.

Helpful Tip: Patients with urea cycle disorders present with a respiratory alkalosis, while patients with organic acidemias and fatty acid oxidation disorders present with a metabolic acidosis.

What additional study would you obtain immediately?
A. Head ultrasound
B. Abdominal ultrasound
C. Echocardiogram
D. Chest x-ray
E. Renal ultrasound

Discussion

The correct answer is **A**. Hyperammonemia causes cerebral edema, and a head ultrasound should be done immediately to look for this life-threatening but treatable complication. A careful neurologic examination should also be performed including assessment of pupils and evaluation for other signs of increased intracranial pressure. Hyperammonemia is not associated with acute cardiac, pulmonary, renal, or gastrointestinal complications.

Objective

1. The differential diagnosis for hyperammonemia in the newborn

CASE 22

You are seeing a 2-year-old male for the first time. He has had frequent visits for otitis media and respiratory infections and recently had tympanostomy tubes placed. A hearing test was postponed until he recovered from his most recent illness. He has mild delays in his language and motor development, which his parents attribute to his being sick "all the time." He has two healthy and normally developing siblings. On physical examination, length and weight are at the 25th percentile, and head circumference is at the 95th percentile. His facial features appear coarse with prominent forehead, thick eyebrows, short/broad nose, and thickened lips. His liver edge extends 5 cm below the costal margin and he has a small umbilical hernia. His neurologic examination is nonfocal.

What is the most likely diagnosis?
A. A chromosomal abnormality
B. A lysosomal storage disorder
C. An organic acidemia
D. A mitochondrial disorder
E. A skeletal dysplasia

Discussion

The correct answer is **B**. This child most likely has a lysosomal storage disorder, such as Hurler syndrome. Individuals with lysosomal storage disorders tend to have short stature with macrocephaly that develops over time. They develop coarse features and organomegaly. Developmental regression is often seen in the lysosomal storage disorders, as material ultimately accumulates in the brain tissue. Some chromosomal abnormalities can result in developmental disabilities with coarse facial features, but hepatomegaly would be unusual. Organic acidemias typically present with significant decompensations associated with an intercurrent illness leading to metabolic acidosis and secondary hyperammonemia in some cases. Mitochondrial disorders can result in developmental delay and multiorgan dysfunction but not typically coarse facial features or organomegaly. Many lysosomal storage disorders result in skeletal changes that can mimic skeletal dysplasias, but organomegaly would be unusual.

What would be the most useful next test for this child?
A. Chromosomal microarray
B. Urine mucopolysaccharide and oligosaccharide analysis
C. Urine organic acids
D. Plasma lactate and pyruvate levels
E. Full skeletal survey

Discussion

The correct answer is **B**. Urine for mucopolysaccharide and oligosaccharide analysis is the most useful screening test for lysosomal storage diseases. While a skeletal survey may be helpful, it is not as useful for determining a specific diagnosis as urine mucopolysaccharide and oligosaccharide analysis. However, skeletal radiographs can demonstrate changes that would be suggestive of a lysosomal storage disorder.

Further laboratory evaluations demonstrate that this child has deficiency of alpha–L-iduronidase, consistent with a diagnosis of Hurler syndrome.

What other specialty referrals would be indicated for this child?
A. Orthopedics and nephrology
B. Hematology and neurology
C. Gastroenterology and ophthalmology
D. Cardiology and otolaryngology
E. Neurosurgery and endocrinology

Discussion

The correct answer is **D**. Children with mucopolysaccharidosis (MPS) type I, also known as Hurler syndrome, develop multiple organ system complications. In the early stages, they present with frequent ear, nose, and throat infections, hearing loss, and upper airway obstruction usually requiring tonsillectomy and adenoidectomy. With progressive accumulation of glycosaminoglycans, patients develop hypertrophic cardiomyopathy, hepatomegaly, severe bone dysplasia (dysostosis multiplex), contractures, corneal clouding, cervical compression, hydrocephalus, and carpal tunnel syndrome. The mainstay of treatment is enzyme replacement therapy and in some cases bone marrow transplantation. Children with MPS type I require a multidisciplinary team for their care. The most important referrals for this patient are cardiology and otolaryngology. Kidney, endocrine, hematologic, and gastrointestinal problems (other than enlarged liver) are not seen or are infrequent in MPS type I. The patient will eventually need an ophthalmology examination and a radiographic bone survey, but his cardiac status and airway status are more pressing.

Objective

1. The common features of the lysosomal storage diseases and their appropriate long-term management

REFERENCES

1. Harper PS. *Practical Genetic Counseling.* 6th ed. London: Oxford University Press Inc.; 2004.
2. Jones KL. *Smith's Recognizable Patterns of Human Malformation.* 6th ed. Philadelphia, PA: Elsevier Inc.; 2006.
3. Scott-Emuakpor AB, Madueke ED. The study of genetic variation in Nigeria: II. The genetics of polydactyly. *Hum Hered.* 1976;26:198–202.
4. Marden PM, Smith DW, McDonald MJ. Congenital anomalies in the newborn infant, including minor variations. *J Pediatr.* 1964;64:357–371.
5. Tsai FJ, Tsai CH, Peng CT. Different race, different face: Minor anomalies in Chinese newborn infants. *Acta Paediatr.* 1999;88:323–326.
6. Leppig KA, Werler MM, Cann CI, et al. Predictive value of minor anomalies: I. Association with major malformations. *J. Pediatr.* 1987;110:531–537.
7. Lin DS, Huang FY, Lin SP, et al. Frequency of associated anomalies in congenital hypoplasia of depressor anguli oris muscle: A study of 50 patients. *Am J Med Genet.* 1997;71:215–218.
8. Adam MP, Hudgins L: The importance of minor anomalies in the evaluation of the newborn. *Neoreviews.* 2003;4:e99–e104.
9. Bull MJ; Committee on Genetics. Health supervision for children with Down syndrome. *Pediatrics.* 2011;128:393–406.
10. Miller DT, Adam MP, Aradhya S, et al. Consensus statement: Chromosomal microarray is a first-tier clinical diagnostic test for individuals with developmental disabilities or congenital anomalies. *Am J Hum Genet.* 2010;86:749–764.
11. Shaw SW, Hsu JJ, Lee CH, et al. First- and second-trimester Down syndrome screening: Current strategies and clinical guidelines. *Taiwan J Obstet Gynecol.* 2008;47:157–162.
12. Malone FD, Canick JA, Ball RH, et al. First-trimester or second-trimester screening, or both, for Down's syndrome. *N Engl J Med.* 2005;53:2001–2011.
13. Nicolaides KH, Syngelaki A, Ashoor G, et al. Noninvasive prenatal testing for fetal trisomies in a routinely screened first-trimester population. *Am J Obstet Gynecol.* 2012;207:374.e1–e6.
14. Newberger DS. Down syndrome: Prenatal risk assessment and diagnosis. *Am Fam Physician.* 2000;62:825–832, 837–838.
15. Frías JL, Davenport ML; Committee on Genetics and Section on Endocrinology. Health supervision for children with Turner syndrome. *Pediatrics.* 2003;111:692–702.
16. McDonald-McGinn DM, Kirschner R, Goldmuntz E, et al. The Philadelphia story: The 22q11.2 deletion: Report on 250 patients. *Genet Couns.* 1999;10:11–24.
17. Gravholt CH, Fedder J, Naeraa RW, et al. Occurrence of gonadoblastoma in females with Turner syndrome and Y chromosomal material: A population study. *J Clin Endocrinol Metab.* 2000;85:3199–3202.
18. Lalatta F, Quagliarini D, Folliero E, et al. Triple X syndrome: Characteristics of 42 Italian girls and parental emotional response to prenatal diagnosis. *Eur J Pediatr.* 2010;169:1255–1261.
19. Beck AE, Hudgins L. Congenital cardiac malformations in the neonate: Isolated or syndromic? *Neoreviews.* 2003;4:e105–e110.
20. Bassett AS, McDonald-McGinn DM, Devriendt K, et al; International 22q11.2 Deletion Syndrome Consortium. Practical guidelines for managing patients with 22q11.2 deletion syndrome. *J Pediatr.* 2011;159:332–339.
21. Andrade SE, Gurwitz JH, Davis RL, et al. Prescription drug use in pregnancy. *Am J Obstet Gynecol.* 2004;191:398–407.
22. Adam MP. The all-or-none phenomenon revisited. *Birth Defects Res A Clin Mol Teratol.* 2012;94:664–669.
23. Farrell T, Neale L, Cundy T. Congenital anomalies in the offspring of women with type 1, type 2 and gestational diabetes. *Diabet Med.* 2002;19:322–326.
24. Adam MP, Hudgins L, Carey JC, et al. Preaxial hallucal polydactyly as a marker for diabetic embryopathy. *Birth Defects Res A Clin Mol Teratol.* 2009;85:13–19.
25. Yang J, Cummings EA, O'Connell C, et al. Fetal and neonatal outcomes of diabetic pregnancies. *Obstet Gynecol.* 2006;108:644–650.

26. Yang P, Zhao Z, Reece EA. Activation of oxidative stress signaling that is implicated in apoptosis with a mouse model of diabetic embryopathy. *Am J Obstet Gynecol.* 2008;198:130. e1–e7.

27. Webster WS, Freeman JA. Prescription drugs and pregnancy. *Expert Opin Pharmacother.* 2003;4:949–961.

28. Tomlinson JK, Morse SA, Bernard SP, et al. Long-term outcomes of surgical tongue reduction in Beckwith–Wiedemann syndrome. *Plast Reconstr Surg.* 2007;119:992–1002.

29. Jacquemont S, Birnbaum S, Redler S, Steinbach P, Biancalana V. Clinical utility gene card for: Fragile X mental retardation syndrome, fragile X-associated tremor/ataxia syndrome and fragile X-associated primary ovarian insufficiency. *Eur J Hum Genet.* 2011;19.

30. Tarleton JC, Saul RA: Molecular genetic advances in fragile X syndrome. *J Pediatr.* 1993;122:169–185.

31. Arsenault ME, Prevost C, Lescault A, et al. Clinical characteristics of myotonic dystrophy type 1 patients with small CTG expansions. *Neurology.* 2006;66:1248–1250.

32. Faivre L, Masurel-Paulet A, Collod-Béroud G, et al. Clinical and molecular study of 320 children with Marfan syndrome and related type I fibrillinopathies in a series of 1009 probands with pathogenic FBN1 mutations. *Pediatrics.* 2009;123:391–398.

33. Wen J, Jian J, Ding C, et al. Birth defects in children conceived by in vitro fertilization and intracytoplasmic sperm injection: A meta-analysis. *Fertil Steril.* 2012;97:1331–1337.e1–e4.

34. Marchesi DE, Qiao J, Feng HL. Embryo manipulation and imprinting. *Semin Reprod Med.* 2012;30:323–334.

35. Bergman JE, Janssen N, Hoefsloot LH, et al. CHD7 mutations and CHARGE syndrome: The clinical implications of an expanding phenotype. *J Med Genet.* 2011;48:334–342.

36. Kee Y, D'Andrea AD. Molecular pathogenesis and clinical management of Fanconi anemia. *J Clin Invest.* 2012;122:3799–3806.

37. Forlino A, Cabral WA, Barnes AM, et al. New perspectives on osteogenesis imperfecta. *Nat Rev Endocrinol.* 2011;7:540–557.

38. Kang L, Marty D, Pauli RM, et al. Chondrodysplasia punctata associated with malabsorption from bariatric procedures. *Surg Obes Relat Dis.* 2010;6:99–101.

39. Magdaleno R Jr, Pereira BG, Chaim EA, et al. Pregnancy after bariatric surgery: A current view of maternal, obstetrical and perinatal challenges. *Arch Gynecol Obstet.* 2012;285: 559–566.

40. Hoogerwaard EM, Bakker E, Ippel PF, et al. Signs and symptoms of Duchenne muscular dystrophy and Becker muscular dystrophy among carriers in The Netherlands: A cohort study. *Lancet.* 1999;353:2116–2119.

Chapter 7
NUTRITION
Patricia W. Denning, MD and Christina J. Valentine, MD, MS, RD

Nutrition and Growth (Fetus)

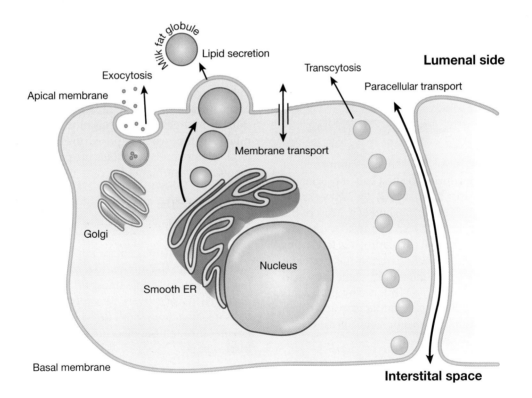

CASE 1

You are examining a 1,700-g 32-week female infant upon admission to the NICU. She was born to a 25-year-old mother after unstoppable spontaneous preterm labor. Prenatal laboratories and pregnancy history were otherwise unremarkable. You determine that she is appropriately sized for gestational age.

Based upon what you know about fetal body composition, about how much of the infant's weight is expected to be comprised of protein?

A. 85 g
B. 170 g
C. 340 g
D. 680 g
E. 1,445 g

Discussion

The correct answer is **B**. The fetus is comprised of approximately 5% protein in the first trimester. This gradually increases to almost 10% by the late second trimester and into the third trimester. Amino acids are actively transported across the placental membrane. The efficacy of placental amino acid transfer is affected by a number of factors including transport capacity, inhibitory effects by drugs such as alcohol and nicotine, uterine blood flow, and transporter capacity.[1]

Helpful Tip: Placental amino acid transport can occur by both sodium-dependent and sodium-independent mechanisms depending on the type of amino acid. For example, branched-chain amino acids such as valine are carried by a sodium-independent transporter.

Based upon what you know about fetal body composition, about how much of the infant's weight is expected to be comprised of fat?
A. 85 g
B. 170 g
C. 340 g
D. 680 g
E. 1,445 g

Discussion

The correct answer is **A**. The fetus is comprised of approximately 0.5% fat during the first half of pregnancy. This gradually increases to about 5% by 32 weeks. By term the fetus is comprised of 15% body fat. Most of the fetus' body fat is deposited between 35 and 40 weeks. The placenta can take up maternal circulating free fatty acids (FFA), and these FFA are able to cross the placental membrane via passive diffusion and by some fatty acid carriers (facilitated transport). While many fatty acids can be synthesized by the fetus, essential fatty acids such as linoleic acid and alpha-linolenic acid must be provided by placental transfer.

Based upon what you know about fetal body composition, about how much of the infant's weight is expected to be comprised of water?
A. 85 g
B. 170 g
C. 340 g
D. 680 g
E. 1,445 g

Discussion

The correct answer is **E**. As the fetus accumulates fat, body water content decreases. The fetus is comprised of over 90% water during the first half of pregnancy. This gradually decreases to about 85% by 32 weeks. By term the fetus is comprised of 75% body water.

In the fetus, glucose does all of the following except
A. Inhibits protein breakdown
B. Increases insulin production and secretion
C. Enters from the placenta due to the transplacental concentration gradient
D. Enters into fetal cells by a family of glucose transporters with Glut-1 being the predominant fetal glucose transporter isoform
E. All of the above are correct

Discussion

The correct answer is **E**. Glucose transport across the placenta is mediated by facilitated transporter proteins such as Glut-1 and Glut-3. In human placenta Glut-1 is the principal transporter at the maternal facing membrane and Glut-3 is found more often on the fetal facing membrane. In the fetus, Glut-1 is found in most fetal tissues, while other isoforms tend to be more tissue-specific such as Glut-2 in hepatocytes and Glut-4 in skeletal muscle and heart. The fetal pancreas develops early second trimester producing measurable insulin concentrations by mid-gestation. While most fetuses do not secrete much insulin, when exposed to diabetic mothers, the fetal pancreas is capable of producing significant amounts of insulin.[61]

Helpful Tip: The fetus has about 9 g of carbohydrate at the 33rd week of gestation, and at birth it rises to 34 g.

Helpful Tip: The placenta is important in the transfer of nutrients from the mother to the fetus. However it is not just an organ of simple transport, but is also able to take up nutrients selectively. The supply of nutrients to the fetus depends upon both the volume of maternal blood flowing through the placenta and the food constituents carried by it.[60]

If this mother had not delivered prematurely, but instead delivered a healthy baby at term, how much more would the infant be expected to weigh?
A. 25% more
B. 50% more
C. 75% more
D. 100% more
E. 200% more

Discussion

The correct answer is **D**. The fetus is expected to double its weight between 32 weeks and term. The fetus grows rapidly over the second half of gestation. Glucose transfer across the placenta must increase to meet the metabolic demands of the growing fetus. The mechanisms responsible for this increased delivery include increases in transport capacity, and a change in concentration gradient as the fetal glucose concentration decreases relative to the maternal glucose concentrations.[60]

Objectives

1. Identify the body composition changes during fetal growth
2. Know nutrient requirements and relative amounts for normal fetal growth
3. Know the maternal, placental and fetal factors, and hormones that affect intrauterine fetal growth

CASE 2

The birthing center calls you in the middle of the night. A mother requires a stat cesarean section for severe preeclampsia. You arrive for the delivery and determine the infant's weight, length, and head circumference as less than fifth percentile.

The infant is described as
A. IUGR
B. SGA
C. AGA
D. LGA

Discussion

The correct answer is **A**. Intrauterine growth restriction can be caused by placental insufficiency, hypoxia, preeclampsia, preterm labor, or undernutrition.[1] Often the terms IUGR and SGA are used interchangeably, but they are not the same. A newborn may be labeled SGA according to a reference population if the newborn is constitutionally small but otherwise normal (e.g., an infant born to parents who are both small and/or born into a population that is smaller than the reference population). In addition, a fetus with delayed growth late in gestation (asymmetric IUGR) may not have a reduction in birth weight significant enough to be classified as SGA. Typically infants <10th percentile are considered SGA for that population and large for gestational age if they are >90th percentile for the reference population. Infants between 10% and 90% are considered appropriate for gestational age (AGA).

You review that normal fetal growth depends on nutrient transport across the placenta during pregnancy. In particular placental and maternal factors can influence the transport of nutrients by influencing the microvillus membrane (MVM) or the basal membrane (BM) of the syncytiotrophoblast. Which nutrients are decreased in transport and most associated with IUGR status?
A. Glucose
B. Lysine and taurine
C. Fatty acids
D. Lipoproteins

Discussion

The best answer is **B**. Decreased lysine and taurine, due to the active transfer across the fetal basal membrane is significantly associated with IUGR.[2] The primary barrier to lysine and taurine transport is the syncytiotrophoblast. Its polarized membranes consist of a microvillus membrane (maternal facing) and the basement membrane (fetal facing). Glucose transport is typically by a maternal–fetal gradient and facilitated diffusion via glucose transporters. Increased IGF-1 can increase BM transport of glucose and can be associated with large for gestational age infants (LGA) and not IUGR. Fatty acids via nonesterified fatty acids and esterified triglycerides are transported with a concentration gradient and fatty acid–binding proteins (FABP). Of interest in maternal diabetes, FABP-1 can be upregulated and increases fat transport and accumulation in the fetus thus most often associated with LGA.[1]

In reading further you discover that hormonal influence for fetal growth is caused by
A. Cortisol
B. Glucocorticoids
C. IGF II
D. Calcitonin
E. PTH

Discussion

The best answer is **C**. Fetal signals from both IGF II and PTH influence placental function.[1] IGF II regulates placental growth, and therefore nutrient transfer ability across the placenta whereas fetal PTH regulates calcium transport by a calcium pump in the BM.[1]

Helpful Tip: Fetal growth is largely controlled by the interaction of genetic programming, with the availability of oxygen and glucose (substrate). As substrate increases or decreases, the endocrine responses vary with their supply. Insulin-like growth factor II (IGF-II), and probably IGF-I, are responsible for modulating fetal growth. Insulin and thyroid hormones are altered by the supply of glucose and oxygen, respectively, and they influence fetal growth, partly via IGF-I.[1] Simply put, fetal growth depends on the mother's nutritional status, the placenta function, and the fetal programming.

In prescribing the appropriate nutrition plan for this IUGR infant you determine based on your reading that the infant will require the following nutrient prescription:
A. Increased calories and protein to achieve catch-up growth above the fifth percentile
B. Adequate calories and protein to remain along the same growth curve
C. Triple the calories and fat to provide adequate brain growth
D. Double the calories to provide catch-up growth
E. Extra calcium and phosphorus to make up for lost stores

Discussion

The best answer is **B**. Adequate calories and protein to achieve similar growth curve to avoid metabolic syndrome later in life.[3] In addition, infants with IUGR are known to have exaggerated jaundice, hypoglycemia, hypothermia, and increased polycythemia.

Which of the following is false regarding fetal growth?
A. Glucose, fat, and protein are all moved across the placenta by facilitated diffusion
B. IUGR babies should not be fed excessive calories to promote catch up weight or they will run the risk of metabolic syndrome later in life
C. Insulin growth factor is important for fetal growth, both by increasing placental growth as well as fetal development
D. Glut-1 is the most abundant glucose transport protein in the fetus
E. The fetus doubles its protein content from the first trimester to late third trimester

Discussion

The correct answer is **A**. Proteins (amino acids) are actually transported by active transport, not passive transport. The fetus actually doubles its protein content from approximately 5% in the first trimester to 10% near the time of delivery. Insulin growth factors I and II are critical for fetal growth. While there are a number of glucose transporters, Glut-1 is in all tissues of the fetus, many of the other glucose transporters are actually tissue-specific, such as Glut-4 in the skeletal muscle.

Objectives

1. Know the postnatal growth patterns for LGA, SGA, and IUGR

2. Know the definitions, causes, and clinical features of SGA and LGA infants
3. Understand the effects of fetal programming and nutrition on the prevalence and types of adult onset disorders

Postnatal Nutrition and Energy Requirements in Preterm Infants

CASE 3

You are managing a stable 3-week-old premature infant who is in room air and on full NG feeds.

What is the expected resting metabolic rate (resting energy expenditure) in this preterm infant?
A. 45 kcal/kg/d
B. 80 kcal/kg/d
C. 110 kcal/kg/d
D. 140 kcal/kg/d
E. Depends upon the gestational age of the infant

Discussion

The correct answer is **A**. Resting energy expenditure (REE) depends upon sleep state and activity levels, thermoregulation requirements, and basal metabolic rate. While this may vary from infant to infant, it is approximately 45 kcal/kg/d in stable infants from 27 weeks to term (based on respiratory calorimetry in a thermoneutral environment).[4] Limited studies indicate that extremely premature infants on ventilators may have REE as high as 90 kcal/kg/d.

ENERGY EXPENDITURE (STABLE PRETERM INFANT)	kcal/kg/d
Basal metabolic rate	40–50
Activity	0–5
Thermoregulation	0–5
Resting energy expenditure	40–60

What is the minimum energy intake required for growth in this preterm infant?
A. 45 kcal/kg/d
B. 80 kcal/kg/d
C. 110 kcal/kg/d
D. 150 kcal/kg/d
E. Depends upon the gestational age of the infant

Discussion

The correct answer is **C**. A minimum of 100 kcal/kg/d is required to provide the energy requirements to meet resting energy expenditure plus deposition of new tissue.[4,5] Assuming 85% to 90% absorption rate of metabolizable energy from enteral feeds, this infant would require 110 to 120 kcal/kg/d of energy intake. Thus, the minimum energy intake requirement is 110 kcal/kg/d. This does not vary with gestational age. Intake of greater than 140 kcal/kg/d does not improve linear growth and may lead to excessive fat deposition. Even if weight gain is inadequate, increasing energy intake above this level is not recommended. Ensuring adequate protein intake (maintaining adequate protein: energy ratio) would be more likely to improve growth.[4]

MINIMUM (RANGE) ENERGY REQUIREMENTS IN PRETERM INFANTS	kcal/kg/d
Resting metabolic rate/resting energy expenditure	45
Deposition of new tissue	55 (55–80)
Total energy requirement	100 (100–125)
Energy losses (stool) Human milk = 85% absorbable energy Formula = 90% absorbable energy	10 (10–15)
Total energy intake requirement	110–140

What are the protein intake requirements in this preterm infant?
A. 1 g/kg/d
B. 3.5 g/kg/d
C. 6 g/kg/d
D. 10 g/kg/d
E. 20 g/kg/d

Discussion

The best answer is **B**. Protein requirements between 3 and 4.5 g/kg/d are safe and adequate. In order to match fetal accretion rates, protein requirements are estimated at 3.5 to 4 g/kg/d. Enterally, protein intake of 3.2 to 4.1 g/kg per 100 kcal intake (in a stable preterm infant) allows for the best match of fetal growth in terms of composition and weight gain. Weight gain rates have been shown to be linearly related to protein intakes up to 4.5 g/kg/d and smaller preterm infants have been shown to accumulate a protein deficit. Since excess protein intake does not appear to cause detrimental effects, but a small deficit can impair growth, smaller preterm infants can benefit from higher protein intake goals. Infants <1,000 g, can benefit from protein intake goals of 4 to 4.5 g/kg/d and 1,000- to 1,800-g preterm infants can benefit from protein intake goals of 3.5 to 4 g/kg/d.[4]

Helpful Tip: Amino acids are classified as indispensable, conditionally essential, and nonessential. Examples of indispensable (cannot be synthesized) are isoleucine, leucine, lysine, methionine, phenylalanine, threonine, tryptophan, and valine, plus histidine. Conditionally essential amino acids include arginine, cysteine, glutamine, glycine, proline, and tyrosine. The other amino acids are nonessential.[4]

What are the fat intake requirements in this preterm infant?
A. 1 g/kg/d
B. 3 g/kg/d
C. 6 g/kg/d
D. 10 g/kg/d
E. 20 g/kg/d

Discussion

The best answer is **C**. Fat provides a major source of energy and should provide 40% to 50% of energy from enteral feedings. Enteral feedings should aim to provide 5 to 7 g/kg/d of fat.[6] There are two essential (poly unsaturated fatty acid) PUFA families, the n–6 and n–3 fatty acids. The parent essential fatty acids (EFAs) of the n–6 and n–3 families are linoleic acid (LA; 18:2n–6) and α-linolenic acid (ALA; 18:3n–3). Essential fatty acid deficiency has been traditionally defined as an elevation in the triene-tetraene ratio. However it may not be as accurate in the preterm population. Essential fatty acid deficiency can also be diagnosed by low serum levels of the essential fatty acid, linoleic acid. Fatty acid deficiency can present as dermatitis, weakness, edema, impaired growth, immune, and mental deficiencies.

What are the carbohydrate intake requirements in this preterm infant?
A. 1 g/kg/d
B. 3 g/kg/d
C. 6 g/kg/d
D. 10 g/kg/d
E. 20 g/kg/d

Discussion

The best answer is **D**. Carbohydrates should provide about 40% to 50% of a preterm infant's caloric intake. Thus, a stable preterm infant should require 10 to 14 g/kg/d of carbohydrate in enteral feeds.[6]

Helpful Tip:

PRETERM INFANT ENTERAL INTAKE REQUIREMENTS	g/kg/d	g/100 kcal	% CALORIC INTAKE
Protein	3–4.5	3.2–4.1	10–20
<1,000-g infant	4–4.5	3.6–4.1	
1,000–1,800-g infant	3.5–4	3.2–3.6	
Fat	5–7	4.4–6	40–50
Carbohydrates	10–14	10.5–12	40–50

Objectives

1. Know the changes in body composition in newborn infants
2. Understand the energy expenditure and caloric requirements for growth
3. Know the protein requirements and the indispensable, essential, and nonessential amino acids
4. Know the fat requirements, the laboratory and clinical manifestations of essential fatty acid deficiency
5. Understand the carbohydrate requirements and the physiology of digestion and absorption

Postnatal Nutrition and Energy Requirements in Term Infants

CASE 4

You are interviewing a mother of a 2-month-old term infant who shows up for a routine well visit. When plotting the infant's growth parameters, you note that the infant seems to be failing to thrive as she was 50% for all parameters at birth and now has dropped to 25%. Your first goal is to assess whether the infant's intake is adequate to meet nutritional needs for growth at this age.

What is the minimum energy intake required for growth in this term infant?
A. 45 kcal/kg/d
B. 95 kcal/kg/d
C. 110 kcal/kg/d
D. 140 kcal/kg/d
E. Depends upon the gestational age of the infant

Discussion

The correct answer is **C**. The recommended energy intake for a term infant ages 0 to 6 months by the WHO is 108 kcal/kg/d. Energy requirements are higher in the

first 6 months of life due to rapid growth. Expert recommendations for energy intake for term infants range from as high as 124 kcal/kg/d at birth to as low as 95 kcal/kg/d by 6 months. Energy intake requirements may be lower for breast-fed infants. The energy intake for the human milk fed infant is estimated to be 100 kcal/kg/d. Thus, the current recommendation for term formulas is to provide 63 to 71 kcal/100 mL.[7]

Helpful Tip: Normal-term neonates generally lose 5% to 8% of birth weight in the days after delivery but regain their birth weight within 2 weeks. Normal weight gain is 14 to 28 g/d until 3 months, with a healthy term infant doubling their birth weight by 5 months, and tripling their birth weight by 12 months.[7]

What is the expected basal metabolic rate in this term infant?
A. 45 kcal/kg/d
B. 90 kcal/kg/d
C. 110 kcal/kg/d
D. 140 kcal/kg/d
E. Depends upon the gestational age of the infant

Discussion

The correct answer is **A**. The basal metabolic rate of a term infant ranges from 43 to 60 kcal/kg/d.[7]

Besides basal metabolic rate, what other factors should be assessed to determine required energy intake for growth?
A. Energy cost of growth (energy content of tissues and energy required for tissue synthesis)
B. Energy required for activity
C. Energy required for thermoregulation
D. All of the above
E. A and B only

Discussion

The correct answer is **E**. Factors that influence the energy intake required for growth include basal metabolic rate, energy cost of growth, energy required for activity, thermic effect of food (energy expended during feeding ~10 kcal/kg/d) and energy excreted (fecal fat losses ~5 kcal/kg/d). Energy required for thermoregulation affects the basal metabolic rate and depends upon the ambient temperature.[7]

What is the expected energy required for activity in the young term infant?
A. 10 kcal/kg/d
B. 20 kcal/kg/d
C. 40 kcal/kg/d
D. 80 kcal/kg/d
E. 120 kcal/kg/d

Discussion

The correct answer is **B**. Energy required for activity has been estimated at 15 to 25 kcal/kg/d.[7]

ENERGY REQUIREMENTS IN TERM INFANTS	kcal/kg/d
Basal metabolic rate	43–60
Feeding	10
Fecal losses	5
Activity	15–25
Energy required for growth	28–33
Total energy requirement	101–133

What are the protein intake requirements for this term infant?
A. 0.1 g/kg/d
B. 0.5 g/kg/d
C. 1 g/kg/d
D. 1.5 g/kg/d
E. 3 g/kg/d

Discussion

The best answer is **D**. Protein intake requirements are significantly affected by growth rate. In the first 3 months of life, 55% of protein intake is used for growth. This decreases to 10% by 8 years of age. The recommended protein intake for term infants is calculated on the basis of the mean intake in healthy breast-fed infants. The average protein intake for a term infant in the first 6 months of life is 1.5 to 2 g/kg/d providing ~7.8% of total caloric intake.[7]

What are the fat intake requirements in this term infant?
A. 1 g/kg/d
B. 3 g/kg/d
C. 6 g/kg/d
D. 10 g/kg/d
E. 20 g/kg/d

Discussion

The best answer is **C**. Fat provides a major source of energy in term infants and should provide about 45% to 60% of energy from enteral feedings. Fat is an important source of concentrated energy in the newborn infant who has high energy requirements due to rapid growth. Fatty acids are also important for constructing cell membranes, as precursors for biometabolites, and facilitate transport and absorption of fat-soluble vitamins. Thus, human milk usually contains 4.6 to 7.8 g/100 kcal to provide ~50% of energy intake. This would equate to enteral feedings that provide ~6 g/kg/d of fat.[6]

What are the carbohydrate intake requirements for this term infant?
A. 1 g/kg/d
B. 3 g/kg/d
C. 6 g/kg/d
D. 10 g/kg/d
E. 20 g/kg/d

Discussion

The best answer is **D**. Carbohydrates should provide about 40% of a term infant's caloric intake. Glucose is the preferred energy source for the brain and estimated requirements are between 8 and 12 g/kg/d in the term newborn. Insufficient carbohydrate intake to meet these glucose demands would require gluconeogenesis resulting in protein/tissue loss. Further, if carbohydrate intake is insufficient to meet energy demands, additional breakdown of fat and protein would be required. Term human milk contains on average 10 g of carbohydrate per 100 kcal to meet these demands.[6]

In assessing nutrition intake for this infant, you ask the mother to bring in the formula she has been feeding the infant. To meet the nutritional needs of a term infant, what is the recommended caloric density of infant formula?
A. 20 kcal/100 mL
B. 24 kcal/100 mL
C. 28 kcal/100 mL
D. 33 kcal/100 mL
E. 67 kcal/100 mL

Discussion

The correct answer is **E**. The mean caloric density of term infant formulas is 67 kcal/100 mL with current recommendations in the range of 63 to 71 kcal/100 mL. Term human milk is also estimated to have a similar caloric density. Caloric densities lower than this range would require high volumes to achieve adequate growth and caloric densities higher than this range could compromise water balance due to lower volume intake.[7]

To meet the nutritional needs of a term infant, what is the recommended protein content of infant formula?
A. 10% of total calories
B. 20% of total calories
C. 40% of total calories
D. 60% of total calories
E. 80% of total calories

Discussion

The best answer is **A**. The recommended minimum protein content of term formula is 1.7 g/100 kcal (6.8% of calories). The protein should be calculated as true protein (excluding nonprotein nitrogen sources). The maximum recommended protein content of term formula is 3.4 g/100 kcal (13.6% of calories). In contrast, preterm formulas are recommended to contain 3.2 to 4.1 g/100 kcal of protein.[7]

To meet the nutritional needs of a term infant, what is the recommended minimum fat content of infant formula?
A. 10% of total calories
B. 20% of total calories
C. 40% of total calories
D. 60% of total calories
E. 80% of total calories

Discussion

The correct answer is **C**. The recommended fat content of term infant formula is 4.4 to 6.4 g/100 kcal which would provide 40% to 57% of calories from fat. The average term formula typically contains ~5.4 g of fat per 100 kcal.[7]

To meet the nutritional needs of a term infant, what is the recommended carbohydrate content of infant formula?
A. 10% of total calories
B. 20% of total calories
C. 40% of total calories
D. 60% of total calories
E. 80% of total calories

Discussion

The correct answer is **C**. The recommended minimum carbohydrate content in term formula is 9 g/100 kcal (36% of total calories). This is based on obligatory needs of the brain (brain oxidation needs estimated at 8 to 12 g glucose/100 kcal and the amount needed to minimize gluconeogenesis. Inadequate carbohydrate intake would result in tissue protein loss from gluconeogenesis. The recommended maximum carbohydrate content in term formula is 13.4 g/100 kcal (53.6% of total calories).[7]

In carbohydrate digestion, the following are true except
A. Sucrase levels are equal in the term infant when compared to the adult levels
B. Glucose transport across the membrane is equal in the term infant to that of the adult
C. Lactase levels are similar to the levels of adults in the term infant
D. Amylase is responsible for hydrolyzing starch
E. Bacteria that ferment nonabsorbed nutrients in the colon to usable energy by the infant is called the colonic salvage pathway

Discussion

The correct answer is **B**. Glucose transport in both the preterm and term infant is reduced compared to levels seen in the adult. Of note all the glucosidases including sucrase are actually at adult levels from about 28 weeks on. The colonic salvage pathway is important when we consider up to 25% of lactose reach the colon. This presentation of lactose along with physiologic changes of the metabolism of these prebiotics results in the growth of commensal bacterial such as lactobacillus and other probiotics.

Helpful Tip: While digestion occurs within the lumen of the GI tract, the actual absorption takes place at the microvillus membrane, where nutrients are moved across the cell to enter the circulation.

Objectives

1. Know the energy, protein, fat, and carbohydrate requirements in the term infant
2. Know the differences in requirements for term versus preterm infants

Parenteral Nutrition

CASE 5

You are admitting a 500-g 24-week premature infant and contemplating whether or not to start early parenteral nutrition.

Which of the following statements are true regarding early parenteral nutrition in this infant?
A. Early protein/amino acid administration is important for growth of lean body mass and brain development
B. As long as enough calories are administered in the first 24 hours, protein administration is not necessary
C. Lipid infusions should be avoided in the first 24 hours for ELBW infants
D. Protein/amino acid administration should be avoided in the first 24 hours for ELBW infants
E. Parenteral nutrition is not necessary if trophic feeds can be initiated in the first 24 hours of life

Discussion

The correct answer is **A**. An increasingly large body of evidence supports the administration of increased amino acid and protein in the first day of life to improve net protein balance, growth of lean body mass (including brain).[8] Protein administration should be started as early as possible to meet recommended intakes for gestational age (3.5–4.0 g/kg/ for <30 weeks' gestational age; 2.5–3.5 g/kg/d for 30 to 36 weeks' gestational age; and 2.5 g/kg/d for >36 weeks' gestational age). The minimum requirement to prevent protein catabolism is 1.5 g/kg/d. Starting early lipid infusions at 0.5 g/kg/d is safe and important to avoid essential fatty acid deficiency.[9] Trophic feeds alone cannot provide enough nutrition for the ELBW infant and thus, parenteral nutrition is necessary.

What are the potential consequences of administering nutrition (adequate calories) with too little protein?
A. Poor growth of lean body mass (muscle, bone, brain tissue)
B. Excess deposition of body fat
C. Poor cognitive development
D. All of the above
E. Only A and B

Discussion

The correct answer is **D**. Preterm infants who have inadequate protein administration are prone to depositing more body fat than would be predicted on the basis of in utero growth, and also deposit less lean body mass (including brain tissue). Studies indicate that this inadequate protein administration could lead specifically to poor cognitive development.[8]

What are the potential consequences of administering adequate calories but with too much protein?
A. Metabolic acidosis
B. Uremia
C. Amino acid toxicity
D. All of the above
E. Only A and B

Discussion

The correct answer is **D**. Metabolic acidosis, uremia, and amino acid toxicity are all possible consequences of too much protein administration. However, studies demonstrating such side effects (which can in turn lead to growth failure and poor neurodevelopmental outcome) in preterm infant populations back in the 1970s occurred with formulas of significantly lesser quality than what is used today, and with double the amount protein as what is recommended for preterm infants today. Thus, clinicians should remain comfortable with administering early protein both enterally and parenterally according to current guidelines.[8]

Which of the following are considered essential amino acids?
A. Leucine
B. Serine
C. Alanine
D. All of the above
E. Only A and B

Discussion

The correct answer is **A**. Essential (or indispensable) amino acids include valine, leucine, isoleucine, threonine, phenylalanine, methionine, lysine, tryptophan, and histidine.[10] Both serine and alanine are nonessential amino acids.

Helpful Tip: While there may not be a specific dietary requirement for nonessential amino acids, they contribute both to the overall nitrogen pool and can be used as substrate to synthesize proteins.

Which of the following are considered nonessential amino acids?
A. Glutamate
B. Cystine
C. Tryptophan
D. All of the above
E. Only A and B

Discussion

The correct answer is **A**. Nonessential (or dispensable amino acids) include glutamate, alanine, serine, aspartate, and asparagine. Conditionally essential (or conditionally indispensable) amino acids include glycine, cystine, glutamine, tyrosine, proline, arginine, and taurine.[10]

CASE 6

You are caring for a 24-week preterm infant who is getting parenteral nutrition for the first time at 12 hours of life. Previous to this, D5W @ 100 mL/kg/d was infusing through his UVC.

Based on your knowledge of protein and amino acid metabolism, you would expect protein catabolism to be at a rate of
A. 0.8 g/kg/d
B. 1.6 g/kg/d
C. 2.4 g/kg/d
D. 3.2 g/kg/d
E. None of the above

Discussion

The correct answer is **A**.[11] To prevent protein catabolism a minimum of 1.5 g/kg/d of protein administration is recommended. However, recent studies indicate that starting protein administration at recommended levels (rather than gradually increasing protein administration) is generally safe. With newer formulations of formula and TPN, early administration of protein at recommended levels does not have a significant risk of causing metabolic acidosis, uremia, or increased metabolic demands in the preterm infant.[8]

The rate of protein breakdown correlates with the rate of synthesis of what?
A. Leucine
B. Phenylalanine
C. Carbon dioxide
D. Urea
E. A and B

Discussion

The correct answer is **E**.[11] Rates of protein breakdown in the body can be determined by measuring the rates of leucine or phenylalanine synthesis. The rate of protein synthesis is severalfold higher than the protein intake, which means that body proteins are constantly being broken down and resynthesized. This is generally referred to as protein turnover. To increase lean body mass, the rate of protein synthesis must exceed that of protein breakdown, resulting in net protein accretion.

The first step in leucine metabolism is performed by what?
A. BCAT (branched-chain amino transferase)
B. BCKDC (branched-chain keto dehydrogenase complex)
C. Branched-chain ketoacid decarboxylase
D. Dihydrolipoamide acyltransferase
E. None of the above

Discussion

The correct answer is **A**. BCAT metabolizes branched-chain amino acids (leucine, isoleucine, valine) to branched-chain alpha-ketoacids. BCAT allows the formation of nonessential amino acids such as glutamine. BCAT plays an important role in redistributing nitrogen pools during protein breakdown and protein building. BCAT activity increases during fasting and decreases during protein accretion.[11]

What is the most abundant dispensable amino acid in the blood and free amino acid pool?
A. Leucine
B. Phenylalanine
C. Glutamine
D. Cystine
E. Taurine

Discussion

The correct answer is **C**. Glutamine is synthesized by almost every organ in the body and is thought to play a key role in the regulation of protein synthesis. Infants with congenital glutamine deficiency die of multiorgan failure. It is believed that enteral glutamine is taken up almost entirely by gut enterocytes and metabolized into glutamate for enterocyte fuel and ammonia (as a byproduct).[11]

What conditionally essential amino acid is thought to play an important role in postnatal neurodevelopment of the preterm infant?
A. Leucine
B. Phenylalanine
C. Glutamine
D. Cystine
E. Taurine

Discussion

The correct answer is **E**. A retrospective analysis showed an association between low-plasma taurine levels during the neonatal period and lower 18-month Bayley scores and lower 7-year WISC-R arithmetic scores.[12] Plasma levels of taurine have been shown to be higher in infants fed human milk compared to infant formulas; thus taurine is routinely added to infant formulas (since mid-1980s).[11,13]

In protein digestion which of the following is false?
A. Proteases such as trypsin are at decreased levels in the preterm infant as well as the term infant
B. Amino acid transport is well-developed even in early life
C. Amino acids are absorbed predominately by the transcellular route
D. Peptidases are at reduced levels in the preterm and term infant
E. The pancreas is the source of many proteases

Discussion

The correct answer is **D**. Peptidases such as dipeptidase are actually at near normal levels even in early life. While amino acids generally enter the body utilizing the transcellular absorptive route, the larger small peptides actually utilize the paracellular route more frequently.[11]

Helpful Tip: The reason preterm formula or breast milk is fortified is that an ELBW would require nearly twice the volume of unfortified breast milk to get the recommended requirement for protein, ~300 mL/kg/d to achieve 3.5 to 4 g/kg/d of protein.

Objectives

1. Distinguish between indispensable, essential, and nonessential amino acids
2. Know the protein requirements for the preterm infant
3. Know the consequences of administering too little or too much protein to an infant
4. Know the physiology of protein digestion

CASE 7

You are caring for a 1-week-old preterm infant for the first time. The infant remains on the ventilator on total parenteral nutrition and phototherapy. Because of the concern of hyperbilirubinemia, no lipid infusion has been started on this infant. The nurse asks you to examine a rash. Upon examination you note a dry, scaly dermatitis around the neck and axillae.

What nutritional deficiency would be most likely to cause this rash?
A. Dehydration (inadequate fluid administration)
B. Essential amino acid deficiency (inadequate protein administration)
C. Hyponatremia (inadequate sodium administration)
D. Starvation (inadequate caloric administration)
E. Essential fatty acid deficiency (inadequate lipid administration)

Discussion

The correct answer is **E**. Essential fatty acid deficiency can occur in as few as 3 days and will definitely occur within 7 days in the preterm infant if dietary fat (enteral or parenteral) is not administered.[9]

Helpful Tip: To avoid essential fatty acid deficiency, the administration 0.50 g/kg/d of 20% intralipid, or 30 to 50 mL/kg/d of breast milk can provide the essential fatty acids required.[9]

What other clinical signs can be associated with this condition?
A. Dehydration
B. Poor growth
C. Infertility
D. All of the above
E. A and B

Discussion

The correct answer is **D**. Essential fatty acid deficiency has been associated with growth retardation, dehydration, scaly rash, and infertility.[14]

What laboratory measurements can confirm the diagnosis?
A. Low-serum linoleic acid (LA) levels
B. High-serum eicosatrienoic acid (ETA) levels
C. Low-serum arachidonic acid (AA) levels
D. All of the above
E. A and B

Discussion

The correct answer is **E**. Essential fatty acid deficiency can be diagnosed by low serum levels of the essential fatty acid, LA. Essential fatty acid deficiency also causes a rise in serum levels of the nonessential fatty acid, ETA. A ratio of ETA:LA of greater than 2 has also been used to diagnose essential fatty acid deficiency. Although serum levels of AA will decrease if dietary fat is withheld, serum AA does not always correct with dietary supplementation and may be deceptively high in the preterm infant with essential fatty acid deficiency. Therefore the traditional definition of essential fatty acid deficiency used in other populations [triene tetraene ratio (ETA:AA) > 0.2] may be an insensitive measure of essential fatty acid deficiency in the preterm infant.[15]

What could have prevented this condition (minimum intake of lipid required)?
A. Early lipid infusion at 0.5 g/kg/d
B. Early lipid infusion at 2 g/kg/d
C. Early lipid infusion at 4 g/kg/d
D. Early lipid infusion at 6 g/kg/d
E. This condition was not preventable

Discussion

The best answer is **A**. Parenteral fat emulsion administration at 0.5 g/kg/d can prevent essential fatty acid deficiency in the preterm infant. Some studies suggest that with adequate caloric intake, the minimal requirement can be as low as 0.25 g/kg/d but with low energy intake requirement can be as high as 1 g/kg/d as fatty acids would then be used for energy instead of fat deposition.[9,15,16]

CASE 8

You are caring for a VLBW preterm infant and are considering a new preterm infant formula being introduced to the NICU.

In assessing the formula composition, what fatty acids should be included in the preterm formula?
A. Arachidonic acid (AA) and docosahexaenoic acid (DHA)
B. Linoleic acid (LA) and alpha-linoleic acid (ALA)
C. Eicosapentaenoic
D. A and B
E. None of the above

Discussion

The best answer is **D**. AA and DHA may have beneficial effects for preterm visual and cognitive development. LA and ALA are essential fatty acids.[6] Eicosapentaenoic is a nonessential fatty acid.

In assessing the formula composition, what are the essential fatty acids that should be provided?
A. Arachidonic acid (AA) and docosahexaenoic acid (DHA)
B. Linoleic acid (LA) and alpha-linoleic acid (ALA)
C. Eicosapentaenoic
D. A and B
E. None of the above

Discussion

The best answer is **B**. While DHA and AA are important for visual and cognitive development, they are not essential fatty acids. Since DHA and AA may be beneficial for the growth and development of preterm infants, they have typically been included at a ratio of 2:1 (similar to the composition in human milk). Since eicosapentaenoic acid competes with AA, and could negatively affect growth, it has been recommended to limit eicosapentaenoic acid levels in preterm formula. LA and ALA are essential fatty acids. LA serves as a precursor for AA. LA intakes of 385 to 1,540 mg/kg/d are recommended. ALA serves as an essential precursor to eicosapentaenoic acid and DHA with recommended intakes at around 55 mg/kg/d. The recommended ratio of LA:ALA in preterm formula is in the range of 5 to 15:1 (by weight).[6]

In assessing the formula composition, what percentage of medium-chain triglycerides (MCT) is optimal?
A. 0%
B. 30%
C. 60%
D. 90%
E. 100%

Discussion

The best answer is **B**. MCT have been shown to facilitate the absorption of fat and calcium. However, since MCT has lower energy content, it is unclear that increased absorption of MCT over long-chain saturated fatty acids will increase availability of metabolizable energy. Studies have yet to demonstrate any positive effect on energy, nitrogen balance, or weight gain. Therefore it is recommended that MCT content of formula should be no more than 40% of total fat content.[4]

CASE 9

You are considering starting feeds on a VLBW 30-week preterm infant on the first day of life.

Based on your knowledge of lipid metabolism in the preterm infant, you would expect decreased gut absorption of lipids for which of the following reason(s)?
A. Low levels of pancreatic lipase
B. Low levels of bile acids
C. Low levels of lingual lipase
D. All of the above
E. A and C only

Discussion

The correct answer is **D**. Low levels of pancreatic lipase, bile acids, and lingual lipase contribute to reduced gut absorption of lipids in the preterm infant at birth.[17]

How might preterm infants compensate for the above defect(s)?
A. Intragastric lipolysis
B. Increased gastric acid secretion
C. With lipases present in human milk
D. All of the above
E. A and C only

Discussion

The correct answer is **E**. Intragastric lipolysis can occur through lingual and gastric lipases which are secreted starting at 25 weeks' gestation. The resulting fatty acids and monoglycerides can form emulsifying lipid mixtures without requiring bile acids. This is why preterm infants fed jejunally do not absorb fat as well as those fed gastrically.[18] Human milk also contains lipases including lipoprotein lipase, bile salt–stimulated esterase, and nonactivated lipase which can continue lipolysis in the intestine.[17] This is why percent fat absorption for preterm and term infants is better when fed human milk.[18]

What compound is required for metabolism of lipids by transporting long-chain fatty acids into the mitochondria?
A. Medium-chain triglycerides
B. Carnitine
C. Bile acid
D. Cholesterol
E. Acetyl-CoA

Discussion

The correct answer is **B**. Clinicians should be aware that preterm infants may be at higher risk for carnitine deficiency because they have decreased ability to synthesize carnitine. Carnitine is present in breast milk and standard infant formulas.[17] The mitochondrial carnitine system plays an obligatory role in beta-oxidation of long-chain fatty acids by catalyzing their transport into the mitochondrial matrix. This transport system consists of the malonyl-CoA sensitive carnitine palmitoyltransferase I (CPT-I) localized in the mitochondrial outer membrane, the carnitine-acylcarnitine translocase, an integral inner membrane protein, and carnitine palmitoyltransferase II localized on the matrix side of the inner membrane.

Helpful Tip: Even though the preterm infant has low levels of bile acids and pancreatic and lingual lipase, essential fatty acid deficiency is rare because of compensation by intragastric lipases and lipases present in human milk.

What is the predominant carbohydrate in human milk?
A. Glucose
B. Sucrose
C. Lactose
D. Glucose polymers
E. Galactose

Discussion

The correct answer is **C**.[17] The predominant carbohydrate in breast milk is lactose accounting for 40% to 50% of caloric content.

Helpful Tip: In human milk there are 30 or more oligosaccharides, all containing terminal Gal-(beta 1,4)-Glc and ranging from 3 to 14 saccharide units per molecule. These may amount in the aggregate to as much as 1 g/100 mL in mature milk and 2.5 g/100 mL in colostrum. Some of these oligosaccharides may function to control intestinal flora because of their ability to promote growth of certain strains of lactobacilli.

You would expect the intestinal lactase activity in this infant to be what percent of expected activity in a term infant?
A. 10%
B. 30%
C. 50%
D. 70%
E. 90%

Discussion

The correct answer is **B**. Preterm infants have relatively low lactase activity. However, lactose intolerance is rare. This may be because preterm infants acquire higher lactase activity than would be expected in utero.[6] Lactase activity reaches adult levels at ~36 weeks' gestation.

The main composition of carbohydrates in preterm formulas is lactose and
A. Glucose
B. Sucrose
C. Lactose
D. Glucose polymers
E. Galactose

Discussion

The correct answer is **D**. Preterm formulas contain approximately 40% to 50% lactose and 50% to 60% glucose polymers. Glucose polymers are readily metabolized by preterm infants who have active glucosidase (specifically glucoamylase) activity.[18] Glucose polymers allow higher caloric density than lactose without increased osmolality.[6]

In what forms can the preterm intestine absorb proteins and their metabolites?
A. As intact protein
B. As tripeptides or dipeptides
C. As single amino acids
D. All of the above
E. B and C only

Discussion

The correct answer is **D**. Neonates can absorb intact food proteins, which is reflected in higher titers of serum antibodies against food antigens. Oligopeptide transporter (Pept-1) in the brush border of the small intestine allows intestinal absorption of tripeptides and dipeptides. Single amino acid transporters have been shown to allow absorption of specific amino acids in the small intestine of fetuses as young as 12 weeks' gestation.[18]

If the mother planned to feed breast milk to this preterm infant, how would you expect her milk to be different from breast milk from a mother of a term infant?
A. Preterm milk contains more fat
B. Preterm milk contains more protein
C. Preterm milk contains more electrolytes
D. Preterm milk contains more carbohydrates
E. B and C

Discussion

The correct answer is **E**. Preterm human milk contains more protein and electrolytes than term human milk but this still does not provide enough nutrients to optimally meet the needs of the preterm infant, which is why human milk fortifiers are recommended. Preterm human milk has been reported to contain 2.5 to 4 g/100 mL of protein in the first week of life (this declines to 0.9 to 1.8 g/100 mL over the first month of life).[19-21] Term human milk contains ~1.6 g/100 mL of protein in early milk and ~0.9 g/100 mL of protein in mature milk but can be as low as 0.5 or as high as 3.2 g/100 mL.[20,22] Protein in term milk content also declines over time.[20] Donor human milk is variable but can often have lower protein levels (possibly due to being obtained longer after delivery); it has been reported to contain 0.6 to 2 g/100 mL of protein (mean values 0.9–1.2 g/100 mL).[21,23,24] Preterm donor human milk can contain on average ~1.36 g/100 mL of protein.[25]

Objectives

1. Understand the indications and utilizations of parenteral nutrition and combined enteral and parenteral nutrition
2. Know the differences of preterm breast milk versus breast milk of a full-term infant
3. Know the distribution of nutrients (protein, fat, and carbohydrate) and how these nutrient requirements are modified for the preterm infant
4. Know the importance of protein and nonprotein nutrients in achieving utilization of energy as well as nitrogen needs

CASE 10

A maternal–fetal medicine physician informs you that they will be delivering an infant that is 35 weeks but symmetrically <10th percentile for weight, length, and head circumference.

This infant's growth status should be defined as
A. IUGR
B. SGA
C. AGA with placental insufficiency
D. Both IUGR and SGA

Discussion

The best answer is **B**. Infants that are less than the 10th percentile compared to their intrauterine counterparts meet this definition and may be due to nonpathologic conditions.[26] Intrauterine growth restriction occurs when a fetus fails to meet its growth potential as a result of intrinsic or environmental factors; it may be symmetric or asymmetric. Small for gestational babies are infants whose birthweight falls less than the 10th percentile.

In understanding of the mechanism related to SGA growth in utero, you realize that the hormone that is NOT involved in utero is
A. Insulin-like Growth Factor-1 (IGF-1)
B. Epidermal Growth Factor (EGF)
C. Insulin
D. Growth hormone (GH)
E. Transforming Growth Factor-Beta (TGF)

Discussion

The best answer is **D**. Growth hormone (GH) receptors are not found in the placenta and do not influence fetal growth; however after birth, GH does have an active role.[27] Maintenance of fetal growth has been attributed to insulin-like growth factor (IGF), epidermal growth factor (EGF), and transforming growth factor beta (TGF-beta).[27]

CASE 11

An infant that is small for gestational age (27 weeks gestation) is admitted to the NICU.

Because the infant is SGA, the team decides to provide:
A. Double the calories and protein to achieve early catch up growth
B. Routine parenteral nutrition to keep the infant on his/her own growth curve
C. Double the calories but not the protein to catch up
D. Parenteral nutrition at 40 kcal/kg so the infant doesn't receive too many calories and growth is limited

Discussion

The best answer is **B**. Adequate nutrition as would be provided in-utero is important[28] but extra nutrition is not recommended for fear of adult onset disease later.[29] Population based, epidemiologic evidence is mounting that SGA infants that are over fed and grow too quickly after delivery have a higher likelihood for hypertension and cardiovascular disease.[30]

CASE 12

An infant is precipitously delivered and weighs 4,300 g at 37 weeks.

The resident plots the infant on The World Health Organization Term growth charts and finds the infant is
A. Large for gestational age (LGA)
B. Appropriate for gestational age (AGA)
C. Small for gestational age (SGA)
D. Intrauterine growth restricted (IUGR)

Discussion

The best answer is **A**. Infants on average are 3,500 g at term. Infants that are LGA can be constitutionally large or are infants of diabetic mothers exposed to excess glucose in utero.[31] By definition LGA is greater than the 90th percentile for the reference population.

As the fellow, you remind the resident that the maternal history is important to see if she had documented elevations in
A. Proteinuria
B. Glucose
C. Magnesium
D. Blood pressure
E. Platelet count

Discussion

The best answer is **B**. The etiology of LGA can be from maternal diabetes resulting in hyperglycemia. The infant produces their own insulin in response to the glucose received and tolerates this but does produce macrosomia.[32] Proteinuria, magnesium, and blood pressure are related to preeclampsia and are often seen in IUGR infants.

Helpful Tip: Up to 10% of infants are affected by abnormalities of glucose regulation in mother (nearly 85% are gestational diabetes). Infants born to moms with glucose intolerance are at increased risk for RDS, hypoglycemia, congenital anomalies, and hyperviscosity due to polycythemia as well as at increased risk for c-section birth.

Besides having the resident ensure the infants glucose is stable postdelivery, you would also check
A. Calcium
B. BUN
C. Sodium
D. Creatinine
E. Chloride

Discussion

The best answer is **A**. An infant that is LGA can experience hypocalcemia in addition to hypoglycemia.[33] The mechanism for low calcium is due to the low blood magnesium levels with type 2 diabetes. This decreased magnesium level is caused by both an excretion from the kidney and increased insulin-mediated magnesium uptake into cells. Low magnesium levels in the infant inhibit the parathyroid gland and decrease the release of PTH in response to low levels of calcium in the baby.

CASE 13

A preterm infant is resuscitated successfully and weighs 750 g.

The mEq/kg requirements for the electrolytes sodium, potassium, and chloride are expected to be how different from the term infant on a daily basis?
A. Double because of the need for growth
B. Triple because of the need for growth
C. ½ to avoid renal insufficiency
D. ¼ to avoid renal failure

Discussion

The best answer is **A**. The fetus accretes electrolytes in a factorial approach in utero and thus if born early and misses the last trimester of fetal life, has tremendous requirements for nutrients involved in the growth velocity required.[34] Infants born preterm also have excess losses of electrolytes.[35]

The dietitian asks you what concentration to provide for sodium in the parenteral nutrition on day of life 3.

You tell her to provide
A. 2 mEq/kg
B. 6 mEq/kg
C. 0.5 mEq/kg
D. 1 mEq/kg
E. None is needed until serum Na is less than 135

Discussion

The best answer is **A**; 2 mEq/kg as a starting point for fetal accretion.[4] Sodium is required for fetal growth with an accretion rate of 1.2 mEq/kg/d between 31 and 38 weeks.[4] Sodium retention is supported by increased aldosterone levels in newborns. However in preterm infants <34 weeks sodium reabsorption is decreased, and the fractional excretion of Na may exceed 5%. Even with the increased fractional excretion of Na, the preterm infant is unable to rapidly increase sodium excretion in response to high sodium loads, so excess Na administration also needs to be avoided.

Helpful Tip: To calculate a sodium deficit, you would use the equation:

$$\text{Na deficit (mEq)} = [\text{Na desired (mEq/L)} \\ - \text{Na observed (mEq/L)}] \\ \times 0.6 \times \text{wt (kg)}$$

CASE 14

The resident comes to you with an elevated alkaline phosphatase >800 and signs of rickets on chest x-ray on a 2-week-old former 24-week infant that has been on parenteral nutrition and minimal enteral nutrition.

The laboratory value *most important to check* for this infant for bone mineralization is
A. PTH
B. Vitamin D
C. Magnesium
D. Phosphorus
E. Calcium

Discussion

The best answer is **D**. Calcium is required at a tremendous level over the last trimester for a total of 30 g but in cases of high alkaline phosphatase in preterm infants it is vital to check phosphorus.[36] In fact a molar ratio of calcium to phosphorus should be 1:1 in the PN to help with this and feedings advanced as possible.[37] Vitamin D and PTH should be evaluated in refractory cases, malabsorption diseases, or with suspicion of congenital disease.

CASE 15

The nurse practitioner is writing parenteral nutrition for the infant that is 26 weeks' gestational age. She is concerned that vitamins in the 5-mL vial may need to be adjusted.

You agree and ask her to order
A. Double the multivitamin infusion for fetal accretion
B. ½ the vial of PN vitamins are adequate
C. ¼ of the vial to ensure renal clearance is not impaired
D. 5 mL is adequate to provide fetal accretion

Discussion

The correct answer is **B**. Typically the preterm infant requires only ½ of the MVI because parenteral absorption is so direct.[38] Current individualization of vitamin orders are not routinely done but intake for each nutrient can be found in the 2014 global consensus recommendations published in the Nutritional Care of Preterm Infants.[39]

CASE 16

A mother has been expressing her milk for her 28-week-old infant in the NICU. The resident is unaware that the mother is a strict vegan.

What water-soluble vitamin deficiency may occur in the infant due to milk inadequacy on a strict vegan diet and what laboratory value would reflect this?
A. Vitamin A; retinol-binding protein
B. Vitamin C; prealbumin
C. B12; CBC
D. Folate; CBC
E. Vitamin D; alkaline phosphatase

Discussion

The best answer is **C**. B12 can be deficient in vegan mother's milk and is not made by the mammary gland and thus should be supplemented in the mother's diet.[40] The CBC will be abnormal with a macrocytic anemia. Other vitamins are usually not deficient in a vegan diet. For reference vitamin A deficiency is thought to play a role in the development of BPD and failure to thrive. Vitamin C deficiency is associated with poor wound healing. Vitamin D is a fat-soluble vitamin associated with bone health, and deficiency is associated with rickets.

Helpful Tip: The fat-soluble vitamins are A, D, E, and K. Water-soluble vitamins are the B-complex vitamins and vitamin C.

CASE 17

You are treating an infant with documented cystic fibrosis in your unit. Despite enzyme supplementation, the team has been struggling with fat malabsorption.

Which fat-soluble vitamin will become deficient and which laboratory value will indirectly represent this limitation?
A. Vitamin E; platelet count
B. Vitamin K and PTT
C. Vitamin D and PTH
D. Vitamin A and CBC

Discussion

The best pair is **A**. An infant with low vitamin E will have often documented thrombocytosis.[41] Vitamin A can also become deficient but would be reflected by prealbumin or retinol levels and not the CBC. Vitamin K deficiency affects the clotting cascade and can be associated with elevated PT (Factors II, VII, IX, and X are affected by vitamin K). Vitamin D deficiency can be the result of inadequate PTH stimulation of the gastrointestinal tract for absorption.

CASE 18

An infant was receiving a double dose of vitamin A per day inadvertently by maternal supplementation.

The infant was admitted through the ER with which adverse sequel from this practice?
A. Blindness
B. Rickets
C. Pseudotumor cerebri
D. Dermatitis

Discussion

The correct answer is **C**.[42] Vitamin A deficiency can result from inadequate intake, fat malabsorption, or liver disorders. Deficiency impairs immunity and hematopoiesis and causes rashes and typical ocular effects (e.g., night blindness). Dermatitis is a sign of essential fatty acid deficiency and not excessive vitamin A administration. Rickets is associated with vitamin D deficiency.

CASE 19

An 25 day-old infant weighing 1,500 g is growing on fortified human milk.

What nutrient may be necessary besides vitamin D as a supplement?
A. Zinc
B. Vitamin E
C. Folate
D. Iron

Discussion

The best answer is **D**. The preterm infant starts to have erythropoiesis 4 to 6 weeks after birth and there is insufficient iron in milk sources and would subsequently require a minimum of 2 mg/kg additional per day of elemental iron.[43]

Helpful Tip: Iron is absorbed primarily in the duodenum and early jejunum. Deficiency of iron leads to a microcytic anemia.

CASE 20

Your dietitian is concerned regarding slow growth in your infant who is on fully fortified human milk with calories, protein, minerals, vitamins, and sodium. This was also a former SGA infant.

What nutrient must you have the dietitian supplement?
A. Copper
B. Potassium
C. Magnesium
D. Zinc

Discussion

The correct answer is **D**. The preterm infants exchangeable zinc pool is low compared to his term counterpart and the SGA infant is even at a higher risk for deficiency.[44] Growth is the major factor used to determine zinc requirements of preterm infants. Calculations of zinc requirements for preterm infants between 24 and 28 weeks of gestational age indicate a requirement of 600 μg/d for the formation of new tissues. The calculation of dietary zinc in order for optimal growth to occur is equivalent to 500 μg/kg/d, for infants weighing approximately 1,000 g at birth (28 weeks gestation); 400 μg/kg/d for newborn infants between 1,500 and 2,000 g (30–32 weeks) and 200 to 300 μg/kg/d for those weighing between 2,500 and 3,500 g (35–40 weeks). Copper deficiency is rare in the neonatal period, but when it is present, it causes hypochromic anemia resistant to iron supplementation, osteoporosis, skin manifestations as well as difficulty in gaining weight.[44]

CASE 21

TPN shortages required the pharmacy to prioritize trace elements in the NICU.

Which trace element besides zinc is important to include early in the parenterally fed low–birth-weight infant not on enteral feeding?
A. Iron
B. Manganese
C. Calcium
D. Selenium

Discussion

The correct answer is **D**. Selenium is a trace element accreted in utero primarily at 36 weeks' gestation and therefore the preterm infant misses this entirely. Selenium is an important component of glutathione peroxidase and is theoretically important in the prevention of BPD.[45] Iron is not required early in the life of a parenterally fed preterm infant. Calcium is not a trace element but is required early on. While manganese is an essential micronutrient component, and is utilized in several enzymes including pyruvate carboxylase and mitochondrial superoxide dismutase, its level is actually high at birth. Blood manganese levels around birth result from in utero accumulation.

The pharmacist on the team is covering from the PICU. She is concerned that the preterm infant in your care that has short bowel syndrome does not have manganese (Mn) in the current order.

You remind her that the Mn contamination alone is plenty and that the following toxic event is more likely if Mn is added?
A. Rickets
B. Neurotoxicity
C. Rhabdomyolysis
D. Cardiac

Discussion

The correct answer is **B**. Neurotoxicity is a problem for the preterm infant on Mn if hepatobiliary function is limited.[46]

The pharmacist is struggling to ensure that nutrients are prioritized accordingly to the NICU patients during shortages. What nutrient in parenteral nutrition is related to glucose tolerance in humans?

A. Vitamin C
B. Vitamin K
C. Copper
D. Chromium

Discussion

The correct answer is **D**. Chromium is involved in the insulin receptor regulation in vivo and enhances insulin action.[47] However, clinical trials are limited. Copper is a cofactor in several metalloproteins, essential for oxidative metabolism, myelination, and the metabolism of several steroid hormones. Vitamin C is thought to be an antioxidant and involved in wound healing. Vitamin K is involved in coagulation.

CASE 22

Your resident knows that an infant with a direct bilirubin over 2 mg/dL requires alteration to the parenteral nutrition.

What two nutrients must be eliminated or reduced?

A. Biotin and calcium
B. Magnesium and chromium
C. Manganese and copper
D. Manganese and zinc

Discussion

The correct answer is **C**. Manganese and copper require hepatic-biliary function for excretion and thus can be eliminated and/or reduced.[45]

Helpful Tip: In addition to elevated direct bilirubin levels, other laboratory values that are elevated in TPN cholestasis include GGT and liver function tests (LFTs). GGT is usually elevated before the rest of the LFTs. Advancing enteral feeds and stopping TPN slowly resolve the TPN cholestasis.

CASE 23

The infant in your care is post cooling for hypoxic ischemic injury. The infant has a very low glomerular filtration rate and is on a fluid restriction.

What nutrient in the parenteral nutrition must be limited to avoid toxicity during this time of renal insufficiency?

A. Calcium
B. Phosphorus
C. Chromium
D. Magnesium

Discussion

The correct answer is **C**. Chromium relies on renal excretion and care should be taken to avoid its use in this scenario.[45]

Objectives

1. Understand minerals and the changing requirements for mineral and electrolyte requirements at different gestational ages
2. Know the requirements for vitamins in the preterm and term infant
3. Know the clinical manifestations of deficiencies of fat- and water-soluble vitamins
4. Understand the trace elements and the clinical presentation and management of iron, zinc, copper, selenium, manganese, and chromium deficiency
5. Know the potential toxicities of element supplementation

CASE 24

You are caring for a "growing" preterm infant in room air and on full-fortified breast milk feeds. Her mother has a limited breast milk supply. She asks you what are the differences between human milk and formula.

You inform her that the protein composition of infant formulas is different from human milk since cow's milk contains

A. More casein than human milk
B. More whey than human milk
C. More lactalbumins than human milk
D. More sulfur-containing amino acids than human milk
E. All of the above

Discussion

The correct answer is **A**. Cow's milk contains more casein than human milk (whey:casein ratio 18:82). Some formulas add cow-milk whey protein to achieve a more whey–casein ratio similar to human milk (60:40). Nevertheless, cow's milk whey protein is predominantly composed of alpha-lactoglobulin while human milk protein is predominantly composed of alpha-lactalbumin. Infant formulas also tend to have a higher overall protein concentration (1.45–1.6 g/dL) when compared to human milk (0.9–1 g/dL).[48]

Helpful Tip: Breast milk is more like a living tissue such as blood rather than just a nutrient source. Breast milk contains immunologic factors such as IgA and lactoferrin, hormones, oligosaccharides, growth factors, antioxidants, as well as numerous other constituents.

You inform her that the fat composition of infant formulas is different from human milk since cow's milk-based formulas contain
A. More fat than human milk
B. Less fat than human milk
C. Less cholesterol than human milk
D. Vegetable oils
E. B, C, and D

Discussion

The correct answer is **E**. While still the major source of calories, fat content is slightly lower in infant formulas when compared to human milk and contains little or no cholesterol. Infant formulas are typically comprised of vegetable oils or a mix of animal and vegetable oils as the source of fat. The vegetable oil composition improves digestion and absorption of fats when compared to cow milk butterfat.[48]

You inform her that the mineral composition of infant formulas is different from human milk since cow's milk-based formulas contain
A. Less calcium than human milk
B. Less phosphorous than human milk
C. More iron than human milk
D. All of the above
E. None of the above

Discussion

The correct answer is **D**. Infant formulas have added iron, calcium, and phosphorous at a concentration greater than that found in human milk.[48]

You inform her that human milk contains immunologic constituents that can benefit her baby that formulas do not. Which of the following are beneficial immunologic constituents in human milk?
A. IgA
B. Lactoferrin
C. Lysozyme
D. Cytokines
E. All of the above

Discussion

The correct answer is **E**. Human milk contains secretory IgA antibodies which can specifically target infections. Human milk also contains lactoferrin and lysozyme, which are antimicrobial. Human milk also contains anti-inflammatory cytokines, such as interleukin-10. In addition, human milk contains oligosaccharides that can prevent bacterial attachment and growth factors which can promote epithelial and nerve growth (epidermal growth factor, transforming growth factor, nerve growth factor).[49]

CASE 25

You are caring for a preterm infant who is starting trophic feeds after treatment for medical necrotizing enterocolitis. However, mother has limited breast milk supply. You are considering ordering donor breast milk.

What are the disadvantages of using donor breast milk?
A. No federal regulations or guidelines
B. Pasteurization required
C. Pooled donor
D. Limited supplies
E. All of the above

Discussion

The best answer is **E**.[6] Donor milk has been advocated by the AAP as an alternative if mother's own milk is not available. Potentially due to the lower protein levels in donor human milk as compared to mother's own milk for premature infants, short-term growth may be compromised with the use of donor milk in preterm infants (compared to formula). However, donor milk has been associated with lower risk of necrotizing enterocolitis if fed to preterm infants instead of formula and there have been no negative effects noted in long-term growth.[50]

A nurse asks you whether the pasteurization process affects the composition of human milk.

Which of the following components of human milk can be affected by pasteurization?
A. IgA
B. Immune cells
C. Enzymes
D. All of the above
E. None of the above

Discussion

The correct answer is **D**. Pasteurization can reduce secretory IgA, number and function of immune cells, and enzymatic activity (amylase, lipase, lactoperoxidase, and lipolytic activity).[51]

In comparison, which of the following components of human milk can be affected by freezing?
A. IgA
B. Immune cells
C. Enzymes
D. All of the above
E. None of the above

Discussion

The correct answer is **E**. Secretory IgA, immune cell number and function, and digestive enzyme activity are stable in frozen human milk.[51]

In comparison, which of the following components of human milk can be affected by microwaving?
A. IgA
B. Immune cells
C. Enzymes
D. All of the above
E. None of the above

Discussion

The correct answer is **D**. Microwave radiation results in significant loss of IgA and lysozyme activity. Microwaving results in higher levels of *Escherichia coli* as opposed to pasteurization which reduces bacterial numbers. Microwave radiation also reduces vitamin C.[51,52]

Objectives

1. Know the differences in composition in human milk and infant formula
2. Know the immunologic constituents in human milk and their effects
3. Recognize the effects of different processing methods of human milk including pasteurizing, freezing, and microwaving
4. Know the advantages and disadvantages of using donor breast milk

CASE 26

You are caring for a preterm infant who is advancing feeding volume successfully with human milk. You inform the mother that it is time to supplement her milk with preterm fortifier. The mother asks whether fortifier can be avoided.

In counseling the mother, you inform her that unfortified human milk may not meet the nutritional needs of her preterm infant.

Which of the following components of human milk are supplemented with fortifier in order to meet the needs of preterm infants?
A. Fat
B. Protein
C. Carbohydrates
D. All of the above
E. None of the above

Discussion

The correct answer is **B**. In addition to protein, human milk fortifiers supplement additional nutrients, minerals, and vitamins to meet the needs of preterm infants.[6]

In counseling the mother, prolonged use of unfortified human milk can lead to which of the following metabolic complications?
A. Hypoproteinemia
B. Osteopenia
C. Zinc deficiency
D. All of the above
E. None of the above

Discussion

The correct answer is **D**.[6] Freshly expressed breast milk has on average 1 g of protein—1.2 g/dL in preterm milk and only 0.9 g/dL in term donor milk and so the preterm 1-kg infant would have to ingest 350 to 400 mL or more to achieve their protein needs without fortification.

CASE 27

You are giving a lecture to the pediatric residents about breast milk production in the NICU.

What are some common problems that physicians should know about?

A. Collection
B. Storage
C. Handling
D. All of the above
E. None of the above

Discussion

The best answer is **D**. Mothers need to be carefully counseled on the proper method of collection, storage, and handling of expressed breast milk. Mothers also should be counseled to start pumping early and regularly in order to encourage breast milk production.[6]

Helpful Tip: Prolactin secretion is important in establishing lactation. During pregnancy estrogen and progesterone levels are elevated and actually inhibit milk production. The subsequent fall of those hormones after delivery allow milk production to increase. Expression of milk is mediated by the hormone oxytocin.

What is (are) the secretory process (es) in the epithelial cell of the lactating mammary gland?

A. Exocytosis
B. Lipid synthesis
C. Transcytosis of proteins
D. Transmembrane transport of ions/fluid
E. All of the above

Discussion

The best answer is **E**.[53] The secretory processes of the epithelial cell of the lactating mammary gland include exocytosis, lipid secretion, transcytosis of proteins, and transmembrane transport of ions, glucose, amino acids, and drugs (from interstitial space to milk).

What is the paracellular transport pathway of the mammary gland?

A. Transports hormones into breast milk
B. Transports molecules between interstitial space and breast milk
C. Bidirectional pathway between interstitial space and breast milk (alveolar lumen)
D. All of the above
E. None of the above

Discussion

The best answer is **C**.[53] This pathway allows for direct bidirectional passage of substances between the alveolar lumen and the interstitial space. This pathway is closed during lactation.

PATHWAY	DESCRIPTION
A. Exocytosis	Primary pathway for alveolar cells to secrete protein, water, lactose, oligosaccharides, calcium, phosphate, and citrate. These substances are transported from the Golgi to the apical membrane via vesicles.
B. Lipid secretion	Lipids are synthesized in the smooth endoplasmic reticulum (ER), form lipid bodies, coalesce, and then are secreted via budding at the apical membrane forming milk fat globules.
C. Transcytosis	Substances are packaged via endocytosis (into endosomes) at the basal membrane and then are degraded in lysosomes or secreted via exocytosis at the apical membrane. Immunoglobulin A, prolactin, and transferrin may be transported through this pathway.
D. Transmembrane transport	Multiple specific transmembrane transport systems/channels for ions, fluid, glucose, amino acids, and drugs.
E. Paracellular transport	Bidirectional flow directly between the lumen and the interstitium (closed during lactation).

CASE 28

You are giving a lecture to the pediatric residents about the use of formulas in the NICU. They ask about the composition of nutrients in term and preterm formulas.

How much protein is in the typical term formula?

A. 2.1 to 2.5 g/100 kcal
B. 2.7 to 3 g/100 kcal
C. 3.5 to 4.5 g/100 kcal
D. 5 to 6 g/100 kcal
E. 10 to 12 g/100 kcal

Discussion

The correct answer is **B**. Term formula contains from 14 to 18 g of protein per liter, which is equivalent to 2.7 to 2.9 g/100 kcal of formula. Term formulas are now designed to try to mimic the growth of breast-fed infants instead of matching the nutrient levels in human milk (since nutrients in formula may not be as bioavailable). Term formulas protein content is almost 50% more than human milk. Human milk contains approximately 9 to 10 g of protein per liter, which is equivalent to 1.4 to 1.6 g/100 kcal of human milk.[22,39]

How much protein is in the typical preterm formula?
A. 2.1 to 2.5 g/100 kcal
B. 2.7 to 3 g/100 kcal
C. 3.5 to 4.5 g/100 kcal
D. 5 to 6 g/100 kcal
E. 10 to 12 g/100 kcal

Discussion

The correct answer is **B**. Preterm formula contains from 22 to 24 g of protein per liter of 24-calorie formula, which is equivalent to 2.8 to 3 g/100 kcal of formula. Note the protein to calorie ratio of term formula and 24-calorie preterm formula is similar. The newer higher protein preterm formulas contain 27 to 29 g of protein per liter of 24-calore formula, which is equivalent to 3.4 to 3.5 g/100 kcal of formula. Transitional formulas contain 19.4 to 21 g of protein per liter of 22-calorie formula, which is equivalent to 2.6 to 2.8 g/100 kcal of formula.[22,39]

How much fat is in the typical term formula?
A. 2.1 to 2.5 g/100 kcal
B. 2.7 to 3 g/100 kcal
C. 3.5 to 4.5 g/100 kcal
D. 5 to 6 g/100 kcal
E. 10 to 12 g/100 kcal

Discussion

The correct answer is **D**. Term formula contains from 35 to 36 g of fat per liter, which is equivalent to 5.3 to 5.6 g/100 kcal of formula. Preterm formula contains from 41 to 44 g of fat per liter of 24-calorie formula, which is equivalent to ~5.1 g/100 kcal of formula. Transitional formulas contain from 39 to 41 g of fat per liter of 22-calorie formula, which is equivalent to ~5.3 to 5.5 g/100 kcal of formula.[22]

How much carbohydrate is in the typical term formula?
A. 2.1 to 2.2 g/100 kcal
B. 2.7 to 3 g/100 kcal
C. 4.9 to 5.1 g/100 kcal
D. 5.3 to 5.6 g/100 kcal
E. 10 to 12 g/100 kcal

Discussion

The correct answer is **E**. Term formula contains from 72 to 76 g of carbohydrate per liter, which is equivalent to ~10.7 to 11.2 g/100 kcal of formula. Preterm formula contains from 86.1 to 90 g of carbohydrate per liter of 24-calorie formula, which is equivalent to ~10.7 to 11.1 g/100 kcal of formula. Transitional formulas contain 77 to 79 g of carbohydrate per liter of 22-calorie formula, which is equivalent to ~10.3 to 10.7 g/100 kcal of formula.[22,39]

How much calcium is in the typical term formula?
A. 30 to 55 mg/100 kcal
B. 60 to 85 mg/100 kcal
C. 85 to 120 mg/100 kcal
D. 150 to 200 mg/100 kcal
E. 200 to 300 mg/100 kcal

Discussion

The best answer is **B**. Term formula contains from 420 to 550 mg/L of calcium, which is equivalent to 62.5 to 81 mg/100 kcal of formula.[22]

How much calcium is in the typical preterm formula?
A. 30 to 55 mg/100 kcal
B. 60 to 85 mg/100 kcal
C. 85 to 120 mg/100 kcal
D. 150 to 200 mg/100 kcal
E. 200 to 300 mg/100 kcal

Discussion

The best answer is **D**. Preterm formula contains from 1,340 to 1,460 mg of calcium per liter of 24-calorie formula, which is equivalent to ~165 to 180 mg of calcium per 100 kcal. Transitional formulas contain from 780 to 890 mg of calcium per liter of 22-calorie formula, which is equivalent to ~105 to 120 mg/100 kcal.[22,39]

How much phosphorous is in the typical term formula?
A. 30 to 55 mg/100 kcal
B. 60 to 85 mg/100 kcal
C. 85 to 120 mg/100 kcal
D. 150 to 200 mg/100 kcal
E. 200 to 300 mg/100 kcal

Discussion

The best answer is **A**. Term formula contains from 245 to 370 mg/L of phosphorous, which is equivalent to ~36 to 55 mg/100 kcal.[22]

How much phosphorous is in the typical preterm formula?
A. 30 to 55 mg/100 kcal
B. 60 to 85 mg/100 kcal
C. 85 to 120 mg/100 kcal
D. 150 to 200 mg/100 kcal
E. 200 to 300 mg/100 kcal

Discussion

The best answer is **C**. Preterm formula contains from 670 to 800 mg of phosphorous per liter of 24-calorie formula, which is equivalent to ~83 to 100 mg/100 kcal. Transitional formulas contain from 463 to 490 mg of phosphorous per liter of 22-calorie formula, which is equivalent to ~62 to 66 mg/100 kcal.[22,39]

How much vitamin D is in the typical term formula?
A. 50 to 100 IU/100 kcal
B. 100 to 200 IU/100 kcal
C. 200 to 300 IU/100 kcal
D. 300 to 400 IU/100 kcal
E. 400 to 500 IU/100 kcal

Discussion

The best answer is **A**. Term formula contains from 400 to 410 IU/L of vitamin D, which is equivalent to ~75 to 95 IU/100 kcal. The AAP recommends 400 IU/d in term infants. Thus, all term infants should be supplemented with vitamin D.[54]

How much vitamin D is in the typical preterm formula?
A. 50 to 100 IU/100 kcal
B. 100 to 150 IU/100 kcal
C. 150 to 300 IU/100 kcal
D. 300 to 400 IU/100 kcal
E. 400 to 500 IU/100 kcal

Discussion

The best answer is **C**. Preterm formula contains from 1,210 to 1,920 IU of vitamin D per liter of 24-calorie formula, which is equivalent to ~150 to 240 IU/100 kcal. Transitional formulas contain from 513 to 590 IU of vitamin D per liter of 22-calorie formula, which is equivalent to ~70 to 80 IU/100 kcal. The AAP recommends 200 to 400 IU of vitamin D daily in preterm infants.[39,55]

Helpful Tip:

NUTRIENT CONTENTS	HUMAN MILK (MATURE)	TERM FORMULA	TRANSITIONAL FORMULA (22 cal)	PRETERM FORMULA (24 cal)	HIGH-PROTEIN PRETERM FORMULA (24 cal)
Energy (kcal/L)	650–700	640–670	740–744	806–812	811–812
Protein (g/L) (g/100 kcal)	8–14 (1.2–1.8)	14–18 (2.7–2.9)	19–21 (2.6–2.8)	22–24 (2.8–3)	27–29 (3.4–3.5)
Fat (g/L) (g/100 kcal)	35 (5.3)	35–36 (5.3–5.6)	39–41 (5.3–5.5)	41–44 (5.1)	41–42 (5.1)
Carbohydrate (g/L) (g/100 kcal)	54–72 (8–10.6)	70–74 (10.4–11)	70–74 (10.4–11)	70–74 (10.4–11)	70–74 (10.4–11)
Calcium (mg/L) (mg/100 kcal)	200–250	420–550 (62.5–81)	780–890 (105–120)	1,340–1,460 (165–180)	1,340–1,460 (165–180)
Phosphorous (mg/L) (mg/100 kcal)	120–140	245–370 (36–55)	463–490 (62–66)	670–800 (83–100)	670–800 (83–100)
Vitamin D (IU/L) (IU/100 kcal)	22	400–410 (75–95)	513–590 (70–80)	1,210–1,920 (150–240)	1,210–1,920 (150–240)

Objectives

1. Know the difference in preterm and term formula mineral content in formula
2. Know the nutritional composition of preterm and term formula

CASE 29

You are caring for a term infant whose parents request the initiation of soy formula. Their first infant had colic which was improved after switching to soy formula.

Which of the following are indications for soy protein–based formula?

A. Term infants with galactosemia or hereditary lactase deficiency
B. Term infants with documented IgE-mediated allergy to cow milk
C. Term infants whose parents are seeking a vegetarian diet
D. All of the above
E. A and C only

Discussion

The correct answer is **D**. The AAP does not recommend starting soy formula in order to prevent colic or allergy. However, infants with documented IgE-mediated allergy to cow milk will usually tolerate soy protein–based formula. In addition, term infants with documented transient lactase deficiency or whose nutritional needs are not being met by current feedings can be switched to soy protein–based formulas.[48]

CASE 30

A preterm infant <1,500 g is delivered and brought to the unit. Because of the infant's immature suck and swallow, a parenteral source of nutrients is required.

To improve growth velocity by discharge, this infant should start on

A. Parenteral glucose alone because of renal immaturity
B. Parenteral glucose and amino acid (starter TPN) therapy
C. Parenteral glucose + amino acids (starter TPN), and enteral trophic (≤15 mL/kg) nasogastric feeding
D. Parenteral glucose and enteral trophic (≤15 mL/kg) nasogastric feeding
E. Parenteral amino acids alone since insulin resistance is high

Discussion

The best answer is **C**. Glucose and amino acids or starter TPN along with trophic enteral feeding by nasogastric tube to provide adequate amino acids for growth and to keep the intestinal tract barrier healthy.[9,56]

CASE 31

When writing the TPN order for a 1,000-g (1 kg) preterm infant, you realize to promote growth, and to avoid excessive carbohydrate calories a balanced nutrient composition is required.

Which of the following is the best composition for your preterm infant?

A. Dextrose 12.5%, 3% amino acids at 130 mL/kg, and 20% intralipid at 20 mL/kg
B. Dextrose 10%, amino acids 4% at 160 mL/kg, and 10% intralipid at 10 mL/kg
C. Dextrose 15%, amino acids 6% at 150 mL/kg, and 20% intralipid at 15 mL/kg
D. Dextrose 17%, amino acids 4% at 150 mL/kg, and 10% intralipid at 15 mL/kg
E. Dextrose 20%, amino acids 4% at 150 mL/kg, and 20% intralipid at 15 mL/kg

Discussion

The correct answer is **A**. Dextrose calories are anhydrous and provide 3.4 kcal/mL, amino acids 4 kcal/mL, and lipids 2 kcal/mL if 20% and 1.1 kcal/mL if 10%. The goal for balancing the ratio of nutrients should be similar to human milk intake: 50% to 60% calories as fat, 40% to 50% carbohydrate, and the remainder as protein.[9,56]

Helpful Tip: To calculate parenteral nutrition, the following formulas are used for answer A as an example:

1. D12.5 at 130 mL/kg/d = 12.5 g/100 mL × 130 mL/kg/d × 3.4 kcal/g = 55 kcal/kg/d
2. 3% amino acids at 130 mL/kg/d = 3 g/100 mL × 130 mL/kg/d = 3.9 g/kg/d × 4 kcal/g = 15.6 kcal/kg/d
3. 20 mL/kg/d lipid (of a 20% solution) = 20 mL/kg/d × 20 g/100 mL × 9 kcal/g = 36 kcal/kg/d

Helpful Tip: Glucose infusion rate (GIR) is given as GIR as mg/kg/min = [(percent dextrose) × (mL/kg/d)]/144. For D10 at 150 mL/kg/d the GIR would be 10 × 150/144 = 10.4 mg/kg/min.

Helpful Tip: A typical GIR is 5–8 mg/kg/min

CASE 32

In both parenteral and enteral nutrition it is important to provide enough calories from nonprotein sources so the protein source can be used for skeletal muscle synthesis and growth.

Which ratio provides the best growth?
A. 1.5 nonprotein:protein calories
B. 2.5
C. 3.6 to 3.8
D. 4.5 to 6

Discussion

The best answer is **C**. This allows nitrogen balance and growth to be optimized.[9,57]

CASE 33

You are rounding with the pediatric residents rotating through the NICU and are double checking their calculations for caloric intake in a preterm infant with advancing feeds. The infant is ordered to have TPN with D10 + 3% amino acid solution @ 120 mL/kg/d and 20% IL @ 15 mL/kg/d.

How many g/kg/d of protein will the infant receive?
A. 1 g/kg/d
B. 2.5 g/kg/d
C. 3 g/kg/d
D. 3.5 g/kg/d
E. 4 g/kg/d

Discussion

The best answer is **D**. A 3% amino acid solution contains 3 g per 100 mL of solution. At 120 mL/kg/d this results in 3.6 g/kg/d of protein (0.03 g/mL × 120 ml/kg/d).

How many g/kg/d of fat will the infant receive?
A. 1 g/kg/d
B. 2.5 g/kg/d
C. 3 g/kg/d
D. 3.5 g/kg/d
E. 4 g/kg/d

Discussion

The best answer is **C**. 20% IL solution contains 20 g IL per 100 mL of solution. At 15 mL/kg/d, this results in 3 g/kg/d of fat (0.2 g/mL × 15 mL/kg/d).

How many total calories will the infant receive?
A. 85 kcal/kg/d
B. 100 kcal/kg/d
C. 110 kcal/kg/d
D. 120 kcal/kg/d
E. None of the above

Discussion

The best answer is **A**. D10 solution contains 10-g dextrose per 100 mL and dextrose contains 3.4 kcal per gram. Thus the infant will receive 41 kcal/kg/d from dextrose (0.1 g/mL × 120 mL/kg/d × 3.4 kcal/g). The infant will receive 4 kcal per gram of amino acid, which is 14.4 kcal/kg/d (3.6 g/kg/d × 4 kcal/g). The infant will receive 9 kcal per gram of fat, which is 27 kcal/kg/d (3 g/kg/d × 9 kcal/g). Thus the total caloric intake being provided by parenteral nutrition ordered for this infant is 82.4 kcal/kg/d.

Helpful Tip: For faster calculations you can use 4 kcal for glucose and 4 kcal for protein, and 10 kcal for fat. This will end up being a slight over estimate and you should look for a value slightly less than your calculation.

How many total calories will the infant receive if the TPN were comprised of D14 with 3.3% amino acid solution at 120 mL/kg/d instead?
A. 90 kcal/kg/d
B. 100 kcal/kg/d
C. 110 kcal/kg/d
D. 120 kcal/kg/d
E. None of the above

Discussion

The best answer is **B**. D14 solution contains 14-g dextrose per 100 mL and dextrose contains 3.4 kcal per gram. Thus the infant will receive 57.1 kcal/kg/d from dextrose (0.14 g/mL × 120 mL.kg/d × 3.4 kcal/g). The infant will receive 4 kcal per gram of amino acid, which is 15.84 kcal/kg/d (0.033 g/mL × 120 mL/kg/d × 4 kcal/g). The infant will receive 9 kcal per gram of fat, which is 27 kcal/kg/d (3 g/kg/d × 9 kcal/g). Thus the total caloric intake being provided by parenteral nutrition ordered for this infant is 99.94 kcal/kg/d.

CASE 34

You are caring for a preterm infant with newly diagnosed necrotizing enterocolitis. When counseling the mother regarding the need for prolonged parenteral nutrition, she asks about the potential complications of such therapy.

Which of the following are potential complications of prolonged parenteral nutrition?
A. Osteopenia
B. Cholestasis
C. Catheter complications
D. Metabolic complications
E. All of the above

Discussion

The best answer is **E**. The concentration of calcium and phosphorus is limited in parenteral nutrition for the nutrients to stay in solution and therefore intrauterine recommendations for calcium and phosphorus are not met, and this can result in osteopenia. In addition, the liver is affected by the source of fatty acids and nutrients unlike enteral provisions and can cause cholestasis and metabolic problems. Finally because intravenous access in a small baby is needed, catheter accidents and infections are a risk.

What is the best calcium to phosphorous ratio (by weight) to maintain in parenteral nutrition solutions in order to minimize the risk of osteopenia?
A. 0.7:1
B. 1:1
C. 1.7:1
D. 2:1
E. None of the above

Discussion

The best answer is **C**. The ideal calcium–phosphorous ratio is 1.7:1 by weight. This will be equivalent to 75 mg/kg/d of elemental calcium and 45 mg/kg/d of elemental phosphorous. Trophamine is also recommended for allowing the maximal calcium and phosphorous content to remain in solution.[58]

What is the first laboratory sign of TPN-associated liver injury?
A. Elevated serum transaminases
B. Elevated serum bile salts
C. Elevated serum alkaline phosphatase
D. Elevated direct hyperbilirubinemia
E. None of the above

Discussion

The best answer is **B**. The first clinical indication is mild hepatomegaly followed by increased serum bile salts, followed by increased serum direct bilirubin, followed by increased serum alkaline phosphatase and transaminases. These changes can occur as early as 2 weeks on TPN.[58]

What is the best treatment for TPN-associated cholestasis?
A. Cycling off TPN for a few hours a day
B. Phenobarbital
C. Enteral feeds
D. Limiting trace elements
E. Limiting lipid infusion

Discussion

The best answer is **C**. TPN-associated liver disease is caused by enteral starvation. Initiating feeds as soon as possible will minimize hepatic complications. Once the patient develops TPN-associated cholestasis, limiting trace elements (copper and manganese), limiting lipid infusion (to no more than 1 g/kg/d) may be wise to limit further injury. Phenobarbital has no role in the treatment of cholestasis.[58,59]

Which of the following may be metabolic consequences of parenteral nutrition administration?
A. Azotemia
B. Metabolic acidosis
C. Aluminum toxicity
D. All of the above
E. None of the above

Discussion

The best answer is **C**. Azotemia is less likely with modern TPN solutions if amino acid administration is limited to ≤4 g/kg/d. Metabolic acidosis caused by TPN has also been less of a concern since modern TPN solutions began using acetate in lysine salts and basic salts of histidine instead of using chlorine. Aluminum is present in some preparations of calcium and phosphorous. Aluminum intake should be monitored and minimized especially for preterm infants or infants with renal dysfunction.[58]

Which of the following are potential catheter complications of parenteral nutrition administration?
A. Pleural/pericardial effusions of parenteral nutrition solution
B. Pneumothorax
C. Hemorrhage
D. Catheter emboli
E. All of the above

Discussion

The best answer is **E**. All of the above are potential complications. Pleural/pericardial effusions of parenteral nutrition solutions can occur with malpositioning of peripherally inserted central catheters (PICCs). Pneumothorax or brachial plexus injuries can occur during placement of subclavian central lines. Hemorrhage can occur during insertion of central lines or associated with erosion of central veins. Other complications include catheter-related sepsis, catheter occlusion (from thrombus, fat deposition, drug precipitation, or calcium–phosphorous precipitation).[58]

Which of the following are signs of a malpositioned PICC line causing effusion into the pleural or pericardial space?

A. Hypoglycemia
B. Acute onset of respiratory distress
C. Cardiac arrest
D. All of the above
E. None of the above

Discussion

The best answer is **D**.[58] Hypoglycemia can signal inappropriate extravasation of parenteral nutrition solution. Effusion of TPN into the pleural space will cause acute onset of respiratory distress. Effusion of TPN in the pericardial space can cause acute cardiac arrest.

Objectives

1. Know how to calculate caloric content, and understand the desired nutrient ratio of TPN
2. Recognize the relationship between calcium and phosphorus and the risk of osteopenia
3. Recognize the association of cholestasis with TPN and understand the management
4. Understand the causes and clinical manifestations of catheter complications
5. Recognize metabolic complications and toxicities associated with TPN

REFERENCES

1. Lager S, Powell TL. Regulation of nutrient transport across the placenta. *J Pregnancy.* 2012;2012:179827.

2. Wladimiroff JW. A review of the etiology, diagnostic techniques and management of IUGR, and the clinical application of Doppler in the assessment of placental blood flow. *J Perinat Med.* 1991;19(1–2):11–13.

3. Lapillonne A, Griffin IJ. Feeding preterm infants today for later metabolic and cardiovascular outcomes. *J Pediatr.* 2013; 162(3 Suppl):S7–S16.

4. Agostoni C, Buonocore G, Carnielli VP, et al. Enteral nutrient supply for preterm infants: Commentary from the European Society of Paediatric Gastroenterology, Hepatology and Nutrition Committee on Nutrition. *J Pediatr Gastroenterol Nutr.* 2010;50(1):85–91.

5. Denne SC, Poindexter BB. Differences between metabolism and feeding of preterm and term infants. In: Thureen PJ, Hay WW, eds. *Neonatal Nutrition and Metabolism.* Cambridge: Cambridge University Press; 2006:437–444.

6. Kleinman RE, Greer FR, eds. Nutritional needs of the preterm infant. *Pediatric Nutrition Handbook.* 7th ed. American Academy of Pediatrics; 2013:83–122.

7. Ratien DJ, Talbot JM, Waters JH. Assessment of nutrient requirements for infant formulas (LRSO Report). *J Nutr.* 1998;128(11 Suppl): i–iv, 2059S–2293S.

8. Hay WW, Thureen P. Protein for preterm infants: How much is needed? How much is enough? How much is too much? *Pediatr Neonatol.* 2010;51(4):198–207.

9. Valentine CJ, Puthoff TD. Enhancing parenteral nutrition therapy for the neonate. *Nutr Clin Pract.* 2007;22(2):183–193.

10. Dupont C. Protein requirements during the first year of life. *Am J Clin Nutr.* 2003;77(6):1544S–1549S.

11. Kalhan SC, Bier DM. Protein and amino acid metabolism in the human newborn. *Annu Rev Nutr.* 2008;28:389–410.

12. Wharton BA, Morley R, Isaacs EB, et al. Low plasma taurine and later neurodevelopment. *Arch Dis Child Fetal Neonatal Ed.* 2004;89(6):F497–F498.

13. Rassin DK, Gaull GE, Heinonen K, et al. Milk protein quantity and quality in low-birth-weight infants: II. Effects on selected aliphatic amino acids in plasma and urine. *Pediatrics.* 1977;59(3):407–422.

14. Essential fatty acid deficiency in premature infants. *Nutr Rev.* 1989;47(2):39–41.

15. Lee EJ, Simmer K, Gibson RA. Essential fatty acid deficiency in parenterally fed preterm infants. *J Paediatr Child Health.* 1993;29(1):51–55.

16. Farrell PM, Gutcher GR, Palta M, et al. Essential fatty acid deficiency in premature infants. *Am J Clin Nutr.* 1988;48 (2):220–229.

17. Martin RJ, Fanaroff AA, Walsh MC. Nutrition and metabolism in the high-risk neonate. In: Pointdexter B, Denne S, eds. *Fanaroff and Martin's Neonatal-Perinatal Medicine.* 9th ed. Vol. 35. St Louis, MO; Mosby, Inc.; 2011;643–65.

18. Kleinman RE, ed. Infant nutrition and the development of gastrointestinal function. *Pediatric Nutrition Handbook.* 5th ed. American Academy of Pediatrics; 2004:3–22.

19. Gross SJ, David RJ, Bauman L, et al. Nutritional composition of milk produced by mothers delivering preterm. *J Pediatr.* 1980;96(4):641–644.

20. Narang AP, Bains HS, Kansal S, et al. Serial composition of human milk in preterm and term mothers. *Indian J Clin Biochem.* 2006;21(1):89–94.

21. Schanler RJ, Oh W. Composition of breast milk obtained from mothers of premature infants as compared to breast milk obtained from donors. *J Pediatr.* 1980;96(4):679–681.

22. Kleinman RE, ed. *Pediatric Nutrition Handbook.* 7th ed. American Academy of Pediatrics. *Elk Grove Village.* 2013.

23. Michaelsen KF, Skafte L, Badsberg JH, et al. Variation in macronutrients in human bank milk: Influencing factors and

implications for human milk banking. *J Pediatr Gastroenterol Nutr*. 1990;11(2):229–239.

24. Wojcik KY, Rechtman DJ, Lee ML, et al. Macronutrient analysis of a nationwide sample of donor breast milk. *J Am Diet Assoc*. 2009;109(1):137–140.

25. Landers S, Hartmann BT. Donor human milk banking and the emergence of milk sharing. *Pediatr Clin North Am*. 2013;60(1):247–260.

26. Chauhan SP, Beydoun H, Chang E, et al. Prenatal detection of fetal growth restriction in newborns classified as small for gestational age: Correlates and risk of neonatal morbidity. *Am J Perinatol*. 2014;31(3):187–194.

27. Ogilvy-Stuart AL, Hands SJ, Adcock CJ, et al. Insulin, insulin-like growth factor I (IGF-I), IGF-binding protein-1, growth hormone, and feeding in the newborn. *J Clin Endocrinol Metab*. 1998;83(10):3550–3557.

28. Tudehope D, Vento M, Bhutta Z. Nutritional requirements and feeding recommendations for small for gestational age infants. *J Pediatr*. 2013;162(3 Suppl):S81–S89.

29. Singhal A, Kennedy K, Lanigan J, et al. Nutrition in infancy and long-term risk of obesity: Evidence from 2 randomized controlled trials. *Am J Clin Nutr*. 2010;92(5):1133–1144.

30. Barker DJ, Osmond C. Infant mortality, childhood nutrition, and ischaemic heart disease in England and Wales. *Lancet*. 1986;1(8489):1077–1081.

31. Sarkar S, Watman J, Seigel WM, et al. A prospective controlled study of neonatal morbidities in infants born at 36 weeks or more gestation to Women with diet-controlled gestational diabetes (GDM-class Al). *J Perinatol*. 2003;23(3):223–228.

32. Lao TT, Wong KY. Perinatal outcome in large-for-gestational-age infants. Is it influenced by gestational impaired glucose tolerance? *J Reprod Med*. 2002;47(6):497–502.

33. Salle BL, Delvin E, Glorieux F, et al. Human neonatal hypocalcemia. *Biol Neonate*. 1990;58(Suppl 1):22–31.

34. Ziegler EE, O'Donnell AM, Nelson SE, et al. Body composition of the reference fetus. *Growth*. 1976;40(4):329–341.

35. Fusch C, Jochum F. Water, sodium, potassium, and chloride. In: Koletzko B, Poindexter B, Uauy R, eds. *Nutritional Care of Preterm Infants*. Basel (Switzerland): Karger; 2014:99–120.

36. Abrams SA. In utero physiology: Role in nutrient delivery and fetal development for calcium, phosphorus, and vitamin D. *Am J Clin Nutr*. 2007;85(2):604S–607S.

37. Koo WW, Tsang RC. Mineral requirements of low-birth-weight infants. *J Am Coll Nutr*. 1991;10(5):474–486.

38. Vanek VW, Borum P, Buchman A, et al. A.S.P.E.N. position paper: Recommendations for changes in commercially available parenteral multivitamin and multi-trace element products. *Nutr Clin Pract*. 2012;27(4):440–491.

39. Koletzko B, Poindexter B, Uauy R, eds. *Nutritional Care of Preterm Infants: Scientific Basis and Practical Guidelines. World Review of Nutrition and Dietetics*. Vol. 110. Basel, Switzerland: Karger; 2014:314.

40. Valentine CJ, Wagner CL. Nutritional management of the breastfeeding dyad. *Pediatr Clin North Am*. 2013;60(1):261–274.

41. Stuart MJ, Oski FA. Vitamin E and platelet function. *Am J Pediatr Hematol Oncol*. 1979;1(1):77–82.

42. Underwood BA. Vitamin A intoxication. *JAMA*. 1985;254(2):232–233.

43. Rao R, Georgieff MK. Iron therapy for preterm infants. *Clin Perinatol*. 2009;36(1):27–42.

44. Krebs NF, Westcott JL, Rodden DJ, et al. Exchangeable zinc pool size at birth is smaller in small-for-gestational-age than in appropriate-for-gestational-age preterm infants. *Am J Clin Nutr*. 84(6):1340–1343.

45. Greene HL, Hambidge KM, Schanler R, et al. Guidelines for the use of vitamins, trace elements, calcium, magnesium, and phosphorus in infants and children receiving total parenteral nutrition: Report of the Subcommittee on Pediatric Parenteral Nutrient Requirements from the Committee on Clinical Practice Issues of the American Society for Clinical Nutrition. *Am J Clin Nutr*. 1988;48(5):1324–1342.

46. Erikson KM, Thompson K, Aschner J, et al. Manganese neurotoxicity: A focus on the neonate. *Pharmacol Ther*. 2007;113(2):369–377.

47. Wang H, Kruszewski A, Brautigan DL. Cellular chromium enhances activation of insulin receptor kinase. *Biochemistry*. 2005;44(22):8167–8175.

48. Kleinman RE, ed. Formula feeding of term infants. *Pediatric Nutrition Handbook*. 7th ed. American Academy of Pediatrics; 2013:61–82.

49. Kleinman RE, ed. Breastfeeding. *Pediatric Nutrition Handbook*. 5th ed. Vol. 3. American Academy of Pediatrics; 2004:55–85.

50. Quigley M, Henderson G, Anthony M, et al. Formula milk versus donor breast milk for feeding preterm or low birth weight infants. *Cochrane Database Syst Rev*. 2007;(4):CD002971.

51. Lawrence RA. Storage of human milk and the influence of procedures on immunological components of human milk. *Acta Paediatr Suppl*. 1999;88(430):14–18.

52. Quan R, Yang C, Rubinstein S, et al. Effects of microwave radiation on anti-infective factors in human milk. *Pediatrics*. 1992;89(4 Pt 1):667–669.

53. McManaman JL, Neville MC. Mammary physiology and milk secretion. *Adv Drug Deliv Rev*. 2003;55(5):629–641.

54. Wagner CL, Greer FR. Prevention of rickets and vitamin D deficiency in infants, children, and adolescents. *Pediatrics*. 2008;122(5):1142–1152.

55. Abrams SA. Calcium and vitamin D requirements of enterally fed preterm infants. *Pediatrics*. 2013;131(5):e1676–e1683.

56. Valentine CJ, Fernandez S, Rogers LK, et al. Early amino-acid administration improves preterm infant weight. *J Perinatol*. 2009;29(6):428–432.

57. Kashyap S. Enteral intake for very low birth weight infants: What should the composition be? *Semin Perinatol*. 2007;31(2):74–82.

58. Kleinman RE, ed. Parenteral nutrition. *Pediatric NutritionHandbook*. 5th ed. American Academy of Pediatrics; 2004:369–389.

59. Klein CJ, Revenis M, Kusenda C, et al. Parenteral nutrition-associated conjugated hyperbilirubinemia in hospitalized infants. *J Am Diet Assoc*. 2010;110(11):1684–1695.

60. Battaglia FC, Meschia G. *An Introduction to Fetal Physiology*. Orlando, FL: Academic Press; 1986.

61. Obenshain SS, Adam PA, King KC, et al. Human fetal insulin response to sustained maternal hyperglycemia. *N Engl J Med*. 1970;283:566–570.

Chapter 8
RENAL FUNCTION
Roshan P. George, MD and Donald L. Batisky, MD

Congenital Anomalies of the Kidneys and Urinary Tract (CAKUT)

CASE 1

A 25-year-old woman at 28 weeks of gestation underwent ultrasonography, which revealed mild bilateral echogenic kidneys in the fetus. The labor and delivery were uneventful. Baby was born at 38 weeks and birth weight was 3.1 kg. There is no family history of renal disease or hypertension. The neonate is 4 days old, feeding well, has a normal physical examination and blood pressure is 82/54 mm Hg. Serum chemistries reveal the following:

LABORATORY TEST	RESULT
Sodium	138 mmol/L
Potassium	5.4 mmol/L
Chloride	103 mmol/L
Bicarbonate	19 mmol/L
Blood urea nitrogen	20 mg/dL
Creatinine	1.0 mg/dL

Renal ultrasound is done and reveals the left kidney to be 4 cm in length with normal echogenicity. Right kidney is 6 cm in length with increased echogenicity and multiple cysts (Fig. 8-1). A voiding cystourethrogram (VCUG) does not show vesicoureteral reflux.

The most likely diagnosis is
A. Bilateral renal dysplasia
B. Multicystic dysplastic kidney disease (MCKD)
C. Autosomal recessive polycystic kidney disease
D. Autosomal dominant polycystic kidney disease
E. Ureteropelvic junction (UPJ) obstruction

Discussion

The correct answer is **B**. Developmental malformations of the kidney and urinary tract constitute a spectrum and have been grouped together as congenital anomalies of the kidneys and urinary tract (CAKUT). The broad classification of these malformations is as follows[1]:

Aplasia or agenesis	Congenital absence of kidney tissue
Hypoplasia	Renal length of less than 2 standard deviation below the mean for age or a reduced number of nephrons and normal renal architecture
	The average length of a term newborn kidney is 4.2–4.3 cm (standard deviation = 0.45 cm).
Dysplasia with or without cysts	Malformation of the tissue elements
Isolated dilation of the collecting system	Hydronephrosis, hydroureteronephrosis
Anomalies of position	Including ectopic and fused (horseshoe) kidney

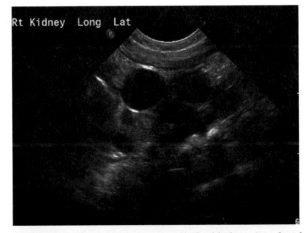

FIGURE 8-1. Note cystic areas in the fetal kidney. (Used with permission of Dr. Ira Adams Chapman.)

CAKUT is the most frequent malformation detected in utero. The incidence of renal and urinary tract malformation identified in fetal ultrasound studies ranges between 0.3 to 1.6 per 1,000 infants (both live born and stillborn).[1]

The MCKD is an extreme form of renal dysplasia in which large polymorphic cysts dominate kidney structure (Fig. 8-1). MCKD is unusally unilateral and the affected kidney is nonfunctional. If it occurs bilaterally, it causes oligohydramnios, pulmonary hypoplasia, Potter sequence, and is fatal. Even if only one kidney appears to be involved, the contralateral kidney should be evaluated carefully as 25% of unilateral MCKD is associated with contralateral abnormalities such as renal hypoplasia, vesicoureteral reflux, or UPJ obstruction.[2]

Blood pressure, though not commonly elevated, should be monitored. The natural history of MCKD is gradual reduction in size of the cysts and involution. Compensatory hypertrophy of contralateral kidney should be evaluated.

The infant in the vignette has a normal left kidney hence bilateral renal dysplasia is not likely. Autosomal recessive and autosomal dominant polycystic kidneys usually show bilateral abnormalities.

Ultrasound evaluation before 48 hours of age may not reveal collecting system dilation due to the relatively volume-contracted state during that period. The serum creatinine concentration at birth is similar to that in the mother. It declines to normal values (0.2–0.4 mg/dL) within approximately 1 week in a full-term infant and in 2 to 3 weeks in preterm infants.

CASE 2

A 28-year-old female, who had no prenatal care had fever and premature rupture of membranes. A male baby was born vaginally without any other complications and is currently 6 days old and currently on antibiotics. For the last 2 days, his urinary output has decreased and he does not have a strong urinary stream. He appears well hydrated. Ultrasonography was done and revealed bilateral hydroureteronephrosis and a thick-walled bladder. Laboratory findings are as follows:

LABORATORY TEST	RESULT
Sodium	140 mmol/L
Potassium	5.6 mmol/L
Chloride	108 mmol/L
Bicarbonate	18 mmol/L
Blood urea nitrogen	17 mg/dL
Creatinine	0.8 mg/dL

The most appropriate next step to confirm the diagnosis would be to
A. Administer intravenous fluid and furosemide
B. Cystoscopy
C. Insert a Foley catheter
D. Perform a radionuclide scan
E. Perform a VCUG

Discussion

The correct answer is **E**. The baby in this case has findings consistent with bladder outlet obstruction and in a male baby the most common cause would be posterior urethral valves (PUV). A VCUG is the imaging study of choice for the diagnosis of PUV. The typical findings include a dilated proximal urethra which narrows distal to the valve, thick-walled and trabeculated bladder. In addition, 30% to 50% of these children may also demonstrate vesicoureteral reflux.[3] Neither cystoscopy or renal scintigraphy will be useful in the initial diagnosis but may be part of the management later. Cystoscopy will help in definitive diagnosis and in management with transurethral resection. 99mTc-mercaptotriglycylglycine (MAG-3) radionuclide scan will be helpful later in determining differential renal function. Temporary drainage of the bladder is important and most often can be accomplished using a soft feeding tube initially rather than a Foley catheter as the internal diameter of the feeding tube is larger providing better drainage and lack of a balloon prevents obstruction at the ureteral orifice.

There are anterior and posterior urethral valves with obstruction of the anterior valve being very rare and found anywhere along the anterior urethra, distal to urinary sphincter. The clinical presentation and management of both anterior and posterior urethral valves are similar. Prenatal ultrasound can detect urethral valve abnormalities as early as 14 to 16 weeks of gestation. This patient most likely has incomplete or partial urethral obstruction as respiratory distress was absent at birth. Fetal cystoscopic treatment of PUV in utero has been tried but remains an investigational procedure.[4]

CASE 3

You are asked to perform an antenatal consult for parents of a male infant who was noted to have bilateral hydronephrosis on a routine ultrasound performed at 20 weeks of gestation.

What additional information from the prenatal ultrasound would be helpful to help provide the

parents with appropriate counseling and recommendations?

A. Appearance of the bladder
B. Severity of hydronephrosis
C. Amniotic fluid volume
D. Appearance of the renal parenchyma
E. All of the above

Discussion

The correct answer is **E**. The widespread use of prenatal ultrasonography has resulted in increased detection of antenatal hydronephrosis. It is important to determine if these findings are mild, moderate, or severe and to also determine if other abnormalities are detected in the fetus. Antenatal hydronephrosis is one of the most commonly diagnosed prenatal abnormalities, detected in approximately 1% to 5% of all fetuses.[4,5] Obstruction in the urinary system typically occurs at transition points in the urinary collecting system including the ureteropelvic junction (UPJ), the ureterovesical junction (UVJ) and PUV. Dilation occurs at all locations proximal to the obstruction, therefore careful evaluation of the ultrasound findings can often help make your diagnosis. Obstruction at the UPJ and UVJ are typically unilateral, however, they can be bilateral. In contrast, obstruction at the PUV typically results in bilateral hydroureteronephrosis in addition to a dilated trabeculated bladder.

PUV occurs in 1:5000 to 1:8000 males and result from abnormal membranous leaflets in the posterior urethra which give a characteristic appearance on ultrasonogra-

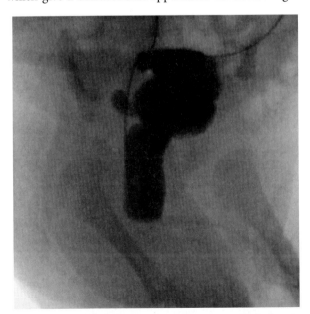

FIGURE 8-2. Radiographic appearance on VCUG showing characteristic appearance of posterior urethral valves showing distended bladder and dilated posterior urethra (*arrow*). (Reproduced with permission from Schlomer BJ, Copp HL. Antenatal hydronephrosis: Assessment and management. *NeoReviews.* 2013;14(11):e551–e561.)

phy (Fig. 8-2). The most common cause of antenatal hydronephrosis is UPJ obstruction which occurs in 1:500–1:1500 births. Unilateral involvement is most common but bilateral UPJ obstruction is reported in 10% to 40% of cases. UVJ obstruction occurs lower in the urinary tract and typically has the appearance on ultrasonography of both hydronephrosis and hydroureter. Unlike PUV which only occurs in males, both male and female infants can have a UPJ or UVJ obstruction. Each type of urinary tract obstruction can be complete or partial. Nonobstructive causes of hydronephrosis include transient dilatation of the renal pelvis and Prune Belly Syndrome.

The ureter begins to develop at the end of the fourth week as a bud from the mesonephric (wolffian) duct as a solid cord but starts to canalize from the midsection and extending to the UPJ and UVJ. Urine flow can be detected in the fetus at 13 weeks of gestation and by 19 weeks of gestation the vast majority of the amniotic fluid is fetal urine. Therefore, prenatal ultrasounds performed near 20 weeks of gestation should detect abnormalities in the genitourinary tract. The presence of oligohydramnios suggests significant obstruction to urinary flow and may contribute to the development of lung hypoplasia. Further evaluation by a maternal fetal medicine specialist is indicated for patients with oligohydramnios to assure fetal well-being and to determine if the fetus is a candidate for prenatal intervention. The integrity of the renal parenchyma, particularly in cases of suspected bilateral severe obstruction, may influence recommendations for postnatal evaluation and management.

Helpful Hint: Other potential causes of lower urinary tract obstruction include the following:

- Anterior urethral valves
- Urethral atresia
- Duplicated collecting system or ureterocele causing mechanical obstruction due to compression of the UJP or UVJ

Helpful Hint: Prenatal intervention to place vesicoamniotic shunt which drains the fetal bladder into the amniotic cavity is a potential option for fetuses with severe hydronephrosis due to obstruction and oligohydramnios. The procedure is performed at special fetal surgery centers by skilled providers. The procedure is associated with complications related to catheter malfunction or migration as well as preterm delivery and fetal loss. Some children who develop the procedure still has chronic renal insufficiency. Patient selection of those most likely to benefit have been difficult to define. Some investigators feel that serial measurements of fetal urine samples may be helpful to identify those most at risk for renal failure. Referrals for further evaluation should occur early in gestation to your regional fetal surgical center.

The infant in the above vignette undergoes PUV ablation. The primary determinant of long-term renal prognosis is which of the following?
A. Creatinine nadir at 1 year of age
B. Strong urinary stream 1 month following the procedure
C. Normal electrolytes at the time of discharge
D. Normal urinary dipstick at 6 months of age

Discussion

The correct answer is **A**. A significant number of infants with PUV will develop impairment of renal function and progress to end-stage renal disease (ESRD). Persistence of elevated creatinine after relief of obstruction is a risk factor for ESRD. Nadir creatinine is the most important determinant of renal prognosis.[6-9] Ongoing assessment of renal function as the infant grows is essential.

CASE 4

The residents present a baby during rounds who was born at 40 weeks of gestation and was noted to have mild unilateral hydronephrosis on prenatal ultrasound performed at 22 weeks of gestation. The infant is breathing comfortably on room air and has had several voids since birth.

The residents ask when and if additional evaluation is recommended for this infant?
A. A renal ultrasound should be performed prior to hospital discharge
B. No additional follow-up is indicated
C. A repeat renal ultrasound should be ordered within 3 to 6 weeks after hospital discharge and consider consultation with a pediatric urologist
D. A VCUG should be ordered prior to hospital discharge

Discussion

The correct answer is **C**. Mild hydronephrosis is one of the most common findings on prenatal ultrasound. It is important for the pediatrician to understand which children need further evaluation for this common ultrasonographic finding. Mild hydronephrosis is often transient and resolves spontaneously in 40% to 80% of cases. It is not recommended to perform the renal ultrasound immediately after birth due to an increased risk of false-

negative findings because the study is performed too soon. A repeat renal ultrasound should be performed 3 to 6 weeks after birth along with consultation from urology. Children with moderate or severe hydronephrosis should be evaluated after birth due to the increased risk of anatomic obstruction. A VCUG should not routinely be performed on the basis of findings from a prenatal ultrasound. The decision for further diagnostic evaluation can be deferred until after the repeat ultrasound for those with mild hydronephrosis.

CASE 5

You are called to attend to delivery of an infant and told that mother is a 27-year-old G3P2 healthy woman who recently moved to the area and has not had the opportunity to establish obstetrical care. She thinks that she is about 34 weeks of gestation, denies any exposures to medications aside from prenatal vitamins, and she has no ongoing medical problems. Her other two children are healthy girls, ages 3 and 6 years.

In the delivery room, the infant is born and has initial respiratory distress. He is noted to be hypotonic, and his physical appearance is shown in Figure 8-3.

What is your initial diagnosis in this infant male?
A. Nephropathic cystinosis
B. Obstructive uropathy secondary to PUV
C. Prune Belly syndrome
D. DiGeorge syndrome
E. Turner syndrome

Discussion

The correct answer is **C**. This infant male presenting with respiratory distress and noted to have lax abdominal musculature and bilaterally undescended testicles has the classic clinical appearance of Prune Belly syndrome. Prune Belly Syndrome is a nonobstructive cause of hydronephrosis. Although initially reported by Frolich in 1839, the name attached to this condition was coined by Osler nearly six decades later. By 1950, a series of nine cases was described by authors who described the eponymous condition Eagle–Barrett syndrome. Typical features of this condition include deficient or absent abdominal musculature, hypotonia, ectasia of the urinary tract, and bilaterally undescended testicles. Similar abdominal wall and urinary tract abnormalities have been described rarely in females, without the cryptorchidism.

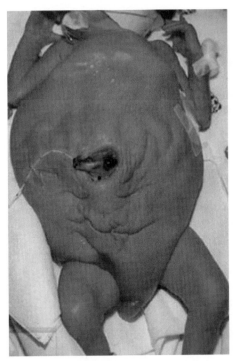

FIGURE 8-3. Physical appearance of the infant in Case 5. (Reproduced with permission from Hassett S, Smith GHH, Holland AJA. Prune belly syndrome. *Pediatr Surg Int.* 2012;28(3):219–228.)

A recent epidemiologic review of male infants with Prune Belly syndrome cited an incidence of slightly less than 4 cases per 100,000 live births.[10] While there have been reports of Prune Belly syndrome occurring in association with trisomy 13, 18, and 21, there have been too few cases to indicate a formal association. There may be a genetic influence, as 12 reported cases of familial Prune Belly syndrome have been reported, and an analysis of these cases suggests a sex hormone influenced autosomal recessive mode of inheritance. This syndrome seems to be more common in both monozygotic and dizygotic twin pregnancies. Yet, in monozygotic twins, both discordance and concordance for Prune Belly syndrome has been reported. Thus implying that genetic mutations alone do not explain the pathogenesis of the Prune Belly syndrome.

Care of these infants requires coordination among many pediatric medical and surgical subspecialists, including pediatric nephrologists, urologists, and general surgeons. Once stabilized, these infants will need to be evaluated in a tertiary care center for ongoing management and chronic care. A recent review by Hassett et al.[11] reviews pathogenesis, diagnosis and management of Prune Belly syndrome, and it underscores the value of a collaborative approach to ongoing management of infants with this condition.

Objectives

1. Known the common causes of urinary tract obstruction in the newborn

2. Know the common causes of congenital abnormalities of the kidney and urinary tract
3. Understand the differences in ultrasound findings based on the level and severity of obstruction
4. Know the recommendations for additional diagnostic testing for neonates with abnormalities noted on prenatal ultrasound involving the genitourinary tract

Hypertension

CASE 6

A 6-week-old baby, born at 32 weeks was observed to have elevated blood pressure (BP: 102/64 mm Hg). He had significant respiratory distress at birth, despite receiving dexamethasone in utero. He received ventilator support and antibiotics for 1 week. He had umbilical venous and arterial lines for the first 7 days of life. The neonate currently is on increasing nasogastric feeds as total parenteral nutrition is being weaned. He is also currently receiving albuterol and furosemide. Physical examination findings are unremarkable. His laboratory findings are as follows:

LABORATORY TEST	RESULT
Sodium	142 mmol/L
Potassium	5.6 mmol/L
Chloride	103 mmol/L
Bicarbonate	30 mmol/L
Blood urea nitrogen	4 mg/dL
Creatinine	0.4 mg/dL

The urine output is >1 mL/kg/hr. Renal ultrasound with Doppler shows slightly increased echogenicity in both kidneys, a normal bladder and patent bilateral renal arteries and veins with normal flow.

Of the following, the most likely reason for this neonate's elevated blood pressure is
A. Multicystic dysplastic kidney
B. Total parenteral nutrition
C. Dexamethasone
D. The umbilical arterial catheterization

Discussion

The correct answer is **D**. The incidence of neonatal hypertension is about 0.2% to 3%.[12] While the etiology of hypertension can be multifactorial, the incidence of renovascular hypertension is reported as high as 33% in infants with a history of umbilical artery catheter use.[13] Hypertension has been reported in infants who underwent umbilical artery catheterization even in the absence of thrombi or abnormalities in doppler studies on renal ultrasound. Risk for renovascular hypertension includes low placement of catheter tip, trauma to the endothelium during placement, and longer duration of catheter use. Renal parenchymal disease (e.g., polycystic dysplastic kidney disease, multicystic dysplastic kidneys), or obstructive renal pathology such as ureteropelvic obstruction can cause elevated blood pressure, but none of these diagnoses are suggested by the ultrasound findings in this patient. Salt and water retention from total parenteral nutrition, though in the differential is less likely cause of hypertension in the patient described in this vignette.

Renal Masses

CASE 7

A 2,850-g male infant was born at 38 weeks of gestation after an uncomplicated pregnancy and delivery. On routine examination in newborn nursery, he had a palpable mass in the right lower quadrant which felt firm. An abdominal ultrasound was performed which showed a well-defined mass with a concentric echogenic ring involving the right kidney. No evidence of hydronephrosis is present and the left kidney appears normal.

What is the most likely diagnosis?
A. Hydronephrosis
B. Wilms tumor
C. Neuroblastoma
D. Mesoblastic nephroma

Discussion

The correct answer is **D**. The most common abdominal mass in a neonate is usually a renal mass which highlights the importance of performing a careful physical examination prior to hospital discharge. Although hydronephrosis is very common in this age group, only those with moderate to severe hydronephrosis will present on clinical examination with a palpable mass. Males with PUV resulting in hydroureteronephrosis as well as a distended bladder may have palpable masses in both flank as well as a firm midline distended bladder on examination. A unilateral solid mass is more likely to be due to a mesoblastic nephroma which accounts for approximately 3% to 6% of all renal tumors in children. Over half of these particular tumors are diagnosed during the neonatal period. These are mesenchymal tumors which macroscopically appear as a solid unencapsulated mass that originates from the

renal hilum and invades the surrounding renal tissues. Calcifications are rare. Histologically, these tumors are composed of connective tissue growing between the nephrons. The most common variant is the classic mesoblastic nephroma which is typically benign. The other variant is the cellular mesoblastic nephroma which is larger, more heterogeneous in appearance grossly and histologically and may have more vascular encasement and metastasis. Abdominal ultrasound is typically diagnostic, however, MRI can provide additional information. Some patients develop hypertension, particularly if there is vascular involvement. Nephrectomy is the treatment of choice and most patients have a favorable outcome and no long-term sequelae. Wilms tumors typically present in older children but are another important cause of renal masses in young children. A neuroblastoma is a tumor involving the adrenal gland and other neural crest tissues rather than the kidney itself. In contrast to the appearance of the mesoblastic nephroma, neuroblastomas are often bilateral, have poorly defined margins and frequently contain calcifications. Patients often present with an abdominal mass, skin lesions, or ocular findings. Neurologic and gastrointestinal symptoms are also common due to the excretion of neuro-exocrine chemicals from the tumor and mass effect from the tumor causing compression on other internal organs. Some children develop tachycardia and hypertension as well. Children frequently have the characteristic findings of bilateral ocular ecchymoses and proptosis due to metastatic lesions to the eye. Metastasis is common with a neuroblastoma therefore full body imaging is necessary to appropriately stage the tumor and determine treatment.

Quick Quiz: Renal Masses in Neonate

Match the following diagnoses with the appropriate image below as seen in Figure 8-4, Figure 8-5 and Figure 8-6.
A. Posterior urethral valves
B. Neuroblastoma
C. Mesoblastic nephroma

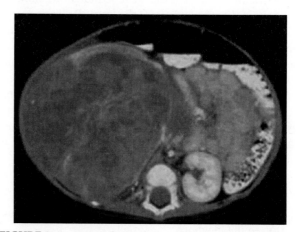

FIGURE 8-4.   Image obtained.

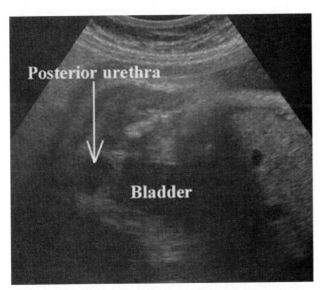

FIGURE 8-5.   Copyright © 2013. The Ultrasound of Life.

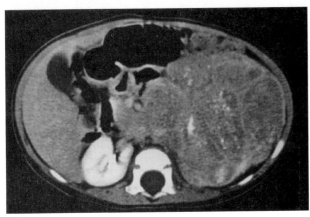

FIGURE 8-6.   Reproduced with permission from Kushner BH. Neuroblastoma: a disease requiring a multitude of imaging studies. *J Nucl Med.* 2004;45(7):1172–1188.

The correct answers are:
Figure 8-4—Mesoblastic nephroma (Answer C)
Figure 8-5—Posterior urethral valves (Answer A)
Figure 8-6—Neuroblastoma (Answer B)

Objectives

1. Know the common causes of abdominal masses in a newborn
2. Recognize the clinical signs and symptoms associated with abdominal masses in a neonate

Renal Vein Thrombosis

CASE 8

A 5-day-old neonate, born at 35 weeks of gestation who is being treated for suspected sepsis was noted to have gross hematuria. Physical examination revealed an afebrile neonate with a blood pressure of 98/66 mm Hg. A UVC was noted to be in position and on examination of the abdomen, you find a palpable right flank mass. Laboratory findings are significant for thrombocytopenia. You suspect renal vein thrombosis and a renal ultrasound with Doppler confirms the diagnosis of right renal vein thrombosis.

What is the next best step in this patient's management?
A. Low molecular heparin
B. Remove UVC
C. Observe
D. Warfarin treatment

Discussion

The correct answer is **B**. Renal venous thrombosis (RVT) may present with the classic triad of flank mass, gross hematuria, and thrombocytopenia. Elevated blood pressure may also be seen. RVT is the most common form of thrombosis not associated with a vascular catheter[14] and may account for approximately 10% of venous thrombosis in newborns. Risk factors associated with RVT include prematurity, perinatal asphyxia, dehydration, sepsis, and maternal diabetes. There is increasing evidence that infants with RVT are more likely to have an inherited prothrombotic condition, such as factor V Leiden mutation, protein C, and S deficiency, compared to the general population.[15] Neonates with RVT have significant mortality and morbidity, particularly with chronic kidney damage that can result in hypertension and renal failure. Unilateral RVT with normal renal function or without extension into the inferior vena cava (IVC) may be managed conservatively with close observation and supportive care.[16] An observational study did not show improved outcome with the use of anticoagulant therapy in unilateral renal thrombosis and it was associated with some bleeding risks.[17] A central catheter in the IVC should be removed if present. Some experts recommend anticoagulation therapy, especially for bilateral RVT or extension into IVC. In this vignette, removing the UVC appears to be the most appropriate next step.

Objectives

1. Know the clinical signs and symptoms and differential diagnosis of renal vein thrombosis
2. Know the management strategies for renal vein thrombosis in the neonate
3. Recognize the risk factors associated with renal vein thrombosis

Normal Development of Kidney

CASE 9

The maximum urinary concentrating capacity of a full-term newborn is around 800 mOsm/kg. By the age of 6 months, the maximum urinary concentrating capacity increases to about 1,200 mOsm/kg.

Of the following, the ability to concentrate urine in a newborn is limited by
A. Low medullary osmolality and decreased responsiveness of collecting duct to arginine vasopressin (AVP)
B. Low levels of AVP
C. Long length of loop of Henle in immature kidneys
D. Low intrarenal prostaglandin (PG) levels

Discussion

The correct answer is **A**. Normal plasma osmolality is approximately 285 mOsm/kg. The urine is concentrated in the inner medullary collecting duct by equilibrating with the high osmolality in the medullary interstitium under the influence of AVP.

Maximum urine concentrations achieved by preterm and full-term infants after fluid restriction are 600 and 800 mOsm/kg, respectively, reaching adult levels of urinary concentration capacity by 6 to 12 months of age.[18]

Normal renal cortical and medullary development is essential in attaining the normal urinary concentrating abilities. Longitudinal growth of the medulla leads to lengthening of loops of Henle (which are short in immature kidneys) enabling these to reach the inner medulla. Longer loops of Henle generate steeper medullary tonicity gradient by greater sodium and urea transport; hence being able to achieve higher urinary concentration. In neonates, there is limited responsiveness of collecting duct cells to AVP, one mechanism being high intrarenal levels of PG which antagonize AVP.[19]

Objectives

1. Understand the normal development of renal function
2. Understand the control of water metabolism in a neonate
3. Know the effects of AVP on sodium and water balance

Medications

CASE 10

A male baby was born at 25 weeks to a 26-year-old primigravida with poor prenatal care. Infant experienced respiratory distress and required surfactant and intubation in the immediate postnatal period. He was also placed on antibiotics. At 3 days of age he was diagnosed with a patent ductus arteriosis (PDA) and received indomethacin. The next day he was noted to have reduced urinary output and creatinine value rose from 0.5 mg/dL to 0.7 mg/dL.

Which of the following statements is true?
A. Indomethacin causes reduction in urinary output and renal impairment which is usually transient
B. Giving furosemide to this patient is recommended as it will help improve urinary output
C. A trial of indomethacin should not have been tried in this premature patient who was at risk for acute kidney injury
D. The hemodynamic benefits of fluid restriction to 100 mL/kg/day will promote PDA closure in this infant and should be tried at this stage

Discussion

The correct answer is **A**. Prostaglandin E_2 (PGE$_2$) maintains ductal patency. Observational and randomized studies have shown that indomethacin, a cyclooxygenase inhibitor, increases the rate of closure of PDA within 24 hours of administration by inhibiting the synthesis of PGE$_2$. However, side effects such as renal impairment, oliguria, gastrointestinal perforation, necrotizing enterocolitis, and platelet dysfunction have been observed. Reduced urinary output and renal impairment are noted in premature infants but are usually transient in nature.[20] Reduction in glomerular filtration rate (GFR) usually returns to normal on cessation of therapy. In fact, it has been postulated that indomethacin may improve renal function by enhancing renal perfusion by mediating PDA closure. However, indomethacin is contraindicated in severe acute impairment of renal function.

Ibuprofen has similar efficacy as indomethacin for PDA closure.[21]

Furosemide is not recommended in this patient who may already be at risk for abnormal fluid balanced on the basis of the extremely immature gestational age. Similarly, severe, fluid restriction does not appear to hasten closure of a PDA and may further compromise renal function and overall fluid balance.

Renal Function and Glomerular Filtration Rate

CASE 11

Mom Monroe was in a motor vehichle accident at 37 weeks gestation. She had onset of profuse vaginal bleeding and was taken to the emergency room. The fetus was noted to have bradycardia therefore an emergency Cesarean delivery was performed. The infant had no spontaneous respiratory effort, was pale in color and had delayed capillary refill. He was intubated and the heart rate improved to 110 beats per minute. A UVC was placed emergently and the baby was given 10 mL/kg of Normal Saline while emergency release blood products were requested. His initial HCT was 7%. At delivery they noted a severe placental abruption.

Of the following, the pathophysiologic response most responsible for maintaining GFR in the initial phase of diminished renal perfusion due to intravascular volume depletion is which of the following
A. Afferent arteriolar dilatation due to intrarenal prostaglandin (PG)
B. Afferent arteriolar constriction due to myogenic autoregulation
C. Efferent arteriolar dilatation due to systemic norepinephrine production
D. Efferent arteriolar constriction due to systemic renin–angiotensin system (RAS) activation
E. None of the above

Discussion

The correct answer is **A**. In a volume-depleted state, mechanisms such as release of norepinephrine and angiotensin II due to the activation of sympathetic nervous system and renin–angiotensin axis, may paradoxically lead to reduced renal perfusion and decrease in GFR. This leads to activation of intrarenal compensatory mechanisms, mainly (1) increase in production of intra-

renal vasodilatory PG and (2) differential effect of intrarenal angiotensin II on afferent and efferent arterioles. Afferent arteriolar dilatation and efferent arteriolar constriction help maintain hydrostatic pressure across the glomerulus. Hence both options (B) and (C) will not be conducive to maintaining GFR.

The intrarenal production of vasodilatory PGE_2 and PGI_2 is mediated by the cyclooxygenase (COX-1 and COX-2) enzymes system. Volume depletion causes upregulation of COX-2 expression in the macula densa and medullary interstitial cells. Nonsteroidal anti-inflammatory medications (such as indomethacin used for the closure of PDA) inhibit this response and when used in the setting of volume depletion can precipitate acute kidney dysfunction.[22]

The systemic RAS helps maintain systemic blood pressure; however the intrarenal RAS regulates glomerular filtration by increasing hydrostatic pressure across the glomerulus. Intrarenal angiotensin II constricts both afferent and efferent arterioles but the effect is more pronounced in the efferent arteriole.[23] Angiotensin-converting enzyme inhibitors (ACEI) can impair this mechanism.[24]

Myogenic autoregulation is activated in response to reduced lateral stretch in blood vessels in a hypoperfused state and causes acute vasodilatation of afferent arteriole (not vasoconstriction). Moreover, the role of this mechanism in volume depletion is unclear. Volume contraction leads to increase in the activity of sympathetic nervous system which plays a key role in increased tubular sodium reabsorption and intrarenal renin secretion.

Objectives

1. Identify the common causes of acute renal failure in the newborn
2. Understand the mechanism of action of commonly used medications on renal function in the newborn
3. Understand the hormonal control of renal function

Fluid and Electrolyte

CASE 12

A 26-year-old G1P0 mother had a pregnancy complicated by polyhydramnios which did not respond to therapeutic amniocentesis. The infant was delivered prematurely at 32 weeks of gestation. The newborn male did not have respiratory distress and did not require any respiratory support. His physical examination and BP were normal. It was noted that the infant had a urine output of >10 mL/kg/hr. By day 4 of life, the infant had lost >20% of his birth weight.

Laboratory studies showed evidence of hyponatremia, hypokalemia, hypercalciuria. The most likely diagnosis is
A. Syndrome of inappropriate anti diuretic hormone secretion (SIADH)
B. Nephrogenic diabetes insipidus
C. Bartter syndrome
D. Mineralocorticoid deficiency

Discussion

The correct answer is **C**. The signs and symptoms of salt wasting, hypokalemia, and hypercalciuria described in this vignette can be attributed to impaired absorption of sodium (Na) in the thick ascending limb of the loop of Henle. The thick ascending loop of Henle is responsible for sodium reabsorption (30% of filtered Na) and for water reabsorption via maintaining medullary hypertonicity. Hence disruption of sodium absorption also leads to water wasting or reduced urinary concentration. Na reabsorption in the thick ascending limb of the loop of Henle occurs via the luminal furosemide-sensitive NKCC2 (sodium–potassium–chloride co-transporter). An inactivating mutation in the NKCC2 causes a disorder called neonatal Bartter syndrome or BS type I.[25] This typically presents in the second trimester with maternal polyhydramnios from fetal polyuria. Premature delivery is common and the neonate typically has significant polyuria after birth. The baby develops salt wasting, hypokalemia, and hyperchloremic metabolic alkalosis. Hypercalciuria may lead to the development of medullary nephrocalcinosis. The proximal tubule and thick ascending limb of loop of Henle are responsible for reabsorption of 90% of the filtered Ca^{2+}. Reabsorption of Ca^{2+} is a passive process and is coupled to Na^+ reabsorption. Defective function of the thick ascending loop of Henle is relevant to Na^+, K^+, and Cl^-, and will thus impair their absorption. This will have a secondary effect on the osmolality of the peritubular space and subsequently reduce the movement of water from the descending limb of the loop of Henle in the direction of the tubular space to the interstitium. The final result of these phenomena is a flooding of the distal tubule with diluted urine that has a high content of Na^+, K^+, Cl^- and Ca^{2+}.

The neonate in this vignette does not have total body volume overload with hyperosmolar urine hence this is not consistent with SIADH. He does have polyuria, but the absence of isosthenuria or hypernatremia makes nephrogenic DI less likely. Hyponatremia with hyperkalemia would have resembled mineralocorticoid deficiency but this baby has hypokalemia. Also, hypercalciuria is absent in mineralocorticoid deficiency.

CASE 13

Baby Girl Morris was born at 23 weeks of gestation and had a birth weight of 510 g. The delivery was precipitous and she was in a footling breech presentation. At delivery she required intubation due to respiratory distress and was noted to have severe bruising of the extremities. The skin was thin and transparent. Baby Girl Morris is stabilized and transferred to the NICU for ongoing care and management.

What are the strategies to decrease insensible water losses as you work to stabilize Baby Girl Morris?
A. Transwarmer in the delivery room
B. Lower the temperature in the delivery room to the comfort level of the attending
C. Humidify the isolette
D. Place hat on infant after delivery
E. All except B

Discussion

The correct answer is **E**. Temperature regulation is a fundamental principle in neonatal resuscitation and is very important for the extremely low–birth-weight infant due to the limited ability they have to regulate insensible water losses. It is extremely important to ensure that the delivery room or operating room is prepared prior to any anticipated preterm delivery. The temperature control should not be lowered to the comfort level of the staff but rather warmed to prevent heat loss from the infant. The resuscitation bed, infant towels, and hat should also be prewarmed if time permits. A hat should be placed on the infant's head shortly after delivery to decrease fluid and heat losses through the scalp. After admission to the NICU, the child should be placed in a thermoregulated isolette. Some isolettes allow you to add additional humidity to the environment to help minimize insensible water losses.

On day of life 2, Baby Girl Morris has laboratory studies obtained which are listed below. Her total fluid intake is being provided through parenteral nutrition at a total fluid volume of 80 mL/kg/day. The dextrose concentration in the TPN is D5% and contains no additional electrolytes. Her urine output over the past 24 hours has been 5 mL/kg/hr. Her net fluid balance is negative 20 mL based on her intake of 41 mL: output 61 mL.

LABORATORY TEST	RESULT
Sodium	154 mmol/L
Potassium	5.0 mmol/L
Chloride	114 mmol/L
CO_2	18 mmol/L
BUN	20 mg/dL
Creatinine	0.8 mg/dL

What would be the most appropriate adjustment to make to your fluid and electrolyte management?
A. Request a nephrology consult
B. Add sodium to the TPN
C. Increase the total fluid intake
D. Repeat laboratory studies in 24 hours

Discussion

The correct answer is **C**. Extremely preterm infants often develop fluid and electrolyte imbalances during the first week of life. They have a limited ability to regulate fluid shifts in the intravascular space. Those who are critically ill may also suffer from additional inappropriate third spacing of fluids. Most sodium abnormalities in the first week of life are more closely related to free water shifts rather than actual sodium intake. Our patient described above has inappropriately high urine output which exceeds her intake resulting in hypernatremia. The most appropriate response would be to increase the total fluid volume. It is often helpful to monitor frequent weights and recheck laboratory studies but this alone would not be an acceptable response. The laboratory values must be interpreted in the context of the overall fluid balance for your patient.

CASE 14

Mrs. Mitchell is a 32-year-old G2P1 hypertensive patient presents to the emergency room complaining of acute onset of severe abdominal pain and vaginal bleeding. She had good prenatal care which was uncomplicated and is now 37 weeks of gestation. External fetal monitoring detects a fetal heart rate of 60 therefore she is taken for an emergency c-section. At delivery the obstetrician detects at 75% placental abruption. The baby is floppy, has no respiratory effort and cyanotic therefore a full resuscitation ensues including intubation, chest compressions, and epinephrine. The Apgar scores are 0, 1, 2, 4 and the infant is taken to the NICU for further care. Full body hypothermia is initiated due to concerns of hypoxic ischemic encephalopathy. Baby Boy Mitchell does not have any urine output for the first 2 days of life. The medical team is monitoring his fluid status closely and adjusting dosing for any potentially nephrotoxic medications. He is receiving clear fluids with D10% plus ¼ normal saline at a rate of 80 mL/kg/day. The morning laboratory studies show the following values:

LABORATORY TEST	RESULT
Sodium	128 mmol/L
Potassium	5.5 mmol/L
Chloride	110 mmol/L
CO_2	15 mmol/L
BUN	18 mg/dL
Creatinine	1.4 mg/dL

Which of the following would be appropriate fluid management?
A. Fluid restriction until urine output improves
B. Add an additional 10 mEq/kg of sodium to the fluids
C. Prescribe Lasix q6 hours
D. Initiate dialysis

Discussion

The correct answer is **A**. Neonates who experience an ischemic insult often exhibit signs of multisystem organ dysfunction, including transient renal insufficiency. Typically the urine output and elevated creatinine values will decrease over time and the ability to regulate acid–base homeostasis is restored. The hyponatremia noted in this patient is dilutional and not a true reflection of the total body sodium content. Excessive amounts of sodium should not be added to the intravenous fluids in this scenario. One may consider addition of a base source to correct the alteration in serum carbon dioxide levels, but as renal function improves, regulation of the pH and serum CO_2 also tend to improve. Dialysis is not yet indicated for this patient. Lasix is frequently attempted as a therapy but is typically not effective.

Helpful Hint: Each of the cases in this series should remind the reader of the various stages of normal renal development and function.[26] In utero, the fluid balance of the fetus is dependent on the placenta. The production and excretion of urine is essential for fetal lung development. At term, the kidney contains approximately 800,000 nephrons. The medullary and juxtamedullary zones are both thicker than the outer cortex at term and the size of the glomeruli are smaller than an older child or adult. GFR increases in a linear fashion throughout gestation due to ongoing nephrogenesis and reaches approximately 3.2 mL/min near term. There is a substantial increase in GFR between 34 and 40 weeks of gestation. Premature infants have a relatively low GFR at birth but this is accelerated relative to gestational age after preterm delivery. Fetal urine is hypotonic relative to the plasma but osmolality increases with gestational age. Preterm infants have a lower urinary concentrating ability and are therefore at risk for significant fluid losses as outlined above. Careful monitoring of fluid status is essential in the management of the extremely low–birth-weight infant.

Urinary sodium clearance is higher in the fetus compared to the term infant. Similarly, urinary excretion of potassium also increases with increasing gestational age. The ratio of urinary sodium to urinary potassium decreases with increasing gestational age. The sodium content of the fetal kidney is approximately 80 mEq/L at 20 weeks of gestation but decreases to 20 to 30 mEq/L at term. Metabolic acidosis is common in the extremely preterm infant due to excessive urinary losses of bicarbonate in the urine. Similar to the other electrolytes, this threshold increases over time but is felt to occur due to the relative high extracellular fluid volume of the fetus and newborn and the limited capacity of the proximal tubule in the immature kidney to reabsorb bicarbonate.

Objectives

1. Understand the etiology of common electrolyte abnormalities in the neonate
2. Know how to manage electrolyte abnormalities in the neonate
3. Understand the hormonal control of renal function
4. Understand the effect of medications commonly used in the sick neonate on renal function
5. Be able to evaluate renal tubular acidosis (RTA) and understand Fanconi syndrome as a generalized form of proximal tubular dysfunction.

Renal Failure and Dialysis

CASE 15

You discuss the patient described in Case 14 during your morning rounds with the pediatric housestaff. Although they understand that this patient is not a candidate for dialysis, they ask you to describe the general indications for dialysis in a neonatal patient.

Which of the following are indications for neonatal dialysis?
A. Refractory electrolyte abnormalities
B. Uremia
C. Fluid overload
D. All of the above

Discussion

The correct answer is **D**. Dialysis is an infrequently used but potentially life saving procedure in the neonate with acute or chronic renal failure. Each of the options listed is an indication for considering dialysis in a neonate. Dialysis in this patient population is often a bridge to renal transplant for patients with chronic renal failure secondary to structurally abnormal kidneys and inadequate intrinsic renal function to allow for growth and nutrition. Common causes of acute renal failure in a newborn are outlined in Table 8-1. Neonates with other severe comorbid conditions such as severe lung hypoplasia, brain injury, or other anomalies not compatible with long-term survival, may not be appropriate candidates for dialysis. Technically, peritoneal or hemodialysis is challenging in a low–birth-weight infant and associated with a higher risk of complications. Relative contraindications for dialysis include patients with severe pulmonary disease, congenital diaphragmatic hernia, abdominal wall defects, multiple extensive abdominal surgeries due to concern for adhesions, vesicostomies, colostomies, Prune Belly syndrome, and necrotizing enterocolitis. Close consultation with the family and your nephrology team is needed before considering dialysis in a neonate.[27]

TABLE 8-1. Causes of Acute Renal Failure in Neonate

PRERENAL
Vasomotor nephropathy
Decreased intravascular volume due to hypoalbuminemia:
• Hepatic failure
• Protein losing enteropathy
• Congenital nephrotic syndrome
• Excessive losses associated with surgery
Decreased cardiac output
INTRINSIC
Acute tubular necrosis
• Hypoperfusion
• Hypoxia
Acute interstitial nephritis
Pyelonephritis
Toxic nephropathy
• Antibiotics (Aminoglycosides, Amphotericin, Vancomycin)
• Renal artery thrombosis
• Renal vein thrombosis
• Malignancy
POSTRENAL
Obstruction of the urinary tract
• Posterior urethral valves
• Prune belly syndrome
• Bilateral ureteropelvic junction obstruction

Reproduced with permission from Lee MM, Chua AN, Yorgin PD. Neonatal peritoneal dialysis. *NeoReviews*. 2005;6(8):e384–e391.

Objectives

1. Understand the causes of acute renal failure and chronic renal failure in the neonate
2. Know the indications for dialysis in a neonate
3. Know the absolute and relative contraindications for dialysis in a neonate

Medication Effects

CASE 16

A male baby was born at 36 weeks of gestation to a G1P0 female with poor prenatal care and history of multiple medical problems including seizure disorder, hypertension, migraine headaches, and recurrent urinary tract infections requiring multiple admissions to several different hospitals for the treatment of urosepsis. She had been on several medications with intermittent compliance and is unable to provide a list of her medications used throughout the pregnancy. The pregnancy was complicated by oligohydramnios. After delivery, the baby has borderline low blood pressures and respiratory distress. He is placed on high flow nasal cannula oxygen which is weaned down quickly to room air. You notice widely open sutures and hypocalvaria. As evaluation and stabilization efforts proceed, it becomes apparent that the baby has renal failure with no urinary output and elevated creatinine of 3.2 mg/dL.

Which medication listed below is the possible cause of the features described in the vignette?
A. Aminoglycosides
B. Angiotensin converting enzyme inhibitor (ACEI)
C. Phenytoin
D. Alcohol

Discussion

The correct answer is **B**. Exposure to teratogens in the environment such as maternal illnesses (e.g., diabetes mellitus), physical agents (e.g., heat exposure), infectious agents (e.g., TORCH infections), or drugs (e.g., antiepileptic), are responsible for causing approximately 4% to 6% of birth defects. The type and sequence of congenital anomalies depend upon the time of antenatal exposure and/or the site of gene action. Formation of the mature heart and kidneys occurs by fetal age of 5 to 7 weeks.

A 2006 epidemiologic study first suggested that angiotensin-converting enzyme (ACE) inhibitors may not be safe in early pregnancy.[28] The adverse fetal renal effects of ACE inhibitors and angiotensin receptor blockers (ARBs) are likely due to their ability to cross the placenta and interfere with fetal renal hemodynamics. Fetal GFR is maintained by high angiotensin II levels and low perfusion pressures. ACE inhibitors and ARBs cause a decline in GFR by lowering angiotensin II levels which in turn lowers intraglomerular pressure. The fetus exposed to in utero ACEI and/or ARBs may have varying degrees of tubular differentiation. Low GFR, manifests as oligohydramnios in utero and anuria after delivery. These medications also cause reduction in normal retinal and cranial vascularization during fetal development, which leads to retinopathy and hypocalvaria.[29,30] Current evidence suggests that all women of childbearing age who are being considered for therapy with ACE inhibitors and/or ARBs should be counseled about their teratogenicity.

Aminoglycoside exposure can lead to progressive decrease in GFR and proximal damage. However, it is usually a nonoliguric or polyuric ATN and bony abnormalities are not present. Orofacial clefts, cardiac malformations, and genitourinary defects are the major anomalies associated with phenytoin use during pregnancy. Alcohol appears to have negative effects throughout pregnancy, including impaired growth, facial dysmorphism, and neurologic anomalies, such as below normal cognitive performance or structural central nervous system abnormalities.

Objectives

1. Understand the actions of the components of the RAS
2. Understand the potential impact of exposure to teratogens to renal development and function

Hydrops Fetalis

CASE 17

A 2.8-kg baby born at 36 weeks of gestation had mild respiratory distress at birth, which resolved by 1 to 2 hours postnatally. It was noted during delivery that the placenta was enlarged, weighing 3.7 kg. Physical examination, laboratory work, and echocardiography were within normal limits. Currently she is 7 days old and over the past 2 days there is noticeable progressive edema of her extremities. Over the last day, she appears to have increasing ascites and overnight she had increasing respiratory distress requiring oxygen via nasal cannula. A sepsis workup was performed including blood and urine cultures. Urine output has decreased to less than 0.2 mL/kg/hr from previous urine output of about 1.5 mL/kg/hr. Urinalysis is positive for 4+ proteins. Laboratory findings show the following:

LABORATORY TEST	RESULT
Sodium	133 mmol/L
Potassium	5.0 mmol/L
Chloride	100 mmol/L
Bicarbonate	21 mmol/L
Blood urea nitrogen	10 mg/dL
Creatinine	0.2 mg/dL
Calcium	7.8 mg/dL
Albumin	1.8 g/dL
Glucose	50 mg/dL
Phosphorus	6.0 mg/dL

What is the most likely diagnosis?
A. AV canal defect
B. Metabolic storage disease
C. Congenital nephrotic syndrome
D. Excessive sodium in IVF
E. Urinary ascites

Discussion

The correct answer is **C**. Congenital nephrotic syndrome (proteinuria, hypoalbuminemia, hyperlipidemia, and edema) appears in the first 3 months of life. Most infants with the congenital nephrotic syndrome have a low birth weight for gestational age and are born prematurely (35–38 weeks). The placenta is enlarged, often being >25% of the total birth weight. The enlarged placenta can lead to flexion deformities of the hips, knees, and elbows in the fetus. Fetal distress is common and widely separated cranial sutures can be seen secondary to delayed ossification. Edema can be present at birth or appear during the first week of life in approximately 50% of the cases. The proteinuria is highly selective initially, however the selectivity is lost later, causing urinary losses of various proteins including immunoglobulins, thyroid binding globulins and proteins involved in the coagulation cascade. This leads to profound hypoalbuminemia, hypogammaglobulinemia, thromboembolic tendencies, and hypothyroidism.

Mutations in genes encoding proteins responsible for the normal structure of the glomerular filtration barrier lead to the congenital nephrotic syndrome. One such gene, NPHS1, which encodes nephrin (a key component of the podocyte slit diaphragm) is responsible for the Finnish-type congenital nephrotic syndrome which is the most common mutation seen. Increase in the amniotic fluid alpha-fetoprotein (AFP) concentration can be

seen, which though nonspecific, can lead to antenatal diagnosis of congenital nephrotic syndrome in high-risk families, especially in the absence of a neural tube defect.[31] The nephrotic syndrome in congenital nephrotic syndrome is resistant to glucocorticoids and immunosuppressive drugs, since this is not an immunologic disease. Standard conservative treatment includes albumin infusion, careful nutrition, low-sodium diet, vitamin, thyroxine supplementation, and prevention of infections and thrombotic complications. Extrarenal manifestations such as genital abnormalities can also be seen in affected males and suggest a WT1 mutation and the diagnosis of Denys–Drash syndrome, which places the infant at risk for Wilms tumor.

Some forms of congenital heart disease are associated with hydrops in the fetal/neonatal period. In our vignette, the neonate developed edema over time but did not present with evidence of hydrops on physical examination at birth. The cardiac lesions most commonly associated with hydrops are atrioventricular septal defect (AVSD), hypoplastic left and right heart, and isolated ventricular or atrial septal defects.

Metabolic or lysosomal storage diseases comprise a heterogeneous group of autosomal recessive disorders that may present with edema and account for 1% to 15% of cases of nonimmune hydrops fetalis. These rare genetic disorders are due to lack of specific enzymes necessary to process various metabolites within the lysosomes. These conditions affect various organs such as the brain, heart, liver, and kidneys. The pathogenesis of edema and ascites is likely related to congestion of abdominal viscera from accumulation of these metabolites, leading to increased hydrostatic pressure, decreased oncotic pressure, and possibly cardiac dysfunction.[32]

Sodium in intravenous fluids and other sources such as flushes and medicines, administered in excess of renal excretory ability, can cause total body volume overload and edema in critically ill neonates, particularly those with impaired renal function.

Urinary ascites can occur from leakage of urine through a ruptured renal pelvis or calyx or through a patent urachus. This can be due to excessive pressure from a lower urinary tract obstruction due to a PUV or less common causes such as a sacrococcygeal tumor.

Objectives

1. Recognize the clinical signs and symptoms of congenital nephrotic syndrome
2. Identify the differential diagnosis of nonimmune hydrops fetalis
3. Understand the genetic abnormalities associated with congenital nephrotic syndrome

Tubular Dysfunction

CASE 18

A 3.6-kg female baby born at 38 weeks of gestation had meconium aspiration syndrome. The baby had required prolonged ventilator support and parenteral nutrition. She is currently 86 days old, and recently discharged home on 0.5 L/min of oxygen via nasal cannula. She is also on full enteral nutrition. It is noted that she is becoming more acidotic over the last several weeks, with a normal anion gap, and she is now requiring increasing amounts of sodium bicarbonate replacement by mouth.

On physical examination, it is noted that her skin and hair are light colored but there are no physical abnormalities detected. Urinalysis reveals 1+ protein and is positive for glucose. The baby has normal serum glucose but low phosphorus and low uric acid levels. You correctly diagnose her with proximal RTA, likely Fanconi syndrome.

Which one of the following tests will reveal the definitive diagnosis for the most common cause of proximal RTA?
A. Cystine content in peripheral blood leukocyte
B. Urine mucopolysaccharides
C. Cystine content in urine
D. Serum very long-chain fatty acid
E. Liver biopsy

Discussion

The correct answer is **A**. This baby has cystinosis, an autosomal recessive metabolic disease of lysosomal storage, characterized by accumulation of cystine in various organs and tissues, leading to potentially severe organ dysfunction.[33] Three forms of cystinosis are described: the infantile (nephropathic) form, the intermediate (adolescent, late-onset) form; and the adult (benign) form. Nephropathic cystinosis, the most common, has been estimated to affect one of every 100,000 to 200,000 children. Cystine is derived from protein degradation within the lysosomes of cells and is normally transported through the lysosomal membrane to the cytosol where it is transformed to cysteine. In cystinosis, there is a defect in the transport system; causing accumulation of cystine inside the lysosomes. The first clinical signs of infantile cystinosis appear around 3 to 6 months of age and are due to impaired proximal tubular reabsorptive capacity, leading to the varied manifestations of Fanconi syndrome (glycosuria, metabolic acidosis, phosphaturia, and aminoaciduria). Biochemical abnormalities

include normal anion gap metabolic acidosis (secondary to proximal renal tubular acidosis), hypokalemia, and hypouricemia. There is progressive decline in the GFR. End-stage renal failure typically occurs by the end of the first decade. The diagnosis of cystinosis can be confirmed by determining the cystine content of peripheral blood leukocyte or fibroblasts. Management of cystinosis consists of symptomatic measures (replace the fluid and electrolyte losses induced by the proximal dysfunction), administration of cysteamine (which directly treats the disease by reducing the intracellular cystine content) and renal transplantation for those progressing to ESRD.

Quantitative urine mucopolysaccharides and oligosaccharides are done to screen for lysosomal storage disorders. Serum very long-chain fatty acids can be assessed to detect peroxisomal disorders, which in neonates present with neurologic abnormalities, such as hypotonia, decreased activity, encephalopathy, seizures or with craniofacial dysmorphism, and skeletal abnormalities (calcific stippling, shortened proximal limbs). Liver biopsy can be done to evaluate the type and location of abnormal storage material once storage disorders are suspected.

Objectives

1. Know the differential diagnoses associated with proximal tubular acidosis in a neonate
2. Know the clinical presentation of cystinosis
3. Know the typical electrolyte abnormalities associated with cystinosis
4. Know the metabolic abnormalities associated with cystinosis
5. Know diagnostic evaluation of patient with proximal RTA

Hematuria

CASE 19

A 5-month-old male infant who was born at 28 weeks of gestation is getting ready for discharge home after a prolonged NICU stay. He had a birth weight of 850 g and required intubation and was mechanically ventilated for a prolonged period of time. Because of the need for prolonged mechanical ventilation, and due to repeated failed attempts at successful extubation, he had a tracheostomy placed. Over the last month, his condition has stabilized to the point of being nearly ready for discharge home and his family is spending more time in the step-down unit preparing for his discharge. His current medications include furosemide, an H_2-blocker for gastroesophageal reflux, and he receives breathing treatments with beta-agonists and an inhaled corticosteroid.

The infant has been clinically well, gaining weight appropriately, and his vital signs have been stable. His physical examination is unchanged, and there are no palpable abdominal masses noted.

While his father is changing a diaper in the nursery, he points out to the infant's nurse that there may be some blood in the diaper?

A likely cause for gross hematuria in this infant would be
A. Urinary tract infection and urosepsis
B. RVT
C. Acute poststreptococcal glomerulonephritis
D. Hypercalciuria
E. Rhabdomyolysis

Discussion

The correct answer is **D**. While acute poststreptococcal glomerulonephritis is the most common form of glomerulonephritis in children, infants seemed to be spared from glomerulonephritis, and this would be a very unlikely cause for gross hematuria at this age. The infant seems relatively well, and there do not seem to be risk factors for the development of rhabdomyolysis such as prolonged seizures or crush injuries. While one must always consider the possibility of urinary tract infection, this infant does not have a foley catheter or any apparent risk factors for either traumatic injury of the urethra or a portal of entry for urinary tract infection. It would certainly be prudent however to send a urinalysis and a urine culture. RVT is usually suspected in the setting of an acutely ill infant and may be associated with a palpable abdominal mass.

Given that this infant is being treated with furosemide, hypercalciuria seems the most likely etiology. Hypercalciuria may be idiopathic, or it may be secondary to risk factors such as immobilization and medication use. Hypercalciuria does appear to be the predominant cause of hematuria in children older than 2 years of age, but there are limited data in younger infants. Former premature infants are felt to be at greater risk for stone formation secondary to a number of exposures during their hospitalizations, including diuretics, corticosteroids, and parenteral nutrition. Corticosteroids are known to increase calcium excretion, and this infant has likely had some exposure to corticosteroids because of his chronic lung disease. Loop diuretics such as furosemide and bumetanide are agents that also increase urinary calcium excretion. Hypercalciuria alone may be associated with gross hematuria but it is also a known risk factor for

the development of renal stones. In this setting it would be prudent to send a spot urine sample for determination of a Ca-to-Cr ratio. The normal range for Ca-to-Cr ratio for this age group is 0.03 to 0.56 mg/mg. It would also prudent to perform a renal ultrasound to look for any evidence of urinary tract stones. A chemistry profile to include electrolytes, Ca, phosphorus level, BUN, and Cr would also be recommended.

Objective

1. Identify potential causes of hematuria in the neonate

Calcium Homeostasis

CASE 20

A baby born at 38 weeks to a diabetic mother with uncomplicated immediate perinatal course was noted to be jittery. The mother had received good prenatal care. There is no family history of seizures. The physical examination for the baby is unremarkable except for increased neuromuscular irritability. A drug screen is also negative. Laboratory values are as below:

LABORATORY TEST	RESULT
Sodium	138 mmol/L
Potassium	5.5 mmol/L
Chloride	108 mmol/L
Bicarbonate	18 mmol/L
Blood urea nitrogen	12 mg/dL
Creatinine	0.3 mg/dL
Calcium	6.8 mg/dL
Albumin	3.6 g/dL
Phosphorus	6.0 mg/dL
Glucose	75 mg/dL

What is the most likely cause for hypocalcaemia?
A. Chronic kidney disease
B. Reduced intake of calcium in breast milk
C. Reduced maternal vitamin D level
D. Transient impairment in parathyroid response

Discussion

The correct answer is **D**. Early neonatal hypocalcemia (presenting in the first 3 days of life) is frequently seen in infants of diabetic mothers and neonates suffering asphyxia. The hypocalcemia is caused by poor parathyroid response, compounded by elevated phosphorus level and hypomagnesemia seen in diabetic pregnant mothers (due to increased urinary loss of magnesium). Late neonatal hypocalcemia (presenting at 5–10 days of life) may result from maternal anticonvulsant use which increases hepatic clearance of vitamin D causing hypovitaminosis in both mother and neonate, leading to poor calcium absorption. Hyperphosphatemia can also lead to delayed hypocalcemia. Other causes include maternal hyperparathyroidism and familial hypocalciuric hypercalcemia, leading to hypercalcemia in mother and fetus, which inhibits fetal PTH production, manifesting as hypocalcemia after birth.[36] Neonates with chronic kidney failure are expected to show hypocalcemia, hyperphosphatemia, elevated PTH, urea nitrogen, and creatinine level, which is not present in this infant. Hyperphosphatemia in a neonate may be due to reduced phosphate excretion by immature neonatal kidneys, transient hypoparathyroidism or higher phosphate intake through milk.

Replacement of calcium in the form of calcium gluconate or as a continuous infusion is the treatment.

Objectives

1. Understand the principles of calcium homeostasis in neonate
2. Know the differential diagnosis of hypocalcemia in the neonate
3. Understand the causes of hypercalcemia in the neonate
4. Understand the causes of hypercalciuria in the neonate
5. Understand the potential complications of hypercalciuria

REFERENCES

1. Rosenblum N. Chapter 73: Malformation of the kidney: Structural and functional consequences. Pediatric nephrology. In: Taal MW, Chertow GM, Marsden PA, et al. *Brenner and Rector's The Kidney.* 2012.
2. Wiesel A, Queisser-Luft A, Clementi M, et al. Prenatal detection of congenital renal malformations by fetal ultrasonographic examination: an analysis of 709,030 births in 12 European countries. *Eur J Med Genet.* 2005;48:131–144.
3. Winyard P, Chitty L. Dysplastic and polycystic kidneys: diagnosis, associations and management. *Prenatal Diagn.* 2001;16:985–992.
4. Blyth B, Snyder HM, Duckett JW. Antenatal hydronephrosis. *J Urol.* 1993;149(4):693–698.
5. Schlomer BJ, Copp HL. Antenatal hydronephrosis: assessment and management. *NeoReviews.* 2013;14(11):e551–e561.
6. Bomalaski MD, Anema JG, Coplen DE, et al. Delayed presentation of posterior urethral valves: a not so benign condition. *J Urol.* 1999;162:2130–2132.
7. Holmes N, Harrison M, Baskin L. Fetal surgery for posterior urethral valves: Long term outcomes. *Pedaitrics.* 2001;108(1):E7.
8. DeFoor W, Clark C, Jackson E, et al. Risk factors for end stage renal disease in children with posterior urethral valves. *J Urol.* 2008;180:1705–1708.
9. Denes ED, Barthold JS, González R. Early prognostic value of serum creatinine levels in children with posterior urethral valves. *J Urol.* 1997;157:1441–1443.
10. Routh JC, Huang L, Retik AB, et al. *Urology.* 2010;76(1):44.
11. Hassett S, Smith GH, Holland AJ. Prune belly syndrome. *Pediatr Surg Int.* 2012;28:219–228.
12. Singh HP, Hurley RM, Myers TF. Neonatal hypertension. Incidence and risk factors. *Am J Hypertens.* 1992;5:51–55.
13. Zubrow AB, Hulman S, Kushner H et al. Determinants of blood pressure in infants admitted to neonatal intensive care units: a prospective multicenter study. *J Perinatol.* 1995;15(6):470–479.
14. Schmidt B, Andrew M. Neonatal thrombosis: report of a prospective Canadian and international registry. *Pediatrics.* 1995;96–939.
15. Kosch A, Kuwertz-Bröking E, Heller C, et al. Renal venous thrombosis in neonates: prothrombotic risk factors and long-term follow-up. *Blood.* 2004;104:1356–1360.
16. Lau KK, Stoffman JM, Williams S, et al. Neonatal renal vein thrombosis: review of the English-language literature between 1992 and 2006. *Pediatrics.* 2007;120:e1278–1284.
17. Messinger Y, Sheaffer JW, Mrozek J, et al. Renal outcome of neonatal renal venous thrombosis: review of 28 patients and effectiveness of fibrinolytics and heparin in 10 patients. *Pediatrics.* 2006;118:e1478–1484.
18. Sujov P, Kellerman L, Zeltzer M, et al. Plasma and urine osmolality in full-term and pre-term infants. *Acta Paediatr Scand.* 1984;73:722–726.
19. Bonilla-Felix M, John-Phillip C. Prostaglandin mediate the defect in AVP-stimulated cAMP generation in immature collecting duct. *Am J Physiol.* 1994;267:F44–F48.
20. Akima S, Kent A, Reynold G, et al. Indomethacin and renal impairment in neonates. *Pediatric Nephrology.* 2004;19(5):490–493.
21. Jones LJ, Craven PD, Attia J, et al. Network meta-analysis of indomethacin versus ibuprofen versus placebo for PDA in preterm infants. *Arch Dis Child Fetal Neonatal Ed.* 2011;96:F45–F52.
22. Heymann MA, Rudolph AM, Silverman NH. Closure of the ductus arteriosus in premature infants by inhibition of prostaglandin synthesis. *N Engl J Med.* 1976;295:530–533.
23. Kastner PR, Hall JE, Guyton AC. Control of glomerular filtration rate: role of intrarenally formed angiotensin II. *Am J Physiol.* 1984;246:F897–F906.
24. Patrono C, Dunn MJ. The clinical significance of inhibition of renal prostaglandin synthesis. *Kidney Int.* 1987;32:1–12.
25. Simon DB, Karet FE, Hamdan JM, et al. Bartter's syndrome, hypokalaemic alkalosis with hypercalciuria, is caused by mutations in the Na-K-2Cl cotransporter NKCC2. *Nat Genet.* 1996;13:183–188.
26. Fanaroff AA, Martin RJ *Neonatal-Perinatal Medicine: Diseases of the Fetus and Infant*
27. Lee MM, Chua AN, Yorgin PD. Neonatal peritoneal dialysis. *NeoReviews.* 2005;6(8):e384–e391.
28. Cooper WO, Hernandez-Diaz S, Arbogast PG, et al. Major congenital malformations after first-trimester exposure to ACE inhibitors. *N Engl J Med.* 2006;354(23):2443–2451.

29. Hård AL, Wennerholm UB, Niklasson A, et al. Severe ROP in twins after blockage of the renin-angiotensin system during gestation. *Acta Paediatr.* 2008;97(8):1142–1144.

30. Barr M Jr, Cohen MM Jr. ACE Inhibitor fetopathy and hypocalvaria: the kidney-skull connection. *Teratology.* 1991;44:485–495.

31. Ryynänen M, Seppälä M, Kuusela P, et al. Antenatal screening for congenital nephrosis in Finland by maternal serum alpha-fetoprotein. *Br J Obstet Gynaecol.* 1983;90(5):437–442.

32. Wraith JE. Lysosomal disorders. *Semin Neonatol.* 2002;7(1): 75–83.

33. Gahl WA, Thoene JG, Schneider JA, et al. *N Engl J Med.* 2002; 347(2):111–121.

34. Alon US, Zimmerman H, Alon M. Evaluation and treatment of pediatric idiopathic urolithiasis-revisited. *Pediatr Nephrol.* 2004;19:516–520.

35. Ammenti A, Neri E, Agistri R, et al. Idiopathic hypercalciuria in infants with renal stones. *Pediatr Nephrol.* 2006;21:1901–1903.

36. Kovacs CS, Kronenberg HM. Maternal-fetal calcium and bone metabolism during pregnancy, puerperium, and lactation. *Endocr Rev.* 1997;18:832–872.

CASE 1

You are present at the delivery of an infant male, born by spontaneous vaginal delivery at 40 weeks of gestation to a healthy 32-year-old G1P1 mother. The infant's APGAR scores at 1 and 5 minutes are 8 and 9, respectively. He weighs 3.05 kg and is 20 in in length. There were no complications with the delivery. On examination, you note a well-appearing, vigorous young male with peripheral cyanosis. On genital examination, he has a normal-appearing phallus (3.5 cm length) and a normal central location of his urethra. Gonads are palpable in a normal-appearing scrotum.

Which of the following is responsible for initiating male gonadal development?
A. SRY gene
B. Dihydrotestosterone (DHT)
C. Anti-mullerian hormone (AMH)
D. Testosterone
E. Luteinizing hormone (LH)

Discussion

The correct answer is **A**. Sexual determination is defined as a series of molecular events that directs the bipotential gonad to develop into a testis or ovary. Due to the expression of a variety of genes, the bipotential gonad develops from the urogenital ridge at approximately 5 weeks of gestation. In the presence of the SRY (sex-determining region on the Y chromosome) gene, the bipotential gonad develops into a testis. In the absence of the SRY gene, the bipotential gonad defaults to an ovary.[1] In the developing male, the wolffian duct forms the internal male genitalia. In the developing female, the mullerian duct forms the internal female genitalia. Once the fetal testis has formed,

Leydig cells produce androgens that promote the development of the wolffian structures (e.g., epididymis, vas deferens, and seminal vesicles) and Sertoli cells produce anti-mullerian hormone (AMH) that inhibits the mullerian duct from forming structures of the internal female genitalia (e.g., uterus, fallopian tubes and upper two-thirds of the vagina). The Leydig cells also produce insulin-like Factor III that causes the testes to descend into the scrotum. In females, a lack of AMH and testosterone, results in the promotion of mullerian duct differentiation and wolffian duct atrophy.[2]

In sexual differentiation of the male, the genital tubercle develops into the head of the penis, the urogenital folds form the ventral aspect of the penis and the urethra, and the labioscrotal folds fuse to form the scrotum. In sexual differentiation of the female, the genital tubercle develops into the clitoris, the urogenital folds form the labia minora, and the labioscrotal folds form the labia majora.[3] The embryologic homologous structures of sexual differentiation are shown in Figure 9-1.

Which of the following is primarily responsible for the development of normal male external genitalia?
A. SRY gene
B. DHT
C. Anti-mullerian hormone
D. Testosterone
E. LH

Discussion

The correct answer is **B**. Sexual differentiation is defined as the hormonal influences that direct the formation of the internal and external genitalia. In the male, once testosterone is produced by the testis, it is reduced to DHT via the enzyme, 5α-reductase II.[1] DHT binds to androgen receptors in the prostate and developing external genitalia and promotes masculinization. DHT is required for

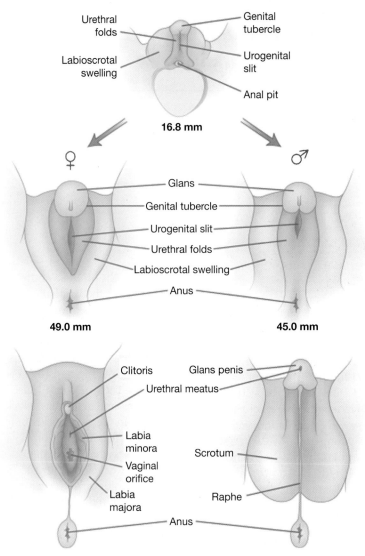

FIGURE 9-1. Reproduced with permission from Hay WW, Levin MJ, Deterding RR, et al. *Current Diagnosis and Treatment: Pediatrics*. 21st ed. New York, NY: McGraw Hill; 2012.

fusion of the urethral and labioscrotal fold, lengthening of the genital tubercle, and regression of the urogenital sinus. Masculinization of the external genitalia is complete by 14 weeks of gestation. In the complete absence of DHT, regardless of sufficient testosterone being produced, the external genitalia will appear female. With partial function of the 5-α reductase II enzyme, the external genitalia will appear ambiguous.

CASE 2

You examine a 48-hour-old newborn who is the product of a normal pregnancy, born at term with a normal birth weight and length, to a healthy, 22-year-old G3P3 mother. On examination, the child is resting comfortably and has no dysmorphic features. He has a phallus 1.5 cm in length and incomplete fusion of the scrotal folds. The gonads are palpable in the inguinal canal.

What would be the next most appropriate step in evaluating this infant?

A. Obtain serum gonadotropin and testosterone levels
B. Obtain serum electrolytes and a serum 17-hydroxy-progesterone (17-OHP) level
C. Obtain a bone age and a serum 17-OHP level
D. Perform a surgical exploration of the gonads and adrenal glands
E. Obtain a karyotype and an abdominal/pelvic ultrasound

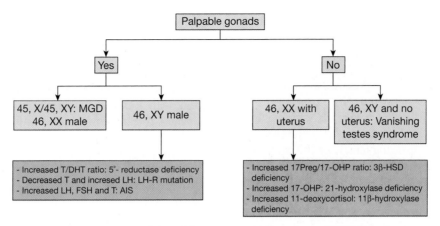

FIGURE 9-2. **MGD:** Mixed Gonadal Dysgenesis; **T:** Testosterone; **DHT:** Dihydrotestosterone; **LH-R:** Luteinizing hormone receptor: **AIS:** Androgen Insensitivity Syndrome; **17Preg:** 17-Pregnenolone; **17-OHP:** 17-hydroxyprogesterone.

Discussion

The correct answer is **E**. This infant has a disorder of sexual development (DSD). There are three categories for infants with a suspected DSD: (1) sex chromosome (Turner syndrome, Klinefelter syndrome variants, and mixed gonadal dysgenesis [MGD]); (2) 46, XY (disorders of testicular development and disorders of androgen synthesis/action); and (3) 46, XX (disorders of ovarian development, androgen excess). Care must be taken to not refer to the infant as a "he," "she," or "it," but instead, as "your baby," or as "your child."

The initial approach is to determine if the child is a virilized female or an undervirilized male. In establishing the diagnosis, the physical examination is important, however, identification of the internal genitalia (via ultrasound) and genotype (via karyotype), are equally important. Particular attention must be given to determining the length and diameter of the phallic structure (if present), location of the urethral opening, degree of fusion of the labioscrotal folds, anorectal distance, and presence or absence of gonads. Measurement of adrenal hormone levels may need to be performed but, after performing a physical examination, the most appropriate next step in the evaluation of this child is to obtain a karyotype and a pelvic ultrasound. The algorithmic approach to evaluating an infant with ambiguous genitalia and symmetric external genitalia is outlined in Figure 9-2.

Collection of a serum 17-OHP level and serum electrolytes are helpful in the evaluation of infants with suspected congenital adrenal hyperplasia (CAH). There are multiple causes of CAH, but 21-hydroxylase (21-OHP) deficiency is the most common. In the classic salt-wasting

form of 21-OHP deficiency, a failure of the conversion of 17-OHP to 11-deoxycortisol, and corticosterone to deoxycorticosterone (DOC), results in elevated 17-OHP levels, low cortisol levels, and low aldosterone levels. The cortisol deficiency leads to hypoglycemia and aldosterone deficiency leads to a low serum sodium level and elevated serum potassium level.

Infants with incomplete androgen insensitivity syndrome (AIS) may have ambiguous genitalia, and increased LH, FSH, and testosterone levels.

A bone age to determine if there is a delay or advancement in skeletal age compared to chronological age is useful in children 2 years of age and older. It would not, however, have any diagnostic value in this situation.

You obtain labs and an imaging study on the infant. Serum electrolytes, a 17-OHP level, and gonadotropin levels are normal. The newborn has a 46, XY karyotype. A pelvic ultrasound confirms the presence of gonads in the inguinal canal and demonstrates the absence of a uterus. The serum testosterone to DHT ratio is elevated.

What is the most likely diagnosis?
A. Androgen insensitivity syndrome
B. Mixed gonadal dysgenesis (MGD)
C. CAH
D. 5α-reductase deficiency
E. Leydig cell receptor mutation

Discussion

The correct answer is **D**. 5-α reductase deficiency is an autosomal-recessive disorder that results in the inability to convert testosterone to DHT, the hormone regulating masculinization of the external genitalia. Gonads are present and palpable and because Sertoli cells develop and function appropriately, AMH is produced and mullerian ducts regress. In the presence of testosterone, wolffian structures develop into the normal internal genital structures of the male. Because infants with complete deficiency of the enzyme have undescended gonads and normal-appearing female genitalia at birth, the diagnosis may be overlooked. During puberty however, with increased testosterone production, the effects of male pubertal testosterone becomes evident with a deepening of voice, increased pubic hair, particularly over the abdomen, face, and chest, and enlargement of the penis and scrotum.[4]

Androgen insensitivity syndrome, also known as testicular feminization syndrome, is an X-linked recessive disorder due to mutations of the androgen-receptor (AR) gene. Although testosterone and other androgens are appropriately produced, without a proper interaction between androgen and its receptor, biologic activity of the androgens does not occur. Therefore, wolffian structures do not develop into internal male genitalia. Mullerian structures, however, will regress due to normal production of AMH, and therefore most of the structures of the internal genitalia do not form. These individuals appear as female infants. During puberty, due to the formation of a blind pouch and absence of internal female genitalia organs, these individuals will not have menstrual cycles. They do, however, have normal breast development, due to the conversion of androgens to estrogens, and likely seek medical attention in the early teenage years. Serum LH, FSH, and testosterone levels will be elevated due to a loss of feedback inhibition at the level of the pituitary gland and uninhibited testosterone production by the testes.[5]

Infants with mixed gonadal dysgenesis may have an abnormal karyotype with a variable clinical phenotype. Defects in ovarian or testicular development or function are the cause for MGD.[6]

CAH can be caused by a variety of enzyme deficiencies, the most common of which is 21-OHP, which is confirmed with an elevated serum 17-OHP level. The diagnosis of CAH may be made sooner in a virilized female because of ambiguous genitalia at birth, whereas, the male, who is normally virilized at birth, may not be identified for more than a week when he becomes lethargic, hypotensive, and hypoglycemic due to aldosterone and cortisol deficiency.[7]

Individuals with an LH-receptor defect have elevated serum LH levels but decreased serum testosterone levels due to the inability of the LH receptor to respond to LH. These individuals have rudimentary wolffian structures with external female genitalia.[5]

CASE 3

You are paged emergently by the obstetrics resident to speak with a mother regarding the sexual assignment of her child. You arrive in the room to find the mother crying hysterically because she does not know whether her child is a boy or a girl. Due to her advanced maternal age, she underwent an amniocentesis to evaluate for potential birth defects. The amniocentesis revealed a 46, XY karyotype with no abnormalities. You examine the child who appears to be a healthy, well-developed female. You repeat the karyotype and confirm that the infant does in fact have a 46, XY karyotype. A pelvic ultrasound demonstrates the presence of a uterus and fallopian tubes.

What is the most likely cause of these findings?
A. LH-receptor defect
B. AR defect
C. SRY gene defect
D. AMH defect
E. Hypopituitarism

Discussion

The correct answer is **C**. The SRY gene, located on the Y chromosome, initiates the process of differentiation of the testis from the bipotential gonad in the developing embryo.[1] Once the testis has formed, Leydig cells release androgens that support wolffian duct formation and the Sertoli cells release AMH, which causes the regression of the mullerian ducts. In the absence of a functioning SRY gene in a 46, XY individual, there is no production of testosterone or AMH, resulting in an infant with fully formed mullerian structures, bilateral streak gonads, and female external genitalia. If these individuals are not detected at birth, they will typically present for evaluation of delayed puberty or amenorrhea. They are at an increased risk of developing a gonadoblastoma, usually after puberty, for which a gonadectomy is recommended.

A 46, XY infant with a defect of the LH receptor, AR, hypothalamus, or pituitary would not present with fully formed mullerian structures because Sertoli cell function and production of AMH is not affected. An infant with a defect in AMH would have mullerian structures, but a 46, XY individual would have a male phenotype due to normal Leydig cell function and production of testosterone.

Objectives

1. Understand the hormonal regulation of sex differentiation

2. Understand the embryology of male and female gonad development
3. Differentiate among disorders of testicular hormone synthesis or action
4. Know the etiology of abnormal sexual differentiation
5. Know the diagnostic approaches to and management of abnormal sexual differentiation
6. Know the etiology of and diagnostic approaches to an infant with ambiguous genitalia
7. Know the clinical manifestations, laboratory features, and therapeutic management of an infant with ambiguous genitalia

CASE 4

You are receiving sign-out in the morning from your colleague who was on call the previous night. Of the many infants on your service, one seems to be of particular interest to you. He is a 2-week-old infant born at 33 weeks of gestation with a birth weight of 1.95 kg to a G2P3 mother. He was admitted to the NICU with difficulty breathing and required supplemental oxygen. His hospital course has been significant for hypoglycemia, difficulty feeding with increased residual volumes, and hypotension. The infant was initially started on dopamine and epinephrine, and recently corticosteroids with improvement in blood pressures. Prior to the start of corticosteroids, a low serum cortisol level (0.5 µg/dL, normal 5–20) and elevated plasma ACTH level (200 pg/mL, normal 10–60) were discovered. A review of laboratory studies over the past few days is remarkable for a low serum sodium level (129 mg/dL), an elevated serum potassium level (6.5 mg/dL), and a low serum OHP level (5 ng/dL, normal 10–200).

What is the most likely diagnosis?
A. Glycogen storage disorder
B. Congenital hypopituitarism
C. Congenital adrenal hyperplasia
D. Autoimmune adrenalitis
E. Adrenal hypoplasia congenita (AHC)

Discussion

The correct answer is **E**. This infant is experiencing symptoms of primary adrenal insufficiency reflecting both glucocorticoid and mineralocorticoid deficiencies, with hypoglycemia, hypotension, hyponatremia, and hyperkalemia. This diagnosis is also supported by a low cortisol with an elevated ACTH level. This infant has adrenal hypoplasia

congenita, also known as congenital adrenal hypoplasia.[8] The most common mode of inheritance is X-linked and is due to mutations in the DAX1 gene, which has also been implicated in Duchenne muscular dystrophy. In adrenal hypoplasia congenita, the definitive zone of the fetal adrenal gland improperly develops and becomes vacuolated.

This infant has adrenal hypoplasia congenita which is a rare inherited disorder. The most common mode of inheritance is X-linked due to a mutation in the DAX1 gene. In some patients, there is a series of contiguous gene deletions resulting in abnormalities in adrenal function, Duchenne muscular dystrophy or gylcerol-kinase deficiency. Affected females will have delayed onset of puberty. In the neonatal period, similar to the patient in the vignette, the children have evidence of primary adrenal failure which presents with hyponatremia, hyperkalemia, metabolic acidosis, elevated ACTH and a decreased or normal 17-OHP level.

Congenital adrenal hyperplasia also presents with adrenal insufficiency in infancy due to a decrease in cortisol production. Depending on the specific enzyme mutation, androgens and mineralocorticoids may be increased or decreased (Fig. 9-3). For an infant with laboratory findings consistent with glucocorticoid and mineralocorticoid deficiency, the most common cause of CAH is 21-OHP deficiency, affecting over 90% of individuals with CAH. In patients with 21-OHP deficiency, the hormone 17-OHP is elevated as it is not converted to 11-deoxycortisol, the precursor to cortisol. Despite hypoglycemia, there are no other indications that this infant has a glycogen storage disorder, such as vomiting and hepatomegaly. Hypopituitarism can present with cortisol deficiency, but this would be due to ACTH deficiency. Autoimmune adrenalitis is typically seen in adult females and is uncommon in neonates.

Objectives

1. Identify the clinical presentation associated with a diagnosis of AHC
2. Understand the diagnostic evaluation of a newborn with a suspected diagnosis of AHC
3. Understand the biochemical alterations present in a patient with AHC

CASE 5

You are present for a high-risk delivery of a 40-year-old G1P1 mother who delivers at 33 weeks of gestation secondary to pregnancy-induced hypertension. The birth

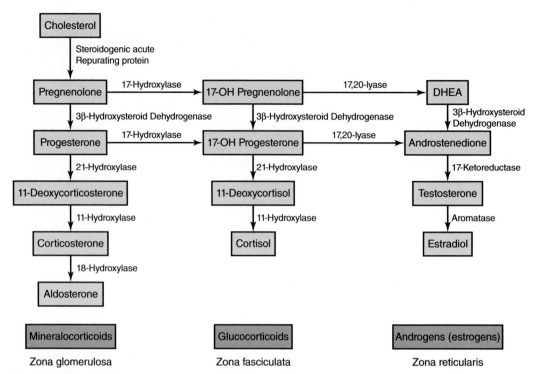

FIGURE 9-3.   Reproduced with permission from Hay WW, Levin MJ, Deterding RR, et al. *Current Diagnosis and Treatment: Pediatrics.* 21st ed. New York, NY: McGraw Hill; 2012.

weight is 2.05 kg and the infant has APGAR scores of 6 and 8, at 1 and 5 minutes, respectively. The mother had an amniocentesis that confirmed that the infant has a 46, XY karyotype. When drying and stimulating the infant, he has a noticeably small phallus and absent gonads in the scrotum. Due to the preterm delivery, the infant is monitored in the step-down NICU. The infant's hospital course is complicated by hypoglycemia that improves with continuous feeds, and jaundice. Newborn screening results collected on the fourth day of life are abnormal with a low TSH (0.01 mIU/L, normal 1.3–16) and a low total T4 (2 μg/dL, normal 2.6–14.0).

What is the most likely diagnosis?
A. Kallman syndrome
B. Central hypothyroidism
C. Panhypopituitarism
D. Primary adrenal insufficiency
E. Isolated gonadotropin deficiency

Discussion

The correct answer is **C**. This infant has clinical findings consistent with multiple pituitary deficiencies, due most likely to hypoplasia of the anterior pituitary gland. The definitive etiology may be unknown, but is most likely due to mutations in transcription factors involved in pituitary development. This infant has

symptoms of growth hormone (GH) deficiency manifested by hypoglycemia, gonadotropin deficiency manifested by a micropenis and cryptorchidism, and hypothyroidism manifested by jaundice and low serum TSH and free T4 levels.[9] This infant should be started on growth and thyroid hormone replacement therapy. Due to hypogonadotropic hypogonadism, this infant will experience delayed puberty and will need testosterone injections to promote further development in the early teenage years.

A micropenis is defined as a stretched phallus length (SPL, measured from pubis to tip of the penis) of 2.5 standard deviations less than the mean age for the group. For infants, this is defined as a SPL of ≤2.5 cm. In the male fetus, placental human chorionic gonadotropin (hCG) stimulates testosterone production from the Leydig cells, which is then converted to DHT that initiates male external genitalia differentiation. Differentiation of the phallus is complete by approximately 12 weeks of gestation. After the first trimester, growth of the phallus is dependent on the fetal androgens that are under fetal pituitary stimulation. Failure of this process after 12 weeks of gestation can result in a micropenis. A neonate may have a micropenis because of hypogonadotropic hypogonadism (e.g., Kallman syndrome, hypopituitarism), hypergonadotropic hypogonadism (e.g., anorchia, gonadal dysgenesis) or, from an idiopathic cause.[10] Kallman syndrome is due to isolated gonadotropin deficiency with anosmia due to failure of the gonadotropin-releasing hormone (GnRH) neurons to migrate from their initial embryologic location in the olfactory bulb to their final location in the hypothalamus.

Evaluation includes the assessment of pituitary function by obtaining serum GH, ACTH, TSH, and if obtained early in infancy, follicle-stimulating hormone (FSH) and LH. An MRI can confirm structural pituitary abnormalities. Testicular function can also be assessed by obtaining serum testosterone, FSH, and LH levels before and after the administration of hCG. A failure to appreciate a post-administration rise in testosterone coupled with a rise in FSH and LH is highly suggestive of testicular absence or failure. Treatment of an infant with a micropenis involves the intramuscular administration of testosterone cypionate (25 mg) monthly for 3 months. Testosterone therapy will need to be restarted and continued for life once the child enters the age of puberty.[10] This therapy schedule is designed to mimic the natural physiologic pattern of testosterone, specifically a rise in testosterone during the first 3 months of life, the so-called "mini-puberty of infancy," followed by a significant decrease to low or undetectable levels in the pre-pubertal period, followed by a secondary rise in levels during puberty.

Objectives

1. Know the clinical signs and symptoms associated with panhypopituitarism
2. Understand the appropriate diagnostic evaluation of a patient with a suspected diagnosis of panhypopituitarism
3. Know the recommended treatment for patient with a diagnosis of panhypopituitarism

CASE 6

A term male infant is born to a 27-year-old G4P4 mother with a birth weight of 2 kg. On examination, you note that the infant's testes are not palpable in the scrotum and that the infant has hypospadias.

What is the most common congenital abnormality to occur in males?
A. Microphallus
B. Chordee
C. Anorchia
D. Hypospadias
E. Cryptorchidism

Discussion

The correct answer is **E**. Cryptorchidism, or undescended testes, is the most common congenital abnormality in males, affecting 2% to 9% of live births. This disorder can be associated with disruption of the hypothalamic–pituitary–gonadal (HPG) axis, low birth weight, or any defect involving testosterone synthesis or action. The diagnosis of undescended testes is made clinically. Management is critical as untreated bilateral undescended testes can increase the risk of sterility and testicular cancer. An hCG stimulation test can be used to confirm the presence of testicular tissue as follows: First, serum testosterone, FSH, and LH levels are measured prior to the administration of hCG. Second, hCG is given intramuscularly for 4 days. Finally, hCG-stimulated hormone levels are collected 24 hours after the last dose of hCG. A low testosterone with an elevated LH and FSH, is highly suggestive of a testicular defect and likely indicates the absence of testicular tissue. A prolonged hCG stimulation test for a period of a few weeks can be used to promote testicular descent. The optimal method of ensuring testicular descent, however, is orchidopexy performed preferably earlier rather than later, between 6 and 12 months of age. Spontaneous descent should not be expected past 6 months of age.[11-13]

Objectives

1. Know the causes of micropenis, including pituitary deficiency
2. Know how to evaluate and manage an infant with micropenis
3. Know how to evaluate and manage an infant with hypospadias and epispadias
4. Know how to evaluate and manage an infant with cryptorchidism

CASE 7

A newborn infant has been admitted to the nursery. The baby was the product of a high risk pregnancy due to advanced maternal age to a 43 year old G1P1 mother. The infant was born at 38 weeks of gestation with a birth weight of 3.2 kg. An amniocentesis confirmed a karyotype of 46, XX. On examination, you notice that the clitoris is enlarged and there is some fusion of the labial folds. Gonads are not palpable. Due to poor feeding and slow weight gain, she remains in the nursery, and on the 10th day of life, she is pale and hypotensive. Laboratory studies are collected revealing a low serum glucose level (30 mg/dL), low serum sodium level (127 mEq/L), and a nonhemolyzed elevated serum potassium level (7.5 mEq/L).

What is the most likely cause of these findings?
A. 17-hydroxylase deficiency
B. 11-β hydroxylase deficiency
C. 3-β hydroxysteroid dehydrogenase deficiency
D. 21-OHP deficiency
E. 17,20-lyase deficiency

Discussion

The correct answer is **D**. This infant is a virilized female with mineralocorticoid and glucocorticoid deficiency, due to classic salt-wasting CAH. The deficient enzyme is 21-OHP. Due to this enzymatic defect, 17-OHP is unable to be converted to 11-deoxycortisol (a precursor of cortisol) and progesterone is unable to be converted to 11-deoxycorticosterone (a precursor of aldosterone), resulting in elevated levels of 17-OHP and corticosterone. Diagnostic laboratory findings in this setting include an elevated 17-OHP level, low cortisol level, low sodium level, and elevated potassium level. A diagnostic newborn screen of 21-OHP deficiency will demonstrate an elevated 17-OHP (Fig. 9-3).[7]

11-β hydroxylase deficiency is the second most common cause of CAH. Deficiency in this enzyme results in failure to convert 11-deoxycorticosterone and 11-deoxycortisol to corticosterone (precursor of aldosterone) and cortisol, respectively. 11-deoxycorticosterone has mineralocorticoid activity. Females with this disorder can also present with virilization, similar to 21-OHP deficiency, but the distinguishing features of 11-β hydroxylase deficiency are hypertension and hypokalemia. Individuals should be treated with glucocorticoid supplementation.[14]

The CYP-17 gene encodes for the 17-hydroxylase enzyme (converts progesterone to cortisol and androgen precursors) and also for 17,20 lyase (converts 17-α hydroxypregnenolone to androgen precursors). Individuals with mutations in this gene have deficiencies of both enzymes, and these precursors (of cortisol and androgens) are shunted to the mineralocorticoid pathway, resulting in volume expansion (Fig. 9.3). 17,20-lyase deficiency results in impaired androgen and estrogen production, as estrogens are formed from aromatization of androgens. Affected males will have normal-appearing external female genitalia or ambiguous genitalia and affected females will have normal-appearing genitalia at birth. If females are not diagnosed early in life with hypertension and electrolyte abnormalities, they usually seek medical attention around the time of expected puberty with failure of breast, pubic hair, and menarche. Due to increased aldosterone production from the loss of negative feedback of cortisol on the hypothalamus

and pituitary, male and female individuals with a CYP-17 gene mutation have hypertension, hypernatremia, hypokalemia, and hypoglycemia. These infants should be treated with glucocorticoid supplementation.[15]

Individuals with 3-β hydroxysteroid dehydrogenase deficiency experience decreased production of cortisol, aldosterone, testosterone, and estrogen (Fig. 9-3). This is a very rare form of CAH. Affected individuals typically present in infancy with symptoms of both cortisol and aldosterone deficiencies (vomiting, hypotension, hyponatremia, and hyperkalemia). Females may have some mild virilization due to excess DHEA, a weak androgen. Males present with varying degrees of genital development including hypospadias to nearly normal-appearing female genitalia. These individuals usually have an elevated DHEA/androstenedione level as well as a very elevated 17-hydroxypregnenolone after ACTH stimulation. Treatment involves the administration of glucocorticoid and mineralocorticoid therapy, and depending on the sex of rearing, testosterone or estrogen therapy at the time of expected puberty.[14]

How would you treat this infant?
A. Salt supplementation; hydrocortisone (20 mg/kg/day) twice a day
B. Hydrocortisone (20 mg/kg/day) twice a day
C. Fludrocortisone (0.1 mg daily); hydrocortisone (20 mg/m^2/day) twice a day
D. Fludrocortisone (0.1 mg daily); hydrocortisone (20 mg/m^2/day) three times a day
E. Fludrocortisone (0.1 mg daily); hydrocortisone (20 mg/m^2/day) three times a day, salt supplementation

Discussion

The correct answer is **E**. This infant has classic salt-wasting CAH and needs supplementation for both glucocorticoid and mineralocorticoid deficiencies. This is best accomplished with hydrocortisone, fludrocortisone, and salt supplementation. Salt supplementation is used primarily in infancy and can eventually be discontinued once the child starts eating table food and receives enough salt from food. The appropriate initial dosing is as follows;[1] hydrocortisone, 20 mg/m^2/day divided three times a day;[2] fludrocortisone, 0.1 mg a day; and[3] salt supplementation, 3 to 4 mEq/kg/day. These should be initiated as soon as the diagnosis of salt-wasting CAH is considered but before serum hormone levels have been collected. These medications will be continued for life and doses will be adjusted on the basis of body surface area, growth velocity, serum electrolyte and hormone levels (sodium, potassium, 17-OHP, and androstenedione), and plasma renin activity levels. Once in childhood, doses of hydrocortisone are usually adjusted to provide ~10 to 15 mg/m^2/day.[7]

CASE 8

A term infant is admitted to the NICU for evaluation. The infant is noted to have hypospadias with labioscrotal fusion. Testes are palpable in the inguinal canal. Further workup reveals a 46, XY karyotype and a pelvic ultrasound does not demonstrate a uterus or ovaries.

What is the most likely diagnosis?
A. 21-OHP deficiency
B. 11-β hydroxylase deficiency
C. 17-β hydroxysteroid dehydrogenase deficiency
D. Persistent mullerian duct syndrome
E. Vanishing testes

Discussion

The correct answer is **C**. 17-β hydroxysteroid dehydrogenase deficiency results in undervirilization of 46, XY fetuses, as this enzyme is located in the testis and catalyzes the conversion of androstenedione to testosterone. Varying degrees of genital development are seen ranging from mild hypospadias to completely normal-appearing external female genitalia. When unrecognized, infants are assumed to be female and reared as females. Diagnostic laboratory findings include increased basal and hCG-stimulated androstenedione to testosterone ratios. Due to extratesticular conversion of androstenedione to testosterone at puberty, progressive virilization can be seen in these individuals.

21-OHP and 11-β hydroxylase deficiencies do not present with undervirilization in 46, XY fetuses. Fetuses affected by persistent mullerian duct syndrome due to AMH deficiency or a defect of the AMH receptor, will present with normal external male genitalia but will often have intertwined male and female internal genitalia structures, resulting in obstruction or nonpatency of the vas deferens or other parts of the male excretory ducts. This can result in infertility, the most serious potential problem caused by this condition. The condition can come to attention because of a bulge in the inguinal canal of a genetically male infant due to herniation of the uterus. The presence of a uterus may be noticed if an ultrasound or MRI of the pelvis is performed to locate the testes.

Vanishing testes, or testicular regression syndrome, are testicular defects that occur after 14 weeks of gestation. Other than absent testes, all internal and external male genitalia structures are present and appear normal. Most of these individuals are presumed to have had a vascular insult to the testes.

All of the following diagnoses can result in an undervirilized 46, XY fetus except
A. Androgen insensitivity syndrome (AIS)
B. 5-α reductase deficiency
C. 3-β-hydroxysteroid dehydrogenase deficiency
D. Placental aromatase deficiency
E. Congenital lipoid adrenal hyperplasia

Discussion

The correct answer is **D**. Placental aromatase converts fetal androgens to estrogens and protects the mother from virilizing effects of fetal androgens. In the absence of fetal aromatase, virilization of both the mother and the female fetus occurs. Although the external genitalia of the female (46, XX) infant may be virilized enough to require a surgical correction, shortly after birth, virilization of both the mother and infant subsides as the placenta is expelled.[14]

Androgen insensitivity syndrome is due to a defect in the AR; androgen activity in the fetus is limited. 5-α reductase converts testosterone to DHT, critical to external male genitalia development. In its absence, 46, XY infants have genital ambiguity or appear as completely normal females. A deficiency of the 3-β hydroxysteroid dehydrogenase enzyme results in testosterone deficiency and undervirilization of the 46, XY fetus. In congenital lipoid adrenal hyperplasia, mutations in the steroidogenic regulatory protein (StAR) result in a defect of the cholesterol transport across the mitochondria to initiate steroidogenesis, resulting in lipid accumulation that alters the cell cytostructure and destroys cells. As a result, there is impaired synthesis of all adrenal and gonadal steroids, causing undervirilization of the 46, XY fetus.[16]

Objectives

1. Recognize the clinical manifestations and laboratory features of the various types of CAH
2. Define the appropriate therapy for the various types of CAH
3. Understand the basic enzymatic defects involved in the various types of CAH

CASE 9

You are called to the delivery room to evaluate a term male infant born via normal spontaneous vaginal delivery to a 25-year-old G1P1 female. In reviewing the mother's medical history, you discover that she was diagnosed with Graves' disease at age 15 years. She was initially treated with methimazole for 2 years but desired definitive therapy, and successfully underwent thyroid ablation with radioactive iodine. Her thyroid function studies have been normal on levothyroxine therapy for the past 8 years. Last week, her thyroid studies were collected and confirmed that she is biochemically euthyroid. The infant appears flushed, has an obvious enlargement of his anterior neck region, and has a heart rate of 160 beats per minute.

Which of the following thyroid function studies are most consistent with this newborn?

	TOTAL T4	FREE T4	TOTAL T3	TSH	TSH-RECEPTOR ANTIBODY
A	↑	↑	↓	↑	Negative
B	↑	↑	↓	↓	Positive
C	↑	↑	↑	↓	Positive
D	↓	↓	↑	↓	Negative
E	↓	↓	↑	↓	Positive

Discussion

The correct answer is **C**. This infant's presentation is most consistent with neonatal Graves' disease, where maternal thyroid-stimulating hormone (TSH) receptor–stimulating antibodies cross the placenta and stimulate production of thyroid hormone from the infant's thyroid gland.[17] Although this mother had appropriate and effective definitive therapy for hyperthyroidism, her TSH receptor–stimulating antibodies persist. Due to the passage of these antibodies, levothyroxine (T4) and triiodothyronine (T3) levels are increased. Through negative feedback (Fig. 9-4), the elevated T4 inhibits both thyrotropin-releasing hormone (TRH) from the hypothalamus and thyrotropin (TSH) from the pituitary gland. The newborn with hyperthyroidism may show signs of irritability, flushing, tachycardia, poor weight gain, and hypertension. On physical examination the newborn may have a goiter, exophthalmos, and jaundice. In rare instances, a newborn with Graves' disease may have thrombocytopenia and cardiac failure.

Given this infant's likely diagnosis, which of the following is the best treatment plan?

A. No therapy because he should improve in less than a week
B. Lugol's solution
C. Propylthiouracil (PTU)
D. Methimazole
E. Synthroid

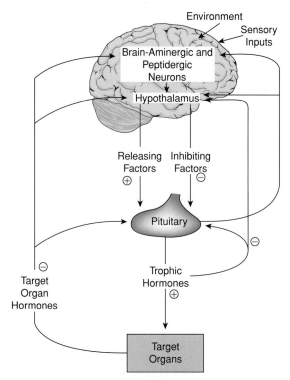

FIGURE 9-4. Reproduced with permission from Rudolph C, Rudolph A, Lister G, et al. *Rudolph's Pediatrics.* 22nd ed. New York, NY: McGraw-Hill Professional; 2011.

Discussion

The correct answer is **D**. This infant has neonatal Graves' disease due to placental transfer of TSH receptor–stimulating antibodies.[17] Iodide (Lugol's solution) or antithyroid medications are given to decrease the production of thyroid hormone. Iodide temporarily inhibits the release of thyroid hormone via the Wolff–Chaikoff effect, an autoregulatory phenomenon that inhibits organification (oxidation of iodide) in the thyroid gland, the formation of thyroid hormones inside the thyroid follicle, and the release of thyroid hormones into the bloodstream. This becomes evident secondary to elevated levels of circulating iodide. The Wolff–Chaikoff effect lasts around 10 days, after which, it is followed by an "escape phenomenon," described by resumption of normal organification of iodine and normal thyroid peroxidase function. "Escape phenomenon" is believed to occur because of decreased inorganic iodine concentration secondary to downregulation of the sodium-iodide symporter on the basolateral membrane of the thyroid follicular cell.

Methimazole and PTU inhibit thyroid peroxidase, the enzyme that facilitates the oxidation of iodide and the organification of thyroglobulin-bound tyrosyl residues to form thyroid hormone. In addition, PTU inhibits the peripheral conversion of T4 to T3. Newborns with Graves' disease usually experience spontaneous resolution, as maternal-stimulating antibodies naturally degrade.

Because the antibodies have a half-life of about 12 days, the infant may experience symptoms of hyperthyroidism for as short as 3 weeks, but as long as 12 weeks.[18] These infants should be started on an antithyroid medication, but this is gradually weaned as tolerated, and eventually discontinued as the infant becomes clinically and biochemically euthyroid.[15] Due to the side effects of PTU, especially in children, methimazole is the preferred antithyroid therapy in all pediatric patients. Levothyroxine is given to patients with hypothyroidism.

CASE 10

During hospital rounds in the neonatal intensive care unit, you examine a 4-day-old male infant, born at 29 weeks of gestation. He is intubated and requires dopamine and epinephrine support to maintain adequate blood pressure and perfusion. The infant is not dysmorphic. His newborn screen reveals a low T4 with a normal TSH. His serum total T4 is low, free T4 is normal, total T3 is low, and TSH is normal.

These laboratory results are most consistent with a diagnosis of
A. Primary congenital hypothyroidism
B. Transient hypothyroxinemia of prematurity (THOP)
C. Central hypothyroidism
D. Iodine deficiency
E. TSH-receptor defect

Discussion

The correct answer is **B**. Premature infants have lower levels of thyroid-binding globulin (TBG) than term infants, and therefore, also have lower total T4 and T3 levels. There is an increased risk of neonatal morbidity associated with nonthyroidal illness (NTI), characterized low total T4 and T3 levels. Both NTI and an immature hypothalamic–pituitary–thyroid (HPT) axis can contribute to transient hypothyroxinemia of prematurity.[19] The effect of THOP on maturation of the brain is still unclear and no studies have demonstrated a definitive benefit of early treatment with thyroid hormone on neurological and cognitive development in childhood. Thyroid studies may be repeated when the infant is considered to be term and is clinically stable.

An infant with primary congenital hypothyroidism or iodine deficiency would present with a low serum FT4 level and an elevated TSH level. Infants with central hypothyroidism may have a brain injury, or physical examination findings suggestive of other hypothalamic or pituitary defects such as GH, GnRH, or adrenocorticotropic hormone (ACTH) deficiencies.

CASE 11

A healthy term infant is born to a G2P2 mother who has a family history of thyroid disease. Prior to this pregnancy, thyroid function tests were performed and all of her levels were within normal limits.

In regard to fetal thyroid physiology, the placenta is impermeable to which of the following?
A. TSH
B. T4
C. T3
D. Iodine
E. TRH

Discussion

The correct answer is **A**. The placenta serves as the main source of nutrition, blood supply, and hormones to the fetus from the mother. Most elements produced by the mother can cross the placenta however; there are some that cannot transfer. By 20 weeks of gestation, the HPT gland axis becomes autonomous in the fetus. The placenta is impermeable to TSH, and is only partially permeable to T4 and T3 with a large maternal-to-fetal gradient present. The fetal thyroid gland competes with the maternal thyroid gland for iodine, which crosses the placenta freely. TRH also crosses the placenta. The placenta produces a pro-TRH molecule and the fetal pancreas produces TRH, both of which are identical to hypothalamic TRH.

The placenta is also permeable to TSH receptor–stimulating antibodies. Women with a history of Graves' disease and who have antibodies can give birth to a newborn with neonatal Graves' disease.[17] Newborns with Graves' disease usually experience spontaneous resolution of hyperthyroidism as maternal-stimulating antibodies naturally degrade, which can take up to 3 months.

CASE 12

A full-term infant is born to a healthy G3P3 mother. As the mother has spent time volunteering in schools for children with disabilities and cared for a child with developmental delays related to unrecognized congenital hypothyroidism. She asks you about the possibility of her child having a neurologic deficit secondary to a hormonal abnormality.

From where does the thyroid gland develop?

A. The upward invagination of the oral ectoderm and downward extension of the neural ectoderm

B. The third and fourth branchial pouches

C. The median anlage from the primitive pharyngeal floor and part of the fourth branchial pouch

D. An outpouching of the ventral wall of the foregut

E. The second and third branchial pouches

Discussion

The correct answer is **C**. The hypothalamus is derived from the lateral wall of the diencephalon. The pituitary gland develops from the midline of the anterior neural ridge. The anterior and intermediate lobes of the gland are derived from oral ectoderm. The posterior pituitary is derived from neural ectoderm. The thyroid gland starts developing within the second week of gestation. By 7 to 8 weeks of gestation, formation of the thyroid gland is complete as it migrates to the anterior neck.[20] The pituitary gland is comprised of the adenohypophysis (develops from Rathke's pouch to oral ectoderm) and the neurohypophysis (develops from infundibulum to neural ectoderm from the floor of diencephalon).[21] The parathyroid glands are derived from the third and fourth branchial pouches. The trachea starts its embryologic development as an outpouching of the ventral foregut. The second branchial pouch gives rise to the middle ear and palatine tonsils (Fig. 9-5).

In 2007, Harris and Pass stated the prevalence of congenital hypothyroidism in the United States as being 1:2,370 births.[22] Congenital hypothyroidism can be permanent or transient. Structural defects (such as ectopic gland, aplasia/hypoplasia of gland) account for the most common cause of congenital hypothyroidism, with dyhormonogenesis (~10–20%) and other causes (such as TSH resistance, and transient causes such as iodine deficiency, maternal antithyroid medication and iodine excess, ~10%) account for the remainder.[23]

Development of the thyroid gland

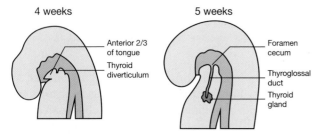

FIGURE 9-5. Used with permission of Motifolio, Inc.

CASE 13

You receive a call from the hospital laboratory regarding the newborn screen of one of your term female infants born to a G2P2 mother with no history of thyroid disease. On physical examination, the infant is mildly jaundiced, has a large anterior fontanelle, and has an umbilical hernia. Her thyroid gland is not enlarged. At 30 hours of life, the TSH is elevated and the T4 is low. You obtain serum studies and confirm that the serum TSH is elevated (>100 mIU/L, normal 1.0–8.0 mIU/L) and the serum free T4 is low (0.5 ng/dL, normal 1.5–2.0 ng/dL).

What is the most likely diagnosis?

A. Thyroid dysgenesis

B. Thyroid dyhormonogenesis

C. Transient hypothyroidism

D. TRH deficiency

E. TSH deficiency

Discussion

The correct answer is **A**. This infant has clinical and biochemical features consistent with primary hypothyroidism. The most common cause of congenital hypothyroidism is thyroid dysgenesis (75–80% of cases) in which the thyroid gland fails to develop (agenesis), partially develops (dysgenesis), or develops in an alternative location (ectopy). The other three less common causes include: (1) thyroid dyshormonogenesis (10–15%), in which the thyroid gland fails to take up iodide, organify iodide, synthesize thyroglobulin, or has impaired iodotyrosine deiodinase activity; (2) transient hypothyroidism (5–10%) due to maternal use of antithyroid medications or maternal TSH receptor–blocking antibodies; and (3) central hypothyroidism (1–5%) due to deficiencies in TRH from the hypothalamus and/or thyrotropin (TSH) from the pituitary gland.[24]

In addition to clinical symptoms consistent with hypothyroidism, an elevated serum TSH and low serum free T4 is diagnostic for primary hypothyroidism. Central causes of hypothyroidism, such as TRH or TSH deficiency, can be ruled out, as infants usually have low or normal range TSH levels. Infants with thyroid dyshormonogenesis would have an elevated serum TSH level in addition to an enlarged, palpable thyroid gland. Infants with thyroid dyshormonogenesis have a thyroid gland, but thyroid hormone synthesis does not occur. Continued stimulation of the thyroid gland results in enlargement of the gland but without thyroid hormone secretion. The infant with thyroid dysgenesis would not have a palpable thyroid gland on examination of the neck.

There is a surge in TSH that occurs in the newborn infant 3 to 5 days postnatally that is subsequently followed by a rise in T4. When a newborn screen is abnormal for thyroid function, it is imperative to obtain serum studies (TSH and free T4). The total T4 measures bound and unbound thyroid hormone. Even in a euthyroid state, with a normal TSH and free T4, T4 can be low due to a benign, TBG deficiency. The classic physical findings of an infant with CH includes a large fontanelle, jaundice, distended abdomen, umbilical hernia, hypotonia, and enlarged tongue. A severe hormonal deficiency left untreated for more than a month, may result in delayed bone maturation and cognitive delay. The goal of treatment is to initiate thyroxine replacement (e.g., levothyroxine) as soon as possible at a dose of 10 to 15 µg/kg/day. The serum free T4 should normalize within 1 to 2 weeks and the TSH within 1 month, after which point thyroid studies can be repeated to ensure adequate treatment on the current dose of medication.

Objectives

1. Know the physiological roles of the hormones and other proteins involved in the regulation of thyroid function
2. Know the relationship between fetal and maternal thyroid physiology
3. Know the embryology and normal physiological function of the thyroid gland
4. Know the proper use of laboratory tests (including screening tests) in the diagnosis of thyroid dysfunction
5. Know the etiology and clinical manifestations of CH
6. Know the laboratory features and approach to therapy of CH
7. Know how to evaluate and manage the causes of transient hypothyroidism in newborn infants
8. Identify the etiology, clinical manifestations, laboratory features, and management of neonatal thyrotoxicosis

CASE 14

A G1P1, 23-year-old mother with poorly controlled gestational diabetes delivers a 4.3-kg term female infant via a c-section. Within the first few hours of life, the blood glucose levels between feeds are consistently low, between 30 and 40 mg/dL. The infant is transferred to the step-down NICU and placed on intravenous fluids. With the exception of a low serum calcium level (7.3 mg/dL), all other serum electrolyte levels are within normal limits.

What is the most likely mechanism of this infant's hypoglycemia?
A. Fetal hyperinsulinism secondary to a pancreatic tumor
B. Fetal hyperinsulinism secondary to increased maternal serum glucose levels
C. Sepsis
D. Stress-induced hyperinsulinism
E. Hypopituitarism resulting in GH deficiency

Discussion

The correct answer is **B**. An infant of a diabetic mother (IDM) has ample glycogen, protein, and fat stores, unlike that seen in an infant who is small for gestational infant. In the setting of poorly controlled gestational diabetes, maternal blood glucose levels are elevated. The increased maternal blood glucose crosses the placenta, and the fetal pancreas responds by secreting insulin, resulting in fetal islet cell hyperplasia and hypertrophy. Prior to delivery of the infant, there is plenty of glucose available to the infant but, after delivery and separation from the placenta, the glucose supply is interrupted. The hypoglycemia develops because of persistent insulin secretion from fetal islet cell hyperplasia and hypertrophy.

Insulin promotes growth and infants of diabetic mothers are typically large for gestational age and are hypoglycemic. Hypoglycemia due to transient hyperinsulinism in an IDM should last no longer than a few days. If hypoglycemia persists, other causes of hyperinsulinism should be considered.[19] Management usually includes the administration of dextrose-containing intravenous fluids at a glucose infusion rate of 8 to 10 mg/kg/min. Most cases of neonatal hypoglycemia due to maternal diabetes are avoidable if appropriate glycemic control is maintained by the mother during her pregnancy.

Hypoglycemia in a neonate is defined as a serum glucose level of ≤50 mg/dL. Symptoms in an infant include cyanotic episodes, apnea, somnolence, respiratory distress, sweating, and seizures. Other causes of hypoglycemia of the neonate include sepsis, hypopituitarism, poor glycogen stores, congenital hyperinsulinism, glycogen storage disease, galactosemia, disorders of gluconeogenesis, and disorders of fatty acid oxidation.

CASE 15

An infant in the nursery has persistent hypoglycemia. After speaking with the endocrinologist, you collect a critical blood sample when the blood glucose of the infant is <30 mg/dL. The serum blood glucose of the infant is 27 mg/dL. The critical sample includes appropriately elevated serum cortisol and GH responses but a measureable serum insulin level. The serum ketones are negative.

What is the most likely diagnosis?
A. Persistent hyperinsulinemic hypoglycemia of infancy
B. Insulinoma
C. Beckwith–Wiedemann syndrome
D. Panhypopituitarism
E. Ketotic hypoglycemia

Discussion

The correct answer is **A**. Persistent hyperinsulinemic hypoglycemia of infancy (PHHI), caused by unregulated insulin secretion, is the most common cause of persistent hypoglycemia in neonates and infants. Physiologically, insulin secretion is inhibited by hypoglycemia. In PHHI, in which mutations of a gene coding for one of the regulatory steps in insulin secretion from the islet cell, insulin is persistently secreted despite hypoglycemia. This infant has measureable insulin levels, which should be suppressed in the setting of hypoglycemia. Insulin also inhibits lipolysis, preventing ketosis. These infants are usually large-for-gestational age birth weight and are hypoglycemic shortly after birth.[24]

Glucose transport into the pancreatic β-cell is facilitated by the glucose transporter, GLUT-2. Once glucose enters the cell, it is phosphorylated by glucokinase, resulting in an increase in the ATP/ADP ratio. This increase causes the potassium-ATP channel (KATP) to close, which depolarizes the cell membrane, and leads to opening of the calcium channel. The influx of calcium promotes the release of insulin from storage granules (Fig. 9-6).

The most common mutations in PHHI affect KATP, which is comprised of two subunits, SUR1 (encoded by ABCC8) and Kir6.2 (encoded by KCNJ11). These loss-of-function mutations are most commonly inherited in autosomal-recessive fashion. In addition to glucose, the amino acid leucine stimulates insulin release through activation of glutamate dehydrogenase, resulting in oxidation of glutamate, which increases the ATP/ADP ratio, closes the potassium channel, depolarizes the membrane, opens the calcium channel, and results in insulin secretion. Activating mutations in the gene encoding glutamate dehydrogenase cause a syndrome of hyperinsulinemia and hyperammonemia. A form of PHHI that classically causes focal islet cell hyperplasia is caused by paternal uniparental disomy.

Short-term treatment involves maintaining blood glucose levels within a normal range initially with intravenous dextrose and frequent enteral feeds. Pharmacologic therapy for long-term management includes diazoxide (a KATP agonist), octreotide (somatostatin analog to inhibit insulin release), or calcium channel blockers (to prevent closure of calcium channel in the β-cell). Response to diazoxide is dependent on the specific mutation causing PHHI. Neonates with ABCC8 or KCNJ11 mutations are less likely to respond to diazoxide because they most commonly cause a diffuse pattern of severe islet cell hyperplasia. Neonates with defects of glutamate dehydrogenase, on the other hand, cause a more benign pattern and are more likely to respond to diazoxide. Should pharmacologic therapy fail, surgery for an identified focal lesion or for diffuse disease, a subtotal pancreatectomy should be considered.[25]

Insulinomas are a rare cause of hypoglycemia in infants. Beckwith–Wiedemann syndrome classically presents as an overgrowth syndrome with features such as macrosomia and macroglossia with a predisposition to

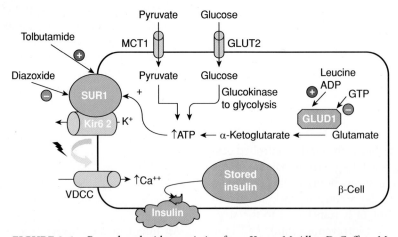

FIGURE 9-6. Reproduced with permission from Kappy M, Allen D, Geffner M. *Pediatric Practice: Endocrinology.* 2nd ed. New York, NY: McGraw-Hill Professional; 2010.

tumor development. Ketotic hypoglycemia usually occurs in older infants who are unable to tolerate a fast and uncommon in neonates.

Most focal lesions are not responsive to diazoxide and are best detected using molecular analysis and 18 F-fluoro-L-DOPA positron emission tomography (18 F-DOPA PET) scans. Identification of these lesions can results in cure with a partial pancreatectomy. Pancreatectomy should also be a consideration in cases where medical treatment is not successful and in all cases, avoidance of near-total pancreatectomy is desired to reduce the risk of postsurgical diabetes.[26]

CASE 16

You are present at the birth of a 34-week-gestation female infant born to a healthy, 31-year-old, G3P2 mother who experienced an uncomplicated pregnancy. The infant is vigorous when placed under the warmer and has APGAR scores of 8 and 9, at 1 and 5 minutes, respectively. Upon arrival to the nursery, the infant's serum glucose is 47 mg/dL. The infant receives her first feed and 1 hour after the feed her serum glucose is 83 mg/dL.

What is the normal glucose production and utilization rate for a preterm infant?
A. 1 to 2 mg/kg/min
B. 5 to 7 mg/kg/min
C. 15 to 20 mg/kg/min
D. 2 to 3 mg/kg/min
E. 10 to 12 mg/kg/min

Discussion

The correct answer is **B**. Physiologic glucose production for term and preterm infants ranges from 4 to 8 mg/kg/min. Adults have a glucose production rate of 1 to 2 mg/kg/min. Any infant requiring >12 mg/kg/min after 3 days of life should be evaluated for a pathologic cause of hypoglycemia. A critical sample collected during an episode of hypoglycemia should be collected. This should be a serum sample as capillary blood glucose can be lower than that seen in plasma.[27]

Which of the following physiologic changes occur in an infant shortly after birth?
A. A decrease in GH levels
B. A decrease in glucagon levels
C. A decrease in free fatty acid levels
D. An increase in insulin levels
E. An increase in epinephrine levels

Discussion

The correct answer is **E**. The fetus does not produce endogenous glucose but rather is dependent on maternal glucose concentration via transfer through the placenta. Fetal insulin and glucagon levels resemble that of the mother, but do not change with acute changes in glucose concentration. At birth there is an acute drop in the fetal glucose concentration with a sluggish responsive decrease in insulin level, and an increase in glucagon and epinephrine levels. Likewise, glucagon, epinephrine, GH, ketone, and free fatty acid levels increase. Free fatty acids and ketones act as an alternate source of energy for muscle and produce factors that are essential for gluconeogenesis, thereby allowing glucose to be utilized for cerebral metabolism. In infants up to 5 weeks of age, the use of cerebral glucose is ~71% to 93% that of an adult. Glucose utilization reaches adult levels by 2 years of age and continues to increase until they peak between 4 to 9 years of age, and then decline to adult levels around the second decade of life.

Breakdown of hepatic glycogen stores is sufficient to meet energy needs for only a few hours, after which, an infant relies on gluconeogenesis from substrates such as amino acids, glycerol, and lactate. Neonates may have less glycogen and muscle protein reserves than adults, but they have an increased rate of glucose consumption due to a larger brain-to-body mass ratio. Prevention of hypoglycemia is mediated through the action of counterregulatory hormones such as epinephrine, GH, glucagon, and cortisol through inhibition of insulin, gluconeogenesis, glycogenolysis, lipolysis, and ketogenesis.[29]

There are multiple causes for hyperglycemia in the neonatal period. Hyperglycemia in a neonate is defined as a blood glucose of >125 mg/dL. Risk factors for hyperglycemia include excess glucose or lipid infusion rate, prematurity, small for gestational age, glucocorticoid administration, and sepsis.

Neonatal diabetes mellitus is a rare cause of hyperglycemia in infancy. The transient form is due to activating mutations in the ABCC8 gene that encodes the SUR1 subunit of the KATP channel in the pancreatic β cell. This keeps the KATP channel open, thereby hyperpolarizing the cell membrane, keeping the calcium channel closed, and preventing insulin secretion. This same mutation can be associated with permanent neonatal diabetes mellitus, but the most common cause is due to activating mutations in the KCNJ11 gene that encodes the Kir6.2 subunit of the KATP channel. Affected infants typically born SGA, have developmental delay, and muscle weakness.[28]

Management of hyperglycemia involves reducing or eliminating the provoking stimuli such as reducing the glucose or lipid infusion rate or decreasing glucocorticoid therapy. For infants with diabetes, the administration of insulin or oral antihyperglycemic agent therapy may be needed.

Objectives

1. Know the amino acid substrates for gluconeogenesis
2. Know the fuels used for brain metabolism
3. Know the relationship of maternal blood glucose to fetal glucose uptake and metabolism
4. Know the normal range of endogenous glucose production in term and preterm infants
5. Know the causes (including hyperinsulinemic hypoglycemia) of neonatal hypoglycemia syndromes
6. Recognize the clinical and laboratory features of neonatal hypoglycemia
7. Recognize the approach to therapy and prevention of neonatal hypoglycemia
8. Know the potential sequelae of neonatal hypoglycemia
9. Know the causes, including genetic disorders and other clinical conditions, of neonatal hyperglycemia, including transient diabetes mellitus
10. Know the clinical and laboratory features and approach to therapy of neonatal hyperglycemia, including transient diabetes mellitus

CASE 17

A 6-day-old term infant who is small for gestational age has a total serum calcium level of 6.8 mg/dL. On physical examination she has hypertelorism, micrognathia, and a cleft palate. A murmur is auscultated and her chest radiograph reveals an absent thymic shadow. An echocardiogram reveals an interrupted aortic arch.

What other finding may be expected in this newborn?
A. Decreased serum thyroxine level
B. Elevated serum parathyroid hormone (PTH) level
C. Elevated urinary calcium/creatinine ratio
D. Elevated serum 25-hydroxy vitamin D level
E. Decreased serum phosphate level

Discussion

The correct answer is **C**. This infant has DiGeorge syndrome due to a deletion of 22q11.2. The defects are due to abnormal embryologic development of the branchial pouches. Each set of pouches leads to development of different anatomical structures. The spectrum of the syndrome is wide because all pouches may not be affected.[29] The four parathyroid glands arise from the third and fourth branchial pouches. A defect in parathyroid gland formation or function will result in insufficient PTH secretion. PTH functions to maintain serum calcium in the normal range directly through bone resorption and kidney reabsorption, and indirectly, by intestinal absorption. In the kidney, PTH reabsorbs calcium in the tubule and excretes phosphate; in the small intestine, PTH indirectly increases absorption of calcium and phosphate by upregulating 1α-hydroxylase and increasing conversion of 25-hydroxy-vitamin D to 1,25-dihydroxy-vitamin D, the major regulator of calcium and phosphate absorption in the small intestine (Fig. 9-7). In a child with physical features suggestive of

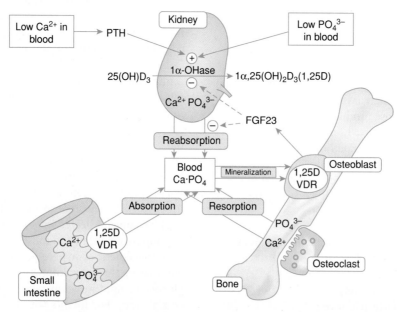

FIGURE 9-7.   Reproduced with permission from Rudolph C, Rudolph A, Lister G, et al. *Rudolph's Pediatrics*. 22nd ed. New York, NY: McGraw-Hill Professional; 2011.

DiGeorge syndrome and hypocalcemia, the most likely cause is due to hypoparathyroidism.

The other features of DiGeorge syndrome are due to other branchial pouch defects. The abnormal facies are likely the result of a defect of the first set of pouches, thymic hypoplasia due to the second set of pouches, and the cardiac abnormalities due to defects in the fourth and fifth pouches. In the absence of PTH, calcium levels remain low and phosphorous high. Because calcium is not reabsorbed from the kidney, there is increased urinary excretion of calcium. 1,25-dihydroxy-vitamin D will be low due to decreased 1α-hydroxylase activity. Thyroid gland development is not usually affected in patients with DiGeorge syndrome.

CASE 18

You are covering the night shift in the NICU and the first admission of the night is a 1-week-old term, AGA female infant born to a G3P2 mother. The infant was born vaginally and went home with the parents on the second day of life. She had been breast-feeding well every 2 to 3 hours but this evening, the parents brought her to the emergency department when they noticed her to have jerking of her upper extremities that lasted for about 2 minutes. In obtaining more detailed maternal and birth histories, you learn that the mother had severe gastroesophageal reflux during her last trimester, and she took a number of antireflux medications. You initiate a workup on the infant and detect an electrolyte abnormality. You start the appropriate therapy. After a week of therapy, the infant is doing much better with no further seizures or abnormal neurologic findings.

What is the most likely cause of this infant's seizure?
A. Hypomagnesemia due to increased maternal use of ranitidine
B. Hyponatremia due to increased fluid intake
C. Hypocalcemia due to increased maternal use of calcium carbonate tablets
D. Hypernatremia due to dehydration
E. Hypoglycemia due to a glycogen storage disease

Discussion

The correct answer is **C**. Increased use of calcium carbonate during pregnancy can cause maternal hypercalcemia. As calcium crosses the placenta to the fetus, the fetal PTH production may be inhibited, decreasing the infant's calcium levels that may lead to tetany or seizures. Infants need to be treated with calcium and possibly

vitamin D supplementation which can gradually be weaned as tolerated. Ranitidine does not result in hypomagnesemia. There is no history to support fluid abnormalities due to feeding difficulties causing disruptions in sodium homeostasis. Similarly, there is no history to support a glycogen storage disease with a child who has no known intolerance of her feeds.

Hypocalcemia in infancy is defined as a total serum calcium level <7.5 mg/dL. The clinical symptoms include irritability, tetany, laryngospasm, and seizures. Hypocalcemia developing in the first 72 hours of life is classified as early neonatal hypocalcemia. The differential includes maternal hypercalcemia, premature or small-for-gestational age infants, asphyxiated infants, and infants of diabetic mothers. This can be due to a delayed response of PTH, extended secretion of calcitonin, or low magnesium. Hypocalcemia occurring after 72 hours of life is classified as late neonatal hypocalcemia and can be due to hyperphosphatemia, hypomagnesemia, hypoparathyroidism, or low vitamin D levels.[30]

The calcium sensing receptor (CaSR) is a G protein-coupled receptor that responds to extracellular ionic calcium changes activating several intracellular signaling systems (phospholipases C, A2, and D) finally inhibiting PTH secretion. In addition to calcium, there are some other agonists and modulators for the CaSR such as magnesium, amyloid β-peptides, and a variety of amino acids. Magnesium helps regulate PTH release (not synthesis) and calcitriol synthesis. Total serum magnesium <1.5 mg/dL can lead to hypocalcemia due to inhibition of PTH release, and occurs in neonates with short gut syndrome, chronic diarrhea states, steatorrhea, Gitelman syndrome, and Bartter syndrome.[30] A neonate with hypocalcemia due to hypomagnesemia may exhibit tetany, seizures, weakness, and prolonged QT interval. Treatment of hypocalcemia in the setting of a serum low magnesium level necessitates magnesium supplementation.

CASE 19

A 5-week-old, former 28-week-gestation premature female infant is intubated for breathing difficulty due to pneumonia. A routine chest x-ray demonstrates a broken rib. You obtain serum electrolytes and determine that serum calcium, phosphorous, and vitamin D levels are low.

Which laboratory finding would be expected?
A. Elevated serum alkaline phosphatase level
B. Decreased serum PTH level

C. Decreased serum magnesium level
D. Increased urine calcium:creatinine ratio
E. Increased urine phosphate level

Discussion

The correct answer is **A**. Accretion rates for calcium and phosphate increase during the third trimester. Accretion rates for preterm infants are as follows: calcium 105 mg/kg/day and phosphate 70 mg/kg/day.[31] Osteopenia of prematurity (OP) is defined as postnatal bone mineralization less than in utero at a concordant gestational age. The condition usually develops in premature infants 1 to 4 months of age.[32] Risk factors include the use of glucocorticoids and loop diuretics, infants of diabetic mothers, and infants small for gestational age. The biochemical features of OP include hypophosphatemia (<3.5 mg/dL, normal 4–8 mg/dL) and hyperphosphatasia (>800 IU/L, normal 100–500 IU/L). The radiographic features are consistent with poor lucency of cortical bone and cupping and fraying of the distal ends of long bones. Management involves providing adequate mineral intake through supplemented breast milk or formula. Calcium and phosphorus intake is optimized through the use of preterm formulas and transitional formulas at hospital discharge. Radiographic changes are considered late findings of OP and are therefore not a sensitive measure for monitoring for this condition.

PTH levels may be decreased due to immature parathyroid gland function in premature infants but are most commonly in the normal to slightly elevated range. Hypomagnesemia is not characteristic of OP. Although low serum calcium and phosphate levels occur in infants with OP, it is most likely due to inadequate intake and not excessive excretion.

CASE 20

A term female infant born to a primiparous woman presents at 3 weeks of age with lethargy. Pregnancy and delivery were both uncomplicated and the birth weight was 3 kg. The infant is breast-fed. The parents note that from 3 days prior to admission, the infant has had a decreased appetite, a weak cry, decreased frequency of stools, and appears to be bloated. Upon physical examination, you notice the baby to be lethargic, hypotonic, pale, and with cool extremities. Her vital signs include a temperature of 36.5 °C, pulse of 139 beats per minute, respiratory rate of 66 breaths per minute, and a blood pressure of 60/48 mm Hg.

You administer a 10 mL/kg normal saline bolus, obtain serum laboratory studies, perform a lumbar puncture, and initiate antibiotics for presumptive sepsis. Spinal fluid analysis and a serum blood count with differential are normal. Upon obtaining a more in-depth history from the parents, they admit to giving a half teaspoon of Milk of Magnesia every day for the past 4 days for constipation.

What electrolyte abnormality is the most likely cause of this infant's clinical presentation?
A. Elevated serum calcium
B. Decreased serum calcium
C. Elevated serum magnesium
D. Decreased serum magnesium
E. Decreased serum glucose

Discussion

The correct answer is **C**. The daily magnesium requirement for an infant is about 1 mmol/L/day. A half teaspoon of Milk of Magnesia daily provides 3.5 mmol/L/day of magnesium, this infant has been receiving over three times the daily requirement. Elevated levels of serum magnesium can cause neuromuscular, respiratory, cardiovascular, and metabolic difficulties in the infant. Infants may present with lethargy, hypotonia, hyporeflexia, respiratory depression, hypotension, and increased bowel motility. The electrocardiogram can show a prolonged QT interval.

The most common causes of hypermagnesemia in the infant are iatrogenic due to the administration of excess magnesium to the infant or magnesium sulfate to the mother prior to delivery. Treatment of hypermagnesemia includes the administration of calcium gluconate to displace magnesium, diuretics to help excrete it through the kidneys, and dialysis. The infant's cardiorespiratory status should be monitored closely.

Excess intake of magnesium does not affect the serum glucose level. Serum calcium levels are usually only affected by hypomagnesemia rather than hypermagnesemia, as magnesium is necessary for PTH secretion.[33,34]

CASE 21

A 5-day-old, former 32-week-gestation female infant has feeding intolerance, constipation, lethargy, and increasing irritability. You conduct an extensive evaluation to determine the etiology of these symptoms including serum electrolytes and a review of the mother's pregnancy history.

This infant is born to a 30 year old G1P1 mother with a history of hypertension, gestational diabetes, and vitamin D insufficiency, for which she was treated with thiazide diuretics and cholecalciferol during pregnancy. The delivery was without complication. She managed her gestational diabetes with diet alone. The mother desires to exclusively breast-feed her infant and does not want to add any form of supplementation to the breast milk.

On physical examination, the infant has no dysmorphic features or abnormalities on physical examination. The only biochemical abnormality is an elevated total serum calcium level (13.4 mg/dL, normal 8.5–11.0).

Which of the following is not a cause of this infant's presentation?
A. IDM
B. Low phosphate content in breast milk
C. Maternal ingestion of thiazide diuretics during pregnancy
D. Large amounts of cholecalciferol in breast milk
E. Secondary hyperparathyroidism

Discussion

The correct answer is **A**. Hypercalcemia in infants is defined as a calcium >11 mg/dL. Infants exhibit symptoms such as decreased appetite, gastroesophageal reflux, hypotonia, and seizures when the total serum calcium level is >13 mg/dL. Potential causes of hypercalcemia are outlined in Figure 9-8. Hypocalcemia, and not hypercalcemia, is typically associated with the IDM, due to a

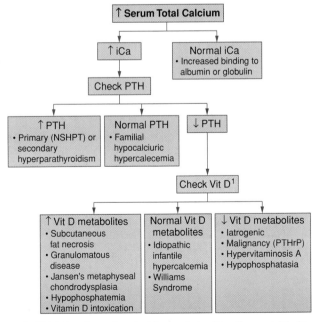

FIGURE 9-8.   Reproduced with permission from Lowry A, Bhakta K, Nag P. *Texas Children's Hospital Handbook and Pediatrics and Neonatology.* New York, NY: McGraw-Hill Professional; 2011.

delayed PTH response in these infants. All the other responses result in hypercalcemia. Preterm infants have increased nutritional requirements compared to term infants and unsupplemented breast milk has a low phosphate content that can cause hypercalcemia. The mother's use of a thiazide diuretic increases absorption of calcium from the renal tubule and decreases phosphate absorption, resulting in hypercalcemia and hypophosphatemia. Increased maternal absorption of vitamin D can result in hypervitaminosis D and subsequent increased serum calcium levels in the breast-fed infant.

Maternal hypocalcemia during pregnancy due to hypoparathyroidism reduces placental transfer of calcium. Fetal sensing of a low calcium state, results in hyperplasia of the fetal parathyroid glands and increased secretion of PTH. This then causes hypercalcemia.

Treatment of hypercalcemia includes the administration of a formula low in calcium but with adequate phosphate. Modestly elevated calcium levels can be improved by administering 0.9% normal saline followed by intravenous furosemide. Other agents that can reduce serum calcium include hydrocortisone, calcitonin, and bisphosphonates.[35]

Objectives

1. Know normal calcium, phosphorous, and magnesium metabolism during the prenatal and postnatal periods, including fetal accretion rates
2. Know the interrelated effects of various hormones on calcium, phosphorus, and magnesium metabolism in the fetus and neonate
3. Know the etiology and clinical manifestations of early and late neonatal hypocalcemia
4. Know the laboratory features and approach to therapy of early and late neonatal hypocalcemia
5. Know the etiology and clinical manifestations of neonatal hypercalcemia
6. Know the laboratory features and approach to therapy of neonatal hypercalcemia
7. Know the etiology, clinical manifestations, radiographic features, and approach to treatment of OP
8. Know the etiology, clinical manifestations, and approach to therapy of hypomagnesemia
9. Know the etiology, clinical manifestations, and approach to therapy of hypermagnesemia

REFERENCES

1. Hughes IA. Minireview: Sex differentiation. *Endocrinology.* 2001;142(8):3281–3287.
2. Rey R, Grinspon RP. Normal male sexual differentiation and aetiology of disorders of sexual development. *Best Pract Res Clin Endocrinol Metab.* 2011;25(2):221–238.

3. Moshiri M, Chapman T, Fechner PY, et al. Evaluation and management of disorders of sex development: multidisciplinary approach to a complex diagnosis. *Radiographics.* 2012; 32(6):1599–1618.

4. Cheon CK. Practical approach to steroid 5α-reductase type 2 deficiency. *Eur J Pediatr.* 2011;170(1):1–8.

5. Witchel SF, Lee P A. Ambiguous genitalia. In: Sperling MA, ed. *Pediatric Endocrinology.* . Saunders Elsevier; 2008: 144–146.

6. Farrugia MK, Sebire NJ, Achermann JC, et al. Clinical and gonadal features and early surgical management of 45,X/46,XY and 45,X/47,XYY chromosomal mosaicism presenting with genital anomalies. *J Pediatr Urol.* 2013;9(2):139–144.

7. Speiser PW, White PC. Congenital adrenal hyperplasia. *N Engl J Med.* 2003;349(8):776–788.

8. Metwalley KA, Farghaly HS. X-linked congenital adrenal hypoplasia associated with hypospadias in an Egyptian baby: a case report. *J Med Case Rep.* 2012;6(1):428.

9. Rosenfeld RG, Pinchas C.Disorders of growth hormone/insulin-like growth factor secretion and action. In: Sperling MA, ed. *Pediatric Endocrinology.* Saunders Elsevier, 2008. 307–308.

10. Wiygul J, Palmer LS. Micropenis. *ScientificWorldJournal.* 2011;11:1462–1469.

11. Dixon J, Wallace AM, O'Toole S, et al. Prolonged human chorionic gonadotrophin stimulation as a tool for investigating and managing undescended testes. *Clin Endocrinol (Oxf).* 2007;67(6):816–821.

12. Macedo A Jr, Rondon A, Ortiz V. Hypospadias. *Curr Opin Urol.* 2012;22(6):447–452.

13. Gapany C, Frey P, Cachat F, et al. Management of cryptorchidism in children: guidelines. *Swiss Med Wkly.* 2008;138(33–34): 492–498.

14. Miller WL, Acherman JC, Fluck C.The adrenal cortex and its disorders. *Pediatric Endocrinology.* Sperling MA, ed. Saunders Elsevier, 2008. 479–480.

15. Fisher DA, Grueters A.Disorders of the thyroid in the newborn and infant. *Pediatric Endocrinology.* Sperling MA, ed. Saunders Elsevier, 2008; 199.

16. Hauri-Hohl A, Meyer-Böni M. Aromatase deficiency due to a functional variant in the placenta promoter and a novel missense mutation in the CYP19A1 gene. *Clin Endocrinol (Oxf).* 2011;75(1):39–43.

17. Harris KB, Pass KA. Increase in congenital hypothyroidism in New York State and in the United States. *Mol Genet Metab.* 2007;91(3):268–277.

18. Polak M, Le Gac I, Vuillard E, et al. Fetal and neonatal thyroid function in relation to maternal Graves' disease. *Best Pract Res Clin Endocrinol Metab.* 2004;18(2):289–302.

19. Committee on Fetus and Newborn, Adamkin DH. Postnatal glucose homeostasis in late-preterm and term infants. *Pediatrics.* 2011;127(3):575–579.

20. Hyman SJ. Perinatal endocrinology: common endocrine disorders in the sick and premature newborn. *Pediatr Clin North Am.* 2011;58(5):1083–1098.

21. Kelberman D, Dattani MT. Hypothalamic and pituitary development: novel insights into the aetiology. *Eur J Endocrinol.* 2007;157 Suppl 1:S3–S14.

22. Olney RS, Grosse SD, Vogt RF Jr. Prevalence of congenital hypothyroidism–current trends and future directions: workshop summary. *Pediatrics.* 2010;125 Suppl 2:S31–S36.

23. LaFranchi, SH. Approach to the diagnosis and treatment of neonatal hypothyroidism. *J Clin Endocrinol Metab.* 2011;96: 2959–2967.

24. Goel P, Choudhury SR. Persistent hyperinsulinemic hypoglycemia of infancy: An overview of current concepts. *J Indian Assoc Pediatr Surg.* 2012;17(3):99–103.

25. Markham L. Persistent hyperinsulinemic hypoglycemia of infancy. *Newborn Infant Nurs Rev.* 2003;3(4):156–165.

26. Yorifuji T. Congenital hyperinsulinism: current status and future perspectives. *Ann Pediatr Endocrinol Metab.* 2014; 19(2):57–68.

27. Cengiz E, Tamborlane W. A tale of two compartments: interstitial versus blood glucose monitoring. *Diabetes Technol Ther.* 2009;11 Suppl 1:S11–S16.

28. De Leon DD, Stanley CA, Sperling MA.Hypoglycemia in neonates and infants. *Pediatric Endocrinology.* Sperling MA, ed. Saunders Elsevier, 2008. 171–175.

29. Al-Tamemi S, Mazer B, Mitchell D, et al. Complete DiGeorge anomaly in the absence of neonatal hypocalcemia and velofacial and cardiac defects. *Pediatrics.* 2005;116(3):e457–e460.

30. Thomas TC, Smith JM, White PC, et al. Transient neonatal hypocalcemia: presentation and outcomes. *Pediatrics.* 2012; 129(6):e1461–e1467.

31. Abrams, SA. Up to Date: Calcium and phosphorous requirements of newborn infants. http://www.uptodate.com/ contents/calcium-and-phosphorus-requirements-of-newborn-infants?source=search_result&search=osteopenia+of +prematurity&selectedTitle=1%7E4#H1. Last update January 16, 2013. Accessed on January 17, 2013.

32. Harrison CM, Johnson K, McKechnie E. Osteopenia of prematurity: a national survey and review of practice. *Acta Paediatr.* 2008;97(4):407–413.

33. Narchi H. The pediatric forum: neonatal hypermagnesemia: more causes and more symptoms. *Arch Pediatr Adolesc Med.* 2001;155(9):1074.

34. Sullivan JE, Berman BW. Hypermagnesemia with lethargy and hypotonia due to administration of magnesium hydroxide to a 4-week old infant. *Arch Pediatr Adolesc Med.* 2000; 154(12):1272–1274.

35. Root AW, Diamond FB. Disorders of mineral homeostasis in the newborn, infant, child and adolescent. *Pediatric Endocrinology.* Sperling MA, ed. Saunders Elsevier; 2008: 699–704.

Chapter 10

NEONATAL IMMUNOLOGY

Nancy A. Louis, MD

CASE 1

A 5-week-old Caucasian female infant is brought in to the pediatrician's office for regularly scheduled appointment. She was born at term, weighing 3.4 kg (75th percentile), with a length of 20 in (75th percentile), and a head circumference measuring 36 cm (75th percentile), and has been fed exclusively breast milk. Her current weight is 3.7 kg (25th percentile), length 21 in (50th percentile), and head circumference 37 cm (50th percentile). Her parents report no history of fever, rash, cough, diarrhea, or vomiting and are only concerned that her umbilical cord remains attached with some surrounding redness, despite daily cleansing with water. On physical examination, she appears wasted without rhinorrhea, conjunctival injection, lymphadenopathy, or rash. Her chest examination is clear, and her abdominal examination is remarkable only for a firmly attached dry umbilical cord with a 2-mm area of induration and erythema around the cord, without any apparent drainage or masses. CBC and blood cultures are sent and the initial results are remarkable for a markedly elevated neutrophil count (6–8× higher than the predicted value for age).

Beyond what age should detachment of the umbilical cord be considered delayed?
A. 3 days
B. 7 days
C. 10 days
D. 3 weeks

Discussion

The correct answer is **D**. The average time for detachment of the umbilical cord is 7 to 10 days with detachment occurring at 3 weeks being considered late.[1,2] While cord detachment may be delayed in the absence of any other anomalies or in the presence of urachal cysts,[2] this patient has dropped growth percentiles since birth, and the presence of erythema around the umbilicus is concerning for omphalitis. The combination of delayed umbilical cord detachment, signs of infection, and failure to thrive raises the question of an underlying immune defect.

Which of the following is true? The most likely defect in the immune function in this patient
A. Represents a defect in acquired immunity
B. Results from a defect in innate immune function
C. Is due to defects in the neutrophil oxidative burst
D. Would not cause any medical problems for the patient after the first 9 months of life

Discussion

The correct answer is **B**. Umbilical cord detachment depends on normal neutrophil function, however, the elevated serum neutrophil count in this patient indicates that the defect is more likely to be one of neutrophil attachment and extravasation, causing neutrophil accumulation within the blood vessels, rather than a defect in the oxidative burst; an important mechanism for bacterial killing (see answer to question 4 below). Neutrophils are important elements of the innate immune response. Innate immune function is critical for the initial activated responses to infection. Mediators of the innate immune response, such as neutrophils, macrophages, and dendritic cells are directed to sites of infection by migration (chemotaxis). These cells are drawn in the direction of increasing concentrations of microbial products or endogenous cytokines or chemokines. Cytokines are immunomodulating agents such as interleukins, interferons, growth factors and tumor necrosis factors, which serve as cellular distress signals and can be peptides, proteins, or glycoproteins.[3]

In contrast, chemokines are a subset of cytokines, which stimulate cellular movement or migration by innate immune cells expressing the corresponding receptor, with migration generally occurring along an increasing concentration gradient with immune cell activation generally occurring at the site of the highest chemokine concentration.[4]

Thus, mechanisms of the innate immune response are site directed but not target specific. In contrast, acquired immunity is a target-specific immune response mediated by B lymphocytes through antibody-mediated (humoral) mechanisms and by T cell subsets through cytotoxic (CD8) or suppressive (CD4) immune responses in response to receptor activating foreign materials.

Helpful Tip: In acquired immunity, the B cells mature within the bone marrow and produce antibodies. These antibodies include: IgA (secretory, found in breast milk and saliva), IgD (important in B cell development), IgE (responsible for allergic response, interacts with mast cells and causes histamine release), IgG (activates complement), IgM (first antibody expressed when presented with new infection).[5]

Helpful Tip: IgG is the only antibody that crosses the placenta.

In addition to omphalitis, which of the following is the most likely diagnosis for this infant?
A. Shwachman–Diamond syndrome
B. Kostmann syndrome
C. Leukocyte adhesion deficiency (LAD)
D. Chediak–Higashi syndrome

Discussion

The correct answer is **C**. Although both cord-care practices and urachal anomalies[2] can lead to delayed cord detachment, the constellation of delayed cord detachment and omphalitis is concerning for the rare disorder of neutrophil chemotaxis, LAD.[6,7] LAD consists of a family of disorders of innate immune functions (LAD I, II, and III). Of these, LAD I is the most common and results from deficiencies in the cell surface adhesion molecule beta-2 integrin CD18, leading to the synthesis of three nonfunctioning proteins (LFA-1, integrin alphaXbeta2, and Mac1/CR3). LAD II involves mutations, which result in defects in fucosylation and processing of integrins, and LAD III results from defects in integrin activation. All three disorders result in deficiencies of neutrophil attachment and migration, which interfere with neutrophil chemotaxis and recruitment to sites of inflammation/infection. Treatment of these disorders involves broad-spectrum antibiotics and bone marrow transplantation.

Unlike LAD, the other listed disorders of neutrophil function all present with some degree of neutropenia. Shwachman–Diamond and Kostmann syndromes are disorders of neutrophil production with their primary immune defect manifested by neutropenia. Chediak–Higashi syndrome is primarily a defect in neutrophil degranulation, leading to ineffective killing of pathogens. However, this ineffective killing in the setting of normal chemotaxis results in more rapid neutrophil consumption. Thus, these patients also present with lower than normal neutrophil counts.

Helpful Tip: Shwachman–Diamond syndrome is characterized by bone marrow dysfunction, pancreatic insufficiency, skeletal abnormalities, malabsorption, and short stature. It is the second most common cause of pancreatic insufficiency in children behind cystic fibrosis.[8]

Helpful Tip: Kostmann syndrome is autosomal recessive and causes severe neutropenia, but usually presents without other prominent physical malformations.[8]

All of the following are functions of neutrophils, except
A. Chemotaxis
B. Phagocytosis
C. Oxidative killing
D. Degranulation
E. Immune memory

Discussion

The correct answer is **E**. Neutrophil function is critical for umbilical cord detachment. In the normal infant, the combined factors of drying, cord infarction, and cell necrosis at the base of the umbilical cord postpartum release signals, which trigger neutrophil adhesion to, and recruitment from the vasculature. This neutrophil recruitment is followed by chemotaxis, or migration in the direction of increasing concentrations of inflammatory mediators and bacterial products. As neutrophils reach the site of the highest concentration of chemoattractant, they release antibacterial mediators through degranulation, phagocytose debris and necrotic cells, and perform oxidative killing of internalized bacteria through the cytochrome b- and NADPH-oxidase–dependent generation of reactive oxygen species (oxidative burst). Thus, neutrophils prevent the establishment of infection and contribute to umbilical cord detachment. Surface bacteria contribute to, and antiseptic cord care actually delays, cord detachment.[9,10] In addition, while the practice of antiseptic cord care is still common, multiple studies have not shown it to be beneficial with respect to the prevention of infection in the immunocompetent host.[11,12]

Which other laboratory results are likely in this infant?

A. An abnormal nitroblue-tetrazolium (NBT) test
B. Deficiency of total immune globulins
C. Abnormal neutrophil migration and phagocytosis
D. Low CD4+ T cell count

Discussion

The correct answer is **C**. The neutrophilia in this patient is a hallmark of LAD. Individuals with LAD present with markedly elevated neutrophil counts due to the inability of their neutrophils to adhere to and exit blood vessels in response to activating stimuli. Thus, neutrophils from a patient with LAD would have abnormally low migration responses. However, these neutrophils are capable of elaborating the oxidative burst and should yield a normal NBT test, unlike patients with chronic granulomatous disease who have a negative NBT test, which results from a deficiency in neutrophil-mediated killing of phagocytosed pathogens. However, due to the inability of their neutrophils to effectively migrate to sites of infection, patients with LAD suffer a lifetime of vulnerability to bacterial infections particularly on mucosal surfaces such as lung, gingiva, and peritoneum.

Helpful Tip: Innate immunity is our quick response system, and first line of defense, it however, is not specific. The elements of innate immunity include skin, natural killer cells (neutrophils, monocytes), basophils, eosinophils, acute-phase reactants, as well as interleukins, interferons, cytokines and TNF.

Helpful Tip: Acquired immunity is specific, and is responsible for memory of past infections. It is made up of T and B lymphocytes. Example for disorders of T lymphocytes include DiGeorge syndrome, Wiskott–Aldrich syndrome, and severe combined immunodeficiency. Disorders of B lymphocytes include X-linked agammaglobulinemia, common variable immunodeficiency, and Job syndrome.

CASE 2

A couple is referred at 18 weeks gestation for prenatal counseling because the female partner had a brother who died of infectious complications of Bruton agammaglobulinemia. Initial anatomic ultrasound screening reveals that the fetus is a male.

What is the basis for the defect in immune globulin synthesis?

A. Interruption of B cell maturation
B. Failed T cell activation of B cells
C. Defect in the preB receptor
D. Deficiency of BLNK

Discussion

The correct answer is **A**. Bruton agammaglobulinemia is an X-linked recessive disorder of the maturation of B lymphocytes resulting from a mutation in the gene encoding the Bruton tyrosine kinase (BTK). The incidence is 1/250,000 males, and female carriers have no clinical signs of the mutation. In a healthy individual, B lymphocytes arise from hematopoietic stem cells within the bone marrow.[5] In an initial stage of B cell maturation, immature B cells develop within the bone marrow evolving through a series of steps in which the genes encoding the chains of the B cell receptor undergo a series of recombination events creating clonal populations of immature B cells, each with its own antigen specificity. These populations are then subjected to clonal deletion through negative selection to eliminate any populations with strong B cell receptor selectivity for self-antigens.

Several humoral immune deficiencies arise as a consequence of defects in the B cell maturation process. In Bruton agammaglobulinemia, deficient or absent target phosphorylation by the Bruton tyrosine kinase results in an arrest in maturation from preB to immature B cells within the bone marrow, blocking all immune globulin production (Fig. 10-1).[5] Other primary immune deficiencies resulting from defects in B cell maturation include hyper IgM syndrome and selective IgA deficiency, which involves a disruption in class switching in the mature B cell, and common variable immunodeficiency which results from a downstream disruption in the maturation of plasma cells and memory B cells.

Together, plasma and memory B cells orchestrate the humoral component of the acquired immune response. Plasma B cells are primarily responsible for antigen-specific antibody production, while memory B cells are longer-lived cells, which are critical for immune memory. Specifically, memory B cells mature in response to, and persist following resolution of, the first inflammatory challenge with the antigen recognized by their surface B cell receptor. The persistence of memory B cells primes subsequent humoral immunity, allowing more rapid immune responses to subsequent challenges with the same antigen.

Bone Marrow

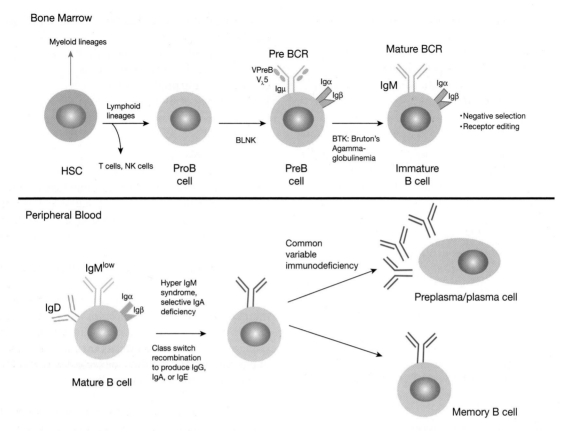

FIGURE 10-1. B cell development. Like T cells, B cells and myeloid lineages all arise from hematopoietic stem cells (HSC) within the bone marrow, and give rise to proB cells. Following activation of phosphorylation of the critical adaptor protein B cell linker (BLNK) critical signaling pathways trigger changes in surface immunoglobulin expression leading to PreB cell development and PreB cell receptor expression. Mutations in BLNK lead to hypogammaglobulinemia and B cell deficiency. BTK, the Bruton tyrosine kinase, catalyzes critical phosphosignaling events necessary for the conversion of PreB cells to immature B cells and surface expression of IgM and a mature form of the B cell receptor. Immature B cells then depart the marrow entering the peripheral blood stream as mature B cells with surface expression of IgD and low IgM. These cells then undergo class switch recombination of immunoglobulins leading to the ability to express surface IgG, IgA, or IgE as memory B cells or to secrete these immunoglobulins as plasma cells. (Adapted with permission from Cunningham-Rundles C, Ponda PP. Molecular defects in T- and B-cell primary immunodeficiency diseases. *Nat Rev Immunol.* 2005;5(11):880–892.)

Which of the following laboratory tests might be valuable for the evaluation of this fetus prior to birth?
A. RT-PCR or direct DNA analysis for the BTK mutation
B. Chorionic villus sampling for immunoglobulin levels
C. Antenatal ultrasound assessment of lymphoid structures
D. A and B

Discussion

The correct answer is **A**. In the fetus, transplacental acquisition of maternal IgG begins after the third month of gestation. This maternal IgG protects affected male infants at birth. However, the presence of maternally derived IgG, combined with a total lack of immune globulin synthesis in even the healthy term newborn, renders quantitative immunoglobulin levels useless for diagnosis of defects in immune globulin synthesis in the fetus or newborn.[13] Levels of maternally acquired IgGs decline beginning at birth, reaching trivial levels by 6 months, by which time these infants are becoming increasingly vulnerable to infections.

At birth, infants have no detectable IgA or IgM, independent of gestational age or birth weight.[14] Exogenous IgA in the newborn period is critical for mucosal immune function and is derived exclusively from maternal breast milk. IgM production begins within the first few weeks, followed within 1 to 2 weeks by the appearance of IgG. However, infant IgG levels remain low, reaching only 60% of adult levels by the end of the first year. Infant synthesis of IgE and IgA follow IgG production, and the total levels of these two immune globulin subclasses also climb slowly throughout the first year. While mean maternal IgG levels detectable in the infant at birth increase along with increasing gestational age, the levels of IgA and IgM are low at birth, independent of gestational age.[15]

In the specific case of Bruton agammaglobulinemia, PCR analysis of fetal blood samples obtained by chorionic villus sampling can be informative, but only when the exact mutation has been identified within the affected family. Fetal blood obtained by umbilical cord sampling can also be analyzed by flow cytometry for CD19+ (mature) B lymphocytes, which normally make up 5% to 20% of peripheral blood lymphocytes, but are essentially absent in affected individuals. However, this procedure poses additional risk to the fetus. Postnatally, the most specific and reliable laboratory finding is a low number, or the total absence of mature B cells in the peripheral blood, as well as low or absent expression of the μ chain of the B cell receptor on the surface of the lymphocyte.

As a result of this deficiency in mature B cells, the secondary lymphoid organs such as the spleen, tonsils, adenoids, intestinal Peyer's patches, and lymph nodes may be small or absent in affected individuals. However, these findings cannot be used reliably for antenatal diagnosis. Final confirmation of the diagnosis is provided by the complete absence of BTK RNA or protein.

What is the likelihood that the fetus is affected?
A. 25%
B. 50%
C. 100%
D. Unable to determine without additional information

Discussion

The correct answer is **D**. The defect in Bruton agammaglobulinemia most commonly results from missense mutations interfering with gene transcription, and two-thirds of the cases are familial, with the remainder representing new mutations. If familial Bruton agammaglobulinemia had been confirmed in this family, there would be a 50% chance that the female partner in this scenario would be a carrier and a 50% chance that, if affected that she would have passed on the mutated X chromosome to her male fetus with a total likelihood of 25% that the fetus would be affected. However, since one-third of the cases represent new mutations, the uncle's condition may not be heritable, and additional information would be required before making this prediction.

Which of the following are not important aspects of management of patients with Bruton agammaglobulinemia?
A. Antibiotics
B. IVIG therapy
C. Vaccination against encapsulated organisms
D. Avoidance of live vaccines
E. Stem cell transplantation

Discussion

The correct answer is **C**. Because patients with either Bruton or autosomal agammaglobulinemia lack mature B cell function, they are incapable of maintaining humoral immune memory, however, they can elaborate intact dendritic cell and T cell responses following inactivated vaccines.[16] Therefore, vaccination against intracellular pathogens may be useful. However, live vaccines such as the oral polio vaccine, should be avoided, as the affected individual is vulnerable to vaccine-associated disease. Monthly IVIG infusions and frequent antibiotics are the mainstays of therapy, and stem cell transplantation from either cord blood or bone marrow is the only curative option currently available.

Helpful Tip: While particularly vulnerable to most viral infections, these patients are uniquely protected from Epstein–Barr virus due to their lack of HLA–receptor-expressing mature B cells normally targeted by this virus. Furthermore, antibody titers cannot be used in these patients to either screen for the presence of infection or to monitor response to therapy. Thus PCR-based screening (or in some cases viral culture) is required for diagnosis and monitoring of illnesses typically monitored by antibody titers, including TORCH infections.

Objectives

1. Understand the developmental biology of the immune system
2. Know the two types of host defense mechanisms (innate and acquired)
3. Understand polymorphonuclear leukocytes (neutrophils). Both development and function as well as diagnosis and management of abnormalities
4. Know the role of cytokines, and the function and activation of T lymphocytes

CASE 3

A 2.9 kg male infant with a prenatal diagnosis of tetralogy of Fallot is born at term and is noted to have persistent cyanosis with postductal saturations of 85%. In addition to a harsh systolic murmur at the left sternal border, the infant is noted to have dysmorphic features including a cleft lip and palate, a short flattened philtrum, micrognathia, hypertelorism, small ears with squared pinnae. The admission chest x-ray reveals diminished pulmonary vascularity and a "boot-shaped" cardiac silhouette with a diminished thymic component. Initial laboratory values revealed normal serum electrolytes with the exception of a serum calcium of 6.5.

Which test would be most likely to yield the definitive underlying diagnosis for this patient's hypocalcemia?
A. Karyotype
B. Chest x-ray
C. Echocardiogram
D. Fluorescence in situ hybridization
E. Parathyroid hormone level

Discussion

The correct answer is **D**. While abnormal parathyroid hormone levels are most likely responsible for this patient's hypocalcemia, the described infant has a combination of physical and clinical findings, which must at least prompt an evaluation for DiGeorge syndrome. DiGeorge syndrome is also described as CATCH-22 for the combined cardiac defects (including truncus arteriosus and tetralogy of Fallot), abnormal facies, thymic hypoplasia, cleft palate, and hypocalcemia.[17] This syndrome results from deletions in the region of 30 to 50 genes referred to as the DiGeorge critical region (DGCR)[18] encoded by chromosome 22q11.2 and is most rapidly diagnosed by fluorescence in situ hybridization. 22q11.2 deletion syndrome has a highly variable range of presentations resulting in alternative nomenclature including velocardofacial syndrome, Shprintzen syndrome, conotruncal anomaly face syndrome, Strong syndrome, and congenital thymic aplasia.[17]

Which of the following immune defects may be associated with this condition?
A. Defective T cell function
B. Abnormal B cell function
C. Compromised innate immunity
D. A and B
E. All of the above

Discussion

The correct answer is **D**. DiGeorge syndrome results from abnormal neural crest cell migration interfering with development of the pharyngeal arches.[17,19] It most commonly involves structures arising from arches 3 and 4, although arches 1 to 6 can be involved. Thus, the heart, thymus, parathyroid, and less commonly, the thyroid glands are affected. The bone marrow is unaffected and normal T and B cell precursors are released into the bloodstream. However, a primary defect in thymus formation interferes with the selection and maturation of T cells. And, due to critical roles for T cells in the maturation of B cells to antibody-producing plasma cells, secondary defects in humoral immunity are also seen.[20] Innate immunity is generally intact.

Development of which of the following lymphoid organs is directly affected by this abnormality?
A. Bone marrow
B. Thymus
C. Peripheral lymph nodes
D. Spleen
E. Liver

Discussion

The correct answer is **B**. Thymic development begins with an epithelial stage formed from the endoderm of the left and right ventral parts of the third pharyngeal pouches from postmenstrual weeks 7 to 8.[21] Mesenchyme accumulates during weeks 9 to 12, with the cortex becoming detectable by week 13 and differentiation of cortex and medulla completed after the 17th to 18th week. Hassall's corpuscles are evident by 13 weeks, but markedly increase in number between the 16th and 18th weeks. Lymph nodes show variable degrees of depletion in paracortical regions, secondary to the extent of thymic aplasia.[8] The liver is unaffected.

The spleen is present in patients with DiGeorge syndrome, although a secondary structural depletion of T cell–dependent regions is noted. The spleen is a lymphoid organ, which serves primarily as a blood filter, removing senescent red blood cells and scavenging hemoglobin. The white pulp of the spleen is also a site of antibody synthesis and site for removal of antibody-coated organisms. Thus, in the absence of splenic function, an individual is particularly vulnerable to infections with encapsulated organisms, which would otherwise be removed.

Study of human abortuses has established the stages of fetal splenic development.[21,22] Splenic development begins with a preliminary stage called the vascular reticular stage, which persists up to the 14th postmenstrual week. Between the 15th and 17th postmenstrual week, splenic lobules consisting of red pulp around central arteries form. Following the onset of lymphoid colonization, white pulp begins to form during the 18th week, and accumulating lymphocytes can be recognized around the central arteries during the 19th and 20th weeks. These lymphoid cells have histologic characteristics of precursor T cells. Primary follicles are first noted around the 23rd week.

Immune evaluation of patients with this diagnosis should include
A. CBC with differential
B. T cell subsets
C. Serum immune globulins
D. Lymphoproliferative responses to mitogens
E. All of the above

Discussion

The correct answer is **E.** Patients have variable degrees of immune compromise related to thymic hypoplasia with a primary finding being abnormal lymphoproliferative responses to mitogens from a deficiency in T cell maturation, which normally occurs in the thymus.[23,24] Due to

the critical role of T cells in B cell maturation, significant numbers of DiGeorge syndrome patients also have defects in humoral immunity with variations in both the severity of immune deficiency and the specific isotype(s) involved.[20,25] Thus, 33% of DiGeorge patients require chronic IVIG therapy.[26]

T cells differ from B cells in that they respond to T cell receptor (TCR) activation to processed antigen presented by antigen-presenting cells within the context of the major histocompatibility complex II on the cell surface. During maturation within the thymus (Fig. 10-2), T cell precursors undergo negative selection with only cells capable of adequate TCR responses to foreign antigen presented within the MHC II surviving.[23,24] Subsequently, T cell precursor clones with strong reactivity to self-antigens are deleted by positive selection. T cell activation results from contact with antigen-presenting cells (macrophages, dendritic cells) which process and present foreign antigen in the context of MHC II on their surface.

The population of mature T cell consists of multiple subsets.[27] These subtypes include CD4+ helper cells, which assist other immune cells, offering critical support to maturing B cells.

CD8+ cytotoxic cells kill infected or tumor cells. Memory T cells may be either CD4+ or CD8+ and allow for

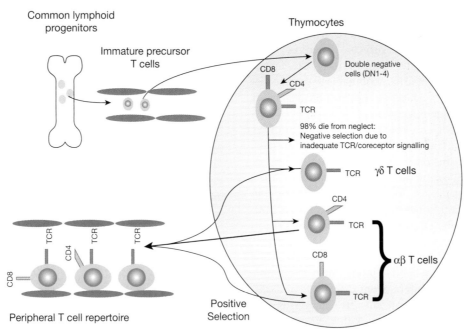

FIGURE 10-2.   T cell development. As depicted in this schematic. T cells are derived from common lymphoid progenitors in the bone marrow and exit the bone marrow as immature precursors, which travel to the thymus. These cells give rise to double negative cells maturing to give rise to lymphocytes, which are double positive for CD8 and CD4, as well as the T cell receptor (TCR). Positive selection then promotes the survival and return to the vasculature of TCR+ γδ T cells, CD4+, TCR+ helper T cells, or CD8+, TCR+ cytotoxic T cells. (Adapted with permission from Skapenko A, Leipe J, Lipsky PE. The role of the T cell in autoimmune inflammation. *Arthritis Res Ther.* 2005;7 Suppl 2:S4–S14.)

more rapid T cell–mediated responses to recurrent challenge with a previously recognized foreign antigen. Regulatory T cells (Treg) are critical for the maintenance of immunologic tolerance, while natural killer (NK) cells respond to glycolipid antigen and can perform cytotoxic or helper functions. γδ T cells, named for their unique TCR, are concentrated in the gut within the intraepithelial lymphocytes. T cells are activated through MHC II–dependent stimulation of the TCR (CD3) complex, which combines a variable αβ (or γδ) heterodimer with nonvariable CD3 components.[28] However, simultaneous presentation of co-stimulatory molecules (such as CD28) by antigen-presenting cells is required for T cell activation, as isolated TCR activation in the absence of the appropriate co-stimulus leads to prolonged failure of that cell to respond to its specific stimulus in a condition known as anergy.

The most common cause of death for patients with this condition is

A. Infection
B. Hypocalcemia
C. Cardiac anomalies
D. Graft-versus-host disease
E. SIDS

Discussion

The correct answer is **C**. DiGeorge syndrome is relatively common, affecting 1/3000 births and present in as high as 5% of infants with cardiac defects.[19] There is an 8% mortality which primarily occurs within the first 6 months of life and is primarily attributable to cardiac disease although both hypocalcemia and immune deficiency can also be life threatening. Although less common than cardiac mortality, DiGeorge patients with severe immune compromise are at significant risk of graft-versus-host disease with transfusion of nonirradiated blood products as well as following bone marrow transplantation. Graft-versus-host disease following PRBC transfusion is such a significant concern that evaluations for both DiGeorge syndrome and immune integrity are critical prior to surgery in the infant with conotruncal anomalies. While undiagnosed DiGeorge syndrome has been reported in rare cases of sudden infant death, the definition of SIDS rules out intercurrent disease or underlying anomalies detectable on autopsy (www.sids.org/ndefinition.htm). Note: Features of this syndrome are also mimicked by fetal exposure to alcohol or isotretinoin.

CASE 4

A 9-week-old male infant whose parents recently arrived from Guatemala is brought to the emergency room with fever and vomiting and decreased movement of his legs. The infant's history is remarkable for poor growth and three episodes of otitis media treated with amoxicillin. His vaccination status is reported verbally as up-to-date with last vaccinations, including oral polio vaccine, administered 10 days prior to the onset of illness. There is no history of sick contacts. The pregnancy history was unremarkable. Family history is remarkable for two maternal great uncles who died of fever in infancy. On presentation, the left leg is flaccid and the infant has no detectable DTRs in that extremity although sensation is intact. Lumbar puncture reveals an elevated protein level and a pleocytosis with a CSF cell count of 100 cells/mm,[3] which are primarily lymphocytes.

What is the most likely immediate cause of the infant's illness?

A. Guillain–Barre syndrome
B. Polio
C. Myasthenia gravis
D. Werdnig–Hoffmann disease

Discussion

The correct answer is **B**. Of the conditions listed, ascending paralysis in the setting of an acute illness is most consistent with poliomyelitis. Vaccine-associated paralysis became recognized as a rare but concerning entity after the introduction of broad-scale vaccination with the live attenuated oral polio vaccine significantly limiting wild-type poliomyelitis. Introduction of the use of an inactivated polio vaccine for use in the household contacts of the immunocompromised failed to address the issue of the first vaccination of a child with an as yet undiagnosed immunodeficiency.[29]

Guillain–Barre syndrome is the most common cause of acute flaccid paralysis or ascending quadriparesis in an infant or child.[30] However, it is usually symmetric, often accompanied by sensory changes, and most commonly presents with pain in children. The severity is variable with some patients revealing a relatively benign course while others become critically ill, requiring intubation and intensive care. Immune therapy (plasmapheresis or IVIG) is indicated for any older child who loses the ability to walk.[31] Congenital myasthenia gravis represents a collection of disorders of the neuromuscular junction, presents with fatigable muscle weakness or hypotonia.[32] Werdnig–Hoffmann disease or spinal

TABLE 10-1. **Primary Defects of Acquired Immunity**

PRIMARY IMMUNODEFICIENCY	CHROMOSOME	IMMUNE DEFECT
X-linked agammaglobulinemia (XLA)	X	Deficiency in Bruton tyrosine kinase necessary for B cell maturation
X-linked hyperimmunoglobulin (Ig) M syndrome (XHIM)	X	Deficiency of CD40 ligand normally expressed on active T cells and required for T cell function, B cell differentiation, and monocyte function
X-linked severe combined immunodeficiency disease (XLSCID)	X	Defect in the IL2 receptor gamma leading to near or complete absence of T cells and NK cells and nonfunctional B cells
Autosomal recessive SCID[35]	Variable	Defect
Reticular dysgenesis	1	Mitochondrial adenylate kinase 2: bone marrow hypoplasia
Adenosine deaminase deficiency (ADA)	20	Impaired purine nucleotide metabolism
RAG1/RAG2 deficiency	11p13	Impaired BCR/TCR recombination
JAK3 deficiency	19	Impaired common γ chain signaling
IL-7Ra deficiency	15	Impaired T cell development
Omenn syndrome (RAG1/2 def with autoimmunity)	11	Impaired BCR/TCR recombination
ZAP-70 kinase	2	Impaired T cell signaling
MHC II deficiency	19	RFXANK deficiency: impaired MHC II gene transcription
P561 ck deficiency	1	T cell development and IL2-dependent T cell signaling
DiGeorge syndrome (DGS)	22 (rarely 10p)	Thymic hypo or aplasia with diminished or absent T cell function leading to impaired cellular and humoral immunity

muscular atrophy (SMA) represents a collection of inherited disorders leading to progressive muscle damage, weakness, and death, and would be unlikely to present as an acute ascending paralysis at 9 weeks.[33]

What underlying immune deficiency is most likely to have predisposed this infant to this infection?
A. SCID
B. IgA deficiency
C. Asplenia
D. Complement deficiency

Discussion

The correct answer is **A**. In this infant, failure to thrive and frequent infections are suggestive of an underlying immune defect, which may have been masked thus far by frequent courses of antibiotics. Specifically, the current illness is concerning for vaccine-acquired paralytic poliomyelitis (VAPP) following the attenuated live oral polio vaccine and is also consistent with an underlying immune defect in T cell function. Of the conditions listed, this presentation is most consistent with severe combined immunodeficiency (SCID). SCID is a primary immune deficiency characterized by severe defects in both T and B cell–mediated acquired immunity.[34] Affected infants generally present with severe infection during the first few months of life. IgA deficiency would

be more likely to manifest as a defect in mucosal immunity and patients with either asplenia or complement deficiencies are more likely to have increased susceptibility to infections with encapsulated organisms.

The most common form of this SCID, accounting for nearly half of the cases, is X-linked, affecting only males, with other forms resulting from recessive inheritance (Table 10-1).[34] X-linked SCID results from a mutation in the interleukin 2 receptor gamma (IL2RG) gene, which encodes the gamma chain subunit common to several interleukin receptors. Less commonly, recessively inherited SCID can result from mutations in JAK3 (chromosome 19), the signaling molecule downstream of the IL2 receptor or through a genetic defect in the gene encoding adenosine deaminase (chromosome 20), leading to the intracellular accumulation of its cytotoxic substrates. Thus, affected individuals are deficient in mature cells of all lymphoid origins.

Which of the following is the definitive treatment for this condition?
A. Monthly IVIG therapy
B. Life-long antibiotic prophylaxis
C. Avoidance of live vaccines
D. Stem cell transplantation from cord blood or bone marrow

Discussion

The correct answer is **D**. While all the listed choices may contribute to the survival of the patient with SCID, along with careful avoidance of exposure to infection, the only definitive therapies are bone marrow or stem cell transplantation. In patients with SCID, there is little or no risk of rejection of the grafts. However, these individuals are at significant risk of graft-versus-host disease in which the donor marrow attacks host tissues.

Pluripotent hematopoietic stem cells are essential for maintaining all lineages of blood cells with clinical uses including reconstitution of bone marrow constituents in patients with either primary deficiencies or following bone marrow ablation for treatment of hematologic malignancies.[36] These cells are present, proliferate and differentiate within hematopoietic organs including fetal liver, bone marrow, thymus, and the spleen, however their site of origin is more controversial. Recent evidence supports multiple potential sites of origin, including pluripotent mesoderm cells in the yolk sac or the aorta, hemangioblasts within these same two sites, or from hemogenic endothelium.

CASE 5

A 5-month-old female infant was brought by her grandmother to a city public health clinic. She was born "around a month early," by vaginal delivery after a "long labor," following a pregnancy with no prenatal care. At birth, she weighed 2.4 kg (50% at 35 weeks), length 46 cm (50%), and head circumference 32 cm. Her grandmother brought the infant in for cough and diarrhea. She reports that the infant only recently started living with her during the past month. The infant's mother has been unwell for months and is currently in jail. The grandmother states that the infant has been coughing for 3 weeks and she does not know how long that the loose stools have been a problem. Currently, the infant weighs 5.5 kg (5%), length 60 cm (25%), and head circumference 41 cm (25%–50%). Vital signs reveal a heart rate of 120 bpm, RR 44 breaths per minute, and a temperature of 99.9°F. The infant is alert, but somewhat wasted in appearance with an intermittent dry, spasmodic cough. White plaque-like exudates are present on the tongue. The chest examination is remarkable for lymphadenopathy of the neck, axilla and groin regions and coarse rales throughout both anterior lung fields. A chest x-ray is obtained and is remarkable for diffuse fluffy opacities. And a CBC is remarkable for a normal white blood cell count with neutrophilia and decreased total lymphocyte count.

The immune defect most likely to be responsible for this infant's condition is
A. Abnormal neutrophil migration
B. Complement deficiency
C. Impaired T cell function
D. Abnormal phagocytic function

Discussion

The correct answer is **C**. The failure to thrive and oral lesions consistent with thrush in this patient are concerning for a chronic underlying immune deficiency in addition to potential acute infection(s) underlying the cough and diarrhea. The lymphadenopathy, particularly in the axillary region is also concerning for more than just a routine viral infection. These findings, along with the absence of prenatal screening, and the mother who is apparently chronically unwell, raise the question in this patient of early presentation of vertically transmitted HIV infection/AIDS. The vast majority of HIV infection in infancy and childhood results from vertical transmission during vaginal birth and the risk of transmission can be significantly reduced by regimens of antiretroviral therapy to reduce maternal viral load prior to or during delivery. AIDS is primarily a defect of acquired or cell-mediated immunity resulting from the HIV retrovirus, which preferentially infects CD4+ T cells and macrophages. CD4+ helper T cells are primarily infected, and these cells are critical for immune activation. Thus, B cell–dependent antibody production is also affected. Neutrophil migration and phagocytosis as well as complement production are generally intact.

Which of the following increase the risk of maternal–child transmission of viral infections?
A. High viral titers
B. Prolonged rupture of membranes prior to delivery
C. Vaginal delivery
D. All of the above

Discussion

The correct answer is **D**. Increased risk of transplacental maternal–child transmission or vertical transmission is associated with a number of factors including factors which control maternal viral load, as well as duration and route of exposure.[37,38] Prenatal factors influencing[38] maternal viral load include timing related to initial versus chronic infection, with viral loads being highest during initial infection prior to immune response and then falling after initial infection until late in the course of HIV infection once the virus has overwhelmed the immune response. Antiretroviral therapy during pregnancy and labor can also substantially reduce the viral load and the risk of infection of the newborn.[39] Additional risks arise from factors increasing fetal exposure to maternal blood, including chorioamnionitis, fetal scalp electrode placement, and vaginal birth, especially in the setting of prolonged rupture of membranes.

In infants with this condition, what is the most common secondary infection at time of diagnosis?
A. Oral candidiasis
B. Pneumocystis carinii pneumonia (PCP)
C. Respiratory syncytial virus
D. Rotavirus

Discussion

The correct answer is **B**. In the case of this infant, the mother appears to have eluded routine health surveillance and preventative care, and the infant is now acutely ill with signs of AIDS. Perinatally exposed infants are asymptomatic at birth and generally develop symptoms within the first 1 to 2 years of life with 15% to 20% dying by age 4. The prognosis is generally worse with earlier presentation. In the United States, the most common infection at the time of presentation is PCP, which develops in the majority of children with untreated HIV between 3 and 6 months. FTT, diarrhea, and candidal esophagitis are also common. Recurrent bacterial infections due to decreased B cell function are also seen as infection progresses and as maternal IgG levels decline from birth to 9 months of age.

Objectives

1. Understand the diagnosis and management of T cell dysfunction, specifically DiGeorge sequence and HIV infection
2. Know the role of the spleen in host defense and the consequences of altered spleen function or asplenia
3. Understand abnormal function of the immune system

CASE 6

A 525 g male infant is born by emergency C-section at 26 weeks gestation to a 34-year-old African-American woman due to worsening preeclampsia following pregnancy-induced hypertension superimposed on baseline essential hypertension. Prenatal care began in the first trimester, and prenatal screens obtained on the first prenatal visit revealed that the mother was rubella immune, hepatitis

B surface antigen negative, HIV negative, RPR nonreactive, and CMV IgG positive. The infant was initially vigorous with spontaneous respiratory effort, and then rapidly developed increased work of breathing with severe intercostal and supraclavicular retractions by 2 minutes of life. The infant was initially managed with bag-valve mask ventilation followed by intubation in the delivery room and treatment with exogenous surfactant via ETT with significantly decreased work of breathing and supplemental oxygen requirement occurring over the next 20 minutes. APGARs were 5 at 1 minute and 7 at 5 minutes. Examination on admission to the NICU revealed a nondysmorphic, intubated premature infant with adequate expansion and aeration on ventilated breaths. The abdomen was soft, nondistended, and nontender to palpation without hepatosplenomegaly. CBC obtained on admission to the NICU was remarkable for a total WBC of 3.0 with 12% neutrophils and 3% bands, hemoglobin of 16.2, and a platelet count of 95,000.

Which of the following arms of the immune system are not impaired in healthy preterm infants relative to those born at term?
A. Neutrophil phagocytosis
B. Antibody production
C. T cell responses to mitogens
D. Neutrophil chemotaxis

Discussion

The correct answer is **C**. Premature infants are compromised in many aspects of immune function. When lymphocytes were harvested from the cord blood of neonates, spontaneous T cell proliferation is higher in premature infants than in those born at term, and T cell responses to most mitogens were not significantly different in premature infants relative to term infants and adults. Furthermore, intrauterine growth restriction had no effect.[40]

With the exception of oxidative killing, most key neutrophil functions, including phagocytosis and chemotaxis are diminished in preterm infants and disproportionately so, in low–birth-weight infants. However, oxidative killing is also impaired in the sick preterm infant.[41] The neutrophil-derived antibacterial peptides BPI, defensins (HNP1–3), and calprotectin are key elements of the innate immune response at mucosal surfaces. While little is known about the effects of prematurity on levels of antibacterial peptides, studies from stool samples[42] and bronchoalveolar lavage of premature infants diagnosed with pneumonia[43] reveal that premature infants are capable of producing them. Beta defensin levels in stool increase with gestational age,[42] however, the significance of this finding with respect to intestinal immunity remains unclear.

Humoral immunity is also impaired in premature infants.[14] IgG levels are determined entirely by transplacental transfer from the mother. As with term infants, IgG synthesis is absent in the preterm newborn. However, the beginning of IgG synthesis is delayed in the preterm infant, with no significant synthesis evident in the first 15 weeks of life of infants born at less than 36 weeks' gestation.[14] Lower gestational ages and birth weights correlate with lower IgG levels. While IVIG therapy effectively boosted serum IgG levels in studies of babies less than 32 weeks,[44] a Cochrane database meta-analysis of IVIG use for prophylaxis of nosocomial sepsis in patients less than 37 weeks gestational age and/or BW <2.5 kg, revealed only a marginal reduction in sepsis without any effect on major outcomes and no support for its further use.[45] Similarly, meta-analyses of numerous clinical trials have failed to establish a clear benefit for IVIG as an adjuvant therapy in suspected or proven sepsis.[46,47]

Helpful Tip: When present in amniotic fluid of women with intact membranes, BPI and HNP1–3 are associated with intra-amniotic inflammation, and shorter time to birth.[48] Furthermore, the combined presence of HNP1 and HNP2 along with calgranulins C and A in amniotic fluid were predictive of neonatal sepsis.[49]

Factors associated with immune compromise in this infant include
A. Low birth weight
B. Prematurity
C. Pregnancy-induced hypertension
D. All of the above

Discussion

The correct answer is **D.** Pregnancy-induced hypertension and preeclampsia are extremely common, with preeclampsia affecting 5% to 8% of pregnancies.[50] Preeclampsia is associated with intrauterine growth restriction and the need for premature delivery as well as neutropenia and thrombocytopenia in the newborn. As discussed above, premature birth is clearly associated with decreases in most aspects of immune function. Intrauterine growth restriction is independently associated with compromised innate immunity including decreased neutrophil number and cytokine production[51]; decreased levels of complement proteins C3, C4, and Factor B; decreased opsonization; and decreased intracellular killing.[52]

Complement pathway activation proceeds through a series of cleavage events (Fig. 10-3), adapted from[53]

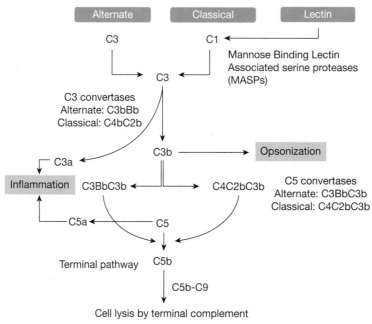

FIGURE 10-3. Complement cascade. Three potential pathways exist for initiation of the complement cascade: classical, alternate, and lectin-mediated activation. Initial activation proceeds through different convertases for the classical pathway and lectin (C4bC2b) pathways relative to the alternative pathways (C3bBb). All three pathways converge with the generation of C3. C3 is then cleaved, releasing C3b. C3b is an opsonin, which is deposited on nearby cell surfaces and particles, facilitating phagocytosis. In the event of further activation, C5 is also cleaved releasing C5b, which can then recruit C6, C7, C8, and C9 to the cell surface where C9 becomes inserted to serve as a pore within the cell membrane mediating cell lysis. C3a and C5a are also released as a result of these cleavage reactions. C3a is potent antimicrobial peptide and both C3a and C5a can trigger anaphylaxis. (Adapted with permission from Zipfel PF, Skerka C. Complement regulators and inhibitory proteins. *Nat Rev Immunol.* 2009;9(10):729–740.)

generating a series of effector molecules which coat and mark particles or microorganisms for phagocytosis.[53] The components of the complement protein cascade are integral to the innate immune response promoting cell integrity and facilitating the removal of dead or modified cells, as well as modulating the intensity of the adaptive immune response. Host cells are protected from the actions of the complement through a series of regulators and inhibitors, and disruption of these protective mechanisms can result in complement-mediated damage.

In addition to alterations in complement function, infants affected by intrauterine growth restriction also demonstrate diminished T and B cell responses[54] with prolonged hypogammaglobulinemia relative to infants whose birth weight are appropriate for gestational age. Infants who are born to mothers with preeclampsia have a 50% incidence of neutropenia,[55] which has been postulated to result from uteroplacental insufficiency and associated inhibition of bone marrow production of myeloid precursors.[56,57] However, this remains to be proved.

Potential etiologies for this patient's neutropenia include all of the following except
A. Deficiency of G-CSF
B. Sepsis
C. Impaired neutrophil chemotaxis
D. Prematurity

Discussion

The correct answer is **C**. While neutrophil chemotaxis is likely to be impaired in this extremely premature, low–birth-weight infant, impairments in migration are not likely to explain this patient's neutropenia. In the absence of other insults, premature infants generally have blood neutrophil counts which are comparable to adults, however, they are vulnerable to bone marrow suppression secondary to multiple factors, and their responses to neutrophil consumption are markedly different from adults due to significantly smaller neutrophil reserves.[58] Although this infant was delivered by caesarian section for maternal indications, sepsis must be considered either as a cause or a consequence of neutropenia in this patient. G-CSF levels are generally lower in preterm infants and contribute in some cases to lower neutrophil counts. However, there has been no established correlation between G-CSF level and neutrophil count,[59] and Cochrane database meta-analysis revealed no evidence of a beneficial effect of G-CSF administration in either the treatment or prevention of neonatal sepsis.[60] Furthermore, follow-up of infants in a large, multicenter trial revealed no impact of G-CSF on adverse outcomes at 2 years of life.[61]

After 48 hours, the patient's blood culture remains negative and he is hemodynamically stable on low ventilatory support. The most appropriate therapy for this patient's neutropenia is
A. Recombinant G-CSF
B. Careful observation and serial monitoring
C. IVIG
D. Granulocyte infusion

Discussion

The correct answer is **B**. While broad-spectrum antibiotics are frequently used in the setting of the critically ill, extremely low–birth-weight infant, growing evidence indicates that their detrimental effects on intestinal flora result in increased risk of necrotizing colitis,[62] and there is also a small amount of in vitro evidence indicating that antibiotic therapy further suppresses antibody production by fetal B cells.[63] In the absence of hemodynamic instability, positive blood cultures, or other infectious risk factors, the best approach is careful observation and continued serial monitoring in this infant.

CASE 7

An African-American male was born at 35 6/7 weeks' gestation to a 26-year-old married primigravida mother, and was referred to the NICU at 4 hours of life for tachypnea. Birth occurred by spontaneous vaginal delivery following a pregnancy complicated only by preterm labor. Available prenatal laboratory studies included that the mother was blood type A+, Hepatitis B surface antigen negative, RPR nonreactive, rubella immune ROM occurred 18 hours prior to delivery with clear fluid. The last 30 minutes of labor were remarkable for a fetal heart rate in the 170s. APGARs were 8 at 1 minute and 9 at 5 minutes. The infant weighed 2.6 kg at birth, had a nonfocal examination by the neonatal nurse practitioner attending the delivery. He was transferred to the postpartum unit with his mother. The mother was noted to have a temperature of 100.2 on arrival in the postpartum unit 30 minutes after delivery.

At 4 hours of life, the infant was noted to be pale and tachypneic with a respiratory rate of 80 breaths per minute. Admission laboratory studies were remarkable for a with a WBC of 18,000 with 25% neutrophils and 10% bands. Hemoglobin was 16.1 and platelet count was 182,000. A serum C-reactive protein was sent and was elevated. Blood culture was sent. Chest x-ray was remarkable for fluid in the right fissure with some streaky densities throughout, and an effusion at the base of the right lung.

Elevated C-reactive protein is consistent with
A. Recent birth
B. Intravascular clot
C. Ongoing infection
D. All of the above

Discussion

The correct answer is **D**. C-reactive protein is an acute-phase reactant which acts as an opsonin to coat microbes, marking them for phagocytosis. C-reactive protein can also be elevated in the setting of any tissue damage or inflammation including tissue damage, recent vaccination, or even just from birth itself. In one study of healthy babies born in Japan, CRP values were low immediately after birth, then increased physiologically during the first few days of life with higher levels associated with vaginal birth.[57]

The acute-phase reactant with the lowest negative predictive value for infection is
A. Serum amyloid P
B. Ceruloplasmin
C. C-reactive protein
D. Ferritin
E. Hepcidin

Discussion

The correct answer is **C**. The principal value of C-reactive protein relative to other acute-phase reactants is that it has the highest negative predictive value such that a negative C-reactive protein test is highly predictive of the absence of infection. A positive or elevated C-reactive protein is harder to interpret.[64]

Acute-phase reactants are most commonly synthesized by the
A. Bone marrow
B. Liver
C. Vasculature
D. Lung
E. Immune cells

Discussion

The correct answer is **B**. Classically, acute-phase reactants are liver-derived glycoproteins found in the plasma in the setting of infection, inflammation, or stress including birth, itself.[65] CRP is most frequently used in the clinical setting as an indicator of infection. Acute-phase reactants can be divided according to whether they are positive acute-phase proteins, in that they function to drive the immune response to the microbe (e.g., CRP, mannose binding protein, complement factors, ferritin, ceruloplasmin, serum amyloid A, or haptoglobin), or as negative acute-phase proteins, which provide feedback inhibition (e.g., serpins, alpha 2-macroglobulin, and coagulation factors).[66] Procoagulant factors may trap microorganisms within clots, increase vascular permeability, and serve as chemotactic agents for phagocytic cells.[67]

Objectives

1. Understand the specific components of the immune system
2. Know the complement system and the role it plays in host defense
3. Understand the inflammatory components and the components of acute inflammation, specifically the role of CRP
4. Know the clinical features of neonates with immune deficiencies, and the tests used to evaluate possible defects

REFERENCES

1. Oudesluys-Murphy AM, Eilers GA, de Groot CJ. The time of separation of the umbilical cord. *Eur J Pediatr.* 1987;146:387–389.
2. Razvi S, Murphy R, Shlasko E, et al. Delayed separation of the umbilical cord attributable to urachal anomalies. *Pediatrics.* 2001;108:493–494.
3. Feldmann M. Many cytokines are very useful therapeutic targets in disease. *J Clin Invest.* 2008;118:3533–3536.
4. Comerford I, McColl SR. Mini-review series: focus on chemokines. *Immunol Cell Biol.* 2011;89:183–184.
5. Cunningham-Rundles C, Ponda PP. Molecular defects in T- and B-cell primary immunodeficiency diseases. *Nat Rev Immunol.* 2005;5:880–892.
6. Guneser S, Altintas DU, Aksungur P, et al. An infant with severe leucocyte adhesion deficiency. *Acta Paediatr.* 1996;85:622–624.
7. Etzioni A. Leukocyte adhesion deficiency (LAD) syndromes. *Orphanet Encyclopedia.* 2005.
8. Good RA. Cellular immunology in a historical perspective. *Immunol Rev.* 2002;185:136–158.
9. Ronchera-Oms C, Hernandez C, Jimemez NV. Antiseptic cord care reduces bacterial colonization but delays cord detachment. *Arch Dis Child Fetal Neonatal Ed.* 1994;71:F70.
10. Pezzati M, Biagioli EC, Martelli E, et al. Umbilical cord care: the effect of eight different cord-care regimens on cord separation time other outcomes. *Biol Neonate.* 2002;81:38–44.
11. Dore S, Buchan D, Coulas S, et al. Alcohol versus natural drying for newborn cord care. *J Obstet Gynecol Neonatal Nurs.* 1998;27:621–627.

12. Evens K, George J, Angst D, et al. Does umbilical cord care in preterm infants influence cord bacterial colonization or detachment? *J Perinatol.* 2004;24:100–104.

13. Esche C, Cohen BA. Novel approach to the evaluation of primary immunodeficiencies. In: Gaspari AA, Tyring SK, eds. *Practical Immunodermatology: Clinical Diagnosis and Management.* London: Springer-Verlag; 2008.

14. Conway SP, Dear PR, Smith I. Immunoglobulin profile of the preterm baby. *Arch Dis Child.* 1985;60:208–212.

15. Salimonu LS, Ladipo OA, Adeniran SO, et al. Serum immunoglobulin levels in normal, premature and postmature newborns and their mothers. *Int J Gynecol Obstet.* 1978;16:119–123.

16. Liu Y, Wu Y, Lam KT, et al. Dendritic and T cell response to influenza is normal in the patients with X-linked agammaglobulinemia. *J Clin Immunol.* 2012;32:421–429.

17. Scambler PJ. The 22q11 deletion syndromes. *Hum Mol Genet.* 2000;9:2421–2426.

18. Desmaze C, Prieur M, Amblard F, et al. Physical mapping by FISH of the DiGeorge critical region (DGCR): involvement of the region in familial cases. *Am J Hum Genet.* 1993;53:1239–1249.

19. Kobrynski LJ, Sullivan KE. Velocardiofacial syndrome, DiGeorge syndrome: the chromosome 22q11.2 deletion syndromes. *Lancet.* 2007;370:1443–1452.

20. Finocchi A, Di Cesare S, Romiti ML, et al. Humoral immune responses and CD27+ B cells in children with DiGeorge syndrome (22q11.2 deletion syndrome). *Pediatr Allergy Immunol.* 2006;17:382–388.

21. Varga I, Pospisilova V, Jablonska-Mestanova V, et al. The thymus: picture review of human thymus prenatal development. *Bratisl Lek Listy.* 2011;112:368–376.

22. Vellguth S, von Gaudecker B, Muller-Hermelink HK. The development of the human spleen. Ultrastructural studies in fetuses from the 14th to 24th week of gestation. *Cell Tissue Res.* 1985;242:579–592.

23. Germain RN. T-cell development and the CD4-CD8 lineage decision. *Nat Rev Immunol.* 2002;2:309–322.

24. Skapenko A, Leipe J, Lipsky PE, et al. The role of the T cell in autoimmune inflammation. *Arthritis Res Ther.* 2005;7(suppl 2):S4–S14.

25. Campbell JM, Knutsen AP. Decreased CD27+ memory B cells in DiGeorge anomaly. *Pediatr Asthma, Allergy & Immunol.* 2008;21:6–13.

26. Boyle ML, Scalchunes C. Impact of intravenous immunoglobulin (IVIG treatment among patients with primary immunodeficiency diseases. *Pharm Policy and Law.* 2008;133–146.

27. Broere F, Apasov S, Sitovsky M, et al. T cell subsets and T cell-mediated immunity. In: FP Nijkamp, MJ Parnham, eds. *Principles of Immunopharmacology.* 3rd ed; revised and extended. Basel: Springer Basel AG; 2011:15–27.

28. Smith-Garvin JE, Koretzky GA, Jordan MS. T cell activation. *Annu Rev Immunol.* 2009;27:591–619.

29. Nkowane BM, Wassilak SG, Orenstein WA, et al. Vaccine-associated paralytic poliomyelitis. United States: 1973 through 1984. *JAMA.* 1987;257:1335–1340.

30. Yuki N, Hartung HP. Guillain-Barre syndrome. *N Engl J Med.* 2012;366:2294–2304.

31. Jones HR Jr. Guillain-Barre syndrome: perspectives with infants and children. *Semin Pediatr Neurol.* 2000;7:91–102.

32. Lorenzoni PJ, Scola RH, Kay CS, et al. Congenital myasthenic syndrome: a brief review. *Pediatr Neurol.* 2012;46:141–148.

33. Lunn MR, Wang CH. Spinal muscular atrophy. *Lancet.* 2008;371:2120–2133.

34. Tasher D, Dalal I. The genetic basis of severe combined immunodeficiency and its variants. *Appl Clin Genet.* 2012;5:67–80.

35. Schwartz R. Pediatric severe combined immunodeficiency. In: Jyonouchi H, ed. *Medscape Reference: Drugs, Diseases, & Procedures.*

36. Cumano A, Godin I. Pluripotent hematopoietic stem cell development during embryogenesis. *Curr Opin Immunol.* 2001;13:166–171.

37. Morrison J, Alp NJ. Vertical transmission of human immunodeficiency virus. *QJM.* 1997;90:5–12.

38. Cao Y, Krogstad P, Korber BT, et al. Maternal HIV-1 viral load and vertical transmission of infection: the Ariel Project for the prevention of HIV transmission from mother to infant. *Nat Med.* 1997;3:549–552.

39. Newell ML. Prevention of mother-to-child transmission of HIV: challenges for the current decade. *Bull World Health Organ.* 2001;79:1138–1144.

40. Pittard WB 3rd, Miller K, Sorensen RU. Normal lymphocyte responses to mitogens in term and premature neonates following normal and abnormal intrauterine growth. *Clin Immunol Immunopathol.* 1984;30:178–187.

41. Al-Hadithy H, Addison IE, Goldstone AH, et al. Defective neutrophil function in low-birth-weight, premature infants. *J Clin Pathol.* 1981;34:366–370.

42. Richter M, Topf HG, Groschl M, et al. Influence of gestational age, cesarean section, and type of feeding on fecal human beta-defensin 2 and tumor necrosis factor-alpha. *J Pediatr Gastroenterol Nutr.* 2010;51:103–105.

43. Tirone C, Boccacci S, Inzitari R, et al. Correlation of levels of alpha-defensins determined by HPLC-ESI-MS in bronchoalveolar lavage fluid with the diagnosis of pneumonia in premature neonates. *Pediatr Res.* 2010;68:140–144.

44. Conway SP, Gillies DR, Docherty A. Neonatal infection in premature infants and use of human immunoglobulin. *Arch Dis Child.* 1987;62:1252–1256.

45. Ohlsson A, Lacy JB. Intravenous immunoglobulin for preventing infection in preterm and/or low-birth-weight infants. *Cochrane Database Syst Rev.* 2004;(1):CD000361.

46. Franco AC, Torrico AC, Moreira FT, et al. Adjuvant use of intravenous immunoglobulin in the treatment of neonatal sepsis: a systematic review with a meta-analysis. *J Pediatr (Rio J).* 2012;88:377–383.

47. Ohlsson A, Lacy J. Intravenous immunoglobulin for suspected or subsequently proven infection in neonates. *Cochrane Database Syst Rev.* 2010;(3):CD001239.

48. Espinoza J, Chaiworapongsa T, Romero R, et al. Antimicrobial peptides in amniotic fluid: defensins, calprotectin and bacterial/permeability-increasing protein in patients with microbial invasion of the amniotic cavity, intra-amniotic inflammation, preterm labor and premature rupture of membranes. *J Matern Fetal Neonatal Med.* 2003;13:2–21.

49. Buhimschi CS, Buhimschi IA, Abdel-Razeq S, et al. Proteomic biomarkers of intra-amniotic inflammation: relationship with funisitis and early-onset sepsis in the premature neonate. *Pediatr Res.* 2007;61:318–324.

50. Saftlas AF, Olson DR, Franks AL, et al. Epidemiology of pre-eclampsia and eclampsia in the United States, 1979–1986. *Am J Obstet Gynecol.* 1990;163:460–465.

51. Troger B, Muller T, Faust K, et al. Intrauterine growth restriction and the innate immune system in preterm infants of ≤32 weeks gestation. *Neonatology.* 2012;103:199–204.

52. Chandra KR, Matsumura T. Ontogenetic development of the immune system and effects of fetal growth retardation. *J Perinat Med.* 1979;7:279–290.

53. Zipfel PF, Skerka C. Complement regulators and inhibitory proteins. *Nat Rev Immunol.* 2009;9:729–740.

54. Singh M, Manerikar S, Malaviya AN, et al. Immune status of low birth weight babies. *Indian Pediatr.* 1978;15:563–567.

55. Mouzinho A, Rosenfeld CR, Sanchez PJ, et al. Effect of maternal hypertension on neonatal neutropenia and risk of nosocomial infection. *Pediatrics.* 1992;90:430–435.

56. Koenig JM, Christensen RD. The mechanism responsible for diminished neutrophil production in neonates delivered of women with pregnancy-induced hypertension. *Am J Obstet Gynecol.* 1991;165:467–473.

57. Backes CH, Markham K, Moorehead P, et al. Maternal pre-eclampsia and neonatal outcomes. *J Pregnancy.* 2011;2011:214365.

58. Del Vecchio A, Christensen RD. Neonatal neutropenia: what diagnostic evaluation is needed and when is treatment recommended? *Early Hum Dev.* 2012;88(suppl 2):S19–S24.

59. Chirico G, Ciardelli L, Cecchi P, et al. Serum concentration of granulocyte colony stimulating factor in term and preterm infants. *Eur J Pediatr.* 1997;156:269–271.

60. Carr R, Modi N, Dore C. G-CSF and GM-CSF for treating or preventing neonatal infections. *Cochrane Database Syst Rev.* 2003;(3):CD003066.

61. Marlow N, Morris T, Brocklehurst P, et al. A randomised trial of granulocyte-macrophage colony-stimulating factor for neonatal sepsis: outcomes at 2 years. *Arch Dis Child Fetal Neonatal Ed.* 2013;98:F46–F53.

62. Cotten CM, Taylor S, Stoll B, et al. Prolonged duration of initial empirical antibiotic treatment is associated with increased rates of necrotizing enterocolitis and death for extremely low birth weight infants. *Pediatrics.* 2009;123:58–66.

63. Cukrowska B, Lodinova-Zadnikova R, Sokol D, et al. In vitro immunoglobulin response of fetal B-cells is influenced by perinatal infections and antibiotic treatment: a study in preterm infants. *Eur J Pediatr.* 1999;158:463–468.

64. Pourcyrous M, Bada HS, Korones SB, et al. Acute phase reactants in neonatal bacterial infection. *J Perinatol.* 1991;11:319–325.

65. Marchini G, Berggren V, Djilali-Merzoug R, et al. The birth process initiates an acute phase reaction in the fetus-newborn infant. *Acta Paediatr.* 2000;89:1082–1086.

66. Gruys E, Toussaint MJ, Niewold TA, et al. Acute phase reaction and acute phase proteins. *J Zhejiang Univ Sci B.* 2005;6:1045–1056.

67. de Boer JP, Creasey AA, Chang A, et al. Alpha-2-macroglobulin functions as an inhibitor of fibrinolytic, clotting, and neutrophilic proteinases in sepsis: studies using a baboon model. *Infect Immun.* 1993;61:5035–5043.

Chapter 11
INFECTIOUS DISEASES

Jumi Yi, Lakshmi Sukumaran, and Joseph A. Hilinski

CASE 1

A full-term 5-day-old male infant presents to your emergency department with a 1 day history of fussiness and fever to 101°F, measured rectally. His parents state that he is not feeding well and is less active than usual. His mother received prenatal care throughout her pregnancy, did not have any complications, and currently feels well. The patient was delivered via normal spontaneous vaginal delivery and APGARs were 9 at 1 minute and 9 at 5 minutes. He was transferred to the newborn nursery and discharged home in a healthy condition 2 days later. Physical examination reveals a rectal temperature of 38.4°C, and a nontoxic, appropriately sized infant. There is a small vesicle in the position of a previous scalp electrode. You decide to admit him for empiric antibiotics while awaiting blood, urine, and cerebrospinal fluid (CSF) cultures.

In addition to your current evaluation, you should also
A. Obtain herpes simplex virus (HSV) culture of the infant's scalp lesion, mucosal surfaces, and skin. Start the patient on empiric acyclovir.
B. Obtain HSV culture of the infant's scalp lesion, mucosal surfaces, and skin. Await culture results before starting acyclovir given its association with nephrotoxicity and risk to the infant.
C. Explain to the patient's mother that the vesicle is likely due to trauma from placement of the scalp electrode and should resolve in several days.
D. Since the patient's mother is not reporting lesions consistent with herpes, her prenatal records should be requested to confirm this information.
E. Discharge the patient and arrange follow-up with a dermatologist for biopsy of the lesion.

Discussion

The correct answer is **A**. Most neonatal HSV infections result from exposure to the maternal genital tract during delivery. Scalp electrode insertion poses a risk since direct inoculation of the virus may occur. Although rare, in utero and postnatal infections may also occur. Mothers with primary infection during their pregnancy are at higher risk of transmitting HSV to their infant than those with recurrent outbreaks, 25% to 50% versus 1%, respectively. Primary genital infections may have nonspecific symptoms and are often subclinical, so there may be no report of active maternal lesions. Neonatal HSV disease is divided into three clinical syndromes which may have some areas of overlap. Skin, eye, mouth (SEM) disease is restricted to the skin, eyes, and mucosa and accounts for about 45% of cases. Disseminated disease, about 25% of cases, involves multiple organs including the lungs and the liver and can be indistinguishable from bacterial sepsis. Central nervous system (CNS) disease, about 30% of cases, may present as seizures, poor feeding, and lethargy. More than half of these children will have moderate-to-severe neurologic abnormalities. Rash is not always present, and the clinician must maintain a high index of suspicion. In addition, prompt initiation of acyclovir is associated with improved morbidity and mortality. This patient should be immediately started on acyclovir while awaiting test results.

Which presentation of HSV disease is associated with the highest risk of death?
A. SEM disease
B. Disseminated disease
C. CNS disease
D. All are associated with equal risk of death
E. Disseminated disease and CNS disease

Discussion

The correct answer is **B**. Risk of death is highest with disseminated disease and may be up to 30% even with appropriate antiviral therapy.

You send a surface culture from the patient's scalp lesion which returns positive for HSV-2. Liver function testing is normal, and CSF studies are normal. CSF HSV polymerase chain reaction (PCR) is negative.

What is the appropriate duration of therapy for this patient?
A. 7 days
B. 14 days
C. 21 days
D. 28 days
E. No further therapy since the infant only has evidence of SEM disease and no evidence of dissemination

Discussion

The preferred answer is **B**. The infant has evidence of SEM disease which warrants a 14-day course of IV acyclovir. Treatment duration for disseminated and CNS disease is 21 days. A lumbar puncture should be performed near the end of the 21-day course in CNS disease if the CSF HSV PCR was initially positive, and acyclovir should be continued until the HSV PCR from the CSF is negative. After completion of IV acyclovir, 6 months of suppressive therapy with oral acyclovir (300 mg/m²/dose PO TID) should be started which has been shown to improve neurodevelopmental outcome in neonates with HSV CNS disease and decrease recurrence of skin lesions with any of the neonatal HSV disease categories (Table 11-1).

TABLE 11-1. **Treatment of Neonatal HSV Disease**

TYPE OF NEONATAL HSV DISEASE	DURATION OF THERAPY	ACYCLOVIR SUPPRESSIVE THERAPY
SEM	14 days	Recommended
Disseminated	21 days	Recommended
CNS	21 days minimum and CSF PCR neg at the end of therapy	Recommended

The infant's mother would like to breastfeed. You advise her that
A. Breastfeeding is allowed as long as she does not have active breast lesions and active lesions elsewhere are covered
B. She should have HSV IgM testing to document that she is longer having active HSV infection. If negative, she may start breastfeeding
C. She should use a breast pump and feed her child with a bottle to avoid HSV transmission by skin contact
D. Breastfeeding is contraindicated since HSV is transmitted through breast milk

Discussion

The correct answer is **A**. HSV-1 and 2 infections are usually a result of direct contact with shedding virus from a lesion or secretions. In addition, the mother should practice careful hand hygiene before and after caring for her infant. While hospitalized, the infant should be on contact precautions.

Objectives

1. Recognize the three subtypes of congenital HSV infections and differentiate between the three groups
2. Identify complications associated with congenital HSV infection
3. Recognize the typical clinical presentation associated with congenital HSV infection
4. Understand recommended evaluation and management for neonates with congenital HSV infection

CASE 2

A small-for-gestational age neonate is born at your hospital. The nurse calls you to the patient's bedside for seizures. Your examination reveals microcephaly, purpura, and a continuous murmur at the left upper sternal border. Ophthalmologic evaluation reveals bilateral microphthalmia and cataracts. The platelet count is 56,000.

Which of the following maternal prenatal laboratory values is likely?
A. Rubella nonimmune
B. Human immunodeficiency virus (HIV) antibody positive
C. RPR positive
D. Hepatitis B immunity positive

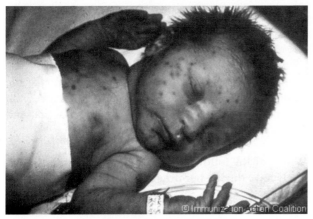

FIGURE 11-1. Congenital rubella – blueberry muffin. (Used with permission of the Immunization Action Coalition.)

Discussion

The correct answer is **A**. This patient exhibits signs of congenital rubella syndrome (CRS). Although rubella elimination was achieved in the United States in 2004, it is endemic in many parts of the world. The Centers for Disease Control and Prevention (CDC) case classification criteria for CRS include presence of signs and symptoms and laboratory criteria consistent with CRS. Signs and symptoms include eye defects (cataracts, congenital glaucoma, pigmentary retinopathy), congenital heart disease, hearing impairment, purpura, hepatosplenomegaly, jaundice, microcephaly, developmental delay, meningoencephalitis, and radiolucent bone disease (Figs. 11-1 and 11-2). Laboratory criteria include isolation of the rubella virus, presence of rubella-specific IgM, or infant rubella antibody level that does not decrease by twofold dilution per month. Infants who are exposed to rubella late in gestation do not have clinical

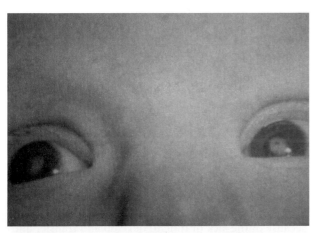

FIGURE 11-2. Congenital rubella – cataract. (Reproduced with permission from the Centers for Disease Control and Prevention.)

manifestations of CRS. However, CRS occurs in 20% of infants whose mothers have had rubella infection within the first 20 weeks of pregnancy.

Which of the following cardiac lesions is most commonly associated with CRS?
A. Tetralogy of Fallot
B. Ventricular septal defect
C. Patent ductus arteriosus
D. Atrial septal defect
E. Total anomalous pulmonary venous return

Discussion

The correct answer is **C**. The most common cardiac manifestations of CRS are patent ductus arteriosus and peripheral pulmonic stenosis.

Which of the following is the most common manifestation of CRS?
A. Hepatosplenomegaly
B. Purpura
C. Glaucoma
D. Sensorineural hearing loss

Discussion

The correct answer is **D**. All of the above are manifestations of CRS. Sensorineural hearing loss is the most common abnormality and occurs in up to 58% of affected neonates. It is the sole manifestation of CRS in approximately 40% of these neonates. Hearing loss can be unilateral or bilateral and may not manifest until the second year of life. It is important to provide appropriate counseling to parents that the infant needs follow-up audiological assessments.

You recommend measles, mumps, and rubella (MMR) vaccination to a patient. She has never had vaccination and does not recall having measles, mumps, or rubella diagnosed as a child. Testing shows no evidence of rubella immunity. She asks you about the risks of receiving MMR and plans to be pregnant in the future.

In regard to the MMR vaccine, you tell her
A. If she receives the vaccine and is pregnant, she should plan for termination of pregnancy due to the high risk of congenital malformations
B. She should have a pregnancy test before receiving the vaccine due to the risk of CRS
C. If she receives the vaccine, she should wait 28 days before becoming pregnant due to the theoretical risk of fetal infection
D. MMR vaccination is contraindicated if she lives with someone with a primary immunodeficiency

Discussion

The correct answer is **C**. Rubella is a component of MMR vaccination and is not recommend for pregnant women due to the theoretical risk of CRS. However, if the vaccine is given by mistake or pregnancy occurs within 28 days of receipt of the vaccination, termination of pregnancy is not indicated based on data from the CDC database, Vaccines in Pregnancy (VIP), which shows that only 1% to 2% of infants whose mothers received MMR during pregnancy had laboratory evidence of infection, and none of the infants had associated congenital malformations. The Advisory Committee on Immunization Practices (ACIP) does not recommend routine laboratory pregnancy screening for women before receiving the rubella vaccine, but women should be asked whether they are pregnant or will likely be pregnant in the 28 days following the date of vaccination.

MMR vaccination is not contraindicated in this setting. MMR vaccination is contraindicated in those with anaphylactic reactions to neomycin, with a history of allergic reaction to any component of the vaccine, who are pregnant or may be pregnant within a 28-day time frame, or certain persons with immunosuppressive conditions.

The ACIP recommends that all women of childbearing age receive the MMR vaccine if they do not have evidence of immunity to rubella, history of laboratory confirmed rubella, or documentation of rubella vaccine. Women who do not have acceptable evidence of rubella immunity should have testing for rubella IgG. Rubella IgM testing is not recommended for evidence of immunity as false-positive and long-persisting IgM can occur.

MMR vaccination is recommended for household and close contacts of immunocompromised persons due to the high risk of severe complications associated with measles.

Objectives

1. Recognize clinical signs and symptoms associated with congenital rubella infection
2. Understand risk of associated cardiac malformations in newborns with congenital rubella infection
3. Know long-term complications associated with congenital rubella infection
4. Know recommendations for maternal immunization after a pregnancy affected by congenital rubella infection

CASE 3

A 32-week-gestation infant is born with noticeable anomalies at birth. On his examination you notice limb hypoplasia with linear scarring, microphthalmia, and microcephaly.

Which of the following illnesses did his mother most likely have during her pregnancy?
A. Chickenpox
B. Fever and ulcerations of her buccal mucosa
C. Nonspecific febrile illness
D. HIV
E. *Mycoplasma pneumoniae* pneumonia

Discussion

The preferred answer is **A**. This infant exhibits physical examination findings consistent with congenital varicella syndrome. The incidence of congenital varicella syndrome is 1% to 2% when infection occurs before 20 weeks' gestation. Fetal infection with varicella can lead to death or congenital varicella syndrome, characterized by limb and muscle hypoplasia that may mimic amniotic band syndrome, cutaneous scarring, eye abnormalities, and CNS damage. Typically, infection is asymptomatic, and the infant may develop zoster early in life without having extrauterine manifestations of varicella. Infants, who have varicella embryopathy but no evidence of active lesions, do not need isolation.

You are asked to evaluate a 2-day-old infant. Her mother had contact with a person with chickenpox about 2 weeks ago, and she has started to notice a generalized, pruritic vesicular rash. The infant is well appearing and afebrile.

When is an infant at highest risk for death due to varicella?
A. 5 days prior to delivery
B. 2 days after delivery
C. 5 days prior to delivery and 2 days after delivery
D. Same for any time period due to the presence of maternal antibodies

Discussion

The correct answer is **C**. Infants with varicella infection are more likely to die if the mother develops varicella infection from 5 days before to 2 days after delivery because of the lack of time to develop and transfer antibody from the mother to the infant, the infant's immature cellular immunity, and direct viral inoculation.

If maternal disease occurs more than 5 days prior to delivery, varicella-specific IgG antibody will be produced which will decrease the severity of disease in the newborn. If however, the infant is premature (<28 weeks) they would not have the benefit of transplacental transfer of maternal antibody.

What is the appropriate therapy for this infant?
A. Acyclovir
B. Intravenous immune globulin
C. Acyclovir and intravenous immune globulin
D. Foscarnet
E. No therapy since the infant does not have evidence of disease

Discussion

The correct answer is **B**. This infant has been exposed to varicella and is at high risk for death associated with varicella. Most infants who are exposed to varicella within this high-risk period are usually initially well appearing. Varicella-zoster immune globulin (VariZIG) if available or IVIG should be given. Prior to the use of varicella-specific immune globulin, about 17% to 30% of newborns born to mothers with varicella developed severe disease, and the risk of death was 31% if a neonate was born to a mother with onset of rash up to 4 days prior to delivery. If the infant develops vesicular lesions, he should be started on intravenous acyclovir.

Objectives

1. Recognize clinical signs and symptoms associated with congenital varicella infection
2. Understand associated morbidity and mortality risks
3. Understand recommended evaluation and treatment of neonate with congenital varicella

CASE 4

A 3-week-old, 27-week gestation male is being cared for in your neonatal intensive care unit. He is currently on a mechanical ventilator due to respiratory failure, had multiple surgeries for necrotizing enterocolitis, and is requiring total parenteral nutrition. Due to his critical status, he is requiring peripheral and central lines. Overall, he has been improving, but for the past 4 days, he had temperature instability, required increasing respiratory and cardiovascular support for hypotension. A lumbar puncture could not be performed because the infant was clinically unstable. *Citrobacter koseri* is identified in the blood culture.

What additional investigation should the patient undergo?
A. Computed tomography of the head with contrast
B. Computed tomography of the abdomen with contrast
C. Lumbar puncture when stable
D. Echocardiogram
E. A and C

Discussion

The correct answer is **E**. The patient has sepsis due to *C. koseri*. Over half of infants with *Citrobacter* septicemia have meningitis, and >80% of those with meningitis may have one or more brain abscesses (Fig. 11-3). Overt signs of meningitis may not be present. Other gram-negative bacilli such as *Cronobacter sakazakii*, *Serratia marcescens*, and *Salmonella spp.* may also cause meningitis and brain abscesses. *Citrobacter* may be vertically or horizontally acquired. Oftentimes, the source of the infection is unclear. Even with appropriate intervention, about 30% of children with *Citrobacter* meningitis will die, and about 50% of survivors will have CNS sequelae.

The most appropriate empiric therapy for this patient is
A. Ampicillin
B. Gentamicin
C. Meropenem
D. Piperacillin/tazobactam
E. Ampicillin and gentamicin

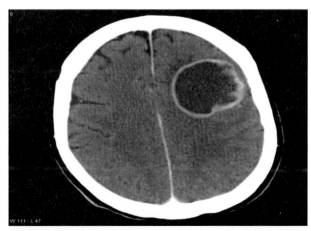

FIGURE 11-3. CNS Abscess secondary to *Citrobacter* infection.

Discussion

The correct answer is **C**. *C. koseri* is resistant to ampicillin. Many species of Citrobacter harbor beta-lactamases that are not inactivated by beta-lactamase inhibitors such as clavulanate and tazobactam. Treatment options include a third-generation cephalosporin plus an aminoglycoside or a carbapenem, such as meropenem. In addition, if an abscess is present, neurosurgical evaluation for possible drainage is important.

CASE 5

A 4-day-old, 35-week gestation infant presents to your emergency department for complaints of fever and decreased activity. On examination, his temperature is 39°C, and he is lethargic and grunting. He is intubated in the ED and receives fluid resuscitation. Blood, CSF, and urine cultures are sent. Complete blood count (CBC) and CSF studies are normal. Aspartate aminotransferase (AST) is 412 IU/L and alanine aminotransferase (ALT) is 456 IU/L. He is started on ampicillin, cefotaxime, and acyclovir. The child continues to do poorly despite aggressive management. Blood, urine, and CSF cultures are negative. HSV PCR from CSF and serum and HSV cultures from skin and mucosa are negative. Upon further discussion with his mother, you learn that around the time of delivery, she had a "head cold." In addition, several members of the household had fever and rash several days prior to the mother's illness. There were no complications during pregnancy or during delivery. The infant was in the neonatal intensive care unit for 2 days.

The most likely cause of this infant's illness is
A. Group B streptococcus
B. Enterovirus
C. Parvovirus B19
D. *Listeria monocytogenes*
E. *Escherichia coli*

Discussion

The correct answer is **B**. In the setting of culture negative sepsis in the neonate, HSV and enterovirus should be considered. In this scenario, the mother and the children of the household exhibit symptoms of a viral infection likely attributable to enterovirus. Enterovirus may be acquired antenatally, intrapartum, or postnatally. Clinical presentations range from asymptomatic disease to sepsis. Common symptoms include fever, lethargy, irritability,

and poor feeding. Rash is nonspecific and may be present in half of infants. Although most infants with enterovirus infection do not present with severe disease, risk factors for severe disease include prematurity, maternal symptoms around the time of birth, onset of symptoms within the first week of life, and absence of serotype-specific antibodies. Complications include myocarditis, hepatitis, hepatic failure, and death. Enteroviruses can be detected through a variety of methods including PCR and culture from clinical specimens. PCR assays for enterovirus RNA are commercially available and are more rapid and sensitive than cell culture. In this scenario, blood and CSF PCR may help establish the diagnosis.

CASE 6

A full-term 2-week-old male presents to your emergency department for fever. He was born via normal spontaneous vaginal delivery and stayed in the newborn nursery for 2 days. His mother was GBS positive and received one dose of penicillin prior to delivery. His mother states that he has not been feeding as well and seems to be sleepier than usual. There are no obvious abnormalities on his physical examination. Blood culture, urine culture, and CSF cultures are sent. He is started on ampicillin and cefotaxime and admitted to the NICU. A Gram stain from his blood and CSF show a Gram-negative rod.

The most likely organism is
A. *E. coli*
B. Group B streptococcus
C. *L. monocytogenes*
D. *Haemophilus influenzae*
E. *Neisseria meningitidis*

Discussion

The correct answer is **A**. *E. coli* is an enteric gram-negative rod, and strains with K1 capsular polysaccharide antigen cause approximately 40% of *E. coli* bacteremia and 80% of *E. coli* meningitis. The patient likely acquired this bacterium through the maternal genital tract. Although *H. influenzae* is a gram-negative rod, meningitis caused by *E. coli* is more common in this age group. Other common early-onset sepsis pathogens in the neonate include Group B streptococcus, a gram-positive coccus, *L. monocytogenes*, a gram-positive rod, and *N. meningitidis*, a gram-negative coccobacillus.

CASE 7

You receive a call from a physician that would like your guidance. He is seeing a 3-day-old, 35-week gestation female who is currently hospitalized in the neonatal intensive care unit for fever and pneumonia. She has not left the hospital since the time of her birth. Her mother recalls having a flu-like illness about 2 to 3 days prior to delivery. The infant currently has organisms resembling "diphtheroids" on Gram stain from the blood. Blood culture results are pending. The physician wonders if this represents skin contamination.

You advise him
A. Skin contamination is common in blood cultures, and the child likely has a viral pneumonia
B. "Diphtheroids" may be confused with *Listeria monocytogenes*, and antibiotics should be continued until culture results are known
C. "Diphtheroids" may be confused with *Escherichia coli*, and antibiotics should be continued until culture results are known
D. "Diphtheroids" may be confused with group B streptococcus, and antibiotics should be continued until culture results are known
E. *Corynebacterium diphtheriae* is a common cause of neonatal meningitis, and sequelae may be devastating if the infection is untreated

Discussion

The correct answer is **B**. *Listeria monocytogenes* is gram-positive bacillus that may be confused with other gram-positive organisms that are usually skin contaminants such as *Bacillus* and *Corynebacterium*. Listeriosis is usually food borne, and foods such as unpasteurized milk, dairy products, soft cheeses, deli meat, smoked or cured fish, undercooked poultry, unwashed raw vegetables, and melons and fruit salads may be implicated in transmission. About 65% of mothers will report a flu-like illness prior to the diagnosis of listeriosis in the infant. Clinical syndromes are divided into early-onset (<1 week of age) and late-onset disease. Early-onset disease typically suggests transplacental acquisition or less commonly, ascending infection. Manifestations include prematurity, sepsis, and pneumonia. In severe early-onset infection, a papular, erythematous rash with granulomas on histology known as "granulomatosis infantisepticum" may be present. Late-onset infection is usually acquired through the birth canal or from the external environment and may manifest as meningitis. Cephalosporins are not active against *Listeria*, and the treatment of choice is ampicillin plus an aminoglycoside.

CASE 8

A 26-year-old G3P2 woman, who did not receive prenatal care, delivers a 24-week gestation male neonate in your hospital. The infant's initial examination is notable for lack of spontaneous breathing, hypotonia, and anasarca. Cardiopulmonary resuscitation (CPR) is initiated, and the child is intubated in the delivery room. He is transferred to the NICU for ventilatory and cardiovascular support. Chest x-ray shows cardiomegaly and diffuse pulmonary edema. Twenty-four hours later, the infant dies. His mother reports that during the end of her first trimester, she had aching of her hands and feet. Her other children had fever and rash that resolved around the time of the mother's illness.

The most likely causative agent of this infant's illness is
A. Parvovirus B19
B. HIV
C. Rubella
D. Group B streptococcus
E. Syphilis

Discussion

The correct answer is **A**. Although all of the above infections may cause fetal and neonatal death, this presentation of heart failure and hydrops is most consistent with congenital parvovirus B19 infection. The mother and her children had symptoms of parvovirus infection during the first trimester of her pregnancy. About 65% of women in North America have serologic evidence of past parvovirus infection, and the incidence of acute parvovirus infection in pregnancy is about 1% to 2%. Symptoms of maternal parvovirus B19 infection include rash, fever, and arthralgia. Risk of fetal transmission is 30% and is highest at the peak of viremia (about 7 days into illness), but most fetal infections are asymptomatic. Infection may result in severe anemia, edema, congestive heart failure, myocarditis, and death. The risk of fetal hydrops is up to 12.5% in those who are infected with the peak incidence occurring at 17 to 24 weeks' gestation. Risk of fetal death is about 2% to 6%, and occurs mainly between 20 and 24 weeks' gestation. Fetal death rarely occurs if maternal infection is beyond the first half of pregnancy.

The most appropriate therapy for this patient is
A. Ribavirin
B. Foscarnet
C. Intravenous immune globulin
D. Supportive care
E. Exchange transfusion

Discussion

The correct answer is **D**. No specific parvovirus-directed therapy is available, and management is supportive care. Intrauterine transfusion can correct fetal anemia and may reduce the risk of intrauterine death.

Objectives—Cases 4–8

1. Recognize common clinical presentations of newborns with various viral and bacterial infection
2. Understand appropriate diagnostic evaluation of a newborn with suspected sepsis
3. Identify common pathogens that cause early-onset and late-onset sepsis in the newborn
4. Identify conditions known to increase the risk for sepsis in the newborn

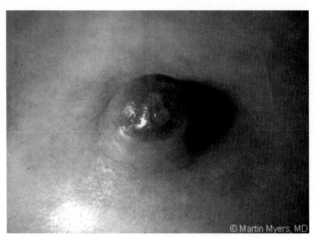

FIGURE 11-4. Omphalitis. (Used with permission of Dr. Martin G. Myers.)

CASE 9

A 9-day-old 33-week gestation female who was born to a G3P2 mother presents to your emergency room for evaluation of fever and decreased oral intake. The birth was notable for persistent fetal decelerations that required an emergency cesarean section. APGARs were 9 and 9 at 1 and 5 minutes, respectively. The infant was admitted to the neonatal intensive care unit for 7 days and received a 7-day course of ampicillin and gentamicin. She was doing well until the day of presentation. On physical examination, you notice that the child is limp and grunting. Abdominal examination shows intact umbilical stump with mild malodorous discharge and surrounding erythema.

The most appropriate course of action is

A. Ask mother if she has obtained her Tdap vaccination during pregnancy since the child has symptoms consistent with tetanus
B. Obtain surgical consult, blood culture, and start broad-spectrum antibiotic therapy
C. Apply topical silver nitrate since the infant likely has an umbilical granuloma
D. Prescribe topical antibiotic ointment to apply to the umbilical stump until the discharge is resolved
E. Inquire further about umbilical cord care and educate the mother

Discussion

The correct answer is **B**. This child is septic and has evidence of omphalitis (infection of the umbilicus) (Fig. 11-4). Symptoms typically start at about 3 days of age. Although

rare, with an incidence of about 0.2%, infants who are of low birth weight and have complicated deliveries are at higher risk of developing omphalitis. Blood culture and culture of the umbilicus are helpful in isolating an organism.

Staphylococcus aureus is the most commonly isolated organism followed by gram-negative rods and anaerobes. Empiric therapy should cover a broad range of organisms and can be narrowed based on culture results. Complications of omphalitis include necrotizing fasciitis, small bowel obstruction, evisceration of the small bowel through the umbilicus, peritonitis, and abscesses.

A 6-week-old infant is diagnosed with omphalitis. You notice that the umbilical stump is still intact and there is minimal erythema surrounding the cord. Her white count is 110,000 with 90% neutrophils.

The most likely underlying disorder is

A. Chronic granulomatous disease
B. Wiskott–Aldrich syndrome
C. Leukocyte adhesion defect
D. Cyclic neutropenia
E. Bruton agammaglobulinemia

Discussion

The correct answer is **C**. Delayed separation of the umbilical cord and omphalitis are usually the first symptoms of leukocyte adhesion defect type 1 (LAD 1). LAD 1 is an autosomal recessive disorder of the gene that encodes for CD 18 on the neutrophil, which is important in adhesion to the endothelium and subsequent migration to infected tissues. Affected patients typically have recurrent bacterial infections, especially of the skin and mucosal surfaces. *S. aureus* and gram-negative enteric bacteria are the most commonly isolated organisms. In acute infections, neutrophil counts are usually greater than 100,000 cells/mL, but because they are not able to migrate to the site of infection, there is no pus formation leading to "cold abscesses." Those who survive infancy have problems with severe gingivitis and periodontitis.

Objectives

1. Recognize the typical clinical presentation of a neonate with omphalitis
2. Know the most likely organisms that cause omphalitis
3. Identify potential underlying conditions that may increase the risk for developing omphalitis

CASE 10

A 28-year-old G3P1 HIV positive mother delivers a 38-week gestation 3,500-g male via spontaneous vaginal delivery. APGARs are 9 at 1 minute and 9 at 5 minutes. The mother's HIV RNA level (viral load) was undetectable and CD4 count was 600 cells/mm³ prior to delivery. Mom received highly active antiretroviral therapy (HAART) during her pregnancy, and her reported adherence is 100%.

Which of the following HIV drug regimens should the infant receive
A. Zidovudine and trimethoprim/sulfamethoxazole (for *Pneumocystis jirovecii* prophylaxis)
B. Zidovudine and nevirapine
C. Zidovudine, nevirapine, and stavudine
D. Zidovudine only
E. No therapy since the risk of mother to child transmission is minimal in this scenario

Discussion

The correct answer is **D**. Prevention of mother to child transmission (PMTCT) of HIV infection involves several important mechanisms. First, HAART, regardless of the mother's viral load, has been shown to reduce risk of transmission. Administration of antiretrovirals at the time of delivery is important in achieving adequate systemic levels of drug in infants during passage through the birth canal, where there is high level of exposure to maternal genital tract virus. Lastly, infant postexposure prophylaxis protects from virus that may have entered the infant's circulation through maternal-fetal transfusion during delivery or from swallowed virus through the genital tract. In this mother, who had undetectable viral load and received HAART during pregnancy, the risk of transmission to the infant is very low (<2%). In this scenario, postexposure prophylaxis with zidovudine is most appropriate as

recommended by the Department of Health and Human Services Panel on Treatment of HIV-Infected Pregnant Women and the Prevention of Perinatal Transmission, a working group of the Office of AIDS Research Advisory Council guidelines (http://aidsinfo.nih.gov/guidelines). HIV DNA or RNA PCR should be tested at the first 14 to 21 days, 1 to 2 months, and 4 to 6 months of age. DNA PCR is preferred for infants on combination ARV prophylaxis or preemptive treatment. HIV antibody testing in the infant would reflect maternal HIV status and should not be used to confirm HIV infection until 18 months of age. For most up to date recommendations for management for maternal exposure prophylaxis, please refer to: http://aidsinfo.nih.gov/guidelines.

How long should this infant receive zidovudine?
A. Until 18 months of age when HIV antibodies are tested
B. 1 week
C. 6 weeks
D. 12 weeks
E. Until HIV DNA PCR is negative

Discussion

The correct answer is **C**. Zidovudine postexposure prophylaxis at doses appropriate for gestation age is generally recommended for 6 weeks. Therapy should be initiated within 6 to 12 hours of birth. A 4-week chemoprophylaxis course can be considered if the mother has received standard combination antiretroviral therapy, has had consistent viral suppression, and there are no concerns about her adherence.

Which of the following is a common side effect of zidovudine?
A. Microcytic anemia
B. Macrocytic anemia
C. Normocytic anemia
D. Anagen effluvium
E. Constipation

Discussion

The correct response is **B**. Typically, infant prophylaxis with zidovudine is associated with minimal toxicity, but may cause significant bone marrow suppression including macrocytic anemia and neutropenia. Macrocytic anemia is most commonly seen and usually resolves by 12 weeks of age. Other side effects include myositis, lactic acidosis, and hepatomegaly. A baseline CBC should be obtained in newborns. Decisions regarding monitoring CBCs are based on baseline hematologic values, gestational age, clinical condition, dose of zidovudine administered, receipt of other antiretroviral drugs and other medications, and maternal antepartum therapy.

Note: The discussion of the following scenarios is based on information up to date as of May 7, 2014. HIV management is an active area of research and recommendations for treatment and prevention are frequently updated. Please refer to the AIDSinfo website for the most current guidelines: http://aidsinfo.nih.gov/guidelines.

CASE 11

A 28-year-old G3P1 HIV positive mother delivers a 38-week gestation 3,500-g male via cesarean section. Rupture of membranes was at the time of delivery. APGARs are 9 at 1 minute and 9 at 5 minutes. The mother's HIV RNA level (viral load) and CD4 are unknown at delivery, and she did not receive antiretroviral therapy during her pregnancy. She received IV zidovudine during delivery.

Which of the following HIV drug regimens should the infant receive?

A. Zidovudine and trimethoprim/sulfamethoxazole (for *P. jirovecii* prophylaxis)

B. Zidovidune and nevirapine

C. Zidovudine, nevirapine, and stavudine

D. Zidovudine only

E. No therapy since the risk of mother to child transmission is minimal in this scenario

Discussion

The correct answer is **B**. This mother's viral load was unknown at the time of delivery. In addition to C section delivery as recommended for women with unknown viral load or viral load >1,000 copies/mL, the child should receive HIV postexposure prophylaxis. An international study, NICHD-HPTN 040/P1043, showed that formula-fed infants whose mothers did not receive antepartum HAART had approximately 50% decreased risk of intrapartum HIV transmission if they received 6 weeks of combination prophylaxis (zidovudine and nevirapine or zidovudine, lamivudine, and nelfinavir) than if they received zidovudine alone. However, the three-drug regimen is associated with greater toxicity than the two-drug regimen and is not currently recommended. This patient should receive zidovudine for 6 weeks and three doses of nevirapine (first dose at birth to 48 hours of life, second dose 48 hours after first dose, and third dose 96 hours after second dose) (Table 11-2).

TABLE 11-2. **Treatment Recommendations for HIV-Exposed Infants**

ALL HIV-EXPOSED INFANTS (INITIATED AS SOON AFTER DELIVERY AS POSSIBLE)		
ZIDOVUDINE	DOSING	DURATION
Zidovudine	≥35 weeks' gestation at birth: 4 mg/kg/dose PO twice daily, started as soon after birth as possible and preferably within 6–12 h of delivery (or, if unable to tolerate oral agents, 3 mg/kg/dose IV, beginning within 6–12 h of delivery, then every 12 h)	Birth through 4–6 weeks[a]
Zidovudine	≥30 weeks to <35 weeks' gestation at birth: 2 mg/kg/dose PO (or 1.5 mg/kg/dose IV), started as soon after birth as possible, preferably within 6–12 h of delivery, then every 12 h, advanced to 3 mg/kg/dose PO (or 2.3 mg/kg/dose IV) every 12 h at age 15 days	Birth through 6 weeks
Zidovudine	<30 weeks' gestation at birth: 2 mg/kg body weight/dose PO (ot 1.5 mg/kg/dose IV) started as soon after birth as possible preferably within 6–12 h of delivery, then every 12 h, advanced to 3 mg/kg/dose PO (or 2.3 mg/kg/dose IV) every 12 h after age 4 weeks	Birth through 6 weeks
Additional antiretroviral prophylaxis agents for HIV-exposed infants of women who received no antepartum antiretroviral prophylaxis (initiated as soon after delivery as possible)		
In addition to zidovudine as shown above, administer NVP	Birth weight 1.5–2 kg: 8 mg/dose PO Birth weight >2 kg: 12 mg/dose PO	Three doses in the first week of life • First dose within 48 h of birth (birth-48 h) • Second dose 48 h after first • Third dose 96 h after second

[a]Six weeks is generally recommended. A 4-week zidovudine chemoprophylaxis regimen may be considered when the mother has received standard antiretroviral therapy during pregnancy with consistent viral suppression and there are no concerns related to maternal adherence. (Reproduced with permission from AidsInfo. Recommendations for Use of Antiretroviral Drugs in Pregnant HIV-1-Infected Women for Maternal Health and Interventions to Reduce Perinatal HIV Transmission in the United States.)

Objectives

1. Understand the risk of mother to child transmission of the HIV virus
2. Understand appropriate treatment recommendations for infants at risk of perinatal HIV transmission
3. Know side effects of commonly prescribed medications for HIV-exposed newborns

CASE 12

An infant is born at 34 weeks' gestation and is admitted to the NICU for prematurity. APGARs are 8 at 1 minute and 9 at 5 minutes, and the infant weighs 2.2 kg. Maternal laboratories are notable for rubella nonimmune and hepatitis B antibody positive.

Which of the following vaccines is recommended at this time?
A. Rubella
B. HiB
C. Rotavirus
D. Hepatitis B
E. Diphtheria, tetanus, acellular pertussis

Discussion

The correct answer is **D**. Hepatitis B vaccine is recommended for all infants at birth weighing >2 kg, regardless of mother's antibody status. MMR is a live vaccine that is generally given after 12 months, and should be given to the mother at this time as she is rubella nonimmune. Rotavirus, DTaP, and HiB are not indicated for infants less than 6 weeks of age.

CASE 13

A full-term gestation infant is born to a G1P0 mother who is hepatitis B surface antigen (HBsAg) positive. She did not receive prenatal care during her pregnancy. The infant's alanine aminotransferase (ALT) is 24 IU/L and aspartate aminotransferase (AST) 22 IU/L. You are called by your resident for advice.

You advise him
A. Because acute hepatitis B virus (HBV) infection in infants rarely leads to chronic infection no intervention except routine HBV vaccination is needed
B. Perinatal transmission of HBV is rare, and no intervention except routine hepatitis HBV is needed
C. Because the infant is at high risk for acquiring HBV infection, he should receive HBV vaccination
D. Because the infant is at high risk for acquiring hepatitis B infection, he should receive HBV vaccination and hepatitis B immune globulin (HBIG)
E. The infant should be carefully monitored. If within 12 hours, the transaminases begin to rise, he should receive HBIG in addition to HBV vaccination

Discussion

The correct answer is **D**. The risk of perinatal transmission is highest when the mother's HBsAg and Hepatitis e antigen (HBeAg) are both positive. Without postexposure prophylaxis, transmission occurs in approximately 70% to 90% of infants. Risk of transmission is 5% to 20% for infants born to HBsAg-positive, HBeAg-negative mothers. Children who acquire HBV perinatally usually have normal ALT, detectable HBeAg, and high HBV DNA for years to decades, which is known as the immune tolerant phase. Prophylaxis with HBIG and HBV vaccine within 12 hours of life can prevent 95% of transmissions.

What percentage of infants (perinatal or <1 year of age) with acute HBV infection will develop chronic HBV infection?
A. More than 90%
B. 50% to 75%
C. 25% to 50%
D. 5% to 10%
E. Less than 1%

Discussion

The correct answer is **A**. Ninety percent of infants with acute HBV infection will develop chronic infection. The risk for chronic infection decreases with age: 25% to 50% of children 1 to 5 years of age will develop chronic infection, and 5% to 10% of older children and adults will develop chronic infection.

CASE 14

An infant in your newborn nursery is born to a mother with chronic hepatitis C virus (HCV) infection. Her HCV RNA at the time of delivery was detectable. She is HIV and hepatitis B negative. She is concerned about the risk of HCV transmission to her child.

You advise her that

A. The risk of perinatal transmission is about 95% and the child should receive HCV immune globulin. Anti-HCV antibody testing should be done at 18 months.

B. The risk of perinatal transmission is about 5%, and the child should receive HCV immune globulin. Anti-HCV antibody testing should be done at 18 months.

C. The risk of perinatal transmission is about 5%, and the child should be tested at 18 months for anti-HCV antibody. Nucleic acid amplification can be done at 1 to 2 months to test for the presence of HCV RNA.

D. The risk of perinatal transmission is about 95% and the child should be tested at 18 months for anti-HCV antibody. Nucleic acid amplification can be done at 1 to 2 months to test for the presence of HCV RNA.

Discussion

The correct answer is **C**. The risk of perinatal transmission is 5% when a mother's HCV RNA is detectable. The infant should have testing done after 18 months for the presence of anti-HCV since maternal antibody may persist. If detected, the patient should be referred to a hepatitis specialist for possible antiviral treatment and clinical monitoring. If desired, nucleic acid amplification testing (NAAT) to detect HCV RNA can be performed at 1 to 2 months of age.

CASE 15

You receive a call from a local pediatrician regarding a hepatitis A virus (HAV) outbreak at daycare that started 1 week ago. This patient is a healthy 6-week-old, and her mother is a daycare worker at the center and she tested positive for HAV IgM. The pediatrician would like your advice regarding prophylaxis for the infant.

You advise her that

A. The infant did not attend the daycare and is not at high risk of HAV infection

B. Since HAV does not cause fulminant liver disease and does not lead to chronic infection, no prophylaxis is needed

C. The infant should receive a dose of HAV vaccination. This vaccine will not count toward the two that is recommended at 12 months and 4 years of age

D. The infant should receive a dose of immune globulin

E. The infant should undergo antibody testing for HAV, and if positive, she should receive a dose of immune globulin

Discussion

The correct answer is **D**. All unimmunized close personal contacts of persons with serologically confirmed HAV infection should receive vaccine or immune globulin within 2 weeks after the most recent exposure. Since the infant is less than 12 months, she should receive HAV IG. If more than 2 weeks have elapsed since the time of exposure, no prophylaxis is indicated. Serologic testing of contacts is not recommended since prophylaxis may be delayed, and there is unnecessary added cost.

Objectives—Cases 12–15

1. Understand the risk of perinatal transmission in Hepatitis A, Hepatitis B, or Hepatitis C

2. Recognize appropriate treatment guidelines for newborns at risk for perinatal transmission of Hepatitis A, Hepatitis B, or Hepatitis C infection

3. Understand how treatment guidelines are modified based on maternal disease status

CASE 16

A 4-week-old, 29-week gestation male presents to his pediatrician's office in December for evaluation. He has had a cough and runny nose for about 3 to 4 days, and on the day of presentation, he started to have trouble breathing. Sick contacts include mom, dad, and a 4-year-old brother with runny nose and cough. On physical examination, temperature is 37.5°F, heart rate 150, respiratory rate 70, and SpO$_2$ at room air is 90%. There is mild nasal flaring, rhinorrhea, and subcostal retractions. On auscultation, there is diffuse wheezing and crackles.

The most likely cause of this patient's illness is
A. *Streptococcus pneumoniae*
B. Respiratory syncytial virus (RSV)
C. Group B streptococcus (GBS)
D. *M. pneumoniae*
E. *Chlamydia trachomatis*

Discussion

The correct answer is **B**. This patient exhibits signs and symptoms of bronchiolitis. RSV is a common cause of bronchiolitis. Other etiologic agents include parainfluenza, influenza, and human metapneumovirus. Most infants have been infected with RSV during the first year of life, and almost all infants have been infected by the second year of life. Although most RSV infections are mild, about 1% to 3% of children within the first year of life will have lower respiratory tract disease. Chlamydial pneumonia may also present with similar symptoms, but congestion or runny nose would not be expected.

The infant is being admitted to the hospital due to tachypnea and hypoxia.

In addition to standard precautions for the hospitalized patient, what other precautions should be in place?
A. Contact
B. Contact and droplet
C. Airborne
D. Contact and airborne
E. Droplet

Discussion

The correct answer is **A**. Contact precautions are recommended for RSV isolation. Transmission of RSV is usually by direct or close contact with secretions (i.e., large particle droplets at distances usually <3 ft and fomites. Parents of all high risk infants should be advised to adhere to strict handwashing policies, particularly during RSV season. There is regional variability for the peak timing and duration of RSV. Pediatricians should be aware of their local environment and/or reference local or national infectious disease surveillance agencies for these data.

This infant has received two previous Synagis injections this winter. The parent asks if he should continue to receive additional injections until the end of RSV season in the community.

How should advise the parents?
A. The child should continue to receive additional Synagis injections throughout the rest of the RSV season

B. The dosage should be increased since the child developed Synagis infection despite the two previous injections
C. The child should not receive additional Synagis doses this year
D. The number of recommended doses increases since the child developed RSV bronchiolitis despite having received Synagis immunization

Discussion

The correct answer is **C**. Guidelines for Synagis prophylaxis were updated in July 2014. These revised guidelines changed the previous recommendation to continue to administer Synagis doses to children who develop RSV disease. The revised guidelines state that no additional doses should be administered due to the very low risk of a second RSV rehospitalization during the same season (<0.5%). All preterm infants <29 weeks are eligible to receive RSV prophylaxis if they are <12 months old at the start of the RSV season. Children with chronic lung disease can be considered for Synagis immunization if they remained on supplemental oxygen >28 days after birth. All infants should receive a maximum of five doses during the RSV season at the standard dosage of 15 mg/kg.

Which of the following is an indication for giving this infant prophylaxis with palivizumab?
A. Infant born in August, the year prior to the onset of this RSV season
B. Infant with a 3-year-old sibling at home
C. Parents plan to send the infant to daycare
D. Patient has a known atrial septal defect
E. Patient has chronic lung disease, treated with diuretics

Discussion

The correct answer is **E**. Palivizumab, a humanized mouse monoclonal antibody is licensed for the prevention of RSV hospitalizations in infants who are at high risk. According to the Red Book, preterm infants 29 and 0 days gestation are eligible to receive a maximum of five doses of palivizumab prophylaxis if they are <12 months old at the start of RSV season. Other infants considered to be at risk for RSV infection are those with chronic lung disease (defined as <32 weeks' gestation and requiring oxygen with $FIO_2 >$ 21% at 36 weeks postconceptual age, bronchodilator, chronic steroid therapy, or diuretic use), therapy (supplemental oxygen, bronchodilator, diuretic, chronic corticosteroid therapy), infants less than 12 months of age with hemodynamically significant congenital heart disease (requiring medication to control congestive heart failure, moderate-to-severe pulmonary hypertension, cyanotic heart disease), and infants with neuromuscular disease or congenital abnormalities of the airway. The time initiation of palivizumab prophylaxis for infants and young children with chronic lung disease of prematurity or congenital heart disease varies by geographic location. The earliest date for initiation of the 5 monthly doses of palivizumab for southeast Florida is July 1, north central and southwest Florida is September 15, and most other areas of the United States is November 1.

CASE 17

Mrs. Jones delivers a 2,800-g male infant with Down syndrome at 35 weeks' gestation on Thanksgiving day. Baby Boy Jones has a cardiac echocardiogram which reveals a secundum atrial septal defect. He does not have any evidence of congestive heart failure and remains on room air throughout his hospitalization. He is not being treated with any diuretics or medications for his heart disease. As you prepare for discharge, the resident asks you if Baby Boy Jones should receive Synagis prophylaxis.

How should you reply to the resident?
A. Baby Boy Jones should receive Synagis prophylaxis because he has Down syndrome
B. Baby Boy Jones should receive Synagis prophylaxis because he has hemodynamically significant congenital heart disease
C. Baby Boy Jones should receive Synagis prophylaxis because he was born premature at 35 weeks' gestation
D. Baby Boy Jones does not meet criteria to receive Synagis prophylaxis

Discussion

The correct answer is **D**. In 2014, the AAP Committee on Infectious Diseases and Bronchiolitis Guidelines updated recommendations for prophylaxis with palivizumab. Immunoprophylaxis is not routinely recommended for children with Down syndrome unless they meet criteria based on preterm gestation <29 weeks or having hemodynamically significant congenital heart disease. Baby Boy Jones has an ASD but has no clinical signs or symptoms suggesting congestive heart failure. He does not have chronic lung disease. Children with asymptomatic atrial septal defects no longer meet criteria for palivizumab.

Helpful Hint: Policy Update: Change in AAP Guidance for Use of Synagis Prophylaxis. The AAP has published a new <u>policy statement</u> and <u>technical report</u>, "Updated Guidance for Palivizumab Prophylaxis Among Infants and Young Children at Increased Risk of Hospi-

talization for Respiratory Syncytial Virus Infection," in the August 2014 issue of *Pediatrics*.

This policy statement and technical report provides updated evidence-based guidance for the use of palivizumab prophylaxis based on new evidence and review of older published literature regarding RSV seasonality, infants at greatest risk of hospitalization, and the pharmacokinetics of palivizumab. Major points of revision include:

• Palivizumab prophylaxis is recommended for infants born at less than 29 weeks' gestation
• Infants with chronic lung disease qualify for prophylaxis only if they require supplemental oxygen for more than 28 days after birth
• With rare exception as defined in this policy statement, prophylaxis is not recommended during the second year of life
• Monthly prophylaxis should be discontinued in any infant or young child who experiences a breakthrough RSV hospitalization

Objectives

1. Understand clinical presentation for RSV bronchiolitis
2. Know guidelines for RSV prophylaxis for preterm infants
3. Know special circumstances for consideration for RSV prophylaxis

CASE 18

You attend the delivery of a 3.8-kg male born at 39 weeks to a healthy 20 G1P0 mother with no relevant medical history. Maternal laboratories, including HIV, RPR, hepatitis B, Rubella, and GBS are negative. Thin meconium was present at delivery. The baby is vigorous, cries spontaneously, and is placed in the warmer. After drying the baby, you place erythromycin ointment on both eyelids.

Which of the following is true regarding the use of erythromycin ophthalmic ointment in the newborn period?
A. It prevents the development of gonococcal infections
B. It prevents the development of Chlamydia infections
C. It prevents the development of congenital lacrimal duct stenosis
D. It prevents the development of infection from exposure to meconium
E. It is only needed if maternal gonorrhea or chlamydia testing was positive during pregnancy

Discussion

The correct answer is **A**. Erythromycin ointment is used to prevent the development of neonatal ophthalmia secondary to *Neisseria gonorrhoeae*. Ophthalmia neonatorum refers to conjunctivitis occurring within the first 4 weeks of life. Up to 40% of cases are due to chlamydia, less than 1% of cases are due to gonorrhea, less than 1% of cases are due to HSV, and 30% to 50% are due to other bacterial etiologies. Chlamydia conjunctivitis is associated with the later development of pneumonia, and both HSV and gonorrhea are associated with the development of disseminated disease. In the case of preventing gonococcal infection, either erythromycin 0.5% or tetracycline 1% is used. Both are less likely to cause irritation than silver nitrate. Prophylaxis can be given up to 1 hour after birth in order to be effective. Topical therapy is not effective against the prevention of chlamydia ophthalmia because it does not prevent colonization of the nasopharynx.

Looking back at the mother's chart you notice a positive gonorrhea culture at 32 weeks' gestation, for which mother had not come back for treatment.

What should you do next?
A. Observe the child in the nursery for 7 days for the development of symptoms of disseminated gonococcal infection
B. Administer a dose of ceftriaxone or cefotaxime IM to the infant
C. Perform eye cultures, surface cultures, and LP to screen for infection
D. Do nothing at this time, but warn parents about signs and symptoms of infection
E. Continue topical erythromycin therapy for 7 days to prevent the progression of disease

Discussion

The correct answer is **B**. Healthy infants born to mothers with untreated gonococcal infection should receive one dose of ceftriaxone (25–50 mg/kg IV or IM, with maximum of 125 mg) or one dose of cefotaxime (100 mg/kg IV or IM). Topical antibiotics alone are inadequate to prevent disseminated infection.

The patient is discharged home and presents back to the emergency room at 4 weeks of life with a repetitive cough and tachypnea. The patient is afebrile and is noted to have diffuse rales on examination. There are no signs of nasal congestion. Chest x-ray reveals diffuse patchy infiltrates and hyperinflation.

What is the most likely diagnosis?
A. Disseminated gonococcal infection
B. *Chlamydophila pneumoniae* infection
C. RSV bronchiolitis
D. *C. trachomatis* infection
E. HSV pneumonitis

Discussion

The correct answer is **D**. The patient is presenting with a staccato cough and hyperinflation on chest x-ray, consistent with *C. trachomatis* pneumonia, secondary to nasopharyngeal carriage of infection acquired at delivery. Treatment recommendations are for oral azithromycin for 5 days or oral erythromycin for 14 days. When the diagnosis is confirmed, both the mother and partner should be treated as well.

What is the rate of transmission of chlamydia from an infected mother to a child born vaginally?
A. 10%
B. 25%
C. 50%
D. 75%
E. 100%

Discussion

The correct answer is **C**. There is a 50% risk of transmission from an infected mother to a newborn infant. The risk of conjunctivitis ranges from 25% to 50% of exposed patients, and the risk of pneumonia is 5% to 20%. Transmission can also occur in some infants who are born via cesarean delivery, even with intact membranes.

Objectives

1. Understand common causes on conjunctivitis in the newborn
2. Understand clinical presentation of Chlamydia pneumoniae
3. Understand risk of perinatal transmission associated with maternal chlamydia or gonococcal infection
4. Know recommended evaluation and treatment for newborns with perinatal exposure to chlamydia or gonorrhea infection

CASE 19

A 2-month-old ex–28-week male infant who has not yet received the 2-month vaccines comes for a well child visit in November. He is followed by ophthalmology for retinopathy of prematurity. His only medications include multi vitamin and iron supplementation. He receives monthly palivizumab injections. His current weight is 2.85 kg.

What vaccinations should be administered at this visit?
A. No vaccines until he reaches a corrected age of 2 months
B. Hepatitis B, HiB, DTaP, IPV, PCV-13, and influenza
C. Hepatitis B, HiB, DTaP, IPV, PCV-13
D. Hepatitis B, HiB, DTaP, IPV, PCV-13, rotavirus
E. HiB, DTaP, IPV, PCV-13

Discussion

The correct answer is **D**. Preterm infants less than 37 weeks are vaccinated with the routinely recommended schedule when medically stable. Gestational age and birth weight are not contraindications to vaccinations. Hepatitis B vaccine can be given to all infants weighing >2 kg. Influenza vaccination should be given to infants starting at 6 months of age with two doses 1 month apart. Rotavirus vaccine can be given to premature infants if there is no history of intussusception or GI disease predisposing to intussusception. Rotavirus vaccine administration must be initiated by 15 weeks of age.

Objectives

1. Understand recommendations for routine immunizations during the neonatal period
2. Recognize specific contraindications for the use of specific immunizations during the neonatal period

CASE 20

A mother presents to you at 38 weeks in labor. Upon reviewing her records, you notice that she had a positive RPR titer of 1:64 earlier in pregnancy that was confirmed with a positive FTA-ABS. You see that she had received three doses of IM penicillin 1 week apart during the first trimester. You do not have records of follow-up titers, and you decide to send them.

Assuming the mother was effectively treated, what RPR minimal value would be consistent with serologic evidence of adequate treatment?
A. ≤1:64
B. ≤1:32
C. ≤1:16
D. ≤1:4
E. Nonreactive

Discussion

The correct answer is **C**. Serologic evidence of adequate treatment is defined as a sustained fourfold decrease in titers, which is equivalent to a change in two dilutions (1:64–1:16). This decrease usually occurs within 6 to 12 months of treatment, and seronegativity usually occurs within 2 years of treatment; however, some patients can have persistently low, stable titers after adequate treatment (RPR less than or equal to 1:4).

The child is born via normal spontaneous vaginal delivery without complications. There are no physical examination abnormalities. Mom's RPR titer is 1:64 and the infant's titer is 1:64.

What should be done next?
A. Measurement of infant FTA-ABS for confirmation
B. Treatment with one dose of Penicillin IM to the infant
C. Evaluation of the infant, including CBC, platelet count, CSF examination for VDRL, long-bone radiography
D. Observation of the infant for development of snuffles
E. The patient can be discharged because physical examination is normal

Discussion

The correct answer is **C**. Because maternal titers are unchanged despite treatment, there is evidence of relapse or repeat infection, and therefore, the child should undergo a full evaluation. If both physical examination and full evaluation are normal, the child should receive one dose of benzathine penicillin IM. If there are any abnormalities on evaluation, the child should receive a 10-day course of IV aqueous penicillin to prevent the long-term effects of congenital syphilis (Fig. 11-5).

Which of the following is not associated with congenital syphilis infections?
A. Nonimmune hydrops
B. Hemolytic anemia
C. Pneumonia
D. Clutton joints
E. Congenital cataracts

Discussion

The correct answer is **E**. The clinical presentation of congenital syphilis can be categorized into early and late outcomes. With adequate treatment of affected infants, late outcomes can be prevented. In utero, outcomes include

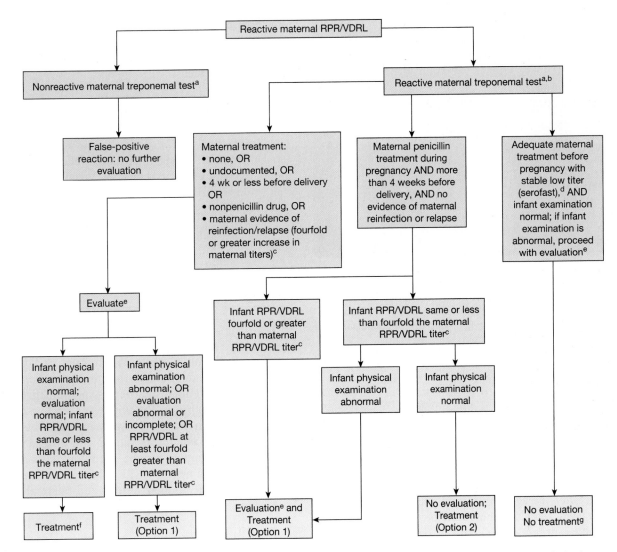

RPR indicates rapid plasma reagin; VDRL, Venereal Disease Research Laboratory; TP-PA, *Treponema pallidum* particle agglutination; FTA-ABS, fluorescent treponemal antibody absorption; TP-EIA, T pallidum enzyme immunoassay; MHA-TP, Microhemagglutination test for antibodies to *T pallidum*.

a TP-PA, FTA-ABS, TP-EIA, or MHA-TP.

b Test for human immunodeficiency virus (HIV) antibody. Infants of HIV-infected mothers do not require different evaluation or treatment.

c A fourfold change in titer is the same as a change of 2 dilutions. For example, a titer of 1:64 is fourfold greater than a titer of 1:16, and a titer of 1:4 is fourfold lower than a titer of 1:16.

d Women who maintain a VDRL titer 1:2 or less or an RPR 1:4 or less beyond 1 year after successful treatment are considered serofast.

e Complete blood cell (CBC) and platelet count; cerebrospinal fluid (CSF) examination for cell count, protein, and quantitative VDRL; other tests as clinically indicated (eg. chest radiographs, long-bone radiographs, eye examination, liver function tests, neuroimaging, and auditory brainstem response).

f Treatment (Option 1 or Option 2, below), with many experts recommending Treatment Option 1. If a single dose of benzathine penicillin G is used, then the infant must be fully evaluated, full evaluation must be normal, and follow-up must be certain. If any part of the infant's evaluation is abnormal or not performed, or if the CSF analysis is rendered uninterpretable, then a 10-day course of penicillin is required.

g Some experts would consider a single intramuscular injection of benzathine penicillin (Treatment Option 2), particularly if follow-up is not certain.

Treatment Options:
(1) Aqueous penicillin G. 50 000 U/kg, intravenously, every 12 hours (1 week of age or younger) or every 8 hours (older than 1 week): or procaine penicillin G. 50 000 U/kg, intramuscularly, as a single daily dose for 10 days. If 24 or more hours of therapy is missed, the entire course must be restarted.
(2) Benzathine penicillin G. 50 000 U/kg, intramuscularly, single dose.

FIGURE 11-5. Algorithm for evaluation and treatment of infants born to mother with reactive serologic tests for syphilis. (Reproduced with permission from Kimberlin DW, Brady MT, Jackson MA, Long SS, eds. *Red Book: 2015 Report of the Committee on Infectious Diseases.* 30th ed. Elk Grove Village, IL: American Academy of Pediatrics; 2015.)

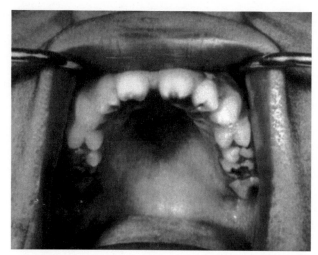

FIGURE 11-6. Hutchinson Teeth. A photograph of Hutchinson teeth resulting from congenital syphilis. Hutchinson teeth is a congenital anomaly in which the permanent incisor teeth are narrow and notched. Note the notched edges and "screwdriver" shape of the central incisors. (Reproduced with permission from the Centers for Disease Control.)

fetal hydrops, stillbirth, and prematurity. Early signs and symptoms include hepatosplenomegaly, snuffles, lymphadenopathy, mucocutaneous lesions, pneumonia, osteochondritis, pseudoparalysis, edema, rash, hemolytic anemia, and thrombocytopenia. These generally occur within the first 4 to 8 weeks of life. Late outcomes occur after the age of two, and affect the CNS, joints, teeth, eyes, and skin. These late outcomes include interstitial keratitis, cranial nerve VIII deafness, Hutchinson triad (Hutchinson teeth (Fig. 11-6) – peg-shaped central incisors, anterior bowing of the shins, and frontal bossing), mulberry molars, saddle nose, rhagades (linear scars at the angle of the mouth), and Clutton joints (symmetric, painful swelling of the knees).

Which of the following maternal infections is a contraindication to breastfeeding?
A. Untreated syphilis without skin lesions
B. Untreated tuberculosis with positive CXR
C. MRSA mastitis
D. Hepatitis B
E. HSV genital lesions

Discussion

The correct answer is **B**. According to the American Academy of Pediatrics, the contraindications to breastfeeding with regard to maternal infection include positive HTLV I or II, untreated brucellosis, untreated tuberculosis, active HSV lesions on the breast, and HIV (in the industrialized world). CMV, hepatitis B, and hepatitis C are not contraindications to breastfeeding. Maternal syphilis can be spread to the infant if mom has active lesions on the breast.

Objectives

1. Understand features associated with congenital syphilis infection
2. Understand management and evaluation for newborns with suspected congenital syphilis infection
3. Understand criteria for adequacy of treatment during pregnancy when mother has documented syphilis infection

CASE 21

A 2-week-old infant presents with cough and difficulty breathing. On examination, the child is febrile, has diffuse lymphadenopathy, hepatosplenomegaly, and abdominal distension. The child was born to a 28-year-old mother with inconsistent prenatal care. She reports having cough and fevers during the pregnancy and had difficulty gaining weight. The infant has a negative HIV PCR and a negative RPR. Chest x-ray reveals diffuse 1 to 2 mm nodular lesions and bilateral pleural effusions.

Which of the following maternal prenatal tests would help reveal the diagnosis in this patient?
A. Tuberculin skin test (TST)
B. HIV antibody testing
C. RPR
D. Hepatitis B
E. Gonorrhea culture

Discussion

The correct answer is **A**. This patient is presenting with congenital tuberculosis with miliary spread. Congenital tuberculosis is rare and can be spread in one of three ways, transplacentally, inhalation of infected amniotic fluid, or direct inoculation from the maternal genital tract at delivery. Neonates can also be infected from postnatal pulmonary exposure, which can often be difficult to differentiate from true congenital cases. In some cases, symptoms are present at birth, but more often they begin around 2 to 3 weeks of life. The majority of children will have chest x-ray findings, and more than half of these children will have miliary disease. Adenopathy and pulmonary infiltrates are common and, cavitary disease is uncommon.

Per recommendations outlined in the Red Book, if congenital tuberculosis is suspected, the following studies should be performed in the infant: TST, Chest x-ray, lumbar puncture, and culture of appropriate sites. Pathology evaluation of the placenta may reveal granulomas and/or acid fast bacilli (AFB). AFB culture should also be sent from the placenta. The mother should be evaluated for pulmonary and extrapulmonary disease, including disease of the uterus. If the maternal examination and chest x-ray findings support the diagnosis of tuberculosis, tuberculosis-directed therapy (isoniazid, rifampin, pyrazinamide, and an aminoglycoside, such as amikacin) should be started promptly. If the lumbar puncture is concerning for meningitis, corticosteroids should also be started. In this infant, a negative TST would not be reassuring as this test is unreliable in children younger than 3 months of age.

What is the most important rationale for the use of BCG vaccine in tuberculosis prevalent settings?
A. Prevention of development of pulmonary tuberculosis in adulthood
B. Prevention of tuberculous meningitis in infancy
C. Prevention of tuberculosis in HIV-infected infants
D. Prophylaxis for a infant born to a PPD-positive mother
E. Prevention of maternal to child transmission during pregnancy

Discussion

The correct answer is **B**. The BCG vaccine is given to infants shortly after birth in tuberculosis prevalent settings. It has approximately 50% efficacy in preventing pulmonary tuberculosis and 64% to 72% efficacy in decreasing tuberculous meningitis and disseminated disease, respectively. The effects are reported to vary, especially since different strains are used in different countries. Duration of protective effect is usually <10 years, but has been reported up to the age of 60 years. BCG vaccine is not recommended for infants with HIV due to the risk of disseminated BCG infection.

Objectives

1. Recognize clinical signs and symptoms of congenital tuberculosis
2. Know diagnostic criteria for congenital tuberculosis
3. Understand the role of Bacillus Calmette–Guérin (BCG) vaccination in areas with high rates of tuberculosis

CASE 22

A mother presents in labor at 39 weeks' gestation. Her membranes are intact. Her GBS screen was positive at 36 weeks.

What is the most appropriate prophylaxis?
A. Vancomycin
B. Clindamycin
C. Gentamicin
D. Penicillin
E. Erythromycin

Discussion

The correct answer is **D**. Both penicillin and ampicillin have been demonstrated to be effective for prevention of early-onset neonatal GBS disease when given >4 hours prior to delivery. An alternative treatment is cefazolin in penicillin-allergic patients. Vancomycin, clindamycin, and erythromycin have not been proven to reach bactericidal levels in the fetal circulation and amniotic fluid, and are not recommended for prophylaxis of GBS. In cases of penicillin anaphylaxis, clindamycin can be given if the isolate shows susceptibility. This test may need to be specifically requested from the laboratory. Alternatively vancomycin can be given; however, neither clindamycin nor vancomycin have proven efficacy. Early guidelines for GBS screening recommended either a risk-based or culture-based screening approach. In the risk-based approach, GBS prophylaxis was administered if delivery was <37 weeks, rupture of membranes >18 hours, or intrapartum temperature >100.4°F. Culture-based screening involved screening all pregnant women at 35 to 37 weeks' gestation for vaginal and rectal GBS. Both approaches offered intrapartum antibiotics if there was history of GBS bacteriuria during the current pregnancy or a history of a previous infant with GBS disease. Data from a large population-based study from 1998 to 1999 showed that culture-based screening was superior to risk-based screening for prevention of early-onset GBS disease. The CDC guidelines for GBS disease prevention were updated to reflect these findings, and currently, universal screening to determine which women should receive intrapartum prophylaxis. In addition, the CDC recommended that women with unknown GBS colonization status should be managed according to risk factors (Table 11-3).

TABLE 11-3. **Indications and Nonindications for Intrapartum Antibiotic Prophylaxis to Prevent Early-onset Group B Streptococcal Disease (GBS)**

INTRAPARTUM GBS PROPHYLAXIS INDICATED	INTRAPARTUM GBS PROPHYLAXIS NOT INDICATED
Previous infant with invasive GBS disease	Colonization with GBS during a previous pregnancy (unless an indication for GBS prophylaxis is present for current pregnancy)
GBS bacteriuria during any trimester of the current pregnancy (not indicated with cesarean delivery is performed prior to onset of labor and amniotic membranes are intact)	GBS bacteriuria during previous pregnancy (unless an indication for GBS prophylaxis is present for current pregnancy)
Positive GBS vaginal–rectal screening culture in late gestation (optimal timing 35 to 37 weeks' gestation) during current pregnancy (not indicated with cesarean delivery is performed prior to onset of labor and amniotic membranes are intact)	Negative vaginal and rectal GBS screening culture in late gestation during current pregnancy, regardless of intrapartum risk factors
Unknown GBS status at the onset of labor and any of the following: 1. Delivery at <37 weeks' gestation 2. Amniotic membrane rupture ≥18 h 3. Intrapartum temperature ≥100.4°F (≥38°C) 4. Intrapartum nucleic acid amplification test (NAAT) positive for GBS	Cesarean delivery performed before the onset of labor on a woman with intact amniotic membranes, regardless of GBS colonization status or gestational age

Reproduced with permission from CDC, Morbidity and Mortality Weekly Report (MMWR): Prevention of Perinatal Group B Streptococcal Disease. Revised Guidelines from CDC, 2010.

The baby is born 2 hours after the first dose of penicillin is given. Maternal rupture was 1 hour prior to delivery and she is afebrile. APGARs are 9 at 1 minute and 9 at 5 minutes and the patient is admitted to the newborn nursery.

What is the next step in management of the infant?
A. Observation for 48 hours
B. Initiation of ampicillin and gentamicin
C. Blood culture, CBC, CRP
D. Blood culture, CBC, chest x-ray
E. Blood culture, urine culture, lumbar puncture

Discussion

The correct answer is **A**. In the case of a mother with no evidence of chorioamnionitis who received inadequate GBS therapy, observation for 48 hours is recommended. No other evaluation is required if the infant is >37 weeks' gestation and had rupture of membranes for less than 18 hours. Ampicillin and gentamicin are recommended after cultures are obtained if there is evidence of neonatal sepsis or maternal chorioamnionitis. If the mother was treated inadequately, and there are high-risk concerns, such as gestation <37 weeks or rupture of membranes >18 hours, then blood culture and CBC with differential and platelets should be obtained, and the infant should be observed for signs of sepsis.

The child has an uneventful course and is discharged home at 3 days of life. At 4 weeks of life, the child presents with decreased movement of the right arm for 1 day.

The patient has been afebrile, and is holding the arm in a flexed position. It is swollen and the infant cries when you attempt to move it. There is no evidence of cellulitis. The rest of the examination is unremarkable. X-ray of the right shoulder and humerus shows soft tissue swelling around the humerus.

What is the most likely diagnosis?
A. Nonaccidental trauma
B. Humeral osteomyelitis
C. Brachial plexus injury
D. Pyomyositis
E. Congenital syphilis

Discussion

The correct answer is **B**. This child is presenting with manifestations of late-onset GBS disease. Late-onset disease occurs from 7 to 89 days postnatally and is not prevented by intrapartum prophylaxis (Fig. 11-7). The incidence and case fatality is reported to be two times lower in late-onset disease than early-onset disease. Late-onset disease most often manifests as bacteremia without a focus, however, meningitis, soft tissue infections (especially facial cellulitis), and osteoarticular infections are also common. The most common osteoarticular infection typically involves the proximal humerus. Septic arthritis most often occurs in the lower extremities, with the hip being the most common location. Both osteomyelitis and septic arthritis are generally not associated with systemic symptoms, although meningitis and sepsis have been reported.

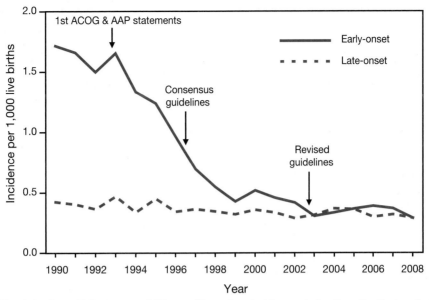

FIGURE 11-7.   Trends in Group B Streptococcal Disease. (Reproduced with permission from the Centers for Disease Control.)

Which of the following infections is the most common cause of late-onset neonatal meningitis?

A. *E. coli*
B. *N. meningitidis*
C. HSV
D. Group B Streptococcus
E. *S. pneumoniae*

Discussion

The correct answer is **D**. Group B streptococcus is the most common cause of neonatal meningitis, accounting for 77% of early-onset cases and about 50% of late-onset cases. *E. coli* accounts for 18% of early-onset cases and 33% of late-onset cases. In preterm infants, *E. coli* is the most common bacteria isolated. Both *S. pneumoniae* and *N. meningitidis* become more common after the first month of life, and persist as the most common cause of meningitis throughout childhood and early adulthood.

Objectives

1. Know trends in incidence of group B streptococcal disease over time
2. Know indications for antibiotic prophylaxis in pregnancies to prevent early-onset group B streptococcal disease
3. Know clinical signs and symptoms associated with early-onset group B streptococcal disease
4. Know recommendations for evaluation and treatment of newborns at risk for early-onset group B streptococcal disease

CASE 23

A 3-week-old previously healthy full-term male infant presents with several days of poor feeding. He has been exclusively breast fed. In addition, his parents report a history of lethargy, poor sucking, and drooling with feeding. He has not had a bowel movement in 4 days. On examination you find a hypotonic infant with poor head control but who is alert appearing. The infant's facial expressions appeared flattened, he has ptosis, and diminished extremity reflexes. He has normal respiratory effort at the time of this examination. His workup is significant for an unremarkable CBC, complete metabolic panel, UA, and lumbar puncture.

What is your initial working diagnosis?

A. Inborn error of metabolism
B. Infantile botulism
C. Spinal muscular atrophy
D. Guillain–Barré syndrome
E. Myasthenia gravis

Discussion

The correct answer is **B**. Infantile botulism fits well with this presentation of cranial nerve dysfunction and hypotonia associated with a normal level of alertness. An inborn error of metabolism will often be accompanied by vomiting, lethargy, or acidosis. Spinal muscular atrophy tends to spare cranial nerves, and typically presents over a longer period of time. Guillain–Barré syndrome typically presents as ascending paralysis, and generally has an elevated CSF protein. Myasthenia gravis tends to present more commonly with a waxing and waning history, and ptosis is typically much more prominent as a sole clinical finding.

In a child with botulism, which finding would not typically be expected at initial presentation?
A. Constipation
B. Dry mouth and pharynx
C. Dehydration
D. Fever
E. Skin flushing

Discussion

The correct answer is **D**. Fever is typically absent in cases of infantile botulism. If fever is present during the initial presentation, other infectious diagnoses should also be considered which may include meningitis, encephalitis, and bacterial or viral sepsis. Constipation is a common presenting finding with botulism, especially in infants. A dry mouth and pharynx and/or skin flushing may be present due to parasympathetic cholinergic blockage. Dehydration may be present due to poor feeding.

What is your initial immediate management for this infant?
A. Admission to ICU setting for management and observation
B. Emergent intubation and ventilation
C. Discharge with parental anticipatory guidance and follow-up in 48 hours
D. Start intravenous peripheral alimentation with intralipids

Discussion

The correct answer is **A**. The child is presently stable with normal respiratory effort, but is at high risk of decompensation. Admission to an ICU setting for close observation is warranted as 50% of infants with botulism will require mechanical ventilation at some point in their course. Discharge to home would not be recommended if infant botulism is suspected given the high probability of continued decline and need for respiratory support. This infant may require supplemental nutrition for continued growth and development while recovering from botulism, but it is generally preferable to use enteral feedings when possible in lieu of intravenous hyperalimentation.

Stool tests are sent to the State Health Department for botulinum toxin assay and *Clostridium botulinum* culture which are both positive.

What definitive therapy do you provide for this patient?
A. Metronidazole and penicillin in combination
B. Immune globulin intravenous (IGIV)
C. Equine botulism antitoxin
D. Botulism immune globulin intravenous (BIG-IV)

Discussion

The correct answer is **D**. BIG-IV has been shown in a randomized controlled trial to reduce mean duration of hospitalization, intensive care, mechanical ventilation, supplemental nutrition, and overall hospital costs. Therapy should be started as early in the course as possible as delay may lead to prolonged need for mechanical ventilation. BIG-IV can be obtained from the California Department of Health Services Infant Botulism Treatment and Prevention Program, which is the sole producer. Standard IGIV would not be indicated as it would not contain sufficient levels of neutralizing antibody to be efficacious. Equine botulism antitoxin would not be indicated as that is used only for the treatment of adult forms of botulism. Antibiotics have not been shown to provide any benefit for botulism infections and should be discouraged unless a secondary infection is present.

Objectives

1. Know the clinical signs of symptoms of newborns with infantile botulism
2. Know appropriate evaluation and management of a neonate with infantile botulism
3. Know common complications associated with infantile botulism infection

CASE 24

You are caring for a 5-week-old ex–24-week gestation infant with a birth weight of 590 g. The infant developed necrotizing enterocolitis at 2 weeks of age and required resection of a small portion of bowel. She completed 2 weeks of broad-spectrum antibiotic therapy. She remains intubated and requires central venous access for hyperalimentation. Yesterday, she developed episodes of poor perfusion accompanied by bradycardia. A sepsis screen was done that was significant for a CBC with a platelet count of 38,000 cells/μL. Broad-spectrum antibiotics were restarted, and she has not clinically improved as of today. You just received a call from the laboratory that the blood culture obtained yesterday from the CVL is growing a yeast. You obtain another set of blood cultures from the CVL as well as peripherally.

What empiric therapy do you start for this presumed fungemia?

A. Fluconazole
B. Amphotericin B deoxycholate (conventional)
C. Liposomal amphotericin B
D. Micafungin
E. 5-FC

Discussion

The correct answer is **B**. Conventional amphotericin B remains the drug of choice for empiric therapy of suspected neonatal candidiasis. The Infectious Diseases Society of America has established consensus guidelines for the treatment of invasive candidal infections in neonates. Fluconazole may be an alternative agent, but the infant's clinical status would argue for choosing the more active agent, amphotericin. Liposomal amphotericin is generally not recommended initially for neonatal infections, unless candidal renal disease has already been excluded, as it may have poor efficacy for treating urinary tract–based infections. The use of echinocandin drugs such as micafungin is generally reserved for refractory cases in neonatal disease rather than an initial empiric choice. 5-FC currently has little to no role in the treatment of neonatal infections given its toxicity, need for oral-only administration, and lack of published data on additive effectiveness.

The following day the laboratory reports that the blood culture isolate has been identified as *Candida glabrata*.

Which among the following is the most true statement regarding C. glabrata?

A. Fluconazole resistance is likely
B. Amphotericin resistance is likely
C. It has a lower associated mortality than other candida species
D. The lipid from intralipid alimentation is a specific growth factor for infection

Discussion

The correct answer is **A**. *C. glabrata* demonstrates dose-dependent resistance to azole antifungals including fluconazole, which may occur at a high level rendering the drug completely ineffective. Although tolerance to amphotericin is occasionally observed, true resistance is uncommon. *C. glabrata* has become the third most common candida species isolated in neonatal and pediatric infections. *Candida albicans* and *Candida parapsilosis* remain the #1 and #2 isolated species, respectively. Recent epidemiologic data on infections in infants and children demonstrates that *C. glabrata* infections may have a higher treatment failure rate and associated mortality

than other candida species. Although hyperalimentation including lipids may be a risk factor for candidal infections in general, the lipid component is typically associated with *Malassezia furfur* as an etiologic agent, which requires a lipid-based medium to grow.

Your patient clinically improves with CVL removal and antifungals. It is now 5 days later. The blood cultures drawn before starting antifungals both grow *C. glabrata* but no subsequent cultures are positive. A pretreatment urine culture was negative.

What is the minimal recommended additional workup for this patient?

A. No further workup unless additional blood cultures positive
B. Echocardiogram
C. Lumbar puncture plus eye examination
D. Lumbar puncture plus eye examination, abdominal/urinary imaging, echocardiogram

Discussion

The correct answer is **C**. There is a high rate of meningitis associated with neonatal candidiasis; therefore, workup should always include a careful evaluation of the CSF as well as an eye examination to look for candidal retinopathy. Given that this patient did not have persistently positive cultures and is clinically improving, the other listed workups could be deferred. Central catheters should be removed as soon as possible. A large prospective study evaluating candidiasis in neonates <1,000 g showed that death was greater and neurodevelopmental outcomes were worse in infants who had >1 day between initiation of antifungals and removal or replacement of central catheters compared to neonates with prompt central catheter removal or replacement.

You have tracked candidal infections over the past 2 years at your institution and note a rate of 15% in premature infants with birth weights <1,000 g.

Which of the following drug interventions would be most appropriate for routine prophylaxis in this high-risk group?

A. Nystatin oral rinse and swallow
B. Amphotericin B dosed three times weekly
C. Voriconazole
D. Micafungin
E. Fluconazole

Discussion

The correct answer is **E**. Fluconazole has been shown in single center randomized controlled trials to be an effective agent to prevent neonatal candidal colonization and infections in nurseries with a high incidence of disease. Nystatin is significantly less effective. There is insufficient evidence to recommend amphotericin, voriconazole, or micafungin for routine neonatal prophylaxis.

Four months later your patient is preparing for hospital discharge. The parent asks if there are any long-term complications in preterm infants who have had a fungal infection in the bloodstream.

How would you most appropriately counsel these parents?

A. All preterm infants who have had fungal sepsis are at higher risk for abnormal neurocognitive functioning in early childhood

B. Preterm infants <750 g who have had fungal sepsis have a higher risk of death and abnormal neurocognitive functioning in early childhood

C. Preterm infants >750 g who have had fungal sepsis have a higher risk of death and abnormal neurocognitive functioning in early childhood compared to those who are <750 g

D. Explain to the parents that their baby does not have an increased risk of abnormal neurocognitive functioning based on having had fungal sepsis during the neonatal period

Discussion

The correct answer is **B**. The NICHD Neonatal Research Network performed a cohort analysis of children being screen for sepsis over a 3-year period to determine predictors for those who had Candida sepsis and/or meningitis and subsequently evaluated neurodevelopmental outcomes at 2 years of age. Candida infected neonates in all birth weight groups had a higher risk of death compared to those with other pathogens causing late-onset sepsis and those who were uninfected. Among survivors, Candida-infected infants had similar rates of neurodevelopmental impairment (NDI) compared to other infants with late-onset sepsis due to other pathogens (31% vs. 31%, $p = $ ns) but higher rates of NDI compared to uninfected preterms who were never screened for sepsis (31% vs. 17%, $p < 0.05$). [1] Preterms infants <750 g had the highest risk for all adverse outcomes, including death and/or NDI.

Objectives

1. Know clinical risk factors associated with an increased risk of Candida infection in the preterm infant
2. Know the implications of retaining central venous catheters in place in preterm infants with Candida sepsis
3. Know the recommended evaluation and treatment options for neonates with Candida sepsis

CASE 25

You are caring for an infant with a suspected congenital infection. This infant was born to a mother with no prenatal care. At delivery, the infant was noted to have macrocephaly, low birth weight for gestational age, and hepatosplenomegaly. Additional workup reveals moderate elevations of hepatic transaminases, chorioretinitis as visualized by dilated ophthalmoscopic examination, and hydrocephalus noted on cranial ultrasound with scattered intracranial calcifications.

What is the most likely working diagnosis?

A. Congenital syphilis
B. Congenital cytomegalovirus infection
C. Congenital toxoplasmosis
D. Congenital rubella
E. Congenital herpes simplex infection

Discussion

The correct answer is **C**. Although several of the listed congenital infections have clinical overlap, the classic triad of chorioretinitis, hydrocephalus, and brain calcifications is highly suggestive of toxoplasmosis, caused by the parasite *Toxoplasma gondii*. Congenital CMV (Fig. 11-8) would more typically present with microcephaly rather than macrocephaly, and more typically has intracranial calcifications located periventricularly rather than scattered. CRS is more typically associated with microcephaly, cataracts, and a heart murmur signifying a cardiac defect. Congenital syphilis infection is typically asymptomatic at birth—although rarely infants are noted to be affected in the delivery room. Although hepatosplenomegaly is common, intracranial calcifications and hydrocephalus are not. True in utero congenial HSV infection is typically associated with microcephaly, ocular dysgenesis, and scarring from skin lesions.

All of the following results would be considered diagnostic of infection in this neonate except?

A. Positive PCR for *T. gondii* from infant's spinal fluid
B. Positive IgM for *T. gondii* from infant blood sample after 5 days of age
C. Positive IgA for *T. gondii* from infant blood sample after 10 days of age
D. Positive IgG for *T. gondii* from infant blood sample after 5 days of age
E. Positive IgM for *T. gondii* from infant's spinal fluid

Discussion

The correct answer is **D**. A positive anti-*Toxoplasma* IgG from the infant's blood at 5 days of age would not

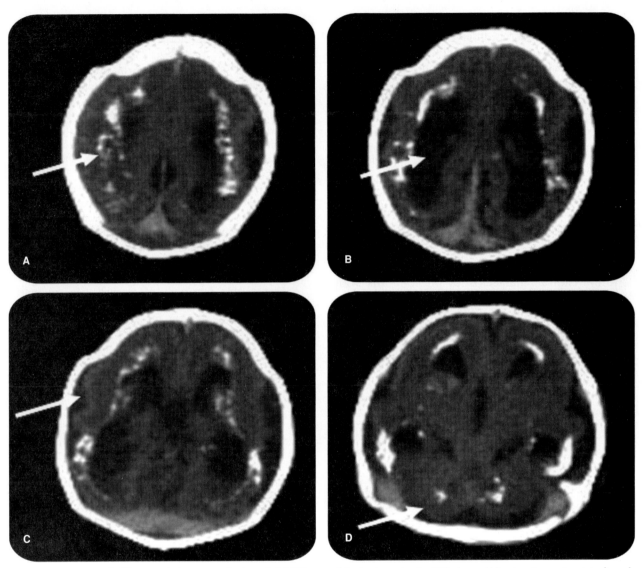

FIGURE 11-8.   Head CT congenital cytomegalovirus. Axial CT scan of the brain at day 1 of life shows (**A**) extensive periventricular calcifications, (**B**) ventriculomegaly, (**C**) reduced cortical sulcation, and (**D**) cerebellar hypoplasia. The arrows indicate the calcifications noted in the CNS. (Reproduced with permission from Dhamija R, Keating G. Teaching neuroimages: CT scan of congenital cytomegalovirus infection. *Neurology*. 2011;76(3):e13.)

by itself be diagnostic of infection or disease, as this result could be due to the influence of transplacental maternal IgG which can remain positive for up to 12 months of life. One could not interpret from that result alone whether the IgG result was due to the mother's antibodies (indicating maternal infection but not necessarily neonatal infection), versus the true antibody response of the neonate. The other results (blood PCR, CSF PCR, neonatal blood and CSF IgM, and neonatal blood IgA) would generally be considered diagnostic for congenital toxoplasmosis infection in the neonate.

The infant is confirmed to have congenital toxoplasmosis infection.

What is the most appropriate management of this infant's disease?

A. Intravenous ganciclovir for 6 weeks
B. Pyrimethamine plus sulfadiazine plus leucovorin orally for 1 year
C. Spiramycin orally for 1 year
D. No therapy indicated but close developmental follow-up is essential

Discussion

The correct answer is **B**. Treatment of congenital toxoplasmosis with a combination of pyrimethamine, sulfadiazine, and leucovorin for 1 year has been showed to significantly and dramatically improve neurodevelopmental outcomes of treated children versus untreated or insufficiently treated historical controls. In addition, treated children have been shown to have significantly less occurrence of eye disease and hearing loss. Intravenous ganciclovir is an antiviral agent that is not active against *T. gondii*. Spiramycin is used for treatment of pregnant women suspected or confirmed of having acquired *T. gondii* infection prior to 18 weeks' gestation for the purpose of preventing fetal infection but is not used for treatment of active disease in neonates. Observation without therapy would not be a reasonable option given the dramatic neurodevelopmental improvements associated with prolonged antimicrobial therapy in congenitally *T. gondii*–infected infants.

Objectives

1. Know clinical characteristics of newborns with congenital toxoplasmosis infection
2. Know recommended diagnostic evaluation for newborns with suspected congenital toxoplasmosis infection
3. Know options for treatment in newborns with suspected congenital toxoplasmosis
4. Know long-term complications associated with congenital toxoplasmosis infection

REFERENCES

1. Abramowsky CR, Gutman J, Hilinski JA. Mycobacterium tuberculosis infection of the placenta: a study of the early (innate) inflammatory response in two cases. *Pediatr Dev Pathol.* 2012;15:132–136.

2. AIDSinfo: Panel on Antiretroviral Therapy and Medical Management of HIV-Infected Children. Guidelines for the Use of Antiretroviral Agents in Pediatric HIV Infection. http://aidinfo,nih.gov/contentfiles/lvguidelines/pediatricguidelines.pdf. Accessed May 7, 2014.

3. AIDSinfo: Panel on Treatment of HIV-infected Pregnant Women and Prevention of Perinatal Transmission. Recommendations for the Use of Antiretroviral Drugs in Pregnant HIV-1-Infected Women for Maternal Health and Interventions to Reduce Perinatal HIV Transmission in the United States. http://aidsinfo.nih.gov/contentfiles/lvguidelines/perinatalgl.pdf. Accessed May 7, 2014.

4. American Academy of Pediatrics. Breastfeeding and the Use of Human Milk. http://pediatrics.aappublications.org/content/129/3/e827.full#content-block, 2012. Accessed August 14, 2014.

5. American Academy of Pediatrics. Parainfluenza viral infections. In: Pickering LK, Baker CJ, Kimberlin DW, eds. *Red Book: 2012 Report of the Committee on Infectious Diseases.* Elk Grove Village, IL: American Academy of Pediatrics; 2012.

6. Arnon SS, Schechter R, Maslanka SE, et al. Human botulism immune globulin for the treatment of infant botulism. *N Engl J Med.* 2006;354:462–471.

7. Benjamin DK Jr, Stoll B, Fanaroff A, et al. Neonatal candidiasis among extremely low birth weight infants: risk factors, mortality rates, and neurodevelopmental outcomes at 18 to 22 months. *Pediatrics.* 2006;117:84–92.

8. Centers for Disease Control and Prevention: case definitions for infectious conditions under public health surveillance. *MMWR Recomm Rep.* 1997;46:1–55.

9. Centers for Disease Control and Prevention: control and prevention of rubella: evaluation and management of suspected outbreaks, rubella in pregnant women, and surveillance for congenital rubella syndrome. *MMWR Recomm Rep.* 2001;50:1–23.

10. Centers for Disease Control and Prevention. *Prevention of Perinatal Group B Streptococcal Disease.* Atlanta, GA: 2010. http://www.cdc.gov/mmwr/preview/mmwrhtml/rr5910a1.htm. Accessed May 8, 2014.

11. Centers for Disease Control and Prevention. *Rubella.* Atlanta, GA: 2012. http://www.cdc.gov/vaccines/pubs/pinkbook/rubella.html. Accessed August 14, 2014.

12. Adams-Chapman I, Bann CM, Das A, et al. Neurodevelopmental outcome of extremely low birth weight infants with Candida infection. *J Pediatr.* 2013;163(4):961–967.e3.

Chapter 12
GASTROENTEROLOGY AND BILIRUBIN

Heidi E. Karpen, MD and Jessica Roberts, MD

CASE 1

The neonatal resuscitation team was asked to attend the delivery of a 33-week preterm female infant born to a 26-year-old mother via spontaneous vaginal delivery. The mother's pregnancy was complicated by polyhydramnios and preterm labor in the third trimester. At delivery, the infant was vigorous. She was warmed, dried and bulb-suctioned, and received Apgar scores of 8 and 8 at 1 and 5 minutes, respectively. However, at 15 minutes of life CPAP was initiated for increased work of breathing and periods of cyanosis that ultimately required intubation. She was also noted to have a full abdomen and copious oral secretions. An attempt to place an orogastric tube for gastric decompression was unsuccessful as the suction catheter was unable to be advanced to the expected length. An x-ray was performed after admission to the special care nursery (Fig. 12-1).

Which of the following is a TRUE statement regarding the infant's diagnosis?

A. Less than 25% of infants with this diagnosis display other associated anomalies

B. Occurs as a result of abnormal development of the embryologic hindgut

C. History and diagnostic workup suggest the presence of an isolated proximal esophageal atresia without tracheoesophageal fistula

D. Anastomotic stricture is a common surgical complication seen after repair of this malformation

E. It is best to intubate infants with this condition in the delivery room to protect the airway

Discussion

The correct answer is **D**. Esophageal atresia/tracheoesophageal fistulas occur in about 1:3,500 live births and are the result of abnormal embryologic development of the foregut structures.[1] The etiology of this abnormal development is not completely understood and is thought to be multifactorial. Other associated anomalies are found in about 50% of cases and in 6% to 10% of cases a unifying genetic diagnosis can be made.[2] Those with isolated esophageal atresia are at the highest risk of other associated anomalies, particularly those of the VACTERL spectrum.[1-3] In cases with other anomalies the organ systems most commonly affected are the cardiovascular (35–45%), gastrointestinal (25%), genitourinary (25%), skeletal (15%), and neurologic (10%).[2] The anatomic descriptions of TEF/EA are of five subtypes or variants. The most common form occurs in 85% of cases and includes a proximal esophageal atresia and a distal tracheoesophageal fistula, as in this case. The anatomic

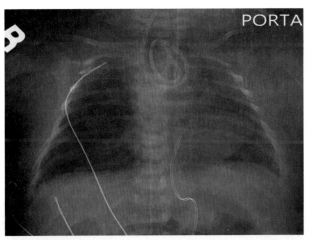

FIGURE 12-1. Abdominal radiograph of infant described in Case 1.

findings in these cases include a dilated esophageal pouch that ends in the neck or upper mediastinum and a distal esophageal segment connected to the stomach that arises from the trachea or bronchus.[2] On x-ray, the dilated air-filled esophageal pouch is usually visible and diagnosis can be confirmed by coiling or termination of an orogastric tube in the pouch. In these cases, an x-ray should also demonstrate air in the stomach and distal bowel, often with gaseous distention of the abdomen on examination (as in Fig. 12-1). The next most common forms of TEF/EA include the isolated esophageal atresia (5–10%) and the isolated TEF or H-type fistula (4–5%) and the rarest forms, each occurring in about 1% of cases, are the proximal fistula with distal esophageal atresia and the double fistula with a separate proximal and distal connection of the esophagus to the trachea.[4] Infants with a proximal esophageal atresia as part of their anatomic malformation are often born to mothers with significant polyhydramnios and with a small or absent stomach on prenatal ultrasonography. After birth, in these infants an inability to swallow oral secretions results in distention of the proximal esophageal pouch with compression of the airway and excessive drooling that can lead to aspiration, respiratory distress and episodes of cyanosis. In those infants with a distal connection between the esophagus and trachea gaseous distention of the stomach and distal bowel is often seen. However, in cases with an isolated esophageal atresia examination will reveal a scaphoid abdomen and x-ray will demonstrate absence of air in the stomach and distal bowel. Diagnosis of the H-type fistula is often delayed and associated with a history of coughing with feedings and sometimes with recurring respiratory infections.

Preoperative management of TEF/EA includes efforts to minimize the risk of aspiration prior to surgical intervention, usually by placing a draining tube put to suction in the proximal esophageal pouch, elevating the infant's head, and allowing for natural respiration if possible to minimize distention of the stomach.[2] The neonate should also be evaluated for other associated congenital anomalies. This evaluation should include a careful physical examination, an echocardiogram, and in some cases a renal ultrasound. Associated vertebral anomalies, if present, are usually detected on x-rays performed to make the initial diagnosis.

The approach to surgical repair depends on several factors including the type of malformation present and the distance between the proximal and distal segments of the esophagus. Those patients with closely approximated esophageal segments can be repaired primarily with an end-to-end anastomosis and ligation of any fistulous

connections via open thoracotomy or thoracoscopically.[5] In those with a large gap between the esophageal segments (generally spanning greater than three vertebral bodies), typically occurring in those with an isolated esophageal atresia without fistula, primary anastomosis may not be possible and the Foker procedure may be utilized to progressively elongate the upper and lower segments of the esophagus before proceeding to surgical anastomosis.[1] Typically a chest tube is placed intraoperatively in case of an anastomotic leak and often a soft nasogastric tube is also placed distal to the anastomotic site by the surgeon to allow enteral feedings to advance while the anastomosis heals.

Postoperatively patients are usually intubated and mechanically ventilated until extubation is likely to be successful. Care should be taken in the postoperative period to avoid inadvertent esophageal intubation and bag-mask ventilation (BMV) that might compromise integrity of the anastomotic site. Gastric acid suppressing therapy and avoidance of manipulation of a surgically placed nasogastric tube are also important considerations for preserving the integrity of the esophageal anastomosis. Contrast esophagram with water-soluble contrast is usually performed after 5 to 7 days to evaluate for anastomotic leak or narrowing. If the esophagram is reassuring, the chest tube can be removed and oral feedings may be initiated.[2]

Long-term survival for infants with TEF/EA is as high as 98% in the lowest-risk group, those greater than 1,500 g at birth and without significant cardiac anomalies.[6] Factors that most influence overall outcome include prematurity and presence of other anomalies, particularly cardiac defects or those associated with chromosomal defects.[1] Complications that contribute to patient morbidity include both those in the immediate postoperative period and those that develop over time. In the immediate postoperative period, anastomotic leaks, most of which are minor and self-resolving, occur in about 10% of patients. Other complicating conditions include clinically significant gastroesophageal reflux, anastomotic strictures (occur in up to 40% of cases in many reports), and recurrent fistula formation which may require further medical or surgical intervention.[6]

Objectives

1. Identify the clinical presentation of patients with TEF/EA
2. Identify the types of TEF/EA
3. Recognize complications associated with and limitations of surgical repair
4. Know anomalies often associated with a diagnosis of TEF/EA

CASE 2

You have been called to the emergency room at the local children's hospital to evaluate a 4-week-old term male infant that is being seen by the ER physician for the second time in 1 week. He was delivered at vaginally at 3,500 g after an uncomplicated pregnancy to a 32-year-old mother and was discharged with her at 48 hours of age. On history the mother reports that initially he had been breast-feeding well with only occasional spits, which have gradually worsened until several days ago when he developed nonbilious vomiting after every feeding. Initially he was feeding well despite the vomiting but now has been less interested in feeding and has not made a wet diaper today. Mother denies loose stools and fever. Family history is significant in that the mother had a similar history of vomiting as a young infant that required surgery. On examination, the infant's weight is unchanged from birth and he appears to be moderately dehydrated. Abdominal x-ray reveals a large gastric air bubble with decreased distal intestinal air and no pneumoperitoneum. Contrast study reveals a large but normally positioned stomach with impaired gastric emptying; shoulder sign is present.

Which of the following is the most likely diagnosis for this patient?
A. Infectious gastroenteritis
B. Gastric volvulus
C. Pyloric atresia
D. Congenital microgastria
E. Hypertrophic pyloric stenosis (HPS)

Discussion

The correct answer is **E**. The differential diagnosis for vomiting in neonates is vast with a wide spectrum of clinical implications from the benign physiologic gastroesophageal reflux seen in many infants to medical and surgical emergencies. Gastric outlet obstruction is a common anatomic etiology for vomiting seen in neonates that typically presents with nonbilious emesis that can be severe enough to result in significant dehydration and electrolyte disturbances. The timing and specific characteristics of the clinical presentation in these cases will depend on specific etiology of the obstruction. HPS is the most common cause of gastric outlet obstruction in infants.[7]

HPS is an acquired condition in which there is a thickening of the muscular layer of the pyloric sphincter, which results in narrowing, and lengthening of the gastric outlet. The incidence of HPS in infants is 2 to 5 per 1,000 live births and is more common in white than black or Asian infants and in boys than girls (4–5:1). Large population studies have suggested a familial or heritable tendency toward the development of HPS. Postnatal erythromycin exposure has also been associated with the condition. A combination of genetic predisposition and environmental factors likely contribute to the development of pyloric thickening.[7]

Infants with HPS usually present with symptoms of high-grade gastric outlet obstruction between 3 and 6 weeks of life. The classic presentation is one with progressive nonbilious projectile vomiting with dehydration and hypochloremic, hypokalemic, contraction metabolic alkalosis with paradoxical aciduria.[2] Laboratory studies may also show hypoglycemia and unconjugated hyperbilirubinemia. Examination classically demonstrates hyperperistalsis and palpation of the hypertrophied pylorus or "olive" in the epigastric area. Palpation of the olive is highly specific for the diagnosis with specificity as high as 97% but can be technically challenging.[8] Diagnosis can be aided with the use of an upper gastrointestinal contrast study or abdominal ultrasound. Findings on a contrast study include a dilated, hyperperistaltic stomach with a narrow line of contrast traversing the pylorus (string sign) and an impression made by the bulging of the thickened pylorus into the contrasted antrum (shoulder sign).[9] Ultrasound findings that suggest the diagnosis include an increased sphincter diameter, increased pyloric wall thickness, and a lengthened pyloric channel.

Operative management of HPS should be delayed until an infant has been adequately rehydrated and any electrolyte abnormalities are corrected. Meanwhile gastric decompression can be achieved with an orogastric tube placed to suction. Surgical treatment, pyloromyotomy, may be done via an open or a laparoscopic technique with similar outcome and incidence of complications, the most common complication being unintentional perforation of the pyloric mucosa. Usually feedings can be initiated soon after surgical correction allowing for discharge after just 24 to 48 hours with excellent outcomes.[2,10]

Neonatal gastric volvulus is a rare condition that can occur as the result of a congenital absence or laxity of the anatomic structures that fix the stomach to the abdominal organs and mesentery. Volvulus may be described as organoaxial or mesentericoaxial depending on which structures are deficient. Gastric volvulus is associated with intestinal malrotation and left-sided diaphragm abnormalities.[2,11] The clinical presentation is usually one of vomiting with or without abdominal distention though in cases of chronic gastric volvulus the presentation may be that of an apparent life-threatening event.[12] Classically, a nasogastric tube may not be able to be passed into the stomach. Radiologic studies demonstrate gaseous distention of the stomach and, with contrast, transverse lie of the stomach with inversion of the greater curvature.[2]

Complete congenital pyloric atresias typically present in the first few days of life with nonbilious emesis and history if maternal polyhydramnios. Gastric distention may be severe enough to lead to respiratory compromise and may lead to perforation. Laboratory findings are typical of those of other causes of gastric outlet obstruction and may include contraction alkalosis and hypoglycemia. There is an association with junctional epidermolysis bullosa and congenital pyloric atresia. However, more common than complete pyloric atresias are membranous pyloric webs. These webs may allow small amounts of gastric juice and air to pass through fenestrations, but may be of inadequate size to allow for complete gastric emptying.[2]

Congenital microgastria is a very rare malformation in which the stomach is small and tubular in shape and abnormally fixed in the abdominal cavity. Often it is associated with other structural anomalies including those of the limbs, malrotation, megaesophagus, and abnormalities of the solid organs of the abdomen. The small size of the stomach results in severe GER symptoms with chronic vomiting and failure to thrive. Infants also often have chronic diarrhea.[2]

Objectives

1. Recognize the clinical presentation of a child with hypertrophic pyloric stenosis
2. Know the differential diagnosis for a child with persistent vomiting
3. Identify the metabolic abnormalities commonly seen in a child with hypertrophic pyloric stenosis
4. Know recommended management and treatment for a child with hypertrophic pyloric stenosis

CASE 3

You are called to evaluate a 6-day-old 37-week gestation male infant who has new-onset respiratory distress and abdominal distention associated with an episode of emesis. The neonate initially required nasal continuous positive pressure for increased work of breathing thought to secondary to mild respiratory distress syndrome but has been on room air for several days; has been receiving oral breast milk feeds. Stooling was noted to be slow for the first several days of life but overnight he had one stool that was noted to be watery and malodorous after an infant suppository. On examination you note a neonate with tachypnea and moderate respi-

ratory distress and temperature of 38.7°C. He has a distended tense abdomen without appreciable bowel sounds. Laboratory studies reveal a WBC count of 19,000 with 40% neutrophils and 18% bands.

Which of the following statements regarding this patient's diagnosis is NOT correct?
A. The underlying cause of this patient's illness is arrest of fetal development of the myenteric nervous system
B. Treatment at this stage would include rectal decompression and broad-spectrum antibiotics
C. It is very unlikely that this infant's parents would have any other children affected by this condition
D. Neonates with this diagnosis often present with intestinal obstruction
E. Biopsy would likely reveal hypertrophy of nerve fibers and absence of ganglion cells

Discussion

The correct answer is **C**. Hirschsprung disease is the most common cause of intestinal obstruction in neonates. Neonates often present with abdominal distention, emesis and failure to pass meconium in the first 24 hours of life. Other presentations of the condition include chronic constipation and complicating enterocolitis (~10%), which can occur both before and after surgical intervention. In all cases functional bowel obstruction occurs as the result of poor peristalsis secondary to absence of ganglion cells in the myenteric (Auerbach) plexus and submucosal (Meissner) plexus of the large intestine. Failure of migration of neural crest cells during the 8th to 10th weeks of gestation leads to aganglionic bowel extending from the anus proximally to include a variable length of bowel.[2]

The incidence of Hirschsprung disease is approximately 1 in 5,000 live births with a male predilection. It is important to both investigate family history and to offer genetic counseling in cases of Hirschsprung disease as there is an overall recurrence risk in siblings of an affected child of ~4%. This risk is modified by gender and length of colonic segment involved.[13] Most often Hirschsprung is found to be an isolated malformation (in ~70%) though in some cases there are other associated malformations, often in syndromic pattern.[14] There are many different syndromic associations but some of the more common associations are trisomy 21, congenital central hypoventilation syndrome, and MEN type 2. The genetic basis of both isolated and syndromic disease continues to be under investigation. The *RET, SOX10, PHOX2B*, and various endothelins are examples of genes involved in Hirschsprung disease.[13]

The vast majority of those with Hirschsprung disease are diagnosed during the newborn period. This diagnosis should be considered in those with delayed passage of meconium and abdominal distention relieved by rectal stimulation. X-ray often reveals a distended small bowel and proximal colon with minimal rectal gas. A contrasted study typically reveals a transitional zone where the narrow aganglionic bowel meets the dilated ganglionic bowel and poorly coordinated motility. Contrast may persist in the rectum for more than 24 hours after the study is completed. Abnormal rectal manometry may also suggest the diagnosis though rectal biopsy remains the gold standard for diagnosis; typically suction but some may require full-thickness biopsy. Biopsy typically reveals hypertrophied nerve fibers with intense acetylcholinesterase staining and absence of ganglion cells. In most cases the aganglionic segment extends from the internal anal sphincter proximally to include the sigmoid. In other more extensive cases more proximal extension may be seen through the splenic flexure or terminal ileum.[13,15]

Decompression is the primary goal of initial medical management of neonates with Hirschsprung disease. This can be done with warm saline irrigations several times a day. If, as in this case, presentation is consistent with Hirschsprung-associated enterocolitis management should include decompression with rectal irrigations, fluid resuscitation, and antibiotic therapy. Surgical management was classically completed in a staged repair but often now the one-stage transanal endorectal pull-through is performed. Early complications of surgical repair may include anastomotic leak, abscess, or obstruction and late complications may include constipation, bowel obstruction/stricture, enterocolitis, or incontinence.[15]

Objectives

1. Recognize the typical clinical presentation of a patient with Hirschsprung disease
2. Know the differential diagnosis for a patient with evidence of lower intestinal tract obstruction
3. Know other anomalies associated with a diagnosis of Hirschsprung disease
4. Identify the genetic mutation associated with this diagnosis
5. Know recommended management and treatment for children with this disorder

CASE 4

You are called to the newborn nursery to evaluate a term infant for several episodes of emesis. His nurse explains that he has no difficulty feeding but has now vomited breast milk after each of his three feedings since birth. The last episode of emesis was described by the mother

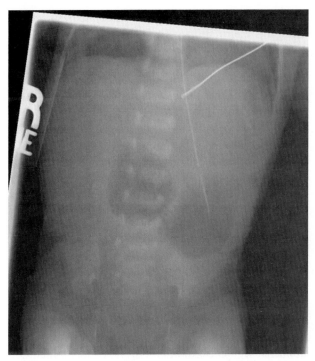

FIGURE 12-2. Abdominal radiograph of infant described in Case 4.

as being green in color. On examination you note a vigorous term infant that is generally well appearing. There is no abdominal distention or apparent tenderness to palpation. You advise the nurse not to feed the infant again and order a plain film of the abdomen (Fig. 12-2).

Which of the following statements regarding this infant's diagnosis is CORRECT?

A. Up to 10% of infants with this diagnosis also have trisomy 21
B. This malformation is rarely associated with other congenital malformations
C. Neonates with this anomaly rarely present with bilious emesis
D. Extrinsic compression of bowel by anomalous structures such cysts of the biliary tree or pancreatic malformations may lead to similar clinical features and radiologic findings
E. You can reassure the infant's mother and nurse that it the infant's symptoms are not suggestive of an acutely worrisome condition

Discussion

The correct answer is **D**. The diagnosis for the infant in the vignette is duodenal atresia. Intrinsic duodenal atresia and stenosis together account for approximately half of all neonatal small bowel atresias with an occurrence of about 1 in 7,000.[2] Extrinsic obstruction of the duodenum can result from several different anomalous structures including malrotation with Ladd bands, preduodenal portal vein, gastroduodenal duplication, cysts of the biliary tree, or pancreas or annular pancreas. Among infants with duodenal atresia or stenosis, trisomy 21 is present in at least 25% and in up to 80% there are other associated congenital anomalies.[2,16] Some other common malformations are congenital heart defect (30%), intestinal malrotation (20%), and imperforate anus (10–20%).[2]

Intrinsic duodenal obstruction is thought to arise from failure of recanalization of the embryonic duodenum after epithelial proliferation obliterates the lumen early in the first trimester. The resultant obstruction is typically morphologically described and classified as one of three types. In type I malformations there is a fenestrated web or intact membrane within the duodenal lumen, which in some cases is described as having a windsock appearance. Type II malformations consist of a fibrous cord that connects a dilated proximal duodenal segment to a narrow distal segment. In type III malformations there is complete discontinuity between the duodenal segments. Another morphologic consideration when describing duodenal atresia/stenosis is the location of the ampulla of Vater and morphology of the common bile duct (CBD), both of which lay within the membrane of a type I malformation, or before or after the site of obstruction. The location of the ampulla of Vater in relation to the site of duodenal obstruction will impact a neonate's presentation, specifically the presence of bilious or nonbilious emesis.[2]

A diagnosis of duodenal stenosis may be suggested while still in utero. Many mothers of infants with duodenal atresia experience a pregnancy complicated by polyhydramnios. Second-trimester prenatal ultrasonography performed to evaluate fetal anatomy may detect the presence of two fluid-filled structures in the fetal abdomen constituting the classically described double bubble and correlating with the air-filled structures seen on postnatal radiography. Other associated anomalies or the presence of trisomy 21 may also be suggested by prenatal testing and imaging.

The clinical presentation of duodenal atresia depends on the completeness of obstruction and the location of the ampulla of Vater in relation to obstruction. Typically the neonate with duodenal atresia presents with emesis without abdominal distention or tenderness in the first 24 hours of life and is otherwise well appearing. In the majority of cases emesis is bilious as obstruction is most often postampullary. In those with complete obstruction radiography typically reveals an air-filled stomach and proximal duodenal bulb without distal air known as the "double bubble" (as in Figs. 12-2 and 12-3), while fenestrated membranes or webs may allow for varying amounts of air to pass into the distal intestine. It is important to

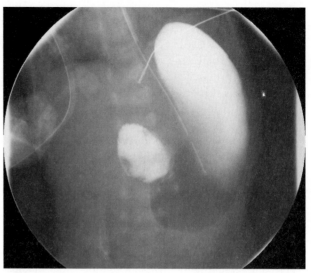

FIGURE 12-3. Contrast study of an infant with bilious emesis and double bubble noted on flat abdominal radiograph. Contrast fills the stomach and the proximal duodenum but fails to pass into the more distal small bowel.

note that the differential diagnosis for bilious emesis and upper gastrointestinal obstruction in the neonate includes the very serious condition of malrotation with midgut volvulus, which is a true neonatal surgical emergency. With compromise of the vascular supply to the intestine which can develop in cases of volvulus associated with malrotation, clinical findings may evolve and include abdominal distention and tenderness, occult or gross hematemesis and signs of systemic decompensation.[2]

Definitive treatment for duodenal atresia is surgical correction. Preoperative medical management includes decompression with a nasogastric drain, fluid resuscitation, and evaluation for other associated anomalies, especially cardiac malformations. Surgical repair often includes the formation of an anastomosis between the two segments of the duodenum, duodenoduodenostomy. Postoperatively neonates with isolated duodenal atresia typically do well and tolerate initiation of advancing feeds 5 to 7 days after surgical intervention. Surgical complications include poor motility and emptying of the proximal GI tract and gastroesophageal reflux. Long-term morbidity and mortality may be related to other associated anomalies.

Objectives

1. Recognize the clinical presentation of a patient with proximal bowel obstruction
2. Know the differential diagnosis of a patient presenting with evidence of proximal small bowel obstruction
3. Recognize the various subtypes of duodenal atresia
4. Know recommended management and treatment guidelines for a child with duodenal atresia

CASE 5

You have been caring for a 36-week female infant who is now 9 days old. She was prenatally diagnosed with gastroschisis and was delivered by cesarean section for fetal distress. She had Apgar scores of 8 and 9 at 1 and 5 minutes, respectively. At 5 days of life her abdominal defect was closed after an incremental reduction of her small bowel using a prefabricated silo. She was extubated on day of life 8 and on examination today her abdomen remains slightly tight and no bowel sounds are appreciated. You are discussing this neonate's case with her parents and the pediatric residents on your team during rounds.

Which of the following statements regarding her case is CORRECT?

A. Preterm delivery is unusual in cases of gastroschisis
B. Issues related to bowel function and nutrition remain the primary concerns for associated morbidity in this patient over the coming weeks to months
C. Extraintestinal anomalies are more commonly found in cases of gastroschisis than in cases of omphalocele
D. Survival in cases of gastroschisis is around 70%
E. Low maternal serum alpha-fetoprotein during second-trimester screening is associated with a diagnosis of gastroschisis in the fetus

Discussion

The correct answer is **B**. Gastroschisis refers to the presence of a defect in the abdominal wall to the right of umbilical stalk that allows herniation of the abdominal contents. The herniated viscera are not covered by the umbilical membrane and typically include a length of small bowel. The pathogenesis of gastroschisis is not precisely understood and is somewhat controversial, but may be the result of a disruption of normally formed tissue, such as an umbilical stalk rupture or a vascular incident, or may be a true malformation as a result of abnormal development. The incidence of gastroschisis is ~1.5 to 4 per 10,000 and has been shown in recent publications to be increasing since the 1980s.[17] Typically, gastroschisis is a sporadic occurrence and is not associated with other syndromic findings. Associated abnormalities are usually isolated to the bowel and often include atretic segments, reported in as many as 25%. Likewise most of the associated morbidity relates to intestinal dysfunction.[17]

Most cases of gastroschisis are diagnosed prenatally with reports of detection by fetal ultrasound as early as 10 to 12 weeks of gestation.[17,18] Other antenatal findings may include elevated maternal serum alpha-fetoprotein and intrauterine growth restriction often associated with oligohydramnios. Serial antenatal testing is often instituted in cases of gastroschisis, as there is an increased risk of premature delivery (occurring in up to 60% of cases) and a classically described risk of third-trimester stillbirth.[17] Prenatal testing is unable to detect the presence of bowel injury, such segmental atresia or serositis that results in intestinal matting or formation of a "peel," that are thought to be caused by exposure to amniotic fluid and mechanical forces in utero.[2]

The challenges of managing a neonate with gastroschisis include water and heat loss. Early management typically includes the placement of a sterile cover over the exposed bowel to limit heat and water loss, a nasogastric tube for decompression, and intravenous line for provision of fluid and nutrients. Reduction of the bowel and surgical closure may be done initially or incrementally in a staged manner with the use of a temporary silo to protect the bowel as the abdominal cavity stretches to accommodate the herniated viscera. In some cases postoperatively there is increased intra-abdominal pressure resulting from the relative inadequacy of the abdominal compartment, which may necessitate a period of mechanical ventilation and careful pain management.[17]

Survival for neonates with gastroschisis is high, 90% to 95%. Much of the mortality is related to perioperative complication including sepsis, necrotizing enterocolitis (NEC), and abdominal visceral ischemia.[2,18] Though all neonates with gastroschisis have obligatory malrotation only rarely do they experience intestinal volvulus after closure. Significant morbidity however does still exist. Much of the morbidity is related to bowel function and nutrition which may be impacted by factors including prematurity, extent of peel formation, and bowel atresias. Intestinal absorption and motility often are abnormal and may result in delayed introduction of enteral feedings, slow feeding advancement, and prolonged use of parenteral nutrition (PN) with its many associated complications including sepsis and cholestasis. Long-term growth may be poor.[2] In contrast to gastroschisis, omphalocele is an abdominal wall defect in which the herniated abdominal contents are contained within the membranous covering of the umbilical cord. Neonates with omphalocele generally have a larger abdominal wall defect and are more likely to have other extraintestinal anomalies. In those with multiple anomalies, chromosomal abnormalities including trisomies and syndromic associations are described (Beckwith–Wiedemann, Pentalogy of Cantrell, VACTERL association). Morbidity and mortality in cases of omphalocele reflect the relative inadequacy of the abdominal cavity in relation to the volume of herniated viscera and to the largest degree the presence and severity of the other associated anomalies.[2]

Objectives

1. Know recommendations for prenatal evaluation of a fetus with gastroschisis
2. Distinguish between a gastroschisis and an omphalocele
3. Know anomalies commonly associated with the types of abdominal wall defect
4. Know recommended management and treatment guidelines for neonates with abdominal wall defects

CASE 6

The resident covering the term nursery is called to evaluate a full-term male infant found by his mother to have meconium coming from the base of the scrotum. The resident evaluates the patient and then calls you to report her findings. The mother's pregnancy and delivery were uncomplicated and the infant has fed twice without difficulty. On examination the resident notes meconium coming from an opening in the scrotum at the midline. The anus appears hypoplastic and anterior displaced. The resident is unable to advance a small catheter into the anus past 0.5 cm. There are no other obvious malformations. You discuss the infant's likely diagnosis and your management plans with the resident.

Which of the following statements regarding a diagnosis of imperforate anus in male infants is CORRECT?

A. Diagnostic workup typically includes abdominal and retroperitoneal ultrasound
B. A detailed physical examination should be carefully completed noting the presence and position of the anal, urethral, and any fistulous openings
C. A fistulous connection between the rectum and the urinary tract may exist at the level of the bladder, prostatic, or bulbar urethra
D. In about half of male infants with imperforate anus without a fistulous connection there is coincident trisomy 21
E. All of the above

Discussion

The correct answer is **E**. Imperforate anus is a diagnosis with many varied anatomical defects with a wide spectrum of severity. The incidence of imperforate anus is 1 in 4,000 to 5,000 neonates with a slight male predomi-

nance. About one-third of anorectal malformations are isolated findings while the remainder are seen in the setting of multiple congenital anomalies. The most common genetic associations are trisomy 21 and 22q deletion syndromes.[2,19]

Diagnosis is usually made on a careful physical examination in the neonate. Particular attention should be paid to the presence and position of the anal, urethral, and fistula openings. Evidence of a fistula may take up to 24 hours to become apparent.[19] In the majority of males with imperforate anus there is a fistulous connection between the rectum and the bladder (rectovesicular) or the urethra (rectoprostatic or rectobulbar). In this case there is a fistulous connection that opens to the perineal skin, which is denoted as a perineal fistula. In the minority of patients with imperforate anus without a fistulous connection the rectum ends in a blind pouch in the pelvis. Greater than 50% of these patients have Down syndrome. Anorectal malformations in females are usually described as either perineal fistulas, vestibular fistulas, or the more complex complete cloacae. Rectovestibular fistula opens in the posterior margin of the introitus outside the hymen and may be mistakenly characterized as a rectovaginal fistula, which is very rare.[2]

The diagnostic workup for anorectal malformations beyond careful physical examination often includes radiographs. The prone cross-table lateral radiograph done at about 24 hours of age may provide information regarding the distance between the most distal colon and the perineal opening for surgical planning. It is typical to do further diagnostic testing to evaluate for other associated anomalies, especially those that may impact surgical correction or anesthesia management. These studies usually include an echocardiogram to evaluate for congenital heart disease. Radiographs may also reveal spinal or vertebral anomalies and may suggest tracheoesophageal fistula with unsuccessful passage of a nasogastric tube. Abdominal/renal ultrasound is usually performed in the initial workup of imperforate anus. The higher the anorectal malformation the more likely an associated genitourinary malformation is present with associated urinary dysfunction and morbidity. For this reason voiding cystourethrogram may eventually be necessary in those with evidence of renal tract anomalies, sacral spine anomalies or frequent urinary tract infections.[19]

Management of anorectal malformation is rarely considered a surgical emergency. Typically in the first 24 hours of life neonates are managed with intravenous hydration, a nasogastric tube and antibiotic coverage while further diagnostic studies are being performed. The presence of other associated urogenital malformations may warrant an earlier intervention. Anorectal malformations may be repaired primarily, particularly those with perineal fistulae, or may require a staged repair with an initial colostomy.[2] The most common cause of long-term morbidity is constipation while some, particularly those with more complex lesions and repairs, may experience some degree of fecal incontinence. Urinary incontinence is also of particular concern in females with complete cloacae malformations.[2,19]

Objectives

1. Recognize the various possible clinical presentations of a neonate with an imperforate anus and understand how this relates to the anatomical abnormalities
2. Understand the differences in presentation and associated issues between neonates with a "high" versus a "low" imperforate anus
3. Recognize other associated anomalies and recommendations for a diagnostic evaluation in a neonate with an imperforate anus
4. Understand the different potential genitourinary tract abnormalities in affected males and females

CASE 7

You are reviewing morning radiographs and come to the film of an 850-g 26-week female preterm neonate that is now 6 days old. She was admitted to the neonatal ICU following preterm labor with maternal fever and a vaginal delivery. Her mother received magnesium sulfate, ampicillin, and a single dose of betamethasone prior to delivery. The neonate was intubated in the delivery room for work of breathing and received a dose of surfactant. After admission umbilical arterial and venous catheters were placed. The infant experienced a brief period of hypotension that resolved with administration of saline and a continuous dopamine infusion. Over the first 72 hours of life she received a second dose of surfactant, was weaned from the ventilator to nasal continuous positive airway pressure with low oxygen requirement, and the umbilical arterial catheter was removed. On day of life four, there is concern that her umbilical venous catheter may have been inadvertently withdrawn by 1 cm. An abdominal radiograph was completed this morning to confirm location of the catheter (Fig. 12-4). After seeing the infant's radiograph you go to the bedside to perform a physical examination. You find a small preterm infant who is active and appears comfortable. Vital signs are normal and her nurse reports that she has not had any episodes of apnea or bradycardia. She is pink with good peripheral perfusion. The abdomen is rounded, soft, and nontender with hypoactive bowel sounds and slight blue discoloration of the right lateral abdominal wall.

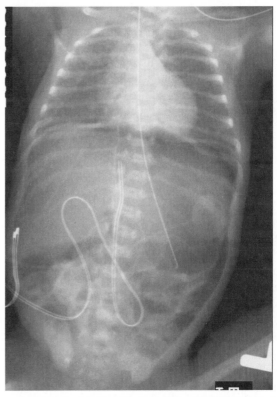

FIGURE 12-4. Abdominal radiograph of infant described in the vignette.

Which of the following statements is MOST accurate regarding the diagnosis and management of this patient?

A. The absence of systemic signs of illness in this neonate is not unusual for those with her current diagnosis
B. The pathology report for the surgical specimen from this infant is likely to show extensive ischemic and coagulative necrosis of the perforated area and the surrounding bowel
C. This diagnosis is usually made in neonates that have been advanced to full volume feeds
D. Laboratory studies drawn now on this infant will likely reveal neutropenia and marked metabolic acidosis
E. The neonate's current condition is unlikely to impact her long-term neurodevelopmental outcome

Discussion

The correct answer is **A**. The premature neonate in the vignette has a spontaneous intestinal perforation (SIP). SIP typically occurs in very low and extremely low–birth-weight preterm neonates. The incidence in these neonates is between 3% and 8%.[20] Several risk factors for SIP have been suggested and the most well established is prematurity. Other published risks have included both antenatal and postnatal factors including antenatal chorioamnionitis and certain drug exposures. Early postnatal steroid administration, particularly dexamethasone, in the first 3 days of life has been shown to increase risk of SIP. The relationship between indomethacin, both antenatal and postnatal administration, and development has been explored. A recent retrospective review of the Neonatal Research Network's general database suggested an increased risk for SIP associated with indomethacin used for the treatment of patent ductus arteriosus but not when used for intraventricular hemorrhage prophylaxis. In this same report, no increased risk of SIP was found in relation to antenatal steroids.[20] Some reports suggest that the use of corticosteroids and nonsteroidal anti-inflammatory drugs together might increase risk. Other risk factors for SIP may include the presence of a hemodynamically significant patent ductus arteriosus and the use of vasopressors.[21]

SIP in premature neonates usually occurs early in life with a median day of onset around 7 days. The intestinal pathology usually consists of a single perforation located in the terminal ileum with localized hemorrhagic necrosis and well-defined margins. The surrounding bowel is usually normal. Histopathologic evaluation of the involved tissue typically does not reveal marked inflammation or mucosal ischemia.[21] Several etiologies have been suggested as causative processes in SIP. Intestinal ischemia may play a role while others have suggested a role for nitric oxide synthase or altered intestinal motility and discordant postnatal development of the layers of intestinal wall.[21,22]

The clinical features of SIP are often considered in contrast with those of NEC. In general, SIP occurs earlier in postnatal life than NEC and at relatively more immature corrected gestational ages, usually 25 to 27 weeks. Affected neonates often have not yet been fed. Neonates with SIP often do not appear acutely ill but some may develop abdominal distention and hypotension. Classically there may be blue-to-black discoloration of the abdominal wall due to meconium staining of the peritoneum. When compared to NEC, classically the presentation of SIP includes fewer signs of systemic illness, although many do develop leukocytosis and several studies have reported the presence of concomitant sepsis with coagulase negative Staphylococcus or Candida. Severe metabolic acidosis is not a typical finding in these cases, perhaps reflecting the absence of extensive intestinal necrosis.[22]

Diagnosis of SIP may be suggested by the above clinical findings but in some cases is diagnosed, as in this case, after pneumoperitoneum is discovered incidentally on a radiograph. Pneumoperitoneum may not be easily detected on a standard supine AP film of the abdomen but may be more easily seen on a supine cross-table lateral or a left lateral decubitus film. Careful examination of the

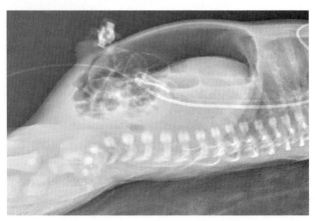

FIGURE 12-5. A large collection of extraluminal air is seen which suggests intestinal perforation.

radiograph from the vignette reveals increased lucency at the lateral margins of the abdomen and beneath the diaphragm, which extends across the midline (see Fig. 12-4). Extraluminal air is more easily detected in the supine cross-table lateral radiograph in Figure 12-5 as a large collection of separates the abdominal wall from the air-filled bowel. In some cases, pneumoperitoneum may not be found but the diagnosis will be suggested by the presence of a gasless abdomen. In all cases, findings such as pneumatosis intestinalis or portal venous gas would suggest a diagnosis of NEC rather than SIP.[22]

Initial medical management of a neonate with SIP includes placement of an oro/nasogastric drain placed to suction to decompress the abdomen and cessation of all enteral feeds. Supportive fluid and antibiotic therapy should also be initiated. Surgical therapy is required for the treatment of infants with SIP and may be managed with primary peritoneal drain or laparotomy. Peritoneal drain with placement of a Penrose drain can be done at bedside and may be a definitive therapy in these patients, many not requiring any subsequent surgical intervention. The drain typically remains in place until there is resolution of pneumoperitoneum and cessation of meconium drainage from the site. Laparotomy may be indicated in some cases particularly in the settings of failed resolution of symptoms, reaccumulation of free air, evidence of bowel obstruction, or fistulous intestinal drainage from the Penrose site.[21,22]

Questions remain regarding the outcome in those with SIP. In the short-term primary peritoneal drain is a definitive therapy for many and they do not require additional abdominal surgery. However, many question the potential for long-term differences in outcome, particularly neurodevelopmental outcome, related to the method of initial surgical management of these neonates.[20,22] Several publications have reported an increased risk of adverse neurodevelopmental outcomes in those with

SIP including a recent publication in which the authors report SIP to be an independent risk factor for adverse neurodevelopmental outcomes at 18 to 22 months in extremely low–birth-weight infants.[20]

CASE 7-A

A 21-day-old male infant born at 26 weeks of gestation has been receiving oxygen via nasal cannula and enteral feedings with premature infant formula. This morning his feeds were discontinued after he had an episode of light green emesis and several apneic and bradycardic events. He was subsequently intubated due to continued cardiorespiratory events and worsening abdominal distention. Abdominal radiographs reveal pneumatosis intestinalis (Fig. 12-6) and he recently had a bloody stool. Laboratory studies reveal thrombocytopenia and an arterial blood gas reveals metabolic acidosis. He is now being managed with intravenous nutrition, a draining orogastric tube to suction, and antibiotic therapy. Serial abdominal radiographs are also ordered.

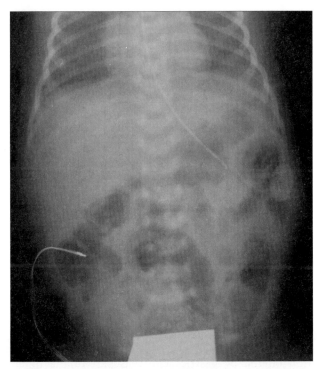

FIGURE 12-6. Several areas of pneumatosis intestinalis are present, most notably in the left lower abdomen.

Which of the following statements regarding the diagnosis of necrotizing enterocolitis is INACCURATE?
A. In general, the more premature the infant, the later this condition occurs after birth
B. Often the subtle and nonspecific nature of the presenting symptoms, and variability in clinical findings, make the diagnosis of necrotizing enterocolitis challenging
C. If found in a term infant, necrotizing enterocolitis is often diagnosed in the first week of life and is more likely to be associated with other predisposing conditions, such as congenital heart disease
D. By the Bell staging system this infant can be diagnosed with stage I necrotizing enterocolitis
E. The pathognomonic findings of this diagnosis on abdominal radiograph are pneumatosis intestinalis and portal venous gas

Discussion

The correct answer is **D**. The patient in the vignette has a presentation typical of that of NEC occurring in premature infants. NEC typically occurs in premature infants after the first week of life with a median age of onset of 15 days. These infants have typically received enteral feedings. Other signs and symptoms might be cardiorespiratory compromise with hemodynamic instability and abdominal wall erythema with signs of peritonitis on examination. The clinical course may display a rapid progression of symptoms though the presenting symptoms can be subtle and nonspecific. The diagnosis is typically established with abdominal radiographs. Radiologic findings might include dilated gas-filled loops of bowel, a paucity of bowel gas, pneumoperitoneum, or the pathognomonic findings of pneumatosis intestinalis and portal venous gas.[21,23]

The presentation and clinical findings in NEC can be variable and several staging systems have been utilized to describe the severity and guide the management of NEC. Because of the variable presentation and progression and the nonspecific nature of many of the findings in early NEC, no classification scheme has proven to be universally helpful. The modified Bell staging system is one such scheme that has been used to classify cases based on a group of clinical parameters which include consideration of systemic findings, gastrointestinal signs, and radiographic evidence.[23,24] Bell stage I characterizes suspected disease and findings include mild nonspecific presenting symptoms such apneic and bradycardic spells, lethargy, and increased gastric residuals.[25] Examination might reveal mild abdominal distention and radiographs mild gaseous distention and ileus. Bell stage II disease is designated proven or definite NEC. Designation of stage II disease requires the presence of pneumatosis intestinalis and is usually associated with increasing systemic

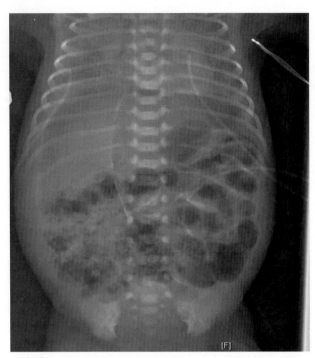

FIGURE 12-7. In this infant with severe necrotizing enterocolitis radiograph reveals extensive pneumatosis intestinalis, pneumoperitoneum, and small lucencies over the liver that suggest portal venous gas.

signs and signs of peritonitis. The more severe stage II disease (stage IIB) is accompanied by mild metabolic acidosis and thrombocytopenia. Advanced or severe NEC is categorized as Bell stage III and includes those cases with ascites or pneumoperitoneum (stage IIIB) (see Fig. 12-7). Infants with Bell stage III NEC typically have severe systemic decompensation with severe acidosis, hemodynamic instability, shock, electrolyte disturbance, and abnormal hematologic parameters. Initial diagnosis may be made at any of these stage designations.[24,26]

Medical management typically includes bowel rest, abdominal decompression, and broad-spectrum antibiotic therapy for 7 to 14 days.[27] Patients also require aggressive intravenous fluid resuscitation and nutrition. It is typical for infants with definite disease to require reintubation and mechanical ventilation. Disease progression may be monitored with serial radiograph examinations. Up to half of patients with NEC require surgical intervention. The development of pneumoperitoneum is a common indication for surgery. Surgical intervention might also be considered for severe systemic decompensation. In some cases a simple peritoneal drain is sufficient but other cases require exploratory laparotomy with resection of necrotic bowel segments and formation of a stoma.[26,28]

CASE 7-B

You are discussing this patient's case with your resident team after rounds. A resident asks about the pathogenesis of NEC. The group engages in a discussion regarding this topic and the potential risk factors present in this infant.

Which of the following statements regarding the suspected pathogenesis of and risk factors for the development of necrotizing enterocolitis is INCORRECT?
A. The vast majority of infants that develop NEC have received enteral feedings
B. The risk of NEC is inversely related to gestational age at birth and birth weight
C. The use of intravenous antibiotics in premature neonates appears to be protective against the development of NEC
D. The development of an abnormal gut flora, including the presence of atypical organisms and an overall decrease in the variety of organisms, likely plays a role in the development of NEC
E. Formula-fed infants are at higher risk for the development of NEC than are those infants fed with expressed maternal breast milk

Discussion

The correct answer is **C**. Clinically there are several identified risk factors for or scenarios associated with the development of NEC.[29] Perhaps the two most strongly associated factors are prematurity and enteral feedings. Infants with NEC are premature in greater than 90% of cases and the risk increases as gestational age and birth weight decrease. Likewise, greater than 90% of neonates that develop NEC have begun enteral feeding. Feeding with commercially available premature formulas is associated with the development of NEC while feeding with expressed maternal breast milk may actually be protective.[30] Previously published evidence also suggests that aggressive feeding advancement may be associated with the development of NEC while early initiation of small volume feeds are safe and may offer benefit in establishing normal gastrointestinal tract function.[31,32]

Several other clinical scenarios have been suggested to increase the risk of NEC in preterm neonates.[33] Other clinical considerations are factors that may disturb the formation of normal intestinal flora, including the prolonged use of intravenous antibiotic therapy, and the use of acid suppressing drugs, which may blunt the protection offered by gastric acidity as part of the innate immune system. The use of probiotic and prebiotic agents are being investigated and some evidence suggests that they may offer a protective benefit in the preterm neonate.[34,35]

The pathogenesis of NEC is incompletely understood and is likely multifactorial. Intestinal immaturity acts as the backdrop for the many other suspected contributing factors. The gastrointestinal tract of the premature infant displays immature motility, digestion, absorption, and immune and barrier defense. Likewise, the enteric circulatory system is poorly regulated. Interplay between these immature elements of the preterm gastrointestinal tract predispose to compromised intestinal integrity and to the development of NEC.[23]

Many elements contribute to the immature gut immunity and barrier defense seen in preterm infants, including a tendency toward an excessive inflammatory response. Published evidence of this exaggerated inflammatory response includes studies that demonstrate elevated levels of proinflammatory cytokines and decreased expression of inflammation regulating cell products. Further complicating this abnormal immunity is the tendency for abnormal microbial colonization of the initially sterile preterm gut.[30] There is evidence that the gut flora of affected preterm infants often includes atypical organisms and decreased variety in species, which may predispose to colonization with pathologic bacterial species. Moreover, this abnormal intestinal flora may stimulate or perpetuate the abnormal inflammatory response seen in premature infants with NEC. Other factors have been suggested to play a role in the development of NEC for which published evidence is sparser. A role for hypoxic–ischemic events has been suggested as well. The pathogenesis may include resultant alterations in modulators of vascular tone, though ischemia alone does not sufficiently account for the pathogenesis of NEC.[23,36,37]

CASE 7-C

The preterm neonate discussed in the previous vignette is initially managed medically with bowel rest and broad-spectrum antibiotic therapy. Bloody stools persist and the infant requires packed red cell and platelet transfusions. On day 3 of illness a follow-up abdominal radiograph demonstrates pneumoperitoneum. With a deteriorating clinical status an exploratory laparotomy is performed. A sizable segment of necrotic small bowel is removed, which includes the entire length of the ileum, and a stoma is formed.

Which of the following statements regarding the complications associated with necrotizing enterocolitis and its management in this and in other patients with NEC is CORRECT?

A. Given that the involved segment of intestine was excised this patient is unlikely to develop post-NEC stricture
B. Bacteremia is a rare early complication of NEC in preterm infants
C. Even with early diagnosis and prompt treatment overall NEC-associated mortality remains at 50%
D. Short-bowel syndrome (SBS) resulting from surgical management of NEC is rarely associated with failure to thrive
E. This infant might be predicted to display symptoms of fat malabsorption and be at risk for vitamin B12 deficiency

Discussion

The correct answer is **E**. The early complications of NEC include many systemic manifestations of disease that make early management of disease challenging. Various infectious complications can occur and include bacteremia, which is found in about one-third of infants, and abscess formation. The hematologic consequences of NEC can result in significant bleeding and disordered clotting which necessitate repeated transfusion of red cells and other blood products. However, the late complications and long-term consequences of NEC pose an equally challenging hurdle and result in significant morbidity. It is many of these early and late complications that impact short- and long-term survival. Overall the mortality associated with NEC remains about 20% to 30% and is highest for those of smaller birth weight and those that require surgical intervention.[27,38]

Stricture formation remains one of the most common late complications of NEC and occurs in 9% to 36% of infants treated for NEC and are thought to occur from scarring in the intestinal wall as affected bowel heals. Intestinal strictures generally occur several weeks to a couple of months after the onset of disease and are not related to the severity of disease. The most common site for stricture is the colon though they can occur in the small bowel and may be single or multiple. Strictures may occur in those that did not undergo surgery initially or after an initial resection and enterostomy. Often patients present with signs of obstruction including abdominal distention and feeding intolerance; Figure 12-8 is an abdominal radiograph of an infant with a history of NEC that developed such symptoms. Contrast enema may help establish the diagnosis of post-NEC intestinal stricture. Often such contrast studies are done prior to reanastomosis in patients with an enterostomy.[23,28]

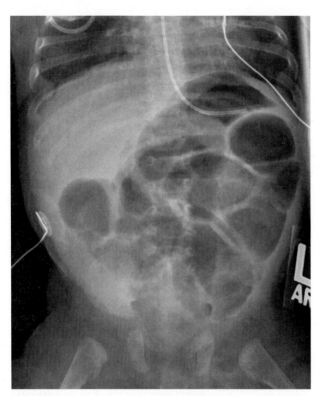

FIGURE 12-8. The radiograph demonstrates very dilated loops of small bowel in a patient with a history of necrotizing enterocolitis suspicious for intestinal obstruction secondary to stricture. Subsequently, on a contrasted study dilated distal small bowel was seen without passage of contrast material into the colon consistent with distal small bowel obstruction.

Bowel resection associated with NEC can result in SBS, which can lead to significant malabsorption, prolonged PN use, and failure to thrive. The severity and character of the malabsorption seen in these patients may reflect the length of intestine remaining and also its absorptive function. Malabsorption from bowel resection may be further complicated by abnormal intestinal motility and the development of bacterial overgrowth of the short bowel. The required prolonged period of PN is associated with an increased risk for sepsis, cholestasis, and ultimately liver failure.[28,39,40]

Some degree of intestinal adaptation after bowel resection may eventually diminish malabsorptive complications associated with NEC surgery. However, the malabsorptive properties of a particular case may be predicted on the basis of characteristics of the remaining bowel and those of the missing segments, particularly in predicting potential nutritional deficiencies. Based on the unique absorptive properties of ileum, particularly the distal ileum, as in this case, one might predict vitamin B12 deficiency without parenteral supplementation. The ileum is also responsible for bile acid and bile salt

resorption, that when impaired, may result in poor fat absorption with steatorrheic diarrhea.[39]

Objectives

1. Identify the typical clinical presentation of a neonate with SIP
2. Identify the typical clinical presentation of a neonate with NEC
3. Understand the underlying pathophysiology resulting in NEC
4. Identify the radiographic appearance of pneumatosis intestinalis
5. Understand associated short- and long-term morbidity associated with a diagnosis of NEC
6. Understand the nutritional implications associated with bowel resection
7. Know recommended treatment and management strategies for patients with a diagnosis of NEC or SIP

CASE 8

You are evaluating an infant on morning rounds who was born at 32 weeks and is now 6 weeks old and working on oral-feeding skills. His course has been typical without major complications. Breast milk feeds began at 2 days of age and were advanced on the basis of unit feeding protocol. He is now receiving both maternal breast milk and premature infant formula as mother's milk supply has diminished. The infant's stooling pattern has been normal until recently as he has developed frequent stools with bright red blood and mucus though he is otherwise well appearing.

Which of the following statements regarding this infant's condition is CORRECT?

A. Expressed maternal breast milk should be discontinued, as it is the likely cause of the infant's symptoms
B. Diagnosis could be confirmed with blood in an in vitro immunoassay (or RAST test) against cow's milk
C. Transition to a soy-based formula in place of the standard preterm infant formula should result in resolution of symptoms
D. Biopsy of the rectum is likely to reveal mild patchy inflammation with large numbers of eosinophils invading the intestinal wall
E. Failure of symptoms to resolve within 72 hours after appropriate dietary intervention has been made should prompt diagnostic evaluation for other causes of hematochezia

Discussion

The correct answer is **D**. The infant in the vignette likely has milk protein proctocolitis of infancy, which commonly presents between 2 and 8 weeks of age with grossly or occultly bloody stools and may be associated with an increased stooling frequency. Frank diarrhea is rare and typically there is a lack of other systemic or constitutional symptoms. Other clinical considerations in an infant with bloody stools may include anal fissure, NEC, volvulus, and other causes of colitis such as infection or that associated with Hirschsprung disease. Biopsy is rarely required but if performed typically reveals mild patchy inflammation involving the rectum and sometimes the distal colon with eosinophilic infiltration of the intestinal wall. Cow's milk protein colitis is not believed to be an IgE-mediated allergy and therefore is not diagnosed with immunoassay or skin prick test. Infants with IgE-mediated allergies to food products typically display systemic symptoms such as hives, vomiting, and wheezing.[41–43]

The management of milk protein proctocolitis requires complete elimination of the problematic protein. Though the condition often occurs in solely breastfed infants, cessation of breast-feeding is not required but rather complete dietary avoidance of cow's milk-based dairy products by the mother should result in eventual resolution of symptoms. In infants receiving cow's milk–based formula a transition to a protein hydrolysate formula should first be attempted. Thirty to forty percent of infants with cow's milk protein intolerance will also demonstrate intolerance of soy protein and 5% to 10% will exhibit intolerance of hydrolysate formulas requiring use of an amino acid–based formula.[44,45]

Response to cow's milk protein avoidance can take up to 2 weeks but often a decrease in grossly bloody stools is seen within 72 hours of avoidance. Occult blood may continue for some time after stools are no longer grossly bloody. Persistence of symptoms in breastfed infants may necessitate further dietary restrictions in the mother, which might include soy and egg protein avoidance. Often infants with milk protein colitis will tolerate reintroduction of the protein after 4 to 6 months of avoidance without difficulty.[45]

Objectives

1. Recognize the clinical presentation of a patient with milk protein protocolitis
2. Know the differential diagnosis for the evaluation of a neonate with bloody stools
3. Understand appropriate management strategies for a patient with milk protein protocolitis

CASE 9

A preterm female infant born at 26 weeks of gestation is now 8 weeks old and is receiving enteral feeds at full volume via nasogastric tube while just beginning oral feeding attempts. Her early course was complicated by respiratory distress syndrome that resulted in a lengthy period of mechanical ventilation and a continued requirement for nasal cannula oxygen to date. Currently she experiences two to three episodes of emesis per day and her nurse perceives her as fussy and uncomfortable after feeds. She has exhibited adequate weight gain on her current regimen with fortified expressed maternal breast milk. Based on the clinical scenario you inform the nurse that the infant's episodes of emesis are likely related to gastroesophageal reflux.

Which of the following statements regarding this infant's condition is CORRECT?
A. Ranitidine would likely result in improvement of the infant's symptoms
B. Metoclopramide should be safe to use in this infant and is effective at reducing reflux-associated symptoms
C. It is likely that this infant's reflux symptoms are responsible for her continued need for respiratory support
D. Treatment should be initiated, as the infant's symptoms are likely to worsen overtime
E. Upper gastrointestinal tract anatomy and transient relaxation of the lower esophageal sphincter are the most important factors contributing to her symptomatology

Discussion

The correct answer is **E**. Gastroesophageal reflux (GER), defined as the retrograde passage of stomach contents into the esophagus, is a physiologic condition that occurs in many healthy infants that resolves with growth and maturation. The diagnosis of gastroesophageal reflux disease (GERD) is typically made in those that display significant morbidities thought to be associated with gastroesophageal reflux. GER is thought to be more common in preterm than in term infants and the clinical morbidities sometimes attributed to GERD in these infants include vomiting, irritability and posturing, failure to thrive, and worsened cardiorespiratory symptoms such apnea, bradycardia, aspiration pneumonia, and worsened chronic lung disease.[46,47]

Several mechanisms for the development of GER have been suggested. Transient lower esophageal sphincter relaxation occurs frequently in preterm infants both with and without GER disease but is thought to be the most important factor contributing to GER disease. The anatomy of the neonatal upper gastrointestinal tract itself likely complicates these transient episodes of lower esophageal relaxation. Infants generally have a shortened segment of intra-abdominal esophagus in relation to the diaphragm and an overall smaller esophageal length and volume. Without a significant segment of intra-abdominal esophagus, esophageal compression by the diaphragmatic crus during inspiration or straining, as seen in older patients, does not occur. Likewise, overall esophageal volume makes reflux of gastric content to the upper esophagus more likely, which may increase the frequency of symptomatic reflux episodes. Other factors that may contribute to the development of GERD include slow gastric emptying and poor esophageal motility. The presence of an orogastric or nasogastric tube may also increase reflux by interfering with lower esophageal sphincter tone and gastric motility.[48,47]

Another consideration is that of comorbid conditions, especially those of apnea and significant respiratory disease such as bronchopulmonary dysplasia. Many studies have attempted to elucidate a causal relationship between apnea in preterm infants and reflux episodes; however, no studies in the recent years have yielded evidence to support this hypothesis. When considering bronchopulmonary dysplasia or chronic lung disease and GERD in preterm infants many believe that there is a reciprocal relationship. Chronic lung disease may contribute to the development of GER as a result of increased work of breathing and resultant changes in intra-abdominal to intrathoracic pressure differentials. GERD is often regarded as an exacerbating factor for chronic lung disease possibly as it results in chronic aspiration of gastric contents into the lungs. For this reason many preterm neonates with chronic lung disease are treated for GERD though there is a lack of experimental evidence that demonstrates improvement in respiratory disease with treatment of GERD.[47,49]

Diagnosing GERD in a preterm infant is complicated by the fact that GER episodes and even associated emesis can be considered normal occurrences in otherwise healthy preterm infants. Moreover, the utility of common diagnostic tests, such as pH probe and impedance monitoring, in establishing the presence of pathologic versus physiologic reflux is often debated. Radiologic tests may help to identify other conditions that may contribute to or masquerade as GERD, such as hiatal hernia, tracheoesophageal fistula, or small intestinal webs or atresias.[47,50]

Treatment of GERD is typically aimed at reducing the frequency and severity of associated symptoms. Often nonpharmacologic interventions are first utilized. These methods may include altered positioning in which prone positioning is preferred over supine and left lateral positioning is preferred over right lateral while an infant is monitored in a nursery. Elevation of the head of the bed is also often attempted. Thickening of feeds is often employed in term infants with reflux symptoms but may prove problematic in preterm infants as it may make oral feeding more difficult and commercial thickeners have not been systematically evaluated for use in preterm infants and may be associated with an increase in adverse events. Frequent, small volume feeds have also been suggested to improve symptoms.[51]

Pharmacologic therapy for GERD has included prokinetic agents and gastric acid lowering drugs. Little evidence exists to support the use of prokinetic agents in premature neonates with GERD and there is considerable apprehension regarding the potential for adverse effects with these drugs. Concern exists regarding potential for adverse neurologic sequelae with the use of metoclopramide and for adverse gastrointestinal sequelae, arrhythmias, and drug interactions with the use of erythromycin. Gastric acid lowering drugs have a role in cases of GERD with associated esophagitis but there is a lack of evidence to support the use of these drugs in reducing perceived reflux symptoms alone. Moreover, there are theoretical disadvantages of profound gastric acid suppression in the premature infant and there is some evidence that suggests the existence of harmful adverse effects associated with the use of these drugs. Many studies have shown improvement in GER symptoms with time irrespective of treatment. With consideration of the anatomical basis for and the natural history of GERD some suggest that time allowed for growth and maturation may be the preferred method of treatment in many cases.[52,53]

Objectives

1. Recognize the clinical presentation of a neonate with GERD
2. Know the differential diagnosis of a neonate with non-bilious vomiting
3. Recognize appropriate management strategies for a neonate with GERD

CASE 10

The neonatal intensive care unit team is rounding on a term infant that was admitted after cesarean section delivery for respiratory distress and is now 36 hours old. His respiratory status has improved and the team would

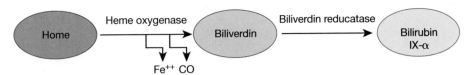

FIGURE 12-9.   Representation of enzymatic metabolism of bilirubin in the reticuloendothelial system.

like to allow the infant to begin breast-feeding. All laboratory studies completed thus far in the infant's course have been within normal limits except for an elevated total serum bilirubin. The resident responsible for the patient asks for about the cause of hyperbilirubinemia in this infant.

Which of the following statements regarding the metabolism of bilirubin in the fetus and neonate in CORRECT?

A. Complete conjugation of bilirubin includes the successive addition of two glucuronide molecules
B. Biliverdin made by the fetus readily diffuses across the placenta and is excreted through the maternal liver
C. Enterohepatic circulation results in the reabsorption of conjugated bilirubin from the intestinal lumen
D. The enzyme UDP-glucuronosyltransferase 1A1 is present and active in the neonate at birth at 25% of adult levels
E. Low levels of Beta-glucuronidase are present on the intestinal mucosa of neonates

Discussion

The correct answer is **A**. Bilirubin is generated in the body from the breakdown of heme molecules, the majority of which are liberated in the catabolism of red blood cells (75–85%).[54] The metabolism of heme includes two steps of enzymatic change in reticuloendothelial cells, then conjugation in the liver, which then permits elimination of bilirubin from the body. This enzymatic process is depicted in Figure 12-9. Of note, both steps in this process require energy in the form of nicotinomide adenine dinucleotide phosphate (NADPH) to be completed. Heme oxygenase also requires oxygen and is the rate-limiting step in this process with byproducts of iron and

carbon monoxide. The product biliverdin is then converted to bilirubin IX-alpha, which at this state is the unconjugated Z, Z isomer of the molecule. During fetal life, bilirubin but not biliverdin is capable of being removed from fetal circulation via the placenta.[54-56]

Unconjugated bilirubin is nearly insoluble in blood and is carried bound primarily to albumin though a relatively small amount is unbound or free in circulation. This unconjugated bilirubin is removed from circulation and taken into liver cells via passive diffusion and transporter mechanisms. Cytoplasmic proteins, such as ligandin, bind this unconjugated bilirubin inside the liver cell. Conjugation of bilirubin then occurs at the endoplasmic reticulum of liver cells to yield a water-soluble molecule that can be excreted in bile into the gastrointestinal lumen and eliminated from the body. The enzyme responsible for conjugation is UDP-glucuronosyltransferase 1A1 or UGT1A1. Complete conjugation of bilirubin includes the successive addition of two molecules of glucuronic acid to each molecule of bilirubin to yield bilirubin diglucuronide. Figure 12-10 depicts the enzymatic conjugation of bilirubin. Of note, in neonates, conjugation is often incomplete resulting in excretion of a significant portion of the monogluronide conjugate of bilirubin. Though there are other minor mechanisms for the processing of bilirubin to allow elimination from the body glucuronide conjugation is most important.[54,55]

Excretion of the now-soluble conjugated bilirubin from the body requires packaging with other hepatocyte cell products into micelles and release in bile, which is an energy-requiring process. Conjugated bilirubin is not absorbable by the intestines but intraluminal processing of bilirubin results in unconjugated bilirubin that is then able to be absorbed and requires further reconjugation by the liver for excretion. Beta-glucuronidase found on the intestinal mucosal surface is primarily responsible

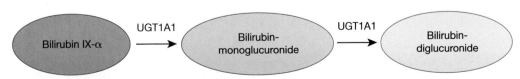

FIGURE 12-10.   Representation of enzymatic conjugation of bilirubin in hepatocytes. Though the complete conjugation of bilirubin-monoglucuronide is primarily carried out by the UGT1A1 enzyme, a more minor contributor may be the enzyme UDP-glucuronate glucuronosyltransferase or transglucuronidase. UGT1A1, uridine diphosphoglucuronate (UDP)-glucuronosyltransferase.

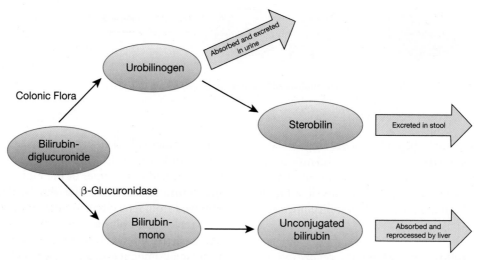

FIGURE 12-11.   Representation of intraluminal processing and excretion of bilirubin after excretion into the intestine.

for hydrolyzing conjugated to unconjugated bilirubin. This process is termed "enterohepatic recirculation of bilirubin." Figure 12-11 depicts the intraluminal intestinal processing of bilirubin after it is excreted in bile.[54,55]

Direct hyperbilirubinemia is usually defined as a level greater than 2 mg/dL and often points to a more serious underlying pathology.[57] Often peak total serum bilirubin levels of 5 to 6 mg/dL around days of life 2 to 4 are observed in neonates and are considered normal, with those of some ethnicities, such as those of Asian descent, displaying higher peak values and longer durations of hyperbilirubinemia. Typically bilirubin levels then fall rapidly over the first week of life and then slowly decline to adult levels in the second week of life. Figure 12-12

lists some contributors to this physiologic jaundice observed in otherwise healthy term neonates. Of note preterm neonates often exhibit higher peak serum bilirubin levels of 10 to 12 mg/dL with a prolonged period of hyperbilirubinemia.[54]

Objectives

1. Understand enterohepatic circulation and how it relates to bilirubin metabolism in the neonate
2. Understand the enzymatic sequences involved in bilirubin metabolism in the neonate
3. Know the differential diagnosis of hyperbilirubinemia in the neonate

Increased bilirubin load	Deficient conjugation	Increased enterohepatic recirculation
High RBC mass (hematocrit often 45–60)	Decreased hepatocyte uptake of bilirubin	High concentrations of intestinal β-glucuronidase
Shortened RBC lifespan (70–90 days)	UGT1A1 levels at 1% of adult levels at birth	High concentrations of bilirubin in meconium
	Tendency toward monoglucuronide form versus diglucuronide form	Tendency toward monoglucuronide form versus diglucuronide form
		Low levels of enteric bacteria flora responsible for converting bilirubin to urobilinogen

FIGURE 12-12.   Factors contributing to the development of physiologic jaundice in neonates. RBC, red blood cell.

CASE 11

A former 31-week preterm African-American male infant in the neonatal intensive care unit is now 3 weeks old. The infant has had an uneventful course other than receiving 4 days of phototherapy for unconjugated hyperbilirubinemia in the first week of life. He has been tolerating full-volume maternal breast milk feedings for 10 days. However, in the last 12 hours the infant has developed an oxygen requirement for desaturations and new short periods of apnea. Examination reveals a small pale infant with jaundice and decreased activity. The team decides to send a complete blood count, urine and blood cultures, blood chemistries, and to start antibiotic therapy. Laboratory studies are significant for an elevated white blood cell count, a low hematocrit of 20%, down from 34% one week ago, with a reticulocyte count of 5.5%, and an total serum bilirubin of 21 mg/dL with a direct fraction of 0.9 mg/dL. At the time of delivery the mother's blood type was reported as B, Rh positive, and indirect Coombs negative.

Which of the following statements regarding this infant's hyperbilirubinemia and likely underlying diagnosis is CORRECT?

A. His hyperbilirubinemia is likely the result of maternal-infant blood type incompatibility

B. The infant is receiving only expressed maternal breast milk and most likely has breast milk jaundice

C. Genetic testing will likely reveal a defect in the promoter region of the uridinediphosphoglucuronate (UDP) glucuronyl transferase gene

D. The infant's underlying diagnosis likely results from a deficiency in a red blood cell enzyme that protects against oxidative injury

E. His newborn screening test is likely positive for galactosemia

Discussion

The correct answer is **D**. The preterm infant in the vignette was found to have glucose-6-phosphate dehydrogenase (G6PD) deficiency and a urinary tract infection. He displayed a rather acute hemolytic anemia and a significant unconjugated hyperbilirubinemia. G6PD is an enzyme responsible for helping to protect the circulating red blood from oxidant stress via the products of the hexose monophosphate pathway. Without the product of this pathway, red blood cells are sensitive to oxidative stress, which results in instability and hemolysis. Many different triggers for acute hemolysis in neonates

have been suggested, such as exposure to certain drugs, directly or through breast milk, development of infection, and exposure to chemicals, such as naphthalene and menthol. However, unconjugated hyperbilirubinemia can occur in those with G6PD deficiency without evidence of significant hemolysis. Glucose-6-phosphate deficiency is an X-linked disorder with a variable phenotype depending on ethnicity and sex.[58]

Gilbert syndrome is a disorder that is relatively common with a typically benign chronic course. The clinical picture results from decreased activity of UDP glucuronyl transferase, a consequence of alterations in the promoter region of its associated gene. This decreased enzyme expression results in unconjugated hyperbilirubinemia. This condition is typically diagnosed outside of the neonatal period but can be detected in some cases, particularly in those with coexistent G6PD deficiency.[58]

Antibody-mediated hemolysis in neonates often results in hyperbilirubinemia shortly after birth. The hemolysis can be quite brisk and the associated hyperbilirubinemia be dramatic with serious consequences. The classically described entity associated with antibody-mediated hemolysis is erythroblastosis fetalis seen in Rh-negative mothers who have been sensitized to the Rh antigen. The ramifications of maternal Rh antibodies can be seen in the fetus while in utero though Rh disease is rare with modern obstetrical management. Other blood group antigens may also be associated hemolytic hyperbilirubinemia. ABO incompatibility jaundice is typically seen in mothers with type O blood who deliver neonates of A or B type. Other minor (lower incidence) red blood cell antigen antibodies, such as anti-Kell or anti-c, found in maternal serum may also result in brisk hemolysis in the neonate and severe neonatal disease.[59]

Breast milk jaundice is less likely to be the cause of this infant's jaundice. Though at 3 weeks of age the timing is typical, breast milk jaundice is not associated with hemolysis. This patient's bilirubin level is higher than typical breast milk jaundice, though in severe cases levels can be markedly elevated.[60]

Objectives

1. Know the differential diagnosis of hemolytic anemia in the neonate
2. Recognize genetic mutations that can cause hemolysis in the neonate
3. Identify metabolic abnormalities associated with neonatal hemolysis
4. Know the laboratory abnormalities typically associated with the various causes of hemolytic anemia in the neonate

CASE 12

A 2.1-kg male infant is born at 37 weeks of gestation to a 35-year-old Asian female. Pregnancy was complicated by IUGR and oligohydramnios. Baby is noted to have mild grunting/retractions at birth and is visibly jaundiced. Initial blood glucose is 30 but responds to D10W bolus and initiation of continuous glucose infusion. On admission to the NICU, the baby is noted to be irritable, in mild respiratory distress with O_2 saturations 95% on NCPAP 6 30%. He markedly jaundiced with bilateral cephalohematomas and subgaleal hemorrhages, as well as diffuse petecchiae. The abdomen is soft and slightly full but is without organomegaly. The examination is otherwise unremarkable and the baby is nondysmorphic. A sepsis evaluation is done which reveals marked thrombocytopenia and modest degree of anemia. LFTs show an AST 87, ALT 54, total serum bilirubin 14.9 with a conjugated fraction of 5.4, an albumin of 1.7 and an ammonia level of 61. The baby is started on empiric antibiotic coverage after cultures are sent, including urine for CMV. A short time later, the nurse calls you to the bedside because the infant has had a large bloody stool. KUB is remarkable only for centralized bowel loops suggestive of ascites. Coagulation studies show a PT 59 with an INR of 6.7, a PTT of 158, and a fibrinogen of 94.

Best next laboratory tests
A. CSF for herpes simplex virus (HSV) PCR
B. Serum amino acids
C. Serum ferritin and iron studies
D. Urine-reducing substances
E. TORCH titers

Discussion

The correct answer is **C**. Serum iron is normal but ferritin is elevated at 5,930 and TIBC is 174%. The baby has increasing abdominal girth with respiratory compromise and is intubated. Blood is suctioned from the ETT and the baby remains coagulopathic despite transfusions of platelets, FFP, and an IV dose of Vitamin K. Ultrasound of the abdomen reveals diffuse ascites and a somewhat small, echogenic liver with elevated hepatic artery resistive indices. The gallbladder is normal with no wall thickening or gallstones.

Of the following, the MOST accurate statement about the disorder affecting this infant
A. Iron studies are pathognomonic
B. It can be diagnosed by amniocentesis
C. Normal liver enzyme tests are reassuring and correlated with recovery

D. The onset of this disorder is during fetal life
E. The mother is to show signs of jaundice and pruritus during pregnancy

Discussion

The correct answer is **D**. Neonatal liver failure (NLF) represents the final common phenotype for a variety of etiologies and portends mortality in excess of 70%. Neonatal hemochromatosis (NH) is a rare disorder that results from the in utero accumulation of massive amounts of intrahepatic and extrahepatic (pancreas, thyroid, heart, and salivary glands) iron deposition, but sparing the reticuloendothelial system. Although rare, NH (also known as neonatal iron storage disease) is one of the most common etiologies for NLF. Previously, it was thought that NH was caused by an error in iron metabolism. Observation that the risk occurrence of NH to subsequent gestations was as high as 90% lead to the suspicion of an alloimmune-mediated process. Accumulating evidence suggests that NH is the final common pathway for gestational alloimmune fetal liver injury mediated by activation of the classical complement pathway. In gestational alloimmune liver disease, the mother becomes sensitized to fetal alloantigens, causing her to form specific reactive antibodies of the IgG class, which are transported across the placenta. This process terminates in hepatocyte necrosis produced by the membrane attack complex (MAC).[61] Iron overload seems to be the result of massive fetal liver injury, rather than the primary disease mechanism.

Metabolic disorders also represent a substantial fraction of NLF, particularly galactosemia, tyrosinemia, mitochondrial disorders, and urea cycle defects. Rapid identification of these disorders is essential, as timely treatment may lead to clinical improvement in the face of fulminant liver failure.[62] Infectious etiologies, particularly viral pathogens such as HSV-1/HSV-2 and enteroviruses, can be particularly damaging to the neonatal liver, causing acute, diffuse necrosis. These usually result from transplacental acquisition of virus in the perinatal period with symptomatic presentation within the first week of life. Shock from any cause, including perinatal asphyxia, cardiac failure, bacterial sepsis, massive hemorrhage, and hemodynamically significant shunts can lead to NLF as well.

Other rare causes of NLF include fatty acid oxidation disorders, bile salt synthetic defects, hereditary fructose intolerance, tumors, other viruses such as adenovirus and parvovirus, TORCH infections, and endocrine abnormalities.[63,62]

Differentiating between timing of liver injury can be helpful in categorizing possible etiologies. Prenatally acquired insults, such as NH, congenital infections, and mitochondrial disorders generally present as chronic hepatic insufficiency. Perinatal forms of NLF, typically secondary to perinatally acquired infectious agents, toxic drug

Etiology of ALF in infants <90 days of age

• **Metabolic disorders:**	18.9%
• Galactosemia	
• Respiratory chain defect	
• Tyrosinemia	
• Niemann-pick type C	
• Mitochondrial disorders	
• Urea cycle defects	
• Ornithine transcarbamylase deficiency	
• **Neonatal hemochromatosis**	13.5%
• **Viral infections**	16.2%
• Herpes simplex virus	
• Enterovirus	
• Cytomegalovirus	
• **Other:**	12.8%
• Shock	
• Hemophagocytic syndrome	
• Escherichia Coli sepsis	
• Hemangioendothelioma	
• Acetaminophen	
• Down syndrome	
• Leukemia	
• Intraventricular hemorrhage	
• **Indeterminate**	37.8%

FIGURE 12-13. Causes of acute liver failure in infants less than 90 days of age. (Adapted with permission from Sundaram SS, Alonso EM, Narkewicz MR, et al. Pediatric Acute Liver Failure Study Group: Characterization and outcomes of young infants with acute liver failure. *J Pediatr.* 2011;159(5):813–818.)

exposures, ischemic injury, and some metabolic disorder, present with acute hepatocyte necrosis as evidenced by significantly elevated transaminase levels. See Figure 12-13.

Despite advances in care, mortality from NLF remains very high (70%) and underscores the need for rapid, accurate diagnosis and therapeutic intervention. Timing and signs/symptoms of presentation vary according the specific etiology, but features common to many forms of NLF include jaundice with elevations of both indirect and conjugated bilirubin, hypoglycemia, coagulopathy with extremely low levels of factors V, VII, and fibrinogen, thrombocytopenia, anemia, hypoalbuminemia, ascites, and oliguria.

Biochemical markers can be very helpful in distinguishing among different etiologies for NLF[64]; results of a study of infants <90 days of age presenting with acute liver failure (ALF) showed significant differences in ALT, AST, fractionated bilirubin, GGT, PT/INR, BUN, and creatinine based on the diagnosis groups (metabolic, viral, NH, indeterminate, and other). Viral causes were associated with highest elevations in aminotransferase levels, severe cholestasis, and coagulopathy compared to NH. In contrast, the biochemical profile of metabolic

disorders shows moderately elevated transaminases, moderate cholestasis, and minimal coagulopathy. The classic biochemical presentation of NH is liver failure out of proportion to minimal elevations in transaminases with a moderate degree of cholestasis.

Initial evaluation of an infant with NLF should include blood chemistries, complete blood count, ammonia, lactate, urine for routine analysis and reducing substances, coagulation panel, ferritin, TIBC, and iron saturation studies. Blood and urine cultures for bacterial and viral pathogens, as well as specimens for viral DNA studies and initiation of empiric antibiotic/antiviral coverage should be implemented. Infants with noninfectious causes of NLF are at high risk of overwhelming bacterial sepsis, which contributes to the overall mortality rate in this population.[63] Maternal labs should be checked for syphilis and HIV status. Initial imaging with screening abdominal ultrasound may be helpful, but if NH is suspected, a contrast MRI is the most appropriate test to evaluate for iron deposition in the liver and pancreas. Salivary gland biopsy may be warranted if MRI results are inconclusive.

If initial studies are not suggestive of NH, further evaluation for metabolic disorders with serum amino acids, urine organic acids, acylcarnitine profile, and succinylacetone are warranted. Because involvement of a pediatric hepatologist and geneticist is essential in rapid evaluation and treatment of these critically ill patients, early transfer to a quaternary care center is warranted.

Treatment and prognosis for NLF predictably varies by etiology. Viral causes, such as neonatal HSV disease and systemic adenoviral infection, carry a grim prognosis, even with adequate treatment. Prompt treatment of metabolic disorders such as galactosemia and urea cycle defects can resolve liver dysfunction. A recent study characterizing etiologies and outcomes of ALF in infants and children showed that spontaneous survival in infants with NLF is about 59%, well below that of older children.[64] Of the infants listed for transplant, only 40% received an organ compared with 66% of the older age cohort. This disparity may reflect a greater severity of illness in young infants, as well as paucity of appropriately sized livers for these small patients. Survival rates for transplanted infants were quite good at 80% overall 5-year survival, which was consistent with that of older children.

Until recently, NH carried a very grim prognosis. As in neonatal alloimmune hemolysis, treatment with exchange transfusion and high-dose IVIG has been shown to attenuate the severity and progression of liver failure in infants NH.[65] Treatment of subsequent pregnancies with high-dose IVIG has shown significantly improved outcomes (15/16 healthy survivors versus 2/16 in previous pregnancies, $p = 0.0009$).[66]

Objectives

1. Know the differential diagnosis of a neonate with liver failure
2. Know differences in clinical presentation and laboratory findings for the various potential causes of neonatal liver failure
3. Know recommended management and treatment guidelines for the evaluation and treatment of neonatal liver failure

CASE 13

A 6-week-old, former 1.5-kg 32-week preterm infant presents to your office for a weight check after hospital discharge. The NICU course was relatively uneventful with a negative sepsis evaluation at birth and 3 days of phototherapy for early jaundice. The mom is a 36-year-old Asian primigravida who has been exclusively breast-feeding and has been reluctant to use formula supplementation. The baby is well appearing, alert, and active with mild scleral icterus. The weight is now 2.3 kg and mom attests that her volume has increased and the baby is feeding well every 2 to 3 hours. Mom feels the baby has been progressing well but her sister, who is a pediatric ER nurse, is concerned that the whites of the baby's eyes are still yellow. Laboratory tests show that the total serum bilirubin is 3.8 with a conjugated fraction of 2.7.

The MOST appropriate response is
A. This is breast milk jaundice and will resolve over the next few weeks
B. Inquire about the color/consistency of the stools
C. Inform her that the blood tests indicate a nondangerous level of bilirubin
D. Arrange for the baby to be admitted for a sepsis evaluation
E. Arrange a Hematology consult

Discussion

The correct answer is **B**.

Which of the following statements is TRUE regarding this patient's diagnosis?
A. Salivary gland biopsy is the gold standard for diagnosis
B. Inheritance is autosomal recessive
C. Stools are likely to be described as foul smelling and greasy
D. Liver enzyme tests are likely to be extremely elevated
E. Early diagnosis is correlated with improved outcome

Discussion

The correct answer is **E**. Neonatal cholestasis is a condition marked by impaired bile formation or obstruction of bile flow that leads to neonatal hyperbilirubinemia. It occurs in 1 in 2,500 live births and manifests itself by persistent jaundice beyond the first 14 days of life. The most common causes of pathologic cholestasis include biliary atresia (BA), neonatal hepatitis, and alpha-1 antitrypsin deficiency. Other causes of persistent jaundice include sepsis, especially gram-negative urinary tract infections, metabolic and endocrine disorders (see Fig. 12-14). Stool color and consistency is a simple, but crucial, diagnostic tool as alcoholic stools and dark urine indicate significant cholestasis and infer defects in biliary excretion. It is impossible by physical examination alone to differentiate between physiologic hyperbilirubinemia or breast milk jaundice and jaundice caused by cholestasis. Persistence of jaundice beyond the typical 2-week well-baby visit should prompt the clinician to initiate a workup beginning with a fractionated bilirubin to determine if a "direct" fraction is present. An elevated direct fraction is always abnormal and can be seen very early in the course of BA. A recent study of patients with isolated BA showed that direct bilirubin levels at 24 to 48 hours of life were significantly elevated compared to normal controls, even with total serum bilirubin levels that were well below phototherapy levels.[67]

BA is a condition unique to infancy and appears to result from inflammatory destruction of the intrahepatic and extrahepatic bile ducts. It is still a disease of largely unknown etiology although many hypotheses such as an aberrant early bile duct development, perinatal viral infection, aberrant immune response, and abnormalities of bile acids have all been suggested as possibly etiologically important. There is a wide variation in incidence of BA across the globe from 1 in 5,000 in Taiwan to 1 in 20,000 live births in Northern Europe, although the reasons for such a disparity remain obscure.

A recent prospective, multicenter observational study categorized BA patients into three groups: Group 1 is isolated BA without associated major malformations (84%), Group 2 is BA without laterality defects but with at least one major malformation (6%), and Group 3 is BA with associated laterality defects.[68] The most commonly associated malformations were cardiovascular, gastrointestinal, and splenic, especially with laterality defects in Group 3. In addition to those malformations, Group 2 patients also displayed a significant incidence of genitourinary anomalies such as hydronephrosis and cystic kidneys. Isolated BA patients were more likely to be older at time of first evaluation, as patients with associated anomalies were more likely to be evaluated for their jaundice. Interesting associations found in this study: gestational diabetes was observed in 9.9%, 11.8%, and 23.3% of infants in Groups

Differential Diagnosis for Neonatal Cholestasis

Biliary tree abnormalities	Biliary atresia
	Choledochal cyst
	Biliary sludge/cholelithiasis
	Congenital hepatic fibrosis/Caroli disease
	Neonatal sclerosing cholangitis
	Non syndromic paucity of bile ducts
	Spontaneous perforation of bile ducts
Infectious	Viral: TORCH, HIV, CMV, Varicella-zoster, Hepatitis B, Parvovirus B19, Human Herpes virus-6, Coxsackie, Adenovirus, Echovirus
	Bacterial: sepsis, urinary tract infection, syphilis
Idiopathic neonatal hepatitis	
Alloimmune	Neonatal Hemochromatosis
Inherited/metabolic disorders	α-1 Antitrypsin deficiency
	Cystic fibrosis
	Alagille syndrome
	Galactosemia
	Tyrosinemia
	Fructosemia
	Niemann-Pick type C
	Progressive familial intrahepatic cholestasis (PFIC)
	Citrin deficiency
	Inborn errors of bile acid metabolism
	ARC syndrome (arthrogryposis, renal tubular dysfunction, cholestasis)
	Zellweger's syndrome
	Dubin-Johnson and Rotor syndromes
	Wolman's disease
	Mitochondrial disorders
	Congenital disorders of glycosylation
	Peroxisomal disorders
Endocrine	Hypothyroidism
	Hypopituitarism
	Adrenal deficiencies
Chromosomal	Trisomy 21, 13, 18; Turner syndrome (45XO)
Toxic	Parenteral nutrition
	Drugs
Vascular	Budd–Chiari syndrome
	Vascular anomalies (hemangiomas)
Systemic	Shock, heart failure
	Perinatal asphyxia
Miscellaneous	Neonatal leukemia
	Erythroblastosis fetalis
	Neonatal lupus erythematosus
	Hemophagocytic lymphohistiocytosis

FIGURE 12-14. Differential diagnosis for neonatal cholestasis.

1, 2, and 3; high incidence of autoimmunity in first degree relatives of all BA groups (average 44%) compared to a national average of 3% to 9%, suggesting that this may be an underpinning of pathogenesis in all groups.

Therapies in neonatal cholestasis are directed toward specific causes and may include medical management as in the case of hepatitis, or early surgical intervention as in the case of BA. Management remains primarily surgical with an attempt to restore bile flow by resection of extra-hepatic biliary remnants and a reconstruction portoenterostomy (the Kasai procedure). Clearance of jaundice to normal values has been achieved in 40% to 55% of cases in large series from around the world, with an expectation of 5-year native liver survival of similar proportions.[69] Patients with BA who are diagnosed after 60 days of age rarely benefit from the Kasai operation and often have advanced liver damage at the time of presentation. These patients proceed to evaluation for liver transplantation (LT) as no other therapeutic options currently exist. Delayed diagnosis of BA and unsuccessful Kasai surgeries lead to LT in nearly half of the BA patients worldwide, making it the leading indication for pediatric LT.[70,71]

Objectives

1. Know the differential diagnosis of neonatal cholestasis
2. Know differences in clinical presentation and associated anomalies for the various causes of neonatal cholestasis
3. Know recommended management and treatment guidelines for the evaluation and treatment of neonatal cholestasis

CASE 14

A 11-day-old former FT infant 2,900 g, mother 26-year-old G6P4AB2, female presents to your office for 2-week weight check. Prenatal US showed and intra-abdominal cyst. US shortly after birth showed liver to be of NL size and echogenicity, a normal gallbladder, aorta, IVC, and pancreas. A 2-cm cystic structure adjacent to the CBD was also identified.

Baby has been feeding Gerber Good Start Soothe formula, 2 ounces every 2 to 4 hours, without difficulty and has regained birth weight. Stools are very pale yellow per mom's report and her urine appears somewhat dark yellow. On examination baby is mildly icteric with icteric sclera. On abdominal examination the infant is nondistended, nontender with no hepatosplenomegaly or palpable masses. T/D bili, 7.2/2.3; GGT, 201; AST, 73; ALT, 54; PT 14.2.

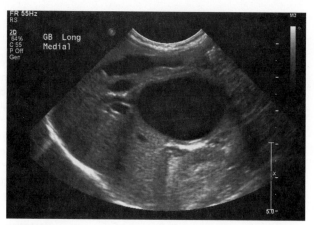

FIGURE 12-15. Ultrasound for patient described in vignette.

US shows dilated CBD but not intrahepatic ductal dilatation. Fusiform type I choledochal cyst (CDC). IOC showed patent hepatic ducts (Fig. 12-15).

Which of the following is a TRUE statement?

A. The most common form of this disorder is associated with multiple intrahepatic cysts
B. Infants with this condition are likely to present with abdominal tenderness and vomiting
C. This disorder is approximately three times more common in males than females
D. The lifetime risk of malignancy related to this disorder is 25% to 40%
E. The developmental pathogenesis of this disorder is related to torsion of the CBD during development

Discussion

The correct answer is **D**. CDC, cystic dilatations of the extrahepatic and/or intrahepatic biliary tree, was first described by Abraham Vater in 1723.[72] Although the precise etiology is not known, it has been shown that the vast majority of CDCs have anomalous insertions of the CBD into the pancreatic duct. This may allow reflux of pancreatic enzymes into the biliary tree leading to ductal dilatation and scarring.[73]

There have been several classification systems put forth, but the one most widely used was described by Todani et al.[74] in 1977. Type I are simple CDCs—this comprises 80% to 90% of all CDCs. Type II are diverticular dilatations of the extrahepatic CBD. Type III is a choledochocele, a malformation of the ampulla of Vater that does not have a high insertion of the pancreatic duct and CBD. Type IV is a CDC associated with other intrahepatic and extrahepatic cysts. Type V is intrahepatic cystic biliary dilatation or Caroli's disease. Types I and IV remain the most common forms of this disease.[75]

The primary differential for CDC is BA with a cyst (Japanese type I cyst). This differentiation is critical because surgical management differs.[76] Intra-op cholangiogram can differentiate between these closely related entities, with CDCs having normal interlobar bile ducts and BA type I cysts having no interlobar bile ducts and bile duct proliferation.[77]

Children less than 1 year typically present with jaundice (72%), hepatomegaly (54%), and clay-colored stools (63%), while older children more typically present with abdominal tenderness and vomiting.[78] There is approximately 3:1 female sex predominance for this disease.

The increased prevalence of routine prenatal ultrasound has resulted in detection of asymptomatic CDCs, raising questions about the optimal timing of surgical repair. Technically, surgical management of these lesions has evolved over the 50 years, with complete cyst excision with Roux-en-Y reconstruction considered the preferred surgical option for Types I and IV cysts. Type II cysts can be managed with cyst resection alone and Type III cysts are amenable to endoscopic sphincterotomy. The advent of minimally invasive procedures has shown that laparoscopic repair of Type I lesions is possible even in the youngest infants.[82] The overall goals of surgery for CDC include relief of biliary obstruction, prevention of cholangitis or pancreatitis, and reduction in the long-term risk of fibrosis and malignancy.

Objectives

1. Know the clinical presentation of a neonate with a choledochal cyst
2. Recognize the various types of choledochal cysts
3. Know the differential diagnosis for a patient with suspected choledochal cyst
4. Know recommended management and treatment guidelines for a patient with a choledochal cyst

CASE 15

On weekly rounds, the nutritionist in your unit notes that one of the preemies on your team has had poor weight gain since birth, less than 10 g/kg in past 2 weeks, and has a lingering conjugated bilirubin of 2.1 mg/dL. The baby was born at 32 weeks of gestation with a birth weight of 1.1 kg and is now 4 weeks old. The baby was initially on NCPAP but weaned quickly to RA. He was begun on trophic feeds on DOL#1 and advanced steadily over the next 10 days to 160 mL/kg/day of fortified EBM.

He has 6 to 8 pale yellow, seedy stools per day. On physical examination, the baby has a prominent forehead with deep-set eyes, scleral icterus, and a high-pitched 2/6 SEM at the LSB that radiates to the axilla and back.

The cause of the murmur is MOST likely to be
A. Peripheral pulmonic stenosis (PPS)
B. Ventricular septal defect
C. PPHN
D. Anemia
E. Coarctation of the aorta

Discussion

The correct answer is **A**.

The vast majority of patients with this disorder are found to have a mutation in which of the following genes
A. PHOXB1
B. NOTCH2
C. JAG1
D. FGFR2
E. Alpha-1 antitrypsin

Discussion

The correct answer is **C**.

Additional findings likely to be seen in this patient
A. Imperforate anus
B. Posterior embryotoxon
C. Polydactyly
D. Wide-spaced nipples
E. Hepatic cysts

Discussion

The correct answer is **B**. Alagille syndrome (AGS) is a genetic cholangiopathy characterized by paucity of intrahepatic bile ducts and defective peripheral branching of the biliary tree. It occurs in approximately 1 out of 30,000 live births and follows an autosomal dominant pattern of inheritance with high penetrance and a variable degree of expression.[83] Approximately 95% of patients with AGS have mutations in *JAG1* gene, located on chromosome 20p12, which encodes the Jagged-1 protein, a NOTCH signaling pathway ligand. Alterations in Jagged-1/Notch-2 interactions result in paucity of intrahepatic bile ducts and defective peripheral branching of the biliary tree.[84] Mutations in the *NOTCH2* gene have been described in AGS as well. It is now believed that AGS occurs as a result of a defect in vasculogenesis, as congenital heart disease and other noncardiac vascular anomalies are frequent in AGS patients. JAG1 signaling controls expansion of the portal vein mesenchyme, which then regulates intrahepatic bile duct development.[85]

The main clinical features of AGS include

- Cardiac abnormalities (85–97%): the most frequent being PPS, but ASD, VSD, pulmonary atresia, and tetralogy of Fallot (TOF) are also seen
- Vertebral anomalies (39–87%); butterfly/hemivertebrae
- Unusual facies (77–98%): triangular facies with pointed chin, broad forehead, deep-set eyes, upslanting palpebral fissures, prominent ears, bulbous nose
- Ocular embryotoxon (60–88%): anterior chamber defects, posterior embryotoxon (prominence of Schwalbe's ring at the junction of the iris and cornea)
- Growth retardation (50–87%) with fat-soluble vitamin deficiencies, metabolic bone disease
- Mental retardation/developmental delay (16–52%)
- Renal disease (40–73%): more common in patients with NOTCH2 than JAG1 defects
- Pancreatic insufficiency (~40%)
- Intracranial (IC) vascular anomalies (16%): often asymptomatic but IC bleeding is the cause of mortality in 34% of AGS patients. May also have vascular anomalies in other parts of the body including renal, abdominal, and carotid vessels
- Hypercholesterolemia with xanthoma formation on extensor surfaces
- Severe pruritus which can be difficult to control

Cholestasis occurs in the neonatal period in 95% of cases and may be mild and clinically unapparent. Those with severe cholestasis may be difficult to distinguish from BA. Given that the outcome for BA is critically dependent on early biliary diversion with the Kasai procedure, it is essential that the correct diagnosis be made in a timely fashion. The associated, nonhepatic features of AGS often help differentiate the two disorders. Biochemically, there is a conjugated hyperbilirubinemia, LFTs up to 10× upper limits of normal and extremely high GGT up to 20× upper limits of normal.[86] Abdominal ultrasound is frequently normal, although occasionally a contracted gallbladder can be seen.

Mortality is estimated at 20% to 30%, most often from cardiac disease, progressive liver disease, or infections. The natural history of this disease is one of cholestasis, which worsens during infancy and remits during early childhood. Maximizing nontransplant therapeutic options is important. LT is ultimately necessary in approximately 10% to 30% of patients, with those presenting cholestasis in the neonatal period having worse outcomes.[87]

Objectives

1. Identify the biochemical findings seen in patients with Alagille syndrome
2. Know the associated anomalies/abnormalities in other organ systems in patients with Alagille syndrome
3. Know the genetic mutations commonly associated with this diagnosis
4. Know the natural history and treatment options for patients with Alagille syndrome

CASE 16

An 850-g, 28-week gestation infant is born via urgent C/S for PTL with footling breech presentation. Mom did not receive antenatal steroids. In the DR, baby was limp, cyanotic with poor respiratory effort, requiring BMV and intubation. Baby required three doses of surfactant as well as dopamine and hydrocortisone for hypotension in the first week of life. Nutritional support began with starter TPN on DOL#1 and progressed to full HAL with 3 g/kg IL by DOL#5. The baby had difficulty progressing past trophic feeds with bilious residuals, intermittent abdominal distention, and irregular stooling. Full feeds were not achieved until DOL#35. Weekly screening nutrition labs showed progressive elevation in conjugated bilirubin, initially normal, which was attributed to a month of TPN exposure. Weight gain has been slow despite feeds which give 125 kcal/kg/day. Stools are bright yellow-green but loose and frequent. At 8 weeks of age, the baby was still clinically jaundiced and a hepatic function panel revealed the following values:

AST	154
ALT	136
Total bilirubin	5.6
Direct bilirubin	4.5
Alkaline phosphatase	652
γ-GT	21
Albumin	2.7
Total protein	4.8

Of the following, the most likely to be TRUE is

A. Liver biopsy is likely to show paucity of bile ducts
B. Abdominal ultrasound shows a large cystic mass adjacent to the porta hepatis
C. Positive maternal history of IV drug use
D. Parents are second cousins
E. Cholestasis is likely to resolve over the next 2 months with enteral feeding and ursodeoxycholic acid (UDCA)

Discussion

The correct answer is **D**.

Which of the following statements is FALSE?

A. Vitamin deficiencies are common
B. Progression to cirrhosis and liver failure before the age of 2 is expected
C. Disease is caused by mutation is in gene encoding an ATP-binding cassette protein located in the proximal small bowel
D. Levels of biliary bile acids are markedly decreased
E. Many mutations in patients are sporadic without a family history of the disease

Discussion

The correct answer is **C**. Progressive familial intrahepatic cholestasis (PFIC) is a group of rare, autosomal recessive disorders that lead to disruption of bile formation and severe, progressive cholestasis. Although collectively PFIC is a rare autosomal recessive condition, with estimates of 1 out of 50 to 100,000 births, it is the etiologic cause and the indication for LT in 10% to 15% of cholestatic children and affects both genders equally. Clinically, these patients present with cholestasis, hepatomegaly, pruritus, growth failure, and fat-soluble vitamin deficiency.[88]

Three types of PFIC have been identified to date and are associated with mutations in hepatocellular transport system genes. PFIC1 and PFIC2 typically display the following features: chronic unremitting cholestasis with onset in infancy, elevated levels of conjugated bilirubin and alkaline phosphatase with low to normal levels of serum gamma-glutamyl transferase (γGT). PFIC3 can be primarily differentiated from the other two forms of PFIC by the significantly elevated GGT levels seen in this type.

PFIC1 (Byler disease) is caused by mutations in the ATP8B1 (FIC1) gene, a P4P-type ATPase belonging to a family of phospholipid-flippases, which are essential for appropriate composition of the bile canalicular membrane and normal bile flow. FIC1 is expressed in liver, pancreas, and kidney, but most highly expressed in the small intestine where it is thought to be involved in enterohepatic recirculation of bile acids.[90] Children with PFIC1 manifest extrahepatic features such as chronic diarrhea (that is not ameliorated by orthotopic LT), pancreatitis, deafness, and persistent short stature, suggesting broader cellular functions of the FIC1 protein. Heterozygous mutations of ATP8B1 have been found in patients with transient neonatal cholestasis and intrahepatic cholestasis of pregnancy type 1 (ICP1), suggesting a dose response in liver disease.[91] Progression to cirrhosis and end-stage liver failure typically occurs in the first few years of life, leaving LT as the only therapeutic option.

PFIC2 is caused by mutations in the bile-salt export pump (BSEP) encoded by the *ABCB11* gene. BSEP is the major bile acid transporter in the hepatocyte, exporting primary bile acids against a steep concentration gradient. Bile acids are the prime determinant of bile flow; decreased bile acid export leads to decreased bile flow, accumulation of toxic bile salts within the hepatocyte leading to severe hepatocellular damage.[92] As in PFIC1, heterozygous mutations in ABCB11 have been identified in patients with transient neonatal cholestasis, drug-induced cholestasis, and ICP2.[93] Patients with BSEP deficiency tend to have a more severe presentation, often in the neonatal period and progress rapidly to end-stage liver disease and cirrhosis in early infancy. They are also at risk for early hepatocellular carcinoma, often in the first year of life.

PFIC3 is caused by defects in the ABCB4 gene encoding the multidrug resistant protein 3 (MDR3), a floppase located in the canalicular membrane of hepatocytes, which translocates phosphatidylcholine to the outer leaflet of the membrane. Phospholipids protect the canalicular membrane against the detergent effects of bile salts; disruption in the export of these phospholipids results in chronic injury to the bile canaliculi and biliary epithelium, eventually leading to cholestasis and development of a cholangiopathy. In contrast to PFIC1 and 2, PFIC3 is rarely seen in the neonatal period, but manifests later in infancy, in childhood or even in young adulthood.[90] Adolescents and young adults with PFIC3 often have symptoms of cirrhosis, such as gastrointestinal bleeding from portal hypertension at the time of presentation. Differentiating features of the PFIC types can be seen in Figure 12-16.

Objectives

1. Identify the typical clinical presentation of a patient with PFIC
2. Distinguish between the clinical presentation of the three subtypes of PFIC
3. Know the natural history of the disease progression for the three subtypes of PFIC
4. Know the genetic mutation associated with each of the three subtypes of PFIC
5. Understand the associated nutritional complications associated with a diagnosis of PFIC

	PFIC1	PFIC2	PFIC3
Inheritance **Chromosome** **Gene/protein**	AR 18q21-22 *ATP8B1/FIC1*	AR 2q24 ABCB11/BSEP	AR 2q24 ABCB11/BSEP
Functional defect	ATP-dependent Aminophospholipid flippase	ATP-dependent bile acid transporter	ATP-dependent bile acid transporter
Other sites of eaxpression	Cholangiocytes, intestine, pancreas	Hepatocytes	Hepatocytes
Age at presentation	Neonatal-infancy	Neonatal-infancy	Neonatal-infancy
Pruritus	Severe	Very severe	Very severe
Extrahepatic symptoms	Diarrhea, pancreatitis, hearing loss, small stature	None	None
Serum ALT	Mildly elevated	Very elevated (>5x normal)	Very elevated (>5x normal)
Serum GGT	Normal	Low-normal	Low-normal
Serum AFP	Normal	Elevated	Elevated
Liver histology	Canalicular cholestasis, mild lobular fibrosis	Canalicular cholestasis, mild lobular fibrosis, giant-cell hepatitis	Canalicular cholestasis, mild lobular fibrosis, giant-cell hepatitis
Diseases associated with **heterozygous defect**	ICP	ICP, drug-induced cholestasis, transient neonatal cholestasis	ICP, drug-induced cholestasis, transient neonatal cholestasis

GGT, gamma-glutamyl transpeptidase; ICP, intrahepatic cholestasis of pregnancy;
LPAC, low-phospholipid associated cholelithiasis syndrome.

FIGURE 12-16. Delineating features of progressive familial intrahepatic cholestasis types 1, 2, and 3.

CASE 17

A 27-week, 960-g preterm infant born to a 25-year-old healthy G2P1 woman for PTL and nonreassuring FHT. One dose of antenatal steroids was given 6 hours PTD. Baby was intubated in delivery room for RDS and given surfactant within 30 minutes of delivery. Baby continued to require significant ventilatory support and clinical course was complicated by recurrent episodes of bilateral pneumothoraces requiring placement of multiple chest tubes, and subsequent development of pulmonary interstitial emphysema. Baby was switched to HFOV and FiO_2 requirement continued to be high at 0.75 to 0.8. Baby weaned off dopamine after the initiation of stress dose hydrocortisone on DOL#8. First CUS performed on DOL#7 showed bilateral Grade III IVH. Baby required phototherapy for indirect hyperbilirubinemia in first week of life, which evolved to conjugated hyperbilirubinemia by DOL#8. Patient was unable to be fed enterally during the first week of life due to pressor requirements and remained on full HAL/IL for nutritional support. Trophic feeds were begun on DOL#9 and advanced slowly to full feeds by DOL#25. On DOL#28, baby was switched back to conventional ventilation but continued to require in excess of 75% oxygen. Examination on DOL#35 revealed hepatomegaly with visible jaundice.

In light of this child's presentation, the correct statement below is

A. This patient's cholestasis is most likely to be related to PN
B. Alpha-1 antitrypsin is most common metabolic disorder resulting in an LT in children
C. There is a high prevalence of hepatocellular carcinoma and cholangiocarcinoma with alpha-1 antitrypsin MM Pi type
D. The gene mutated in this patient displays autosomal recessive inheritance
E. Alpha-1 antitrypsin is a very rare cause of cholestasis in infants

Discussion

The correct answer is **B**. Alpha-1 antitrypsin (A1AT) is a serum glycoprotein, synthesized and secreted from the liver, which acts to inhibit a variety of serine proteases. It is present in most tissues in the body, but its main function is to protect alveolar tissue from proteolytic damage by enzymes such as neutrophil elastase. A1AT deficiency is caused by mutations in the *SERPINA1 gene* and displays autosomal codominant inheritance. Incidence is estimated at 1:2,500 live births, making it the most common inherited metabolic cause of liver disease in infants, and one of the most commonly inherited diseases worldwide with frequency similar to cystic fibrosis.[94]

A1AT alleles from each parent are independently expressed, leading to autonomous function of each A1AT protein produced by those alleles. Serum isoelectric focusing reveals the type of allelic deficiency, Pi typing (protease inhibitor) present in a particular patient, and generally correlates with serum A1AT levels.[95] Normal Pi type is MM and is associated with normal serum concentrations of AAT. Although more than 100 A1AT variants have been described, the S (E264 V) and Z (E342 K) alleles represent 95% of A1AT deficient alleles and result in low serum A1AT levels.[96] Clinically apparent lung disease is found in association with Pi Null, Pi SZ and ZZ, although liver disease is only seen in the Pi ZZ phenotype.[97]

Clinical manifestations of the ZZ phenotype vary widely from asymptomatic to fatal liver and lung disease. Pulmonary symptoms of pneumothorax and pulmonary interstitial emphysema relate to the unmitigated effects of protease inhibitors, such as neutrophil elastase, on the fragile alveoli. Liver disease is thought to occur as a result of accumulated of abnormally folded A1AT molecules in the endoplasmic reticulum of hepatocytes. Neonatal hepatitis occurs in a small percentage of newborns with the ZZ phenotype and is characterized by prolonged conjugated hyperbilirubinemia, elevated liver enzymes, and bleeding tendency. Presentation in later childhood or adulthood is the one typified by a cirrhotic response of progressive fibrosis and an elevated risk of hepatocellular carcinoma and cholangiocarcinoma. Treatment with ursodeoxycholic acid may provide some biochemical and clinical improvement in a percentage of patients with ZZ-associated liver disease.[98] LT with an MM-type liver restores A1AT levels to normal and reverses many of the extrahepatic manifestations of the disease.

Objectives

1. Identify the genetic mutations that result in A1AT deficiency and pattern of inheritance
2. Understand the cause for associated lung disease in some patients with A1AT deficiency
3. Identify the clinical presentation of patients with A1AT deficiency
4. Understand treatment options for patients with A1AT deficiency

CASE 18

A 12-week-old former 28-week, 892-g male infant with history of NEC at 3 weeks of age, resulting in intestinal resection of 85 cm with a jejunostomy and midcolonic mucous fistula. The baby continues to be supported on full HAL via PICC line. He had been on slowly advancing enteral feeds but recently developed increasing feeding intolerance and abdominal distention—blood culture was positive for GNR. On examination, his skin is a deep bronze color, icteric sclera; abdomen is full and round with liver palpated at level of umbilicus and spleen 2 cm below the LCM. There are visible veins on the abdominal wall.

Of the following, which statement is TRUE?
A. There is no reason to pursue other diagnoses, as this is a clear case of parenteral nutrition-associated liver disease (PNALD)
B. The risk of PNALD is higher in infants with surgical NEC than with medical NEC
C. Abdominal US Doppler is likely to show a low resistance to flow in the hepatic arteries
D. SGA infants are at decreased risk of developing TPN cholestasis than AGA infants
E. It is common for PNALD to begin at less than 14 days of age in premature infants

Discussion

The correct answer is **B**.

Of the following, the most accurate statement is
A. Reduction of PN lipid emulsion to 1 g/kg/day is associated with essential fatty acid deficiency
B. Fish oil–based emulsions are enriched in anti-inflammatory omega-6 fatty acids
C. Patients with cholestasis require increased copper and manganese supplementation
D. Although cycling PN may reduce the incidence of cholestasis in neonates, many infants require some enteral nutrition to avoid hypoglycemic episodes
E. Fish-oil emulsions promote resolution of cholestasis and prevent ongoing cirrhosis in patients with PNALD

Discussion

The correct answer is **D**. By 16 weeks of age, the baby has undergone surgical reanastomosis of the remaining intestine, which is estimated to leave 55 cm of small bowel remaining. Laboratory studies show the conjugated bilirubin level to be 15.2 mg/dL, PT 19.2.

Of the following which is MOST accurate statement?
A. Residual intestinal length is of greater predictive value for enteral autonomy than presence of the ICV.
B. This patient's cholestasis is expected to resolve within a few weeks after achieving full enteral feeds and discontinuation of PN.
C. Vitamin deficiencies are rare in these patients if they are fed hydrolyzed formulas.
D. Enteral long-chain fats are ideal for these patients as they are broken down more slowly in the intestine.
E. Risk of mortality is not related to peak conjugated bilirubin concentration.

Discussion

The correct answer is **A**. The introduction of PN in the early 1970s revolutionized the care of critically ill neonates by providing a solution containing a combination of concentrated glucose, amino acids, micronutrients, vitamins, and minerals that could support weight gain and growth. This provided the possibility of survival for the most fragile infants in whom enteral feeding was not possible.[99] Infants who are unable to achieve significant enteral nutrition, however, are at risk for developing an acquired cholestasis and progressive liver disease related to long-term PN. Parenteral-nutrition associated liver disease (PNALD) is likely a multi-factorial disorder with contributions from PN components, such as soy-derived lipid emulsions, hepatic immaturity, sepsis, inadequate intestinal function, and toxicity of hydrophobic bile acids.

PNALD is almost exclusively a disease of neonates, underscoring the role of immaturity and inadequate hepatic adaptive mechanisms. The infants at highest risk of developing PNALD are preterm infants <750 g, those with NEC, gastroschisis, and intestinal atresias. Of infants with surgical NEC, approximately 70% will go on to develop PNALD, with additional independent risk factors of small bowel resection, creation of jejunostomy, and duration of time on PN.[40] SGA has also been shown as an independent risk for the development of PNALD in preterm infants.[100]

Of all risk factors for PNALD, however, time on PN appears to carry the greatest risk. A recent, large prospective study of nearly 1,000 infants showed that only 20% of infants required PN for longer than 14 days.[101] Of those neonates, however, the incidence of conjugated hyperbilirubinemia (direct bilirubin >2.0 mg/dL) was directly related to time on PN, with the development of cholestasis uncommon in infants treated with PN for less than 14 days (see Fig. 12-17).[101]

PNALD is an important, independent risk of mortality. Infants with PNALD have a 30% incidence of mortality compared to a 3% risk in infants on PN for >14 days who do not develop cholestasis. A study of infants with SBS showed a far greater probability of death for infants who developed early, persistent jaundice compared to those who did not develop early jaundice.[102] Risk of mortality in patients with PNALD has also been correlated

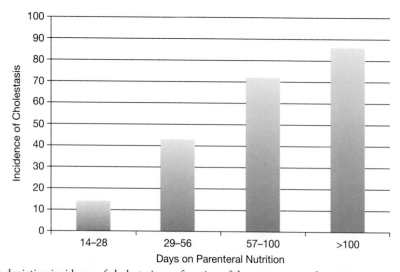

FIGURE 12-17. Graph depicting incidence of cholestasis as a function of days on parenteral nutrition.

with peak conjugated bilirubin concentration, with a fivefold increase in mortality for those with conjugated bilirubin levels >10 mg/dL.[103]

Clinically, PNALD may be indistinguishable from other causes of neonatal cholestasis with jaundice, conjugated hyperbilirubinemia and hepatomegaly, making it a diagnosis of exclusion after more pressing diagnoses such as BA, metabolic disorders, and genetic causes of cholestasis have been ruled out. Timing and level of conjugated hyperbilirubinemia can give useful diagnostic information. A high conjugated bilirubin in the first week of life is always abnormal and is unlikely to be related to PN. Initial studies in a cholestatic infant should include liver enzyme tests, including a GGT, protime, fibrinogen, ammonia, serum glucose, serum amino acids, urine organic acids, succinylacetone, acylcarnitine profile, blood and urine cultures, A1AT Pi typing, and a baseline liver ultrasound with Doppler to evaluate blood flow.

Resolution of PNALD is related to enteral autonomy, peak conjugated bilirubin concentration, and time off PN, particularly the lipid fraction. Patients with established PNALD have been shown to have improvement, and even resolution, of conjugated hyperbilirubinemia after changing from soy-based lipids to a fish-oil emulsion.[104,105] In the United States, fish-oil emulsions are limited to centers that hold an IND for compassionate use, limiting access for many infants. These protocols limit usage to 1 g/kg/day, due to concern for bleeding complications at higher doses. Several studies have shown similar resolution of PNALD with limitation of soy-based emulsions to a dosage of 1 g/kg/day, as compared to the standard 3 g/kg/day.[106,107] There have also been two reports of progressive cirrhosis in patients treated with fish-oil emulsions, despite resolution of cholestasis, underscoring the complex nature of PNALD.[108,109] Newer, blended lipid emulsions containing a mixture of soy-based lipid, olive oil, medium-chain triglycerides, and fish oil are approved for use in Europe and have shown great promise in the treatment and prevention of PNALD in infants.[110–112] These newer lipid formulations have not yet been studied in the United States and are not available for use. Other strategies for management of PN, including cycling, have shown weak evidence of benefit and possible harm to neonates, especially preterms, due to risk of hypoglycemia if they are not able to achieve even partial enteral nutrition.[113]

Infants with high peak conjugated bilirubin levels often require 2 to 6 months off PN to completely resolve their cholestasis.[103] Enteral feeding with breast milk or elemental formulas with a high MCT content are associated with a shorter duration of PN and time to full feedings in patients with SBS.[114] UDCA, a hydrophilic chenodeoxycholic acid derivative, has been shown to be of some benefit in cholestatic patients. It acts to displace the more toxic, hydrophobic bile acids, improving bile flow, and lowering serum bilirubin levels in patients with SBS and cholestasis.[115] As these patients wean off PN, they are at increased risk for fat-soluble vitamin deficiencies, as delivery of bile salts to the intestine is essential for effective absorption of these vitamins and many of these compounds are metabolized or utilized in the liver.[116] Although breast milk and hydrolyzed formulas may produce improved feeding tolerance, they place infants at increased risk for vitamin K deficiency and hemorrhagic complications.[117] The vast majority of cholestatic infants receiving standard vitamin supplements will develop fat-soluble vitamin deficiencies, which can be prevented by supplementation with additional oral solutions containing vitamins A, D, E, and K.[118]

Objectives

1. Identify risk factors associated with development of PNALD
2. Understand the natural progression of disease in patients with PNALD
3. Know associated metabolic and nutritional abnormalities found in patients with PNALD

CASE 19

A 3.8-kg male infant born at 39 weeks of gestation born by cesarean section for failure to progress. Mother develops fever just before delivery and is treated with IV antibiotics for several days for presumed chorioamnionitis. Baby has screening blood culture, which is negative after 48 hours, and does not receive antibiotics. Discharged at 4 days of life, mom feels that he is sleepier than the other baby was. The baby was seen by the pediatrician at 6 days of age for follow-up and has lost 10% of birth weight. Mom is an experienced breast feeder and attest to good milk supply. TSB is 12.8 and DB is 1.8 at that time. On DOL#7 baby presents to ED pale, lethargic with frequent apneic spells. The baby is intubated, started on dopamine for hypotension after several volume boluses, and sepsis evaluation is done before empiric antibiotic coverage is begun. The nurse reports that the baby is bleeding from stick sites. Laboratory values are as follows:

LABORATORY TEST	RESULT
White cell count	3,700
Hemoglobin	12.6 g/dL
Hematocrit	36.9
Platelets	43,000
PT	45 seconds
PTT	>190 seconds
Fibrinogen	73
AST	15,800
ALT	8,560
Alkaline phosphatase	1,612
GGT	110
Total bilirubin	6.8
Conjugated bilirubin	2.3
Albumin	1.7
NH$_3$	580
Glucose	23

Of the following, the MOST accurate statement is

A. Mother is likely to have a history of HSV in past
B. Risk of transmission of HSV disease to a neonate is highest with HSV-1
C. HSV-1 causes a more severe clinical phenotype with an increased incidence of systemic disease
D. 14% of women with a history of recurrent genital HSV infections will develop at least one recurrence during pregnancy
E. The vast majority of infants with systemic HSV disease have lesions at some point in their course

Discussion

The correct answer is **B**.

Of the following statements, which is FALSE?

A. Neonatal HSV is the second most common cause of acute NLF
B. 70% of infants with skin–eye–mouth (SEM) HSV disease will progress to CNS or disseminated disease if left untreated
C. The accuracy and rapidity of PCR have largely begun to replace culture as the diagnostic method of choice in neonates
D. Systemic HSV disease is associated with higher aminotransferase levels, more severe cholestasis, and coagulopathy compared to other causes of NLF
E. The majority of neonatal HSV disease is caused by HSV-2

Discussion

The correct answer is **E**. HSV disease can be acquired *in utero*, during delivery or postnatally, all resulting in

significant morbidity and mortality. Intrauterine infection occurs in a small percentage of patients (~5%) and is considered one of the TORCH infections. It is associated with teratogenic results, including preterm birth, growth restriction, scarring skin lesions, limb deformities, CNS and ophthalmologic abnormalities, and fetal demise.[119,120] A small number of NHSV cases may occur from postnatal transmission of HSV-1, presumably from contact with oral lesions/saliva of a caregiver shedding virus and may present as late as 31 to 45 days of life. The vast majority of NHSV, however, occurs as a result of perinatal transmission of virus due to viral shedding in the female genital tract.

A recent study from a New York City surveillance project showed the incidence of neonatal HSV disease to be approximately 13/100,000 live births with an annual incidence of 1,500 cases per year in the United States.[121] Risk of transmission is higher with HSV-1 than HSV-2 (HSV-1 transmission rates in both primary and secondary infections) but the clinical outcomes do not differ by serotype. Roughly half of NHSV disease is caused by HSV-1, a percentage that appears to be rising, perhaps due to a higher rate or oral–genital contact.

The risk of perinatal acquisition of virus does vary, however, by the type of maternal infection with HSV and is divided into the following categories:[122]

- First-episode primary genital infection by HSV-1 or HSV-2 (i.e., no prior infection with either virus as documented by the absence of antibodies to both serotypes): *risk of transmission 50% to 60%*
- First-episode nonprimary HSV (genital infection with a different serotype of HSV as compared to prior genital or extragenital infection; maternal antibodies to other HSV serotype): *risk of transmission 25%*
- Recurrent genital HSV infection (maternal antibodies match the serotype of the virus she is shedding): *risk of transmission <2%*

Other factors that contribute to risk of transmission of HSV to the neonate:

- Mode of delivery (vaginal vs. cesarean section)
- Duration of rupture of membranes
- Invasive fetal monitoring or instrumented delivery
- Type of HSV (HSV-1 vs. HSV-2)

Up to 90% of women who acquire genital HSV infection are either asymptomatic or have nonspecific symptoms. Because of the lack of recognized symptoms, most mothers of infants with NHSV have no history. Even in relationships where both parents have had only one partner, the woman can asymptomatically shed HSV-1 from oral–genital contact. Among women with a history of genital herpes, 75% have at least one recurrence during pregnancy but only 14% have prodromal symptoms or lesions at the time of delivery.

At the time of presentation, infants can be classified into the following categories:

- SEM disease (~45% of cases): 70% of these infants will progress to CNS or disseminated disease if left untreated
- CNS disease (~30% of cases): infants may present with lethargy, seizures, or temperature instability. Up to a third will never develop herpetic skin lesions
- Disseminated disease (~25% of cases): infants typically present with a severe sepsis syndrome due to a combination of liver, lung, and CNS involvement. Approximately half of these infants will never develop herpetic skin lesions

Viral replication results in morphologic changes in the infected hepatocyte, including microvesicular and macrovesicular steatosis, apoptotic bodies, and ballooning of hepatocytes. Rapid progression to hepatic failure is due to massive necrosis and apoptosis of hepatocytes within the liver.[123]

Prompt pharmacologic treatment is essential, as antiviral treatment cannot reverse tissue destruction caused by the virus.[124] This underscores the need for a high index of suspicion, rapid detection of the virus, and empiric treatment until confirmative studies are available. The diagnosis of NHSV infection can be made from cultures of fluid from skin lesions, if present, or on swabs from the eye, oropharynx, urine, stool or rectum, and blood cultures.[125] The accuracy and rapidity of PCR, though, has largely begun to replace culture as the diagnostic method of choice.

A recent study of NLF documented NHSV as the second leading cause of NLF, preceded only by NH.[64] Viral-induced NLF, especially due to disseminated NHSV disease, is associated with extremely high aminotransferase levels, severe cholestasis, and coagulopathy compared to other causes of NLF. As NH and HSV disease represent the two largest cohorts of infants presenting with NLF, it is imperative to exclude these diagnoses first, using the aminotransferase levels to help distinguish between these diagnoses. Of infants who survived NLF without transplant, only 10% were in the NHSV group, underscoring the overall poor prognosis for infants with disseminated NHSV disease.

Objectives

1. Identify the clinical signs and symptoms associated with neonatal HSV infection
2. Understand the classification for type of neonatal HSV infection

3. Understand risk of transmission with the various serotypes of HSV infection and timing of infection
4. Identify associated teratogenic findings commonly associated with neonatal HSV infection
5. Know the metabolic abnormalities and laboratory findings associated with hepatic failure associated with neonatal HSV infection

CASE 20

A 947-g, 32-week preterm infant born with petechiae, purple macules on chest, abdomen and extremities, hepatosplenomegaly. HC is below 5% and cranial US shows ventriculomegaly with periventricular calcifications. Urine culture is positive for CMV.

Of the following, the most ACCURATE statement is
A. Transmission rate is highest from reactivated maternal disease
B. More than 50% of infants are symptomatic at birth.
C. Hearing screen before discharge is predictive of long-term hearing potential
D. Treatment with gancyclovir is associated with improved long-term growth
E. Hepatitis is the most common finding in neonates with symptomatic CMV disease

Discussion

The correct answer is **E**. Cytomegalovirus (CMV) is a large, ubiquitous virus belonging to the herpes virus family, which also includes roseola, varicella-zoster (VZV), HSV-1 and HSV-2, and Epstein–Barr virus (EBV). The species of CMV known to infect humans also goes by the name human herpes virus 5 (HHV-5). CMV is widespread with the vast majority of adults being seropositive by 40 years of age. The virus is typically transmitted through breast-feeding, sexual contact, and spread from children by contact with infected secretions such as saliva, blood, genital secretions, urine, and breast milk. After acute infection, the virus establishes latency in the monocytes and granulocytes and can be reactivated in the immunocompromised host.

CMV infection can occur during the fetal, perinatal, and postnatal periods. Timing of infection and the mother's serologic status can alter the risk of transmission and clinical outcome of the infant. The overall incidence of congenitally acquired CMV is 0.5% to 2.2% of all life births in developed countries, with higher incidences in third world areas. It is estimated that 1% to 4%

of seronegative women will become infected during pregnancy and approximately a third of these will result in fetal transmission of the virus. In contrast, 10% to 30% of women seropositive for CMV will experience a reinfection or reactivation of CMV during pregnancy, although only 1% to 3% of them will transmit virus to the fetus, with preformed antibodies conferring some degree of protection. Fetal infection with CMV has also been documented in women who have undergone organ transplantation and have either primary or reactivation of CMV disease due to immunosuppression.[126] As the kidney is the primary site of CMV viral replication in the fetus, viral shedding is highest in the urine making it the easiest fluid to culture postnatally.[127]

Fetal infection with CMV results in symptomatic infections in only 10% of all cases of congenital CMV. Classical symptoms include:[128]

- Intrauterine growth restriction (IUGR): 50%
- Hepatosplenomegaly: 60%
- Conjugated hyperbilirubinemia (>2 mg/dL): 81%
- Hepatitis with elevated ALT (>80 units/L): 83%
- Petechiae: 76%
- Thrombocytopenia: 77%
- Pneumonitis: 15%
- Microcephaly: 53%
- Periventricular calcifications: 55%
- Seizures: 7%
- Chorioretinitis: 10%
- Sensorineural hearing loss (SNHL): 56%

In addition, findings of bone abnormalities, abnormal dentition, and hypocalcified dental enamel can also be seen.

Hepatosplenomegaly seen with symptomatic CMV disease is often partially due to extramedullary hematopoiesis.[129] Liver pathology typically reveals multifocal hepatic necrosis with giant cell transformation, inflammation, bile stasis, and bile duct proliferation. The presence of intracytoplasmic inclusion bodies within the hepatocytes and large nuclear inclusions, also called owl's eye inclusions, in hepatocytes and biliary epithelium confirms the diagnosis.[130] Laboratory studies show evidence of mild-to-moderate liver dysfunction with elevated transaminases and alkaline phosphatase in the majority of patients.

Treatment with gancyclovir is recommended for infants with evidence of CNS disease and should be considered in infants with other end-organ disease (hepatitis, pneumonia, thrombocytopenia). Gancyclovir is a synthetic nucleoside analog, similar to acyclovir, which requires phosphorylation for antiviral activity. It is generally well tolerated in neonates, with neutropenia being the most common side effect of long-term therapy. Gancyclo-

vir does not reverse CNS injury, but has been shown to preserve hearing[131] and improve neurodevelopmental outcomes at 6 and 12 months.[132] Treatment with a newer agent, valgancyclovir, an oral prodrug of gancyclovir appears to have equal efficacy in treatment of symptomatic CMV infections, without the need for indwelling central line access typically required for the 6-week treatment course.[133] Longer-term treatment studies aimed at assessing the risks/benefits of 6-week versus 6-month treatment courses is currently ongoing.

Hepatomegaly and cholestasis usually resolve in the first year of life, but some of these patients go on to develop portal hypertension without evidence of cirrhosis. Almost 90% of infants surviving symptomatic congenital CMV infection will go on to display long-term neurologic sequelae, the most common of which is SNHL, with very few children displaying normal intellect.[134] Other findings include visual deficits, mental retardation, seizure disorders, cerebral palsy, and developmental delay. Hearing loss after CMV infection, in both symptomatic and asymptomatic infants, is progressive and may not present until later in childhood, underscoring the need for frequent evaluations in early childhood.

Objectives

1. Identify the classic signs and symptoms associated with congenital CMV infection
2. Understand risk of transmission based on timing of infection
3. Understand how CMV infection can affect the liver
4. Treatment options for neonates with congenital CMV infection
5. Long-term complications associated with congenital CMV infection

CASE 21

A 980-g, 28-week preterm infant born via C/S for maternal fever with transverse lie to a 34-year-old G1P0 woman with PPROM× 3 days. Mother's labs show that she is A+/antibody negative/rubella immune/serology nonreactive/hepatitis B negative/HIV negative. Baby cried vigorously at delivery and was placed on NCPAP. Sepsis evaluation at birth was negative and antibiotics were discontinued at 48 hours. Baby was started on trophic feeds with maternal EBM on DOL#2 and advanced easily to full feeds by DOL#14. Mom's milk supply is excellent and she frequently pumps at the bedside while visiting. On DOL#34, baby develops respiratory distress with increasing apnea, requiring intubation. Sepsis screen in performed and baby is placed on empiric antibiotics. KUB is unremarkable and there is no history of feeding intolerance. CBC shows a WBC 5.6, HCT of 31%, and a platelet count of 57,000. Baby is noted to be jaundiced with petechiae scattered over chest and abdomen, the liver is 3 cm below the RCM and a spleen tip is palpable. LFTs are obtained which show AST 346, ALT 534, alkaline phosphatase 453, total bilirubin 4.3/direct bilirubin 3.5, and albumin 2.3.

Of the following, which is most likely to be true?
A. Mother has a history of IV drug abuse
B. Organism isolated is an obligate intracellular pathogen
C. Abdominal ultrasound shows an occlusive clot at the junction of the inferior vena cava and hepatic veins
D. Urine culture is positive for *Escherichia coli*
E. Presence of trophozoites on peripheral blood smear

Discussion

The correct answer is **B**. Hepatitis panel is negative, HSV PCR is negative, urine culture is positive for CMV. Breast milk sample is found to be positive for CMV on PCR with a viral copy number estimated to be $>1 \times 10^5$/cc.

The following statement is TRUE
A. Infants with symptomatic postnatally acquired CMV infection have an increased risk of progressive SNHL
B. CMV can only be isolated from the cellular fraction of breast milk
C. Infants born at 32 weeks' gestational age or with a birth weight <1,500 g may be at higher risk of developing symptomatic postnatal CMV disease
D. Freezing at −20°C or colder prevents transmission of CMV from breast milk
E. The risk of postnatal acquisition of CMV from human milk is 40% in VLBW infants

Discussion

The correct answer is **C**. Postnatally, CMV is most often transmitted through virus-containing breast milk, although other sources include transfusion of infected blood products and horizontal transmission from close contact. Most postnatal CMV infections in term infants are mild, often asymptomatic, and self-limited. Transmission of protective antibodies to CMV begins after the 28th week, placing preterm infants at particular risk for postnatally acquired CMV infection. Symptomatic infants typically present with a sepsis-like syndrome (SLS) including respiratory distress, apnea, thrombocytopenia, neutropenia, and petecchiae. In addition, they often display hepatitis with elevated transaminases, hepatosplenomegaly, and cholestasis.

CMV can be isolated from both the cellular and whey fractions of breast milk and is commonly found in milk from seropositive women. CMV excretion into breast milk begins shortly postpartum and peaks at 1 to 2 months after delivery, declining thereafter. A recent meta-analysis of CMV transmission from breast milk in preterm infants estimates the rate of CMV transmission from untreated breast milk to be 6.5% with only 1.4% developing SLS. The risk of acquiring CMV infection from frozen breast milk is decreased compared to fresh breast milk, but the rate of CMV–SLS in these infants is not reduced. Holder pasteurization (62.5°C [144.5°F] for 30 minutes), which is standard procedure for most US milk banks, has been shown to reliably inactivate HIV and CMV and eliminate or substantially decrease titers of most other viruses. Milk acquired from milk-sharing sites is not pasteurized and would be expected to represent a risk of CMV transmission.

The benefit of breast milk feeding in preterm infants appear to outweigh the risks of severe disease from breast milk–acquired CMV infection in the neonatal period, as this has not been definitively associated with developmental delays or SNHL as seen with congenital CMV infection.[135–137] This stance has been recapitulated in the 2012 statement from the AAP on breast-feeding and use of human milk. A recent study of VLBW infants with breast milk–acquired postnatal CMV infection, however, does generate some concern about long-term outcomes in these infants. Although school age cognitive and motor function scores of the infected infants were in the normal range, they were not as high as uninfected VLBW infant controls.[135]

REFERENCES

1. Kunisaki SM, Foker JE. Surgical advances in the fetus and neonate: esophageal atresia. *Clin Perinatol.* 2012;39:349–361.
2. de Jong EM, Felix JF, de Klein A, et al. Etiology of esophageal atresia and tracheoesophageal fistula: "mind the gap". *Curr Gastroenterol Rep.* 2010;12:215–222.
3. Solomon BD. VACTERL/VATER association. *Orphanet J Rare Dis.* 2011;6:56.
4. La Placa S, Giuffrè M, Gangemi A, et al. Esophageal atresia in newborns: a wide spectrum from the isolated forms to a full VACTERL phenotype? *Ital J Pediatr.* 2013;39:45.
5. Borruto FA, Impellizzeri P, Montalto AS, et al. Thoracoscopy versus thoracotomy for esophageal atresia and tracheoesophageal fistula repair: review of the literature and meta-analysis. *Eur J Pediatr Surg.* 2012;22:415–419.
6. Spitz L. Esophageal atresia. Lessons I have learned in a 40-year experience. *J Pediatr Surg.* 2006;41:1635–1640.
7. Otjen JP, Iyer RS, Phillips GS, et al. Usual and unusual causes of pediatric gastric outlet obstruction. *Pediatr Radiol.* 2012; 42:728–737.

8. Godbole P, Sprigg A, Dickson JA, et al. Ultrasound compared with clinical examination in infantile hypertrophic pyloric stenosis. *Arch Dis Child*. 1996;75:335–337.

9. Hernanz-Schulman M. Infantile hypertrophic pyloric stenosis. *Radiology*. 2003;227:319–331.

10. Dutta S, Albanese CT. Minimal access surgery in the neonate. *NeoReviews*. 2006;7:e400–e409.

11. McIntyre RC, Bensard DD, Karrer FM, et al. The pediatric diaphragm in acute gastric volvulus. *J Am Coll Surg*. 1994;178:234–238.

12. Okada K, Miyako M, Honma S, et al. Discharge diagnoses in infants with apparent life-threatening event. *Pediatr Int*. 2003;45:560–563.

13. Amiel J, Lyonnet S. Hirschsprung disease, associated syndromes, and genetics: a review. *J Med Genet*. 2001;38:729–739.

14. Kapur RP. Practical pathology and genetics of Hirschsprung's disease. *Semin Pediatr Surg*. 2009;18:212–223.

15. Haricharan RN, Georgeson KE. Hirschsprung disease. *Semin Pediatr Surg*. 2008;17:266–275.

16. Freeman SB, Torfs CP, Romitti PA, et al. Congenital gastrointestinal defects in Down syndrome: a report from the Atlanta and National Down Syndrome Projects. *Clin Genet*. 2009;75:180–184.

17. Holland AJA, Walker K, Badawi N. Gastroschisis: an update. *Pediatr Surg Int*. 2010;26:871–878.

18. Islam S. Advances in surgery for abdominal wall defects: gastroschisis and omphalocele. *Clin Perinatol*. 2012;39:375–386.

19. Herman RS, Teitelbaum DH. Anorectal malformations. *Clin Perinatol*. 2012;39:403–422.

20. Wadhawan R, Oh W, Vohr BR, et al. Spontaneous intestinal perforation in extremely low birth weight infants: association with indometacin therapy and effects on neurodevelopmental outcomes at 18–22 months corrected age. *Arch Dis Child Fetal Neonatal Ed*. 2013;98:F127–F132.

21. Gordon PV, Attridge JT. Understanding clinical literature relevant to spontaneous intestinal perforations. *Am J Perinatol*. 2009;26:309–316.

22. Blakely ML, Gupta H, Lally KP. Surgical management of necrotizing enterocolitis and isolated intestinal perforation in premature neonates. *Semin Perinatol*. 2008;32:122–126.

23. Neu J, Walker WA. Necrotizing enterocolitis. *N Engl J Med*. 2011;364:255–264.

24. Caplan MS, Jilling T. The pathophysiology of necrotizing enterocolitis. *NeoReviews*. 2001;2:e103e–e109.

25. Bell MJ, Ternberg JL, Feigin RD, et al. Neonatal necrotizing enterocolitis. Therapeutic decisions based upon clinical staging. *Ann Surg*. 1978;187:1–7.

26. Raval MV, Lawrence Moss R. Surgical necrotizing enterocolitis: a primer for the neonatologist. *NeoReviews*. 2013;14:e393–e401.

27. Dimmitt RA, Moss RL. Clinical management of necrotizing enterocolitis. *NeoReviews*. 2001;2:e110–e117.

28. Kastenberg ZJ, Sylvester KG. The surgical management of necrotizing enterocolitis. *Clin Perinatol*. 2013;40:135–148.

29. Sharma R, Hudak ML. A clinical perspective of necrotizing enterocolitis: past, present, and future. *Clin Perinatol*. 2013;40:27–51.

30. Calder PC, Krauss-Etschmann S, de Jong EC, et al. Early nutrition and immunity – progress and perspectives. *Br J Nutrition*. 2006;96:774–790.

31. Gephart SM, Hanson CK. Preventing necrotizing enterocolitis with standardized feeding protocols: not only possible, but imperative. *Adv Neonatal Care*. 2013;13:48–54.

32. Bell EF. Preventing necrotizing enterocolitis: what works and how safe? *Pediatrics*. 2005;115:173–174.

33. Stritzke AI, Smyth J, Synnes A, et al. Transfusion-associated necrotising enterocolitis in neonates. *Arch Dis Child Fetal Neonatal Ed*. 2013;98:F10–F14.

34. Lin HC, Hsu CH, Chen HL, et al. Oral probiotics prevent necrotizing enterocolitis in very low birth weight preterm infants: a multicenter, randomized, controlled trial. *Pediatrics*. 2008;122:693–700.

35. Chen CC, Allan Walker W. Probiotics and the mechanism of necrotizing enterocolitis. *Semin Pediatr Surg*. 2013;22:94–100.

36. Zhang HY, Wang F, Feng JX. Intestinal microcirculatory dysfunction and neonatal necrotizing enterocolitis. *Chin Med J*. 2013;126:1771–1778.

37. Watkins DJ, Besner GE. The role of the intestinal microcirculation in necrotizing enterocolitis. *Semin Pediatr Surg*. 2013;22:83–87.

38. Gephart SM, McGrath JM, Effken JA, et al. Necrotizing enterocolitis risk: state of the science. *Adv Neonatal Care*. 2012;12:77–87.

39. Gutierrez IM, Kang KH, Jaksic T. Neonatal short bowel syndrome. *Semin Fetal Neonatal Med*. 2011;16:157–163.

40. Duro D, Mitchell PD, Kalish LA, et al. Risk factors for parenteral nutrition–associated liver disease following surgical therapy for necrotizing enterocolitis: a Glaser Pediatric Research Network Study [corrected]. *J Pediatr Gastroenterol Nutr*. 2011;52:595–600.

41. Bakirtas A, Turktas I, Dalgic B. Cow milk allergy presenting as colitis. *Eur J Pediatr*. 2003;162:653; .

42. Dhaheri Al W, Diksic D, Ben-Shoshan M. IgE-mediated cow milk allergy and infantile colic: diagnostic and management challenges. *BMJ Case Rep*. 2013;1;2013.

43. Vandenplas Y, Gottrand F, Veereman-Wauters G, et al. Gastrointestinal manifestations of cow's milk protein allergy and gastrointestinal motility. *Acta Paediatr*. 2012;101:1105–1109.

44. Vandenplas Y, Steenhout P, Planoudis Y, et al; Althera Study Group. Treating cow's milk protein allergy: a double-blind randomized trial comparing two extensively hydrolysed formulas with probiotics. *Acta Paediatr*. 2013;102:990–998.

45. Koletzko S, Niggemann B, Arato A, et al. Diagnostic approach and management of cow's milk protein allergy in infants and children: ESPGHAN GI Committee practical guidelines. *J Pediatr Gastroenterol Nutr*. 2012;55:221–229.

46. Birch JL, Newell SJ. Gastrooesophageal reflux disease in preterm infants: current management and diagnostic dilemmas. *Arch Dis Child Fetal Neonatal Ed*. 2009;94:F379–F383.

47. Jadcherla SR, Rudolph CD. Gastroesophageal reflux in the preterm neonate. *NeoReviews*. 2005;6:e87–e98.

48. Martin RJ, Hibbs AM. Diagnosing gastroesophageal reflux in preterm infants. *Pediatrics*. 2006;118:793–794.

49. Sindel BD, Maisels MJ, Ballantine TV. Gastroesophageal reflux to the proximal esophagus in infants with bronchopulmonary dysplasia. *Am J Dis Child*. 1989;143:1103–1106.

50. van der Pol RJ, Smits MJ, Venmans L, et al. Diagnostic accuracy of tests in pediatric gastroesophageal reflux disease. *J Pediatr*. 2013;162:983–987.e1–e4.

51. Malcolm WF, Cotten CM. Metoclopramide, H2 blockers, and proton pump inhibitors: pharmacotherapy for gastroesophageal reflux in neonates. *Clin Perinatol*. 2012;39:99–109.

52. Ward RM, Kearns GL. Proton pump inhibitors in pediatrics: mechanism of action, pharmacokinetics, pharmacogenetics, and pharmacodynamics. *Paediatr Drugs*. 2013;15:119–131.

53. Czinn SJ, Blanchard S. Gastroesophageal reflux disease in neonates and infants: when and how to treat. *Paediatr Drugs*. 2013;15:19–27.

54. Wong RJ, Stevenson DK, Ahlfors CE, et al. Neonatal jaundice: bilirubin physiology and clinical chemistry. *NeoReviews*. 2007;8:e58–e67.

55. Hansen TWR. Core concepts: bilirubin metabolism. *NeoReviews*. 2010;11:e316–e322.

56. Schulz S, Zhao H, Wong RJ, et al. Heme oxygenase biology: part 2: neonatal disorders. *NeoReviews*. 2012;13:e158–e165.

57. McKiernan P. Neonatal jaundice. *Clin Res Hepatol Gastroenterol*. 2012;36:253–256.

58. Bhutani VK. Jaundice due to glucose-6-phosphate dehydrogenase deficiency. *NeoReviews*. 2012;13:e166–e177.

59. Ross MB, de Alarcon P. Hemolytic disease of the fetus and newborn. *NeoReviews*. 2013;14:e83–e88.

60. Preer GL, Philipp BL. Understanding and managing breast milk jaundice. *Arch Dis Child Fetal Neonatal Ed*. 2011;96:F461–F466.

61. Pan X, Kelly S, Melin-Aldana H, et al. Novel mechanism of fetal hepatocyte injury in congenital alloimmune hepatitis involves the terminal complement cascade. *Hepatology*. 2010;51:2061–2068.

62. Saenz MS, Van Hove J, Scharer G. Neonatal liver failure: a genetic and metabolic perspective. *Curr Opin Pediatr*. 2010;22:241–245.

63. Shanmugam NP, Bansal S, Greenough A, et al. Neonatal liver failure: aetiologies and management–state of the art. *Eur J Pediatr*. 2011;170:573–581.

64. Sundaram SS, Alonso EM, Narkewicz MR, et al. Pediatric Acute Liver Failure Study Group: Characterization and outcomes of young infants with acute liver failure. *J Pediatr*. 2011;59:813–818.e1.

65. Rand EB, Karpen SJ, Kelly S, et al. Treatment of neonatal hemochromatosis with exchange transfusion and intravenous immunoglobulin. *J Pediatr*. 2009;155:566–571.

66. Whitington PF, Hibbard JU. High-dose immunoglobulin during pregnancy for recurrent neonatal haemochromatosis. *Lancet*. 2004;364:1690–1698.

67. Harpavat S, Finegold MJ, Karpen SJ. Patients with biliary atresia have elevated direct/conjugated bilirubin levels shortly after birth. *Pediatrics*. 2011;128:e1428–e1433.

68. Schwarz KB, Haber BH, Philip R, et al. Extra-hepatic anomalies in infants with biliary atresia: results of a large prospective North American multi-center study. *Hepatology*. 2013;58(5):1724–1731.

69. Davenport M. Biliary atresia: clinical aspects. *Semin Pediatr Surg*. 2012;21:175–184.

70. Sokol RJ, Shepherd RW, Superina R, et al. Screening and outcomes in biliary atresia: summary of a National Institutes of Health workshop. *Hepatology*. 2007;46:566–581.

71. Mieli-Vergani G, Vergani D. Biliary atresia. *Semin Immunopathol*. 2009;31:371–381.

72. Herman TE, Siegel MJ. Neonatal type 1 choledochal cyst. *J Perinatol*. 2007;27:453–454.

73. Makin E, Davenport M. Understanding choledochal malformation. *Arch Dis Child*. 2012;97:69–72.

74. Todani T, Watanabe Y, Narusue M, et al. Congenital bile duct cysts: classification, operative procedures, and review of thirty-seven cases including cancer arising from choledochal cyst. *Am J Surg*. 1977;134:263–269.

75. Savader SJ, Benenati JF, Venbrux AC, et al. Choledochal cysts: classification and cholangiographic appearance. *Am J Roentgenol*. 1991;156:327–331.

76. Zhou LY, Guan BY, Li L, et al. Objective differential characteristics of cystic biliary atresia and choledochal cysts in neonates and young infants: sonographic findings. *J Ultrasound Med*. 2012;31:833–841.

77. Rozel C, Garel L, Rypens F, Viremouneix L, Lapierre C, Décarie JC, et al. Imaging of biliary disorders in children. *Pediatr Radiol*. 2011;41:208–220.

78. Mishra A, Pant N, Chadha R, et al. Choledochal cysts in infancy and childhood. *Indian J Pediatr*. 2007;74:937–943.

79. Ruiz-Elizalde AR, Cowles RA. A practical algorithm for accurate diagnosis and treatment of perinatally identified biliary ductal dilation: three cases that underscore the importance of an individualised approach. *J Matern Fetal Neonatal Med*. 2009;22:622–628.

80. Diao M, Li L, Cheng W. Timing of surgery for prenatally diagnosed asymptomatic choledochal cysts: a prospective randomized study. *J Pediatr Surg*. 2012;47:506–512.

81. Tanaka N, Ueno T, Takama Y, et al. Diagnosis and management of biliary cystic malformations in neonates. *J Pediatr Surg*. 2010;45:2119–2123.

82. Yamataka A, Lane GJ, Cazares J. Laparoscopic surgery for biliary atresia and choledochal cyst. *Semin Pediatr Surg*. 2012;21:201–210.

83. Vajro P, Ferrante L, Paolella G. Alagille syndrome: an overview. *Clin Res Hepatol Gastroenterol*. 2012;36:275–277.

84. Guegan K, Stals K, Day M, et al. JAG1 mutations are found in approximately one third of patients presenting with only one or two clinical features of Alagille syndrome. *Clin Genet*. 2012;82:33–40.

85. Penton AL, Leonard LD, Spinner NB. Notch signaling in human development and disease. *Semin Cell Dev Biol*. 2012;23:450–457.

86. Hartley JL, Gissen P, Kelly DA. Alagille syndrome and other hereditary causes of cholestasis. *Clin Liver Dis*. 2013;17:279–300.

87. Kamath BM, Loomes KM, Piccoli DA. Medical management of Alagille syndrome. *J Pediatr Gastroenterol Nutr*. 2010;50:580–586.

88. Suchy FJ, Burdelski M, Tomar BS, et al. Cholestatic liver disease: working group report of the first world congress of pediatric gastroenterology, hepatology, and nutrition. *J Pediatr Gastroenterol Nutr*. 2002;35(Suppl 2):S89–S97.

89. Paulusma CC, Groen A, Kunne C, et al. Atp8b1 deficiency in mice reduces resistance of the canalicular membrane to hydrophobic bile salts and impairs bile salt transport. *Hepatology*. 2006;44:195–204.

90. Davit-Spraul A, Gonzales E, Baussan C, et al. Progressive familial intrahepatic cholestasis. *Orphanet J Rare Dis*. 2009;4:1.

91. Jacquemin E, Malan V, Rio M, et al. Heterozygous FIC1 deficiency: a new genetic predisposition to transient neonatal cholestasis. *J Pediatr Gastroenterol Nutr*. 2010;50:447–449.

92. Jacquemin E. Progressive familial intrahepatic cholestasis. *J Gastroenterol Hepatol*. 1999;14:594–599.

93. Jacquemin E. Progressive familial intrahepatic cholestasis. *Clin Res Hepatol Gastroenterol*. 2012;36(Suppl 1):S26–S35.

94. Hughes MG, Khan KM, Gruessner AC, et al. Long-term outcome in 42 pediatric liver transplant patients with alpha 1-antitrypsin deficiency: a single-center experience. *Clin Transplant*. 2011;25:731–736.

95. Brantly M, Nukiwa T, Crystal RG. Molecular basis of alpha-1-antitrypsin deficiency. *Am J Med*. 1988;84:13–31.

96. Greene DN, Procter M, Krautscheid P, et al. α1-antitrypsin deficiency in fraternal twins born with familial spontaneous pneumothorax. *Chest*. 2012;141:239–241.

97. Fregonese L, Stolk J. Hereditary alpha-1-antitrypsin deficiency and its clinical consequences. *Orphanet J Rare Dis*. 2008;3:16.

98. Lykavieris P, Ducot B, Lachaux A, et al. Liver disease associated with ZZ alpha1-antitrypsin deficiency and ursodeoxycholic acid therapy in children. *J Pediatr Gastroenterol Nutr*. 2008;47:623–629.

99. Dudrick SJ. Innovation, persistence, and proficiency in parenteral nutrition. *Nutr Clin Pract*. 2009;24:436–440.

100. Robinson DT, Ehrenkranz RA. Parenteral nutrition-associated cholestasis in small for gestational age infants. *J Pediatr*. 2008;152:59–62.

101. Christensen RD, Henry E, Wiedmeier SE, et al. Identifying patients, on the first day of life, at high-risk of developing parenteral nutrition-associated liver disease. *J Perinatol*. 2007;27:284–290.

102. Quirós-Tejeira RE, Ament ME, Reyen L, et al. Long-term parenteral nutritional support and intestinal adaptation in children with short bowel syndrome: a 25-year experience. *J Pediatr*. 2004;145:157–163.

103. Willis TC, Carter BA, Rogers SP, et al. High rates of mortality and morbidity occur in infants with parenteral nutrition-associated cholestasis. *J Parenter Enteral Nutr*. 2010;34:32–37.

104. Gura KM, Lee S, Valim C, et al. Safety and efficacy of a fish-oil-based fat emulsion in the treatment of parenteral nutrition-associated liver disease. *Pediatrics*. 2008;121:e678–e86.

105. de Meijer VE, Gura KM, Le HD, et al. Fish oil-based lipid emulsions prevent and reverse parenteral nutrition-associated liver disease: the Boston experience. *J Parenter Enteral Nutr*. 2009;33:541–547.

106. Rollins MD, Ward RM, Jackson WD, et al. Effect of decreased parenteral soybean lipid emulsion onhepatic function in infants at risk for parenteral nutrition-associated liver disease: a pilot study. *J Pediatr Surg*. 2013;48:1348–1356.

107. Cober MP, Killu G, Brattain A, et al. Intravenous fat emulsions reduction for patients with parenteral nutrition-associated liver disease. *J Pediatr*. 2012;160:421–427.

108. Mercer DF, Hobson BD, Fischer RT, et al. Hepatic fibrosis persists and progresses despite biochemical improvement in children treated with intravenous fish oil emulsion. *J Pediatr Gastroenterol Nutr*. 2013;56:364–369.

109. Soden JS, Lovell MA, Brown K, et al. Failure of resolution of portal fibrosis during omega-3 fatty acid lipid emulsion therapy in two patients with irreversible intestinal failure. *J Pediatr*. 2010;156:327–331.

110. Tillm`an EM. Review and clinical update on parenteral nutrition-associated liver disease. *Nutr Clin Pract*. 2013;28:30–39.

111. Angsten G, Finkel Y, Lucas S, et al. Improved outcome in neonatal short bowel syndrome using parenteral fish oil in combination with ω-6/9 lipid emulsions. *J Parenter Enteral Nutr*. 2012;36:587–595.

112. Vanek VW, Seidner DL, Allen P, et al. A.S.P.E.N. position paper: clinical role for alternative intravenous fat emulsions. *Nutr Clin Pract*. 2012;27:150–192.

113. Rangel SJ, Calkins CM, Cowles RA, et al. Parenteral nutrition-associated cholestasis: an American Pediatric Surgical Association Outcomes and Clinical Trials Committee systematic review. *J Pediatr Surg*. 2012;47:225–240.

114. Andorsky DJ, Lund DP, Lillehei CW, et al. Nutritional and other postoperative management of neonates with short bowel syndrome correlates with clinical outcomes. *J Pediatr*. 2001;139:27–33.

115. Amin SC, Pappas C, Iyengar H, et al. Short bowel syndrome in the NICU. *Clin Perinatol*. 2013;40:53–68.

116. van Hasselt PM, de Koning TJ, Kvist N, et al. Prevention of vitamin K deficiency bleeding in breastfed infants: lessons from the Dutch and Danish biliary atresia registries. *Pediatrics*. 2008;121:e857–e863.

117. van Hasselt PM, de Vries W, de Vries E, et al. Hydrolysed formula is a risk factor for vitamin K deficiency in infants with unrecognised cholestasis. *J Pediatr Gastroenterol Nutr*. 2010;51:773–776.

118. Shen YM, Wu JF, Hsu HY, et al. Oral absorbable fat-soluble vitamin formulation in pediatric patients with cholestasis. *J Pediatr Gastroenterol Nutr*. 2012;55:587–591.

119. Marquez L, Levy ML, Munoz FM, et al. A report of three cases and review of intrauterine herpes simplex virus infection. *Pediatr Infect Dis J*. 2011;30:153–157.

120. Robinson JL, Vaudry WL, Forgie SE, et al. Prevention, recognition and management of neonatal HSV infections. *Expert Rev Anti Infect Ther*. 2012;10:675–685.

121. Handel S, Klingler EJ, Washburn K, et al. Population-based surveillance for neonatal herpes in New York City, April 2006–September 2010. *Sex Transm Dis*. 2001;38:705–710.

122. Brown ZA, Wald A, Morrow RA, et al. Effect of serologic status and cesarean delivery on transmission rates of herpes simplex virus from mother to infant. *JAMA*. 2003;289:203–209.

123. Prétet JL, Pelletier L, Bernard B, et al. Apoptosis participates to liver damage in HSV-induced fulminant hepatitis. *Apoptosis*. 2003;8:655–663.

124. Benador N, Mannhardt W, Schranz D, et al. Three cases of neonatal herpes simplex virus infection presenting as fulminant hepatitis. *Eur J Pediatr*. 1990;149:555–559.

125. Verma A, Dhawan A, Zuckerman M, et al. Neonatal herpes simplex virus infection presenting as acute liver failure: prevalent role of herpes simplex virus type I. *J Pediatr Gastroenterol Nutr.* 2006;42:282–286.

126. Laifer SA, Ehrlich GD, Huff DS, et al. Congenital cytomegalovirus infection in offspring of liver transplant recipients. *Clin Infect Dis.* 1995;20:52–55.

127. Brown HL, Abernathy MP. Cytomegalovirus infection. *Semin Perinatol.* 1998;22:260–266.

128. Boppana SB, Pass RF, Britt WJ, et al. Symptomatic congenital cytomegalovirus infection: neonatal morbidity and mortality. *Pediatr Infect Dis J.* 1992;11:93–99.

129. Boyer TD, Michael P, Manns MD, et al. *Zakim and Boyer's Hepatology.* W. B. Saunders Company; 2011.

130. Suchy FJ, Sokol RJ, Balistreri WF. *Liver Disease in Children.* Cambridge University Press; 2007.

131. Kimberlin DW, Lin CY, Sánchez PJ, et al. Effect of ganciclovir therapy on hearing in symptomatic congenital cytomegalovirus disease involving the central nervous system: a randomized, controlled trial. *J Pediatr.* 2003;143:16–25.

132. Oliver SE, Cloud GA, Sánchez PJ, et al. Neurodevelopmental outcomes following ganciclovir therapy in symptomatic congenital cytomegalovirus infections involving the central nervous system. *J Clin Virol.* 2009;46(Suppl 4):S22–S26.

133. del Rosal T, Baquero-Artigao F, Blázquez D, et al. Treatment of symptomatic congenital cytomegalovirus infection beyond the neonatal period. *J Clin Virol.* 2012;55:72–74.

134. Nassetta L, Kimberlin D, Whitley R. Treatment of congenital cytomegalovirus infection: implications for future therapeutic strategies. *J Antimicrob Chemother.* 2009;3:862–867.

135. Bevot A, Hamprecht K, Krägeloh-Mann I, et al. Long-term outcome in preterm children with human cytomegalovirus infection transmitted via breast milk. *Acta Paediatr.* 2012; 101:e167–e172.

136. Plosa EJ, Esbenshade JC, Fuller MP, et al. Cytomegalovirus infection. *Pediatr Rev.* 2012;33:156–163.

137. Kurath S, Halwachs-Baumann G, Müller W, et al. Transmission of cytomegalovirus via breast milk to the prematurely born infant: a systematic review. *Clin Microbiol Infect.* 2010; 16:1172–1178.

Chapter 13
DERMATOLOGY

Leslie Potter Lawley, MD and Zakiya Pressley Rice, MD

CASE 1

A 3-day-old Hispanic infant girl is transferred to your neonatal intensive care unit. Her mother received routine prenatal care. Her birth weight was 3,120 g and Apgar scores at 1 minute of 8 and 5 minutes of 9. She was noted at birth to have multiple red to purple firm papules scattered over the face, trunk, and extremities (Fig. 13-1). Per transfer report she has experienced some low-grade fevers but has been sucking and swallowing well. On your examination, you find a well-appearing newborn girl in no acute distress. Her head is normocephalic and atraumatic. Her pupils are equal and reactive to light. Within the oropharynx she has one 3-mm shallow erosion on the

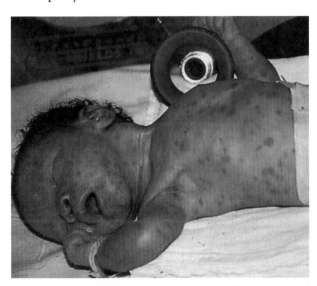

FIGURE 13-1. Red-purple firm papules on face, trunk, and extremities. (Reproduced with permission from Weinberg S, Prose N, Kristal L. *Color Atlas of Pediatric Dermatology.* 3rd ed. New York, NY: McGraw-Hill; 1998.)

hard palate. She has normal work of breathing and lungs are clear to auscultation. Her heart has a regular rate and rhythm with no murmurs, gallops, or rubs. Her abdomen is soft, nontender. She has normal active bowel sounds, her liver is 3 cm below the costal margin. On cutaneous examination, she has multiple firm 3- to 9-mm erythematous to purple firm nodules scattered on the face, trunk, upper, and lower extremities. There is no lymphadenopathy. You also note some waxy scale on the scalp and shallow postauricular erosions. She has mild erythema of the labia and inguinal folds.

What is the most appropriate next step?
A. Complete metabolic panel
B. TORCH serologies
C. Otolaryngology consult
D. Liver ultrasound
E. Stool guaiac

Discussion

The correct answer is **B**. For an infant with multiple firm erythematous to purple nodules on the skin, infection should be considered first and of the above options TORCH serologies ordered. TORCH serologies traditionally include screening tests for toxoplasmosis, syphilis, rubella, cytomegalovirus, and herpes simplex virus (HSV) as these are infections which may present in similar fashion in the newborn with rash as well as ocular findings.[1] Other infections may also create this clinical picture of the "blueberry muffin" baby including varicella virus, Coxsackie B2, and parvovirus B19.[2] When testing for such infections it may be reasonable to selectively test for infections depending on clinical findings and history. In an infant whose mother received good prenatal care then rubella and syphilis are unlikely as these are standard screenings during pregnancy. An infant with CMV or HSV may be asymptomatic at birth. The complete metabolic panel, otolaryngology consult, liver ultrasound, and stool guaiac tests are not the most appropriate next step.

Which of the following tests is not part of the workup for a "blueberry muffin" baby?
A. Peripheral blood count and hemoglobin
B. Calcium level
C. Viral cultures
D. Coombs test
E. Skin biopsy

Discussion

The correct answer is **B**. Of the above options for tests, only the calcium level would not be indicated in this child. This test would be indicated in the setting of subcutaneous fat necrosis of the newborn. Blueberry muffin baby was first described with congenital rubella and represents persistent dermal erythropoiesis. It may occur with other infections including cytomegalovirus, coxsackie B2, and parvovirus B19 as discussed above. Blood dyscrasias (Rh incompatibility, maternal-fetal ABO incompatibility, spherocytosis, and twin transfusion syndrome) may present with dark blue nodules of the skin as well. The peripheral blood count, hemoglobin, and Coombs test will screen for these etiologies.[2] The clinical picture of "blueberry muffin" baby has also been described in the setting of malignancies such as neuroblastoma, rhabdomyosarcoma, myelogenous leukemias, and Langerhans cell histiocytosis. A skin biopsy will help delineate these etiologies.

In this female infant, viral serologies were normal. Her white blood count was 10.2, hemoglobin 14.2 g/dL, hematocrit 43%, platelets 188,000, and Coombs test negative. A skin biopsy is performed and reveals a dense dermal infiltrate of uniform cells with abundant eosinophilic cytoplasm and reniform nuclei which are S-100 and CD1a positive. These findings are consistent with a histiocytic process such as Langerhans cell histiocytosis (LCH).

Which of the following tests should be considered first?
A. Pulmonary function tests
B. Hepatic function tests
C. Chest x-ray
D. Bone marrow biopsy
E. A and B
F. B and C

Discussion

The correct answer is **F**. In the setting of LCH, an evaluation to determine systemic involvement should be performed as the majority of children with early onset LCH do have multisystem disease. This evaluation should include hepatic function tests, urine osmolality, complete skeletal radiographic survey, chest radiography in addition to complete blood count, and coagulation studies. If there are positive findings further studies may include bone marrow biopsy, pulmonary function tests, lung biopsy, liver biopsy, dental films, CT or MR of the CNS, and endocrine evaluation.[3]

While in the unit undergoing evaluations, you notice the infant's skin lesions are improving day to day. Tests results continue to return with normal findings. What is the probable diagnosis?
A. Dermal erythropoiesis
B. Congenital self-healing reticulocytosis
C. Parvovirus B19 infection
D. Maternal autoimmune thrombocytopenia

Discussion

The correct answer is **B**. The most plausible diagnosis is congenital self-healing reticulohistiocytosis also referred to as congenital self-healing Langerhans cell histiocytosis (CSHLCH). While the other options can present with cutaneous purpura or blueberry muffin lesions, this infant is otherwise well and tests for such diagnoses have been normal. In addition, the histopathology was consistent with LCH.

In one review of infantile LCH, it was noted that of the five infants presenting with blueberry muffin lesions, four spontaneously resolved and only one had systemic involvement of LCH.[4] Those infants with cutaneous only LCH and spontaneous resolution are diagnosed as having Hashimoto-Pritzker disease or CSHLCH. CSHLCH is now considered a mild variant of LCH. CSHLCH is characterized as having congenital cutaneous lesions in an otherwise well infant which spontaneously involute and histopathology consistent with a Langerhans cell process.[5] In these infants, skin lesions typically resolve over weeks to months with complete resolution by 12 months of age.[6] Because there have been reports of later onset of systemic involvement in some cases, long-term monitoring for development of multisystem disease such as bone involvement or diabetes insipidus is warranted.[5,7] Infants with multisystem LCH are treated with chemotherapy or even bone marrow or stem cell transplants therefore distinguishing between multisystem LCH and CSHLCH is important to prevent potentially adverse therapies in an otherwise healthy infant with cutaneous only disease.

True dermal erythropoiesis spontaneously fades resolving in 3 to 6 weeks. Treatment is directed at the underlying cause.

CASE 2

A newborn black male has been admitted to the neonatal intensive care unit with tetralogy of Fallot. He was the product of an uncomplicated pregnancy and normal spontaneous vaginal delivery. On day 2, he is noted to have randomly scattered pustules on the buttocks, lower back, abdomen, and thighs (Fig. 13-2A). There is no surrounding erythema. He has had no fevers. Despite his cardiac abnormalities he is otherwise well.

Which of the following tests is most likely to provide the diagnosis?
A. Blood cultures
B. Chest x-ray
C. Gram stain
D. Tzanck smear
E. Complete blood count

Discussion

The correct answer is **C**. A Gram stain of a pustule is a quick and easy investigative tool to gather information and can be diagnostic in cases of common neonatal eruptions. Other than the tetralogy of Fallot, this child is healthy without signs of systemic disease or sepsis, therefore blood cultures are not indicated and would take days for results to finalize. Chest radiography is not indicated with this skin eruption. If the lesions are grouped and if there are erosions with scalloped edges on examination you could also consider a Tzanck smear to rule out herpes simplex or varicella viral eruptions, however in this case the child has discrete pustules. A complete blood count may provide diagnostic clues but is not as likely to give the diagnosis.

In this case, you first perform a Gram stain of a pustule since it is a quick and easy test. The slide reveals neutrophils and few eosinophils and no organisms.

What is the probable diagnosis?
A. Congenital candidiasis
B. Erythema toxicum neonatorum
C. Transient neonatal pustular melanosis (TNPM)
D. HSV
E. Staphylococcus pustulosis

Discussion

The correct answer is **C**. A Gram stain revealing neutrophils and few eosinophils without organisms is consistent with expected findings for TNPM. The majority of cases of TNPM occur in term black infants however it has been reported in infants with lighter skin as well. Typically pustules are present at birth but may not arise until the first few days. Pustules are fragile and break easily leaving a collarette of scale followed by a hyperpigmented macule. The macules slowly fade over months. No treatment is necessary as spontaneous resolution is the rule.[8] Congenital candidiasis presents at birth or in the first day of life with many scattered erythematous macules, papules, and papulovesicles that transform into pustules over several days. The organism is acquired from the mother in the birth canal. Affected neonates are generally otherwise well and the rash is self-limited, however there is risk of systemic infection including sepsis in

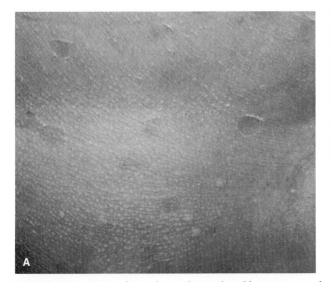
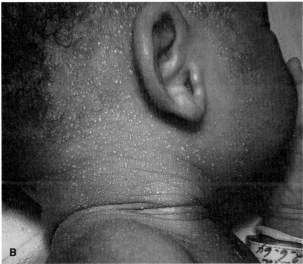

FIGURE 13-2. Scattered pustules on the trunk and hyperpigmented macules with collarette of scale. **(A)** Multiple pinpoint papulo-pustules on the head and neck. **(B)** (Reproduced with permission from Weinberg S, Prose N, Kristal L. *Color Atlas of Pediatric Dermatology*. 3rd ed. New York, NY: McGraw-Hill; 1998.)

low–birth-weight infants, especially those under 1,000 g.[9] A potassium hydroxide (KOH) preparation from a representative pustule would show pseudohyphae and spores. Diagnosis can also be made by fungal cultures which typically grow *Candida albicans*, but other species of *Candida* may also present in this manner.[10] Congenital candidiasis differs from neonatal candidiasis in timing and presentation. Neonatal candidiasis appears after the first week of life typically as thrush or diaper dermatitis. Erythema toxicum neonatorum is a very common neonatal eruption developing in the first 1 to 3 days of life. Poorly defined discrete erythematous macules and wheals with white to yellow papules, papulovesicles, and pustules arise scattered on the face, trunk, and extremities. Individual lesions have irregular shapes and wax and wane typically resolving spontaneously in 1 week. A Gram stain of a representative pustule demonstrates numerous eosinophils with few neutrophils. The patient may also have eosinophilia.[8] Neonatal or perinatal herpes simplex infection presents with small clustered vesicles with surrounding erythema on cutaneous or mucosal surfaces typically in the first 1 to 2 weeks of life. Individual vesicles become pustules then develop crusts. Neonates may also have signs of sepsis or encephalitis. A Tzanck smear demonstrates multinucleated giant cells typical for viral infection. A direct immunofluorescent antibody test or viral culture can differentiate herpes simplex from varicella. Intravenous acyclovir is the appropriate treatment.[11] Staphylococcus pustulosis presents as small pustules on the abdomen and groin which may rupture easily resulting in a collarette of scale. Pustules are often on an erythematous base with or without honey-colored crusts. It typically appears in the first few days to weeks of life. A Gram stain would reveal neutrophils and gram-positive cocci in clusters. A bacterial culture would be diagnostic. Widespread eruptions require systemic antibiotics.[12]

At day of life 17, a new eruption of small erythematous papules and papulopustules develops on the face, neck, and upper trunk (Fig. 13-2B). You note increased number of the papulopustules clustered at sites of cardiac monitor leads. Again you perform a Gram stain and KOH which reveal lymphocytes and few neutrophils, but no eosinophils or organisms.

What is your treatment?
A. Clotrimazole cream
B. Benzoyl peroxide wash
C. Intravenous clindamycin
D. Cooler environment
E. Hydrocortisone 2.5% ointment

Discussion

The correct answer is **D**. With the description of a newborn at 2 to 3 weeks of age in the neonatal intensive care unit with a new erythematous papulopustular eruption concentrated on the upper body and especially at the sites of adhesives, the diagnosis of miliaria rubra or candidiasis should be considered. The Gram stain and KOH described above is consistent with miliaria and thus providing a cooler environment would be the appropriate treatment. Miliaria represents an occlusion of the immature eccrine ducts and often appears in newborns who are overheated or febrile.[13] Clotrimazole cream would be appropriate treatment for localized candidiasis or neonatal cephalic pustulosis. The former would reveal pseudohyphae and spores on KOH and the latter may show spores of *Malassezia*. Neonatal cephalic pustulosis is also typically restricted to the face. Benzoyl peroxide wash treats neonatal acne which is also typically restricted to the face and often presents with open and closed comedones.[13] Intravenous antibiotics are not indicated in an afebrile infant with no organisms on the Gram stain. Topical corticosteroids would treat eosinophilic pustular folliculitis which would show neutrophils and eosinophils on Gram stain.[8]

CASE 3

An 8-day-old term female neonate is transferred to your unit for evaluation of a violaceous growing mass on the right leg (Fig. 13-3). Her birth weight was 3,217 g. Her mother had normal prenatal care and an ultrasound at 37 weeks' EGA did not show any abnormality of the right leg. The mass was apparent at birth and grew significantly during the first week of life. Outside records indicate thrombocytopenia at <10,000. On examination she is well appearing, in no acute distress and afebrile. There is a large erythematous to violaceous firm tumor encompassing the entire right thigh with extension to the right proximal calf, lower abdomen, mons pubis, and right labia majora. She has an ulceration measuring 1.5 cm within the mass on the right thigh. There is no thrill upon palpation of the entire tumor, and no bruits on auscultation. Laboratories upon admission include white blood count 4,000, hemoglobin 13.5, platelets <10,000, PT 17.6, fibrinogen 78, and D-dimer 10,000.

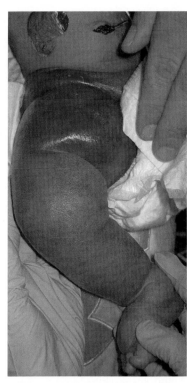

FIGURE 13-3. Confluent violaceous firm edematous tumor involving the right leg and distal trunk. (Used with permission of Leslie P. Lawley, MD.)

Prior to a biopsy of the tumor, what transfusion would be appropriate?
A. Packed RBCs
B. Platelets
C. Fresh-frozen plasma
D. A and B
E. B and C

Discussion

The correct answer is **C.** Fresh-frozen plasma would be appropriate prior to biopsy to reduce the risk of bleeding with the procedure. The case described above is consistent with Kasabach–Merritt phenomenon (KMP) in which a growing vascular tumor traps platelets resulting in a consumptive coagulopathy. The thrombocytopenia associated with KMP is severe as compared to thrombocytopenia described with vascular malformations which would be much milder. It is important in situations of KMP to avoid transfusions with platelets if possible as they are quickly consumed by the expanding vascular tumor. It is thought that abnormal blood vessel endothelium in the tumor activates the platelets.[14] Transfusions with fresh-frozen plasma and cryoprecipitate are preferred. At this time point the neonate is not severely anemic therefore packed red blood cells are not indicated.

After a transfusion of fresh-frozen plasma a skin biopsy from the right thigh is obtained. The pathologist reports a vascular tumor with features of capillaries and lymphatics. Given the clinical scenario, which of the following diagnoses is most likely?
A. Infantile hemangioma (IH)
B. Kaposiform hemangioendothelioma (KHE)
C. Rhabdomyosarcoma
D. Congenital hemangioma
E. Pyogenic granuloma

Discussion

The correct answer is **B.** KHE is a rare vascular tumor that most often presents in infancy as red-brown stain that thickens and becomes purpuric. It may affect multiple levels including the dermis, subcutis, muscle, fascia, and bone. A recent review of patients with KHE suggests that more extensive or deeper involvement of the tumor and earlier age of onset imparts higher risk of developing KMP.[15] Many patients present with the features of KMP along with the growing vascular tumor. On histopathology, KHE has ill-defined large lobules of capillaries and interspersed spindle cells and thin-walled vessels. Narrow slit-like vessels filled with erythrocytes are present around the spindle cells similar to Kaposi sarcoma hence the given name. Stains for lymphatic markers, LYVE-1, and Prox-1 are positive. This same pattern is present in the histopathology of tufted angiomas which some argue is a variant of KHE.[16] Although initially described in association with "hemangiomas," KMP has been shown in the literature to associate with KHE and tufted angiomas distinct vascular tumors from infantile hemangiomas and congenital hemangiomas. IHs are occasionally present at birth but more often appear in the first 4 weeks of life. IH are the most common benign tumor of infancy. They have a typical course with initial rapid growth over the first 3 to 4 months followed by slow growth up to 1 year of age.[17] The tumor then slowly involutes over 5 to 10 years. On histopathology, IHs show plump capillaries in a lobular distribution and may be distinguished by Glut-1-positive staining. A congenital hemangioma is fully formed at birth and does not demonstrate a proliferative phase. On histopathology it will have features more typical of a vascular malformation and Glut-1 -negative staining. While a congenital hemangioma may be associated with thrombocytopenia it is usually transient and not severe and progressive as seen with KMP.[18] Pyogenic granulomas more commonly appear later in life as friable vascular tumors although they have been reported at birth. On histopathology multiple capillary lobules are present and Glut-1 negative. It is not associated with typical KMP.[19]

You render a diagnosis of KMP in the setting of kaposiform hemangioendothelioma. The neonate is now 12 days old and the tumor continues to enlarge. Her platelets remain <10,000, fibrinogen low, and D-dimers elevated. Her hemoglobin is now 9.2. What is considered first-line therapy?
A. Vincristine
B. Interferon-α
C. Propranolol
D. Sirolimus
E. Radiation

Discussion

The correct answer is **A**. While vincristine, interferon-α, propranolol, sirolimus, and radiation have all been reported as treatment for KHE, several sources cite vincristine with or without systemic corticosteroids as the first intervention.[20,21] Kasabach–Merritt phenomenon is a medical emergency and treatment typically involves multiple disciplines and multiple therapies including corticosteroids, vincristine, interferon-a, ticlopidine plus aspirin, surgical excision, arterial embolization, and radiotherapy. The decision of treatment modalities considers associated risks and toxicities.[18] The combination of vincristine, ticlopidine, and aspirin has been reported successful in treating KMP with KHE and TA.[22] Recently, propranolol, which has been well reported to treat IH, has been suggested as adjuvant therapy for Kaposiform hemangioendothelioma and Kasabach–Merritt phenomenon in combination with vincristine.[23] Sirolimus has been reported to provide a rapid response in KHE and associated Kasabach–Merritt phenomenon.[20] Mortality has been reported in up to 30% of patients with Kasabach–Merritt phenomenon.[15]

CASE 4

A newborn Caucasian girl is admitted to the neonatology unit for monitoring of possible sepsis and intravenous antibiotics. Her mother arrived at the hospital fully dilated and she was delivered vaginally without complication however her mother's Group B Streptococcal (GBS) screen had been positive and no antibiotics were given during labor or delivery. Her Apgar scores were 6 at 1 minute and 7 at 5 minutes. On physical examination in the NICU blood pressure 82/45, pulse 168, axillary temperature 36.5, respiratory rate 28, height 55 cm, weight 3.67 kg, head circumference 35.5 cm, and SpO$_2$

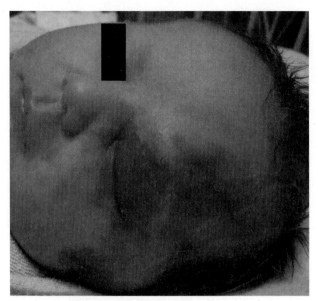

FIGURE 13-4. Well delineated red patch involving the left side of the face. (Used with permission of Leslie P. Lawley, MD.)

95%. She has a well-delineated red patch on the left forehead, eyelid, and cheek (Fig. 13-4). It blanches slightly with pressure but is not warm or indurated and does not appear to be tender. There is no pulsation or bruit. Her eyelids open equally and pupils are equal round and reactive to light.

What is your working diagnosis?
A. Cellulitis
B. Capillary vascular malformation
C. Nevus simplex
D. Birth trauma
E. Infantile hemangioma

Discussion

The correct answer is **B**. GBS infection is one of the most common forms of septicemia in neonates and may present in one of two forms: early or late onset. Early onset disease occurs in the first 7 days of life, often presenting at birth or soon after with signs of infection. Late onset disease develops anywhere from 7 days to 3 months of life and may present with cellulitis most often affecting the mandibular areas of the face. Cutaneous GBS infection is rare and most often occurs in late onset GBS but may be present at birth. Although the case infant has been exposed to GBS and may be bacteremic or septic, the facial patch described is not consistent with cellulitis in that it has no warmth, edema, induration, or tenderness.[12] A capillary vascular malformation ("port-wine stain") would be present at birth and well delineated. Nevus simplex ("angel kiss" or "stork bite") is also present at birth but is typically symmetric in distribution and located in the midline. It may be lighter in color than a capillary vascular malformation and fades over 1 to 2 years whereas port-wine stains persist through life becoming darker and thicker over time. A capillary vascular malformation may have extracutaneous manifestations in association with syndromes which would be rare with nevus simplex.[18] Prolonged labor or use of instrumentation during delivery may be associated with birth trauma which typically manifests as ecchymoses with multiple colors, edema, and tenderness. While infantile hemangiomas often appear and proliferate in the first few weeks of life, up to 50% to 60% of patients have subtle skin changes in the affected area at birth. It can be difficult to distinguish an early infantile hemangioma from a capillary vascular malformation.

Which of the following tests would you order first?
A. MRI of the head and neck
B. Ultrasound of the skull
C. Ophthalmology examination
D. Skin biopsy for cultures
E. Plain films of the face

Discussion

The correct answer is **C**. On examination of this infant, the erythematous patch is most consistent with a vascular birthmark, either a capillary malformation ("port-wine stain") or a precursor to an infantile hemangioma. For a capillary malformation in the cranial nerve V1 distribution, approximately 10% may develop Sturge–Weber Syndrome (SWS) a combination of facial port-wine stain, ipsilateral eye abnormalities, and leptomeningeal and brain abnormalities. If there is bilateral involvement of V1 segments or multiple segments in a unilateral distribution (i.e., V1, V2, and V3) this risk increases to 25% for manifestations of SWS. The capillary malformation almost always involves the V1 segment in SWS.[24] While there are no reports of SWS in the setting of a port wine stain only affecting the V3 area, there are rare reports of Sturge-Weber Syndrome with V2 capillary malformations. The eyelid has been shown to be a "watershed" area with some overlap of V1 and V2. An ophthalmology examination would be the appropriate first test for this child. Serial ophthalmology examinations are recommended for infants at risk of Sturge-Weber Syndrome with glaucoma representing the most common manifestation. An early MRI or CT is not indicated in an infant without any neurologic or ophthalmologic deficits since a negative scan at this age does not rule out future neurologic disease.[24] When there are neurologic signs, MRI is the most useful imaging modality. It is not clear at what age a negative MRI negates existence of Sturge-Weber Syndrome as normal MRI has been reported as late at 9 months of age in infants who later developed manifestations of Sturge-

Weber Syndrome.[25] Ultrasound is not likely to diagnose findings associated with Sturge-Weber Syndrome. As discussed previously this case does not fit infectious etiology of the facial patch or traumatic injury.

Following 10 days of IV antibiotics the infant is doing well and you are preparing her discharge. On final examination the erythematous patch has become brighter red in color and there are several discrete 2- to 3-mm papules within the patch. The initial patch still involves the left forehead, eyelid, and cheek and there are additional bright red plaques along the mandible and chin. The left eyelid is edematous and there is slight ptosis. Her eyes fix and follow and pupils are equal round and reactive to light. She has normal work of breathing without retractions and there are subtle inspiratory and expiratory stridorous sounds on auscultation. Her heart has a regular rate and rhythm without murmurs.

Given the new findings what is your next step?
A. Discharge the baby home with reassurance this is typical thickening expected for a capillary malformation (PWS)
B. Consult otolaryngology for evaluation
C. Order MRI/MRA/V of the head and neck
D. Consult cardiology for evaluation
E. Consult dermatology for a skin biopsy

Discussion

The correct answer is **B**. The changes described brighter red color, new papules, involvement of the mandible, would be expected if the vascular birthmark is an infantile hemangioma. The thickening and darkening of capillary malformations typically does not occur until puberty. The involvement of the hemangioma along the jawline suggests that the stridor is due to airway hemangioma. Otolaryngology consult would be appropriate to evaluate for airway involvement and would be the next step. Positive findings would determine necessity for earlier intervention. MR imaging and cardiology consultation are part of the evaluation of patients with large segmental facial hemangiomas at risk of PHACE syndrome (posterior fossa malformation, hemangioma, arterial anomalies, coarctation of the aorta and cardiac defects, and eye abnormalities). This patient will need evaluation from cardiology and MR imaging of the head and neck the timing of which would be determined by the laryngoscopy findings. If the infantile hemangioma has a typical appearance then skin biopsy is not necessary.

The laryngoscopy reveals hemangiomas near the vocal cords resulting in narrowing of the airway. What is your treatment of choice?
A. Prednisolone
B. Aspirin
C. Interferon-a
D. Propranolol
E. Vincristine

Discussion

The correct answer is **D**. Most recently the literature supports first line use of propranolol to treat hemangiomas including PHACE syndrome and airway hemangiomas with better efficacy when compared to systemic corticosteroids.[26,27] A patient with PHACE syndrome should undergo evaluation for arterial and cardiac anomalies to assess the risk for stroke before initiating propranolol.[28] If arterial anomalies are present and the patient is at higher risk of stroke, aspirin for stroke prophylaxis may be used. Second-line treatments for hemangiomas include interferon and vincristine.

CASE 5

A 10-day Caucasian male infant is transferred to your neonatal intensive care unit for evaluation and treatment of blisters. Per transfer report, he was 39 weeks and 2 days EGA at birth, the product of an uncomplicated pregnancy to a healthy 23-year-old G1P1 woman. There was no known family history of skin disease. Blisters were present at birth on the hands, wrists, and chin. He was started on intravenous ampicillin, gentamicin, and acyclovir. At 2 days of life additional blisters began to appear all over his body on erythematous plaques. He was afebrile and feeding well. Given the additional rash the ampicillin was replaced with vancomycin. Cultures and Gram stain from the vesicles were negative. Blood cultures × 2 were negative, parvovirus IgG (+), parvovirus IgM (−), CMV negative, clostridium difficile negative. He continued to have new blister formation and hence transferred to your center. On your examination he is a well-appearing infant male in no acute distress weighing 3,410 g. Head was normocephalic and atraumatic. There were large coalescing erythematous plaques with overlying keratotic papules and vesicles scattered on the face, scalp, neck, trunk, upper extremities, and lower extremities. The plaques demonstrated a rounded and swirling pattern on the face and trunk and linear patterns on the extremities (Fig. 13-5A–C). A complete blood count

showed WBC 22, Hgb 15.1 g/dL, HCT 45.1 g/dL, PLT 316,000, Seg 26, band 1, Lymph 41, Mono 14, Eos 18. Skin biopsy revealed epidermal necrosis, mild eosinophilic spongiosis with epidermal dyskeratosis and an eosinophilic pustule.

What is your diagnosis?
A. HSV infection
B. Epidermolysis bullosa (EB)
C. Incontinentia pigmenti
D. Linear and whorled hypermelanosis
E. Bullous impetigo

Discussion

The correct answer is **C**. Incontinentia pigmenti (IP) is a genetic disease with manifestations in the skin, teeth, central nervous system, and eyes. There are four distinct phases in the skin which may not all appear, and these phases often overlap: inflammatory, verrucous, hyperpigmented, and hypopigmented or atrophic.[29] In 90% of patients, inflammatory vesicles and pustules develop in the skin in the first 2 weeks of life. New lesions appear in crops especially after infection, immunizations, or physical trauma.[30] The second stage consists of warty verrucous papules arising in linear streaks starting as early as 1 to 2 weeks of life and clearing by 6 months in 80% of patients.[29] Hyperpigmented macules in irregular shapes often referred to as "Chinese letter writing figures" form in the third stage. In two-thirds of patients these macules fade by adolescence. The final stage reveals atrophic hypopigmented plaques. During the first stage (inflammatory) there is marked increase in eosinophils in the epidermis and peripheral blood.[31] Skin pathology reveals spongiotic vesicles containing eosinophils, dyskeratotic cells, and whorls of squamous cells.[32] In all stages, lesions are distributed in the lines of Blaschko: linear and whorled patterns reflecting embryologic development of the skin.[31] Peripheral eosinophilia occurs in over 70% of patients with IP.[33] Linear and whorled hypermelanosis presents as hyperpigmented patches also in the lines of Blaschko. It would not show vesicles. Herpes simplex in the neonate reveals vesicles in clusters but not in the lines of Blaschko. These infants may develop systemic signs of sepsis or encephalitis but cutaneous manifestations may appear first. Rapid diagnosis can be made with a Tzanck smear or direct fluorescence antibody test.[11] EB is a genetic mechanobullous disease. Vesicles and bulla appear soon after birth at sites of friction. It does not follow the lines of Blaschko. Bullous impetigo should not be present at birth but can develop in the first few days. Discrete vesicles and pustules that rupture and form honey-colored crusts appear most often at the diaper or periumbilical area. Gram stain would show neutrophils

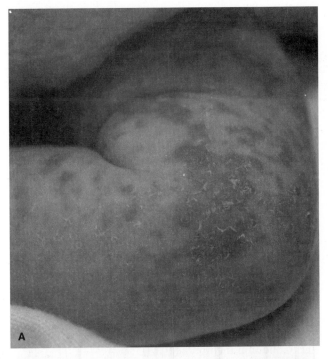

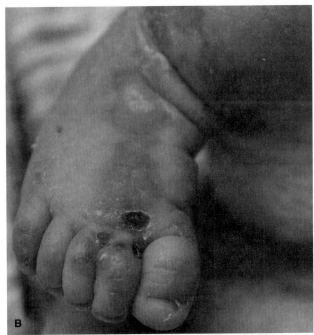

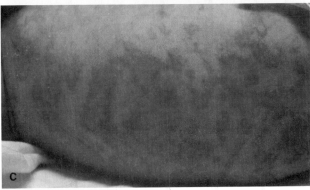

FIGURE 13-5. **(A)** Erythematous plaques with keratotic papules in linear distribution on the left leg. **(B)** Erythematous plaques with keratotic papules and crusted vesicles in linear distribution on the foot **(C)** Erythematous plaques in linear distribution on the back. (Used with permission of Leslie P. Lawley, MD.)

and gram-positive cocci in chains or clusters depending on the inciting bacteria.

In this case of incontinentia pigmenti, what is the genetic inheritance pattern?
A. Autosomal dominant
B. Autosomal recessive
C. X-linked dominant
D. X-linked recessive
E. Mosaicism

Discussion

The correct answer is **C**. Most cases of IP (98%) are X-linked dominant in transmission and therefore lethal to males prenatally while females survive due to random X-inactivation. The mutated gene at Xq28 encodes NF-κB essential modulator (NEMO) which regulates within the pathway for NF-κB. NF-κB is a nuclear activator for chemokines, adhesion molecules, and cytokines and leads to increased apoptosis. Boys described to have IP either have Klinefelter syndrome (XXY) or a postzygotic mutation resulting in somatic mosaicism.[34]

Genetics is consulted for further evaluation and testing. The infant is overall well despite the continued new vesicles and now hyperkeratotic papules. The parents are comfortable with his skin care but are curious about other manifestations.

What additional workup should be considered at this time point?
A. Dental examination
B. Ophthalmology examination
C. MRI
D. Lumbar puncture
E. Complete metabolic panel

Discussion

The correct answer is **B**. IP potentially may affect multiple systems: skin, eyes, central nervous system, and teeth. While previous studies have suggested up to 95% of patients may show dental anomalies a recent meta-analysis of the literature reported 54% of patients affected, most often with shape anomalies (conical or pegged teeth) or hypodontia.[35] A formal dental examination is not recommended in the neonatal period but should be considered by age 2 years. Ophthalmology examination is recommended in the first month of life and frequently during the first year. Reported associations include retinal ischemia, retinal neovascularization with bleeding, retinal detachment, optic atrophy, microphthalmos, cataracts, conjunctival pigmentation, corneal changes, iris hypoplasia, uveitis, phthisis, nystagmus, strabismus, myopia, and whorl-like keratitis which present in 20% to 77% of patients.[31] Up to 30% of patients with IP develop neurologic manifestations most commonly seizures, developmental delay, and paresis.[30] Unless there are neurologic deficits or signs on examination then MRI is not necessary. In IP patients with neurologic disease neuroimaging may reveal cerebral atrophy, porencephaly, hemorrhagic necrosis, hydrocephalus, and white matter disease.[30] Lumbar puncture and complete metabolic panel are not indicated.

CASE 6

A 1-day-old, estimated gestational age 39 weeks, African-American male is transferred to your unit for care. His gestational period was unremarkable. His birth weight was 3,012 g, with Apgar scores of 6 at 1 minute and 7 at 5 minutes. At the time of your initial examination, vital signs are temperature 37°C, respiratory rate 66 breaths/min, heart rate 110 bpm, and mean arterial blood pressure of 40 mm Hg. What is immediately notable is that he is completely wrapped in thick yellow waxy scale with significant ectropion (outward turning of the eyelid margin) and eclabium (outward turning of the lips) (Fig. 13-6). It is also noted that he is in mild respiratory distress; however, his lungs are clear to auscultation. His heart has a regular rate and rhythm with no murmurs, gallops, or rubs. His abdomen is soft, nontender with normal active bowel sounds with no hepatosplenomegaly. All distal extremities had normal capillary refill.

These cutaneous findings are most concerning for which of the following entities?
A. Congenital candidiasis
B. Staph-scalded skin syndrome
C. TORCH syndrome
D. Trisomy 21
E. Collodion membrane (CM)

Discussion

The correct answer is **E**. A collodion membrane (CM) is a shiny tight skin resembling parchment or casing that covers the entire body. In rare cases, a localized CM may occur.[36] The CM presents at birth, as it forms in utero and is secondary to abnormal desquamation. The name "collodion baby" (CB) is the name given to a baby who is born in a CM. The tautness of the skin of the CB may distort features of their face and extremities resulting in ectropion, eclabium, sparse scalp, and eyebrow hair, and pseudocontractures. In addition, the CM may initially cause restrictive pulmonary ventilation and respiratory distress, until expansion of the chest with breathing

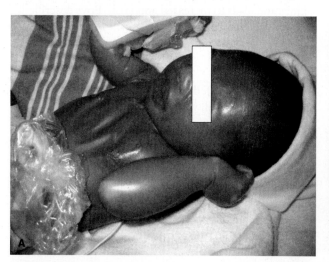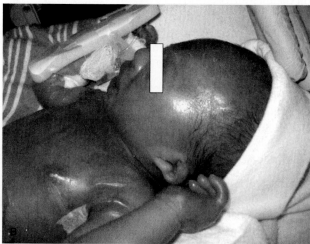

FIGURE 13-6. Generalized erythema with overlying thick waxy scale and blanching over joints; eclabium and ectropion. (Used with permission of Zakiya P. Rice, MD.)

results in tears of the membrane in the first few days of life. Gradually after 2 to 3 weeks of life the CM undergoes complete desquamation. Most CBs are born at term and appropriate size for gestational age, a slight male predominance of unclear significance has been found in the literature.[37–39] These cutaneous findings above are not consistent with congenital candidiasis, staph-scalded skin syndrome, TORCH syndrome, or trisomy 21.

Which of the following etiologies could be an underlying cause for this presenting entity?
A. Lamellar ichthyosis (LI)
B. Ectodermal dysplasia
C. Congenital ichthyosiform erythroderma (CIE)
D. A and C
E. B and C

Discussion

The correct answer is **D**. CM is an initial presentation of several genodermatoses. Once the CM desquamates, the resulting phenotype depends on the underlying genodermatosis, and may present with varying degrees of severity depending on penetrance. The most common underlying genodermatoses are lamellar ichthyosis (LI) and congenital ichthyosiform erythroderma (CIE) both autosomal recessive congenital ichthyoses. Lamellar ichthyosis results in large, dark plate-like scales in flexures, persisting ectropion, and palmoplantar keratoderma secondary to mutations in transglutaminase 1 (TGM1) gene. TGM1 gene mutations result in interference with normal cross linking of structural proteins in the protein lipid envelope around the keratinocytes of the upper dermis, leading to defective desquamation.[40] Congenital ichthyosiform erythroderma results in generalized erythroderma with fine white scale of flexures and larger scale on extensor surfaces and these changes are also secondary to mutations in TGM1, as well as mutations in ALOXE3 and ALOX12B which encode proteins with similar function to TGM1.[41–43] Other rare conditions presenting with a collodion membrane include Sjögren–Larsson syndrome, Gaucher disease type 2, trichothyodystrophy, Netherton syndrome, and neutral lipid storage disease. Up to 10% of collodion babies have normal underlying skin—also known as "self-healing" CB.[44,45] The ectodermal dysplasias are a large and complex group of genodermatoses with genetic mutations that result in abnormalities of the hair, nail, teeth, and sweat glands. Infants with ectodermal dysplasia are not born with collodion membrane.

Which of the following laboratory abnormalities is most commonly seen with this entity in the neonatal period?
A. Hyponatremia
B. Hypoglycemia
C. Hypernatremia
D. Hypokalemia
E. Pancytopenia

Discussion

The correct answer is **C**. Hypernatremia is the most common laboratory abnormality associated with a CM. This hypernatremia is secondary to increased permeability of the CM, resulting in a transepidermal water loss (TEWL) up to seven times greater than normal skin.[46] Increased TEWL is also associated with temperature instability and subsequently with increased caloric loss.[47] Initial high TEWL improves in parallel with desquamation of the CM and overall skin improvement. In the interim, placement of the CB in a high humidity incubator and close monitoring of temperature, caloric needs, and fluid intake, as measured by daily weights, and electrolytes are a critical component of neonatal care of the CB. Other systemic complications in the CB include infection and percutaneous toxicity secondary to increased permeability of the CM, as well as pneumonia secondary to aspiration of squamous material in the amniotic fluid.[48] Hyponatremia, hypoglycemia, hypokalemia, and pancytopenia are not routinely seen in the CB.

CASE 7

A 2-day-old, estimated gestational age 35 weeks, Hispanic female, born to a 29-year-old mother who is G1P0→1, is transferred to your unit for evaluation and management of intermittent seizures. Her pregnancy was uncomplicated. Her birth weight was 2,400 g, with Apgar scores of 7 at 1 minute and 8 at 5 minutes. At the time of your initial examination, vital signs are temperature 37°C, respiratory rate 33 breaths/min, heart rate 110 bpm, and mean arterial blood pressure of 40 mm Hg. On cutaneous examination, she has a large tan and hyperpigmented brown plaque with several inlying papules and plaques of varied colors and morphologies covering the upper half of the back and neck (Fig. 13-7). Also there are approximately 50 satellite papules and nodules. She is not in any respiratory distress and her lungs are clear to auscultation bilaterally. Her heart has a regular rate and rhythm with no murmurs, gallops, or rubs. Her abdomen is soft, nontender with normal active bowel sounds with no hepatosplenomegaly. All distal extremities have normal capillary refill. Of note, she has a full anterior fontanel and overall increased neurologic tone.

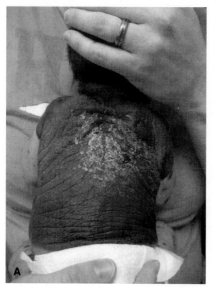 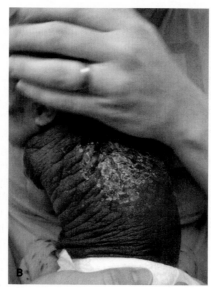 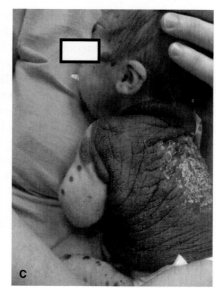

FIGURE 13-7. Tan and hyperpigmented plaque on the upper back with several plaques of varied colors. (Used with permission of Leslie P. Lawley, MD.)

These cutaneous findings described and pictured are most concerning for which of the following entities?
A. Congenital melanocytic nevus
B. Congenital neuroblastoma
C. Tuberous sclerosis
D. Neurofibromatosis
E. Nevus of Ito

Discussion

The correct answer is **A**. Congenital melanocytic nevi (CMN) are present at birth and result from a proliferation of benign melanocytes in the dermis, epidermis, or both. CMN are present in 1% to 2% of newborn infants and are thought to develop between the 9th and 20th weeks of gestation. One small study in Spain found a higher prevalence of CMN in preterm infants, females, and nonwhite infants, whereas maternal age, number of previous pregnancies, and birth weight did not appear to influence the prevalence.[49] Occasionally there are nevi that appear during the first 2 years of life and are not present at birth. When they are biopsied they are histologically identical to congenital nevi. These type of nevi are referred to as congenital nevus tardive.[50] The etiology of CMN remains unclear. The melanocytes of the skin originate in the neuroectoderm, although the specific cell type from which they derive remains unknown. One hypothesis is that pluripotential nerve sheath precursor cells migrate from the neural crest to the skin along paraspinal ganglia and peripheral nerve sheaths and differentiate into melanocytes upon reaching the skin. Another explanation for the presence of CMN is that an external insult results in a mutation in c-Met proto-oncogene and/or overexpression of hepatocyte growth factor/scatter factor during early embryogenesis that affects the morphogenesis of the embryonic neuroectoderm and migration of precursor cells to the skin. One study found that the melanocortin-1-receptor (MC1R) genotype, which corresponds to a red-haired genotype and a tendency to increased birth weight, was overrepresented in a cohort of CMN-affected Northern European patients. How MC1R variants promote growth of CMN and the fetus itself is unknown as is the application of this finding to non-European and more darkly pigmented races.[51–57] CMN have been stratified into three groups according to expected size in adulthood: (1) small congenital nevi are less than 1.5 cm in greatest diameter; (2) medium congenital nevi are 1.5 to 19.9 cm in greatest diameter; and (3) large or giant congenital nevi (GCN) are greater than 20 cm in greatest diameter. GCN are often surrounded by several smaller satellite nevi as discussed in this clinical vignette. The cutaneous presentation is not consistent with congenital neuroblastoma, tuberous sclerosis, neurofibromatosis, or nevus of Ito.

An MRI of the brain of this infant would show which of the following findings?
A. Tram-track calcifications
B. Dandy–Walker malformation
C. Cortical tubers
D. Chiari type 1 malformation
E. Neurocutaneous melanosis

Discussion

The correct answer is **E**. CMN may also be seen as a component of neurocutaneous melanosis (NCM), a rare congenital syndrome characterized by the presence of

CMN and melanotic neoplasms of the central nervous system. The current diagnostic criteria for NCM are[37] (1) large (>20 cm) or multiple (>3) congenital nevi in association with meningeal melanosis or melanoma,[51] (2) no evidence of meningeal melanoma except in patients in whom cutaneous lesions are histologically benign, and[2] (3) no evidence of cutaneous melanoma except in patients in whom meningeal lesions are histologically benign. In a study of 394 patients, there was a 5.1-fold increased risk of NCM with GCN on the posterior axis with large satellites.[58] Clinically, patients may present with signs of increased intracranial pressure, increased tone, full anterior fontanel or seizures, due to hydrocephalus or a mass lesion. The prognosis of patients with symptomatic NCM is very poor, even in the absence of malignancy. In another study of 39 reported cases of symptomatic NCM, death occurred in more than half of the patients within 3 years of the onset of neurologic symptoms, and most deaths were in patients younger than 10 years.[59] Tram-track calcifications are pathognomonic for Sturge–Weber syndrome, Dandy–Walker malformations (partial or even complete absence of cerebellar vermis) may be associated with PHACE(s) syndrome, cortical tubers are pathognomonic with tuberous sclerosis, and Chiari type 1 malformation is classically associated with neurofibromatosis.

Mutation in which of the following genes has been proven to be most often associated with the onset of melanoma within the lesion?
A. p53
B. NRAS
C. HRAS
D. CDKN2 A
E. Mel-A

Discussion

The correct answer is **B**. Mutations in *NRAS* in congenital melanocytic nevi can cause mitogen-activated protein kinase activation and may represent early events in melanoma development.[60] GCN place individuals at an increased risk for the development of melanoma at the site of the nevus. For GCN, the risk of developing melanoma has been reported to be as high as 5% to 7% by age 60 years. One study suggests that the risk of melanoma may be greater in those with GCN with more satellite lesions or a larger diameter. Another suggests multiple satellite nevi alone or with associated posterior midline location of GCN is linked with this increased risk melanoma. In addition, melanoma developing within GCN may develop during childhood and occur deeper in the

tissue where it is harder to detect clinically. While the general consensus regarding smaller nevi is that they pose a greater risk for the development of melanoma than normal skin, this risk has not been quantified. Also suggested is that melanoma developing within smaller congenital nevi usually occurs at puberty or later and develops more superficially in the skin, where it is easier to detect clinically.[61–64] Gene mutations in p53, HRAS, CDKN2 A, and Mel-A are seen in other melanoma syndromes.

Which of the following treatments is the best choice for reducing the risk of melanoma arising in this lesion?
A. Curettage
B. Laser
C. Excision
D. Chemotherapy
E. Radiation

Discussion

The correct answer is **C**. Surgical excision of GCN, depending on the size and location of the lesion, may be challenging. Often, the size of the lesion necessitates a staged excision. Tissue expanders, tissue grafts, and tissue flaps are often necessary to close the large defects following excision.[65] Cultured skin replacements have also been used in the closure of surgical wounds. Because the melanocytes may extend deep into underlying tissues (including muscle and bone) removing the cutaneous component may not eliminate the risk of malignancy.[66–68] Curettage of the lesions may be performed during the neonatal period, but long-term studies suggest the nevus will, in part, recur. This is likely due to those components of the epidermis that are deep to the level of curettage. Furthermore, curettage is less likely to eliminate the risk of malignancy than surgical excision.[69] Laser treatment of the lesions has been performed with a number of different types of lasers. However, due to of the lack of penetrance to deeper tissue levels, long-term recurrence and eliminating the risk of malignancy is also an issue with laser techniques. Laser treatment of CMN also remains controversial for a variety of other reasons. The effects of sublethal laser on the risk of malignant transformation of melanocytes are uncertain. In addition, while the destruction of more superficial melanocytes may improve cosmesis, if melanoma does develop in a laser-treated lesion, it may be more likely to occur deeper in the tissue where it may evade clinical detection until it reaches a more advanced stage.[70] Radiation and chemotherapy have not been shown to reduce the risk on melanoma arising in a GCN.

CASE 8

A neonate of uncertain gestational age is born precipitously to a 36-year-old, G1P0→1 mother. Forceps were required to deliver the infant. The right lower extremity is noted immediately to have a large defect similar to an erosion (Fig. 13-8). The right and left legs are of equal length and demonstrate good mobility. Per delivery records there were no other erosions, cutaneous defects, or anomalies noted with the initial assessment after birth. Both the maternal and paternal medical histories were unknown. The mother did not have any prenatal care.

What is the diagnosis?

A. Birth trauma
B. Aplasia cutis congenita (ACC)
C. Goltz syndrome
D. Adams–Oliver syndrome
E. Amniotic band syndrome

Discussion

The correct answer is **B**. ACC is part of a heterogeneous group of disorders characterized by the absence of a portion of skin in a localized or widespread area at birth. It most commonly (70%) manifests as a solitary defect on the scalp but may occur anywhere on the body, as shown in this clinical vignette on the leg.[71-73]

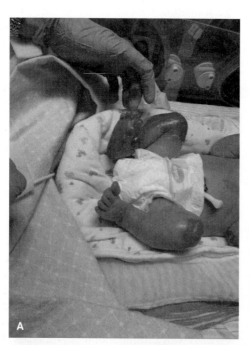
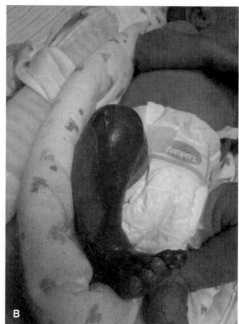
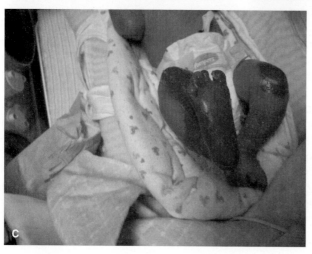

FIGURE 13-8. Right leg with well demarcated denuded plaque. (Used with permission of Zakiya P. Rice, MD.)

While forceps were reportedly used in delivery, the location of the defect on the leg is not consistent with forceps injury which would be most likely to appear on the head. Infants with Goltz syndrome may present with ACC associated with streaky plaques of atrophy within the lines of Blaschko. Adams–Oliver syndrome presents with a large scalp ACC in association with limb reduction abnormalities, cranial bone defects, and cutis marmorata telangiectatica. The infant described did not have any other anomalies. Neonates with amniotic band syndrome present with constriction or amputation-like scaring defects.

Which of the following medications could the mother have taken during gestation that would most increase the risk of this ACC occurring?
A. Thalidomide
B. Tetracycline
C. Methimazole
D. Lithium
E. Ethanol

Discussion

The correct answer is **C**. The most common medication associated with ACC is methimazole, which was historically used in the treatment of maternal thyrotoxicosis during pregnancy. Carbimazole, misoprostol, and valproic acid have also been associated with ACC.[74-77] The other medication answer choices are teratogens but with the following pathognomonic associations: Thalidomide—phocomelia; Tetracycline—hypoplasia of teeth enamel; Lithium—cardiac abnormalities, Ethanol—fetal alcohol syndrome.

On your examination of the neonate upon admission to the NICU, in addition to the area of ACC on the lower right leg, you find vesicles and a few erosions scattered on the face, trunk, and extremities. Which of the following in utero infections would increase the risk of these lesions occurring?
A. Varicella zoster virus
B. Cytomegalovirus
C. HSV
D. A and C
E. B and C

Discussion

The correct answer is **D**. ACC may be associated with varicella zoster virus (VZV) and HSV. A direct fluorescence antibody test for antigens associated with VZV or HSV can be performed to distinguish between these two etiologies quickly as viral cultures require days to result. Since both of these infections can have devastating consequences it is important to test and treat appropriately. In the congenital form of both HSV and VZV chorioretinitis and/or microphthalmia may also occur. Low birth weight, cataracts, seizures, cortical atrophy, encephalomyelitis, developmental delays, limb hypoplasia, and varied other anomalies of the eyes, central nervous system, musculoskeletal system, gastrointestinal or genitourinary tract may be associated with congenital varicella.[78] In addition to chorioretinitis and microphthalmia, congenital herpes may also present with microcephaly, hydranencephaly, and abnormal brain CT findings.[79] Cytomegalovirus is not associated with ACC.

The neonate is otherwise healthy without any additional anomalies or significant findings noted on examination. His weight is 3,410 g. Tests for HSV and VZV are negative. During the first few days of admission new blisters on a nonerythematous base continue to form near the diaper area and scattered on the arms, legs, and trunk. He has a few erosions on the lips, tongue, and palate.

What is the most appropriate next step in management?
A. Cardiology consult
B. Orthopedic consult
C. Ophthalmology consult
D. Neurology consult
E. Dermatology consult

Discussion

The best answer is **E**. Initial reports of ACC occurring on the lower extremities were described in combination with EB, known as Bart syndrome.[80-82] EB is a group of inherited bullous disorders that result from mutations in genes that encode proteins that are responsible for adherence of the epidermis to the dermis or the basement membrane zone. Clinically EB is characterized by blister formation in response to mechanical trauma. Historically, EB subtypes have been classified according to skin morphology but more recently have been based on underlying genetic defects. EB may be classified as simplex, junctional, or dystrophic types. Within these categories there are several forms which vary in severity of disease and therefore prognosis. In the neonatal and infantile period it may be impossible to distinguish the subtype of EB, however the diagnosis of EB may be made by a dermatologist with the aid of routine histopathology, direct immunofluorescence, and electron microscopy. In addition to the pediatrician or neonatologist, the dermatologist may provide guidance not only in diagnosis but also in wound care and disease-specific concerns. Other specialists may be part of the care team depending on the subtype. Given the fragile nature of the skin in EB, it is important that these infants are handled with caution and with avoidance of adhesives and unnecessary trauma to the skin to minimize new blister formation. Infants with EB need monitoring for wound healing, secondary infections, pain control, and proper nutrition.

CASE 9

A 14-day-old, 40-week Caucasian male is directly admitted to your neonatal care unit from his primary pediatrician's office for evaluation and management of a severe dermatitis of unclear etiology. His gestational period and birth were unremarkable. He was born via a natural spontaneous vaginal delivery, Apgar scores of 8 at 1 minute and 9 at 5 minutes, birth weight 3,800 g, and he was discharged home to his parents within 48 hours, breastfeeding well. On the seventh day of life he developed an asymptomatic rash on his scalp which rapidly progressed to cover his entire body over the next 7 days. On your initial examination, his vital signs are temperature 37°C, respiratory rate 35 breaths/min, heart rate 112 bpm, mean arterial blood pressure of 42 mm Hg, and weight is 3,788 g. On cutaneous examination he has diffuse confluent erythematous scaly plaques covering approximately 90% body surface area, sparing distal extremities as well as the palms and soles (Fig. 13-9). He

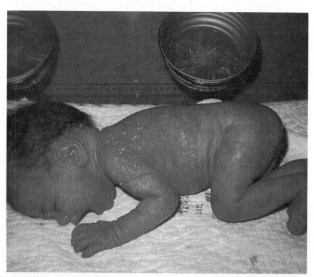

FIGURE 13-9. Diffuse erythematous scaly plaques. (Reproduced with permission from Weinberg S, Prose N, Kristal L. *Color Atlas of Pediatric Dermatology*. 3rd ed. New York, NY: McGraw-Hill; 1998.)

is not in any respiratory distress and his lungs are clear to auscultation bilaterally. His heart has a regular rate and rhythm with no murmurs, gallops, or rubs. His abdomen is soft, nontender with normal active bowel sounds with no hepatosplenomegaly. All distal extremities had normal capillary refill.

This patient is presenting with cutaneous findings most concerning for which of the following entities?
A. Erythroderma
B. Calcinosis cutis
C. Leukemia cutis
D. Congenital syphilis
E. TORCH syndrome

Discussion

The correct answer is **A**. Erythroderma is an inflammatory cutaneous disorder consisting of erythema and scaling affecting more than 90% of the body surface area. Neonatal and infantile erythroderma or 'the red scaly baby' is a rare condition; its frequency is unknown. In one study, an incidence of 0.11% of neonatal and infantile erythroderma was noted out of 19,000 pediatric patients treated over 6 consecutive years.[83] Overall, it is important to recognize this dermatological entity as the prognosis is poor with a mortality of 16%.[84] Clinical features of calcinosis cutis, congenital syphilis, leukemia cutis, and TORCH syndrome are not featured in this vignette.

Which of the following underlying abnormalities for this presentation needs to be considered?
A. Seborrheic dermatitis
B. DiGeorge syndrome
C. Biotin deficiency
D. A and C
E. A, B, and C

Discussion

The correct answer is **E**. The differential for neonatal erythroderma is very broad. In general, it may be divided into four categories: (1) Primary cutaneous; (2) metabolic (disorders of biotin and zinc metabolism, essential fatty acid deficiencies); (3) infectious (staph-scalded skin syndrome, toxic shock syndrome, staph pustulosis); or (4) immunodeficiency syndromes (Omenn syndrome, graft versus host, hypogammaglobulinemia, DiGeorge syndrome, severe combined immunodeficiency, cutaneous T-cell lymphoma). The two most common primary cutaneous etiologies are atopic dermatitis and seborrheic dermatitis; the other etiologies include psoriasis, pityriasis rubra pilaris, and diffuse mastocytosis.[85] It is recommended that a dermatologist is involved in the care of an infant presenting with neonatal erythroderma in order to secure the diagnosis and prevent mismanagement. The etiology of neonatal and infantile erythrodermas is difficult to establish and is often delayed, due to the poor specificity of clinical and histological signs. In one study, the mean age to determine the cause of erythroderma was 11 months after onset; furthermore, in 10% of patients the underlying cause was never determined.[84]

What is the next best next step in management?
A. Obtain complete blood cell count
B. Chest x-ray
C. Electrocardiogram
D. Echocardiogram
E. MRI of brain

Discussion

The correct answer is **A**. Mortality in neonatal erythroderma is secondary to hypernatremic dehydration, infections, failure to thrive, or due to severity of skin disease and the underlying disease process.[84] A chest x-ray may be useful if there is a cough or positive findings on pulmonary examination to suggest secondary infectious processes. There is not a role for electrocardiogram, echocardiogram, or MRI at this time. Given the risks of adverse events or even mortality, careful initial management of erythroderma should include excellent supportive care, specifically the monitoring of vital signs and electrolyte levels, adequate oral or parenteral fluid intake, caloric and protein intake, and prevention and treatment of infection.

CASE 10

A 1-day-old, 31-week gestation female delivered by routine vaginal delivery to a 17-year-old G1P0→1 female is in your care for a rash that presented at delivery (Fig. 13-10A). The mother received routine prenatal care, with a history of a vesicular eruption noted on the left knee that spontaneously resolved at week 18. On examination, her vital signs are temperature 35.5°C, respiratory rate 30 breaths/min, heart rate 100 bpm, mean arterial blood pressure of 38 mm Hg. On cutaneous examination there were scattered circular erosions that were Tzanck test positive. She is not in any respiratory distress and her lungs are clear to auscultation bilaterally. Her heart has a regular rate and rhythm with no murmurs, gallops, or rubs. Her abdomen is soft, nontender

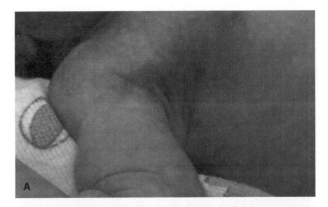
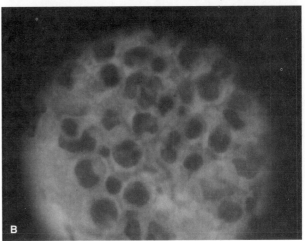

FIGURE 13-10. (**A**) Round erosions and one discrete vesicle on the trunk. (**B**) Tzanck cells (multinucleated giant cells). (Used with permission of Allyson Spence-Shishido, MD.)

with normal active bowel sounds but with notable hepatosplenomegaly. Initial laboratory values revealed normal electrolytes; however, aspartate aminotransferase and alanine aminotransferase were elevated at 500 U/L (normal 14–70 U/L) and 312 U/L (normal <54 U/L), respectively, with normal alkaline phosphatase 146 U/L and normal total bilirubin 2.8 mg/dL, and low albumin 1.4 g (normal 3.7 g/dL.) The white blood cell count was elevated at 16,000/mL (normal <14,000/mL) with 2% polymorphonuclear neutrophils; 23% bands; 66% lymphocytes; 2% monocytes. Hematocrit and platelets were normal at 47% and 155,000/mL. Cerebrospinal fluid from the lumbar puncture reveals a lymphocyte predominate pleocytosis. The total CSF protein was 700 mg/dL (65–150 mg/dL) and glucose 75 mg/dL (normal, 24–63 mg/dL.) Chest x-ray was unremarkable. Blood, urine, and cerebrospinal fluid cultures were sent. A computerized tomographic scan of the brain revealed ventricular enlargement, a thin cortical mantle, and very little supratentorial matter.

Please select the correct underlying infectious etiology:
A. *Staphylococcus aureus*
B. *Treponema pallidum*
C. Rubella
D. HSV
E. Parvovirus B19

Discussion

The correct answer is **D**. This neonate has a HSV infection. A Tzanck prep, is a bedside histopathologic test where the base of an ulcer, erosion, or unroofed vesicle is scraped and placed on a glass slide with a counter stain applied to look for multinucleated giant cells (Tzanck cells, Fig. 13-10B). A positive Tzanck test may be found in lesions infected with HSV.[86] Tzanck tests may also be positive in cases involving varicella zoster virus as well as cytomegalovirus. Negative Tzanck tests would be found in the case of skin lesions of *Staphylococcus aureus*, the pathogenic agent implicated in staph-scalded skin syndrome, *Treponema pallidum* the pathogenic agent implicated in syphilis, rubella one of the pathogenic agents implicated in the "blue berry muffin baby," and parvovirus B19 which is rarely causative in "blue berry muffin baby."

What was the most likely mode of transmission in this presenting case?
A. Transplacental
B. Perinatal
C. Postnatal
D. Iatrogenic
E. Genetic

Discussion

The correct answer is **A**. The majority of cases (85%) of neonatal herpes virus infection (NHSV) occur during delivery through an infected birth canal. The second most common transmission of HSV in NHSV is in the postnatal period when a neonate comes in contact with an infected individual. In postnatal neonatal herpes virus infection, the most common cause is HSV-1, "oral" HSV infection. However, 5% of cases NSHV occur when the fetus is in utero and there is acquisition of HSV due to maternal viremia through transplacental spread.[87,88] The most common cause of perinatal and transplacental NHSV is HSV-2.[89] Of note, transplacental neonatal herpes virus infection is often termed *congenital herpes* (CHSV) to highlight this as a specific entity. CHSV in comparison to neonatal herpes virus infection usually presents at birth or within the first 24 to 48 hours, whereas perinatal neonatal herpes virus infection presents after 48 hours and postnatal NHSV occurs 48 hours to 28 days after birth. Furthermore, CHSV may also present with chorioretinitis, microphthalmia, microcephaly, and abnormal brain CT findings.

What is the correct treatment for this etiology?
A. Ceftriaxone
B. Acyclovir
C. Gentamycin
D. Phenytoin
E. Observation

Discussion

The correct answer is **B**. Reduction in morbidity and mortality in NHSV is due to the use of antiviral treatments.[90] However, morbidity and mortality still remain high due to delayed diagnosis of disseminated and CNS HSV, as 20% to 40% of infected neonates have no visible lesions. Nonetheless, prevention is still a mainstay of NHSV care. Pregnant women with a known history of HSV may be managed by antiviral therapy. Pregnant women with active genital HSV lesions at the time of labor should be delivered by caesarean section.

REFERENCES

1. Epps RE, Pittelkow MR, Su WP. TORCH syndrome. *Semin Dermatol.* 1995;14:179.
2. Baselga E, Torrelo A. Inflammatory and purpuric eruptions. In: Eichenfield LF, Frieden IJ, Esterly NB, eds. *Neonatal Dermatology.* 2nd ed. Philadelphia, PA: Saunders Elsevier; 2008:330.
3. Satter EK, High WA. Langerhans cell histiocytosis: A review of the current recommendations of the Histiocyte Society. *Pediatr Dermatol.* 2008;25:291.
4. Popadic S, Brasanac D, Arsov B, et al. Congenital self-healing histiocytosis presenting as blueberry muffin baby: A case report and literature review. *Indian J Dermatol Vernereol Leprol.* 2012;78:407.
5. Longaker MA, Frieden IJ, LeBoit PE, et al. Congenital "self-healing" Langerhans cell histiocytosis: The need for long-term follow-up. *J Am Acad Dermatol.* 1994;31:910.
6. Hashimoto K, Bale GF, Hawkins HK, et al. Congenital self-healing reticulohistiocytosis (Hashimoto-Pritzker type). *Int J Dermatol.* 1986;25:516.
7. Jensen ML, Bygum A, Clemmensen O, Fenger-Gron J. Congenital self-healing reticulohistiocytosis–an important diagnostic challenge. *Acta Paediatr.* 2011;100:784.
8. Van Praag MC, Van Rooij RW, Folkers E, et al. Diagnosis and treatment of pustular disorders in the neonate. *Pediatr Dermatol.* 1997;14:131.
9. Darmstadt GL, Dinulos JG, Miller Z. Congenital cutaneous candidiasis: Clinical presentation, pathogenesis, and management guidelines. *Pediatrics.* 2000;105:438.
10. Smolinski KN, Shah SS, Honig PJ, et al. Neonatal cutaneous fungal infections. *Curr Opin Pediatr.* 2005;17:486.
11. Friedlander SF, Bradley JS. Viral infections. In: Eichenfield LF, Frieden IJ, Esterly NB, eds. *Neonatal Dermatology.* 2nd ed. Philadelphia, PA: Saunders Elsevier; 2008:193.

12. Dinulos JG, Pace NC. Bacterial infections. In: Eichenfield LF, Frieden IJ, Esterly NB, eds. *Neonatal Dermatology*. 2nd ed. Philadelphia, PA: Saunders Elsevier; 2008:173.

13. Lucky AW. Transient benign cutaneous lesions in the newborn. In: Eichenfield LF, Frieden IJ, Esterly NB, eds. *Neonatal Dermatology*. 2nd ed. Philadelphia, PA: Saunders Elsevier; 2008:86.

14. Hall GW. Kasabach-Merritt syndrome: Pathogenesis and management. *Br J Haematol*. 2001;112:851.

15. Croteau SE, Liang MG, Kozakewich HP, et al. Kaposiform hemangioendothelioma: Atypical features and risks of Kasabach-Merritt phenomenon in 107 referrals. *J Pediatr*. 2013; 162:142.

16. Le Huu AR, Jokinen CH, Rubin BP, et al. Expression of prox1, lymphatic endothelial nuclear transcription factor, in Kaposiform hemangioendothelioma and tufted angioma. *Am J Surg Pathol*. 2010;34:1563.

17. Tollefson MM, Frieden IL. Early growth of infantile hemangiomas: What parent's photographs tell us. *Pediatrics*. 2012; 130:e314.

18. Enjolras O, Garzon MC. Vascular stains, malformations, and tumors. In: Eichenfield LF, Frieden IJ, Esterly NB, eds. *Neonatal Dermatology*. 2nd ed. Philadelphia, PA: Saunders Elsevier; 2008:343.

19. Browning JC, Eldin KW, Kozakewich HP, et al. Congenital disseminated pyogenic granuloma. *Pediatr Dermatol*. 2009; 26:323.

20. Blatt J, Stavas J, Moats-Staats B, et al. Treatment of childhood kaposiform hemangioendothelioma with sirolimus. *Pediatr Blood Cancer*. 2010;55:1396.

21. Drucker AM, Pope E, Mahant S, et al. Vincristine and corticosteroids as first-line treatment of Kasabach-Merritt syndrome in kaposiform hemangioendothelioma. *J Cutan Med Surg*. 2009;13:155.

22. Fernandez-Pineda I, Lopen-Guiterrez JC, Ramirez G, et al. Vincristine-ticlopidine-aspirin: An effective therapy in children with Kasabach-Merritt phenomenon associated with vascular tumors. *Pediatr Hematol Oncol*. 2010;27:641.

23. Hermans DJ, van Beynum IM, van der Vijver RJ, et al. Kaposiform hemangioendothelioma with Kasabach-Merritt syndrome: A new indication for propranolol treatment. *J Pediatr Hematol Oncol*. 2011;33:e171.

24. Piram M, Lorette G, Sirinelli D, et al. Sturge-Weber syndrome in patients with facial port-wine stain. *Pediatr Dermatol*. 2012;29:32.

25. Melancon JM, Dohil MA, Eichenfield LF. Facial port-wine stain: When to worry? *Pediatr Dermatol*. 2012;29:131.

26. Izadpanah A, Izadpanah A, Kanevsky J, et al. Propranolol versus corticosteroids in the treatment of infantile hemangioma: A systematic review and meta-analysis. *Plast Reconstr Surg*. 2013;131(3):601–613.

27. Loizzi M, De Palma A, Pagliarulo V, et al. Propranolol as first-line treatment of a severe subglottic haemangioma. *Eur J Cardiothorac Surg*. 2013;43:187.

28. Metry D, Frieden IJ, Hess C, et al. Propranolol use in PHACE syndrome with cervical and intracranial arterial anomalies: Collective experience in 32 infants. *Pediatr Dermatol*. 2013; 30:71.

29. Landy SJ, Donnai D. Incontinentia pigmenti (Bloch-Sulzberger syndrome). *J Med Genet*. 1993;30:53.

30. Hadj-Rabia S, Froidevaux D, Bodak N, et al. Clinical study of 40 cases of incontinentia pigmenti. *Arch Dermatol*. 2003; 139:1163.

31. Itin P. Genodermatosis: Incontinentia pigmenti (Bloch-Sulzberger). In: Schachner LA, Hansen RC, eds. *Pediatric Dermatology*. 4th ed. Mosby, MI: Elsevier; 2011:391.

32. Kwan TH. Spongiotic dermatitis. In: Barnhill RL, ed. *Textbook of Dermatopathology*. New York, NY: McGraw-Hill; 1998:30.

33. Paller AS, Mancini AJ. Disorders of pigmentation. In: Paller AS, Mancini AJ, eds. *Hurwitz Clinical Pediatric Dermatology*. 4th ed. Elsevier Saunders; 2011:248.

34. Pacheco TR, Levy M, Collyer JC, et al. Incontinentia pigmenti in male patients. *J Am Acad Dermatol*. 2006;55:251.

35. Minic S, Trpinac D, Gabriel H, et al. Dental and oral anomalies in incontinentia pigmenti: A systematic review. *Clin Oral Investig*. 2013;17:1.

36. Mazereeuw-Hautier J, Aufenvenne K, Deraison C, et al. Acral self-healing collodion baby: Report of a new clinical phenotype caused by a novel TGM1 mutation. *Br J Dermatol*. 2009;161:456.

37. Akcakus M, Gunes T, Kurtoglu S, et al. Collodion baby associated with asymmetric crying facies: A case report. *Pediatr Dermatol*. 2003;20:134.

38. Larreque M, Ottavy N, Bressieux JM, et al. Collodion baby: 32 new case reports. *Ann Derm Venereol*. 1986;113:773.

39. Van Gysel D, Lijnen RL, Moekti SS, et al. Collodion baby: A follow-up study of 17 cases. *J Eur Acad Dermatol Venereol*. 2002;16:427.

40. Huber N, Rettler I, Bernasconi K, et al. Mutations in keratinocyte transglutaminase in lamellar ichthyosis. *Science*. 1995; 267:525.

41. Choate KA, Williams ML, Khavari PA. Abnormal transglutaminase 1 expression pattern in a subset of patients with erythrodermic autosomal recessive ichthyosis. *J Invest Dermatol*. 1998;110:8.

42. Harting M, Brunetti-Pierri N, Chan CS, et al. Self-healing collodion membrane and mild nonbullous congenital ichthyosiform erythroderma due to 2 novel mutations in the ALOX12B gene. *Arch Dermatol*. 2008;144:351.

43. Vahlquist A, Bygum A, Ganemo A, et al. Genotypic and clinical spectrum of self-improving collodion ichthyosis: ALOX12B, ALOXE3, and TGM1 mutations in Scandinavian patients. *J Invest Dermatol*. 2010;130:438.

44. Raghunath M, Hennies HC, Ahvazi B, et al. Self healing collodion baby: A dynamic phenotype explained by a particular transglutaminase-1 mutation. *J Invest Dermatol*. 2003;120:224.

45. Theiler M, Mann C, Weibel L. Self-healing collodion baby. *J Pediatr*. 2010;157:169.

46. Buyse L, Graves C, Marks R, et al. Collodion baby dehydration: The danger of high transepidermal water loss. *Br J Dermatol*. 1993;129:86.

47. Moskowitz DG, Fowler AJ, Heyman MB, et al. Pathophysiologic basis for growth failure in children with ichthyosis: An evaluation of cutaneous ultrastructure, epidermal permeability barrier function, and energy expenditure. *J Pediatr*. 2004;145:82.

48. Prado R, Ellis L, Gamble R, et al. Collodion baby: An update with a focus on practical management. *J Am Acad Dermatol.* 2012;67:1362.

49. Monteagudo B, Labandeira J, Acevedo A, et al. Prevalence and clinical features of congenital melanocytic nevi in 1,000 Spanish newborns. *Actas Dermosifiliogr.* 2011;102:114.

50. Clemmensen OJ, Kroon S. The histology of "congenital features" in early acquired melanocytic nevi. *J Am Acad Dermatol.* 1988;19:742.

51. Ansarin H, Soltani-Arabshahi R, Mehregan D, et al. Giant congenital melanocytic nevus with neurofibroma-like changes and spina bifida occulta. *Int J Dermatol.* 2006;45:1347.

52. Cramer SF. The melanocytic differentiation pathway in congenital melanocytic nevi: Theoretical considerations. *Pediatr Pathol.* 1988;8:253.

53. Cruz MA, Cho ES, Schwartz RA, et al. Congenital neurocutaneous melanosis. *Cutis.* 1997;60:178.

54. Kinsler VA, Abu-Amero S, Budd P, et al. Germline melanocortin-1-receptor genotype is associated with severity of cutaneous phenotype in congenital melanocytic nevi: A role for MC1R in human fetal development. *J Invest Dermatol.* 2012;132:2026.

55. Kos L, Aronzon A, Takayama H, et al. Hepatocyte growth factor/scatter factor-MET signaling in neural crest-derived melanocyte development. *Pigment Cell Res.* 1999;12:13.

56. Silfen R, Skoll PJ, Hudson DA. Congenital giant hairy nevi and neurofibromatosis: The significance of their common origin. *Plast Reconstr Surg.* 2002;110:1364.

57. Takayama H, Nagashima Y, Hara M, et al. Immunohistochemical detection of the c-met proto-oncogene product in the congenital melanocytic nevus of an infant with neurocutaneous melanosis. *J Am Acad Dermatol.* 2001;44:538.

58. Marghoob AA, Dusza S, Oliveria S, et al. Number of satellite nevi as a correlate for neurocutaneous melanocytosis in patients with large congenital melanocytic nevi. *Arch Dermatol.* 2004;140:171.

59. Kadonaga JN, Frieden IJ. Neurocutaneous melanosis: Definition and review of the literature. *J Am Acad Dermatol.* 1991; 24:747.

60. Blokx WA, van Dijk MC, Ruiter DJ. Molecular cytogenetics of cutaneous melanocytic lesions - diagnostic, prognostic and therapeutic aspects. *Histopathology.* 2010;56:121.

61. Bett BJ. Large or multiple congenital melanocytic nevi: Occurrence of cutaneous melanoma in 1008 persons. *J Am Acad Dermatol.* 2005;52:793.

62. Hale EK, Stein J, Ben-Porat L, et al. Association of melanoma and neurocutaneous melanocytosis with large congenital melanocytic naevi–results from the NYU-LCMN registry. *Br J Dermatol.* 2005;152:512.

63. Lovett A, Maari C, Decarie JC, et al. Large congenital melanocytic nevi and neurocutaneous melanocytosis: One pediatric center's experience. *J Am Acad Dermatol.* 2009;61:766.

64. Rhodes AR, Wood WC, Sober AJ, et al. Nonepidermal origin of malignant melanoma associated with a giant congenital nevocellular nevus. *Plast Reconstr Surg.* 1981;67:782.

65. Warner PM, Yakuboff KP, Kagan RJ, et al. An 18-year experience in the management of congenital nevomelanocytic nevi. *Ann Plast Surg.* 2008;60:283.

66. Demirseren ME, Ceran C, Demirseren DD. Treatment of a congenital melanocytic nevus on the forehead with immediate tissue expansion technique: A three-year follow-up. *Pediatr Dermatol.* 2012;29:621.

67. Hoffman D, Ratner D. Diagnosis and management of a changing congenital melanocytic nevus. *Skinmed.* 2006;5:242.

68. Margulis A, Adler N, Bauer BS. Congenital melanocytic nevi of the eyelids and periorbital region. *Plast Reconstr Surg.* 2009;124:1273.

69. De Raeve LE, Roseeuw DI. Curettage of giant congenital melanocytic nevi in neonates: A decade later. *Arch Dermatol.* 2002;138:943.

70. Michel JL. Laser therapy of giant congenital melanocytic nevi. *Eur J Dermatol.* 2003;13:57.

71. Caksen H, Kurtoglu S. Our experience with aplasia cutis congenita. *J Dermatol.* 2002;29:376.

72. Frieden IJ. Aplasia cutis congenita: A clinical review and proposal for classification. *J Am Acad Dermatol.* 1986;14:646.

73. Moros Pena M, Labay Matias M, Valle Sanchez F, et al. Aplasia cutis congenita in a newborn: Etiopathogenic review and diagnostic approach. *An Esp Pediatr.* 2000;52:453.

74. Izhar R, Ghani T. Aplasia cutis congenita and antithyroid drugs. *J Pak Med Assoc.* 2002;52:526.

75. Karg E, Bereg E, Gaspar L, et al. Aplasia cutis congenita after methimazole exposure in utero. *Pediatr Dermatol.* 2004;21:491.

76. Mandel SJ, Brent GA, Larsen PR. Review of antithyroid drug use during pregnancy and report of a case of aplasia cutis. *Thyroid.* 1994;4:129.

77. Nakamura S, Nishikawa T, Isaji M, et al. Aplasia cutis congenita and skull defects after exposure to methimazole in utero. *Intern Med.* 2005;44:1202.

78. Birthistle K, Carrington D. Fetal varicella syndrome–a reappraisal of the literature. *J Infect.* 1998;36:25.

79. Riley LE. Herpes simplex virus. *Semin Perinatol.* 1998;22:284.

80. Benvenuto C, Kraemer CK, Kruse RL, et al. Familial epidermolysis bullosa with aplasia cutis congenita: Bart's syndrome? *Skinmed.* 2003;2:319.

81. Bigliardi PL, Braschler C, Kuhn P, et al. Unilateral aplasia cutis congenita on the leg. *Pediatr Dermatol.* 2004;21:454.

82. McCarthy MA, Clarke T, Powell FC. Epidermolysis bullosa and aplasia cutis. *Int J Dermatol.* 1991;30:481.

83. Sarkar R, Basu S, Sharma RC. Neonatal and infantile erythrodermas. *Arch Dermatol.* 2001;137:822.

84. Pruszkowski A, Bodemer C, Fraitag S, et al. Neonatal and infantile erythrodermas: A retrospective study of 51 patients. *Arch Dermatol.* 2000;136:875.

85. Hoeger PH, Harper JI. Neonatal erythroderma: Differential diagnosis and management of the "red baby". *Arch Dis Child.* 1998;79:186.

86. Solomon AR, Rasmussen JE, Varani J, et al. The Tzanck smear in the diagnosis of cutaneous herpes simplex. *JAMA.* 1984; 251:633.

87. Hutto C, Arvin A, Jacobs R, et al. Intrauterine herpes simplex virus infections. *J Pediatr.* 1987;110:97.

88. Sarkell B, Blaylock WK, Vernon H. Congenital neonatal herpes simplex virus infection. *J Am Acad Dermatol.* 1992;27:817.

89. Glover MT, Atherton DJ. Congenital infection with herpes simplex virus type 1. *Pediatr Dermatol.* 1987;4:336.

90. Kimberlin DW, Lin CY, Jacobs RF, et al. Safety and efficacy of high-dose intravenous acyclovir in the management of neonatal herpes simplex virus infections. *Pediatrics.* 2001;108:230.

Chapter 14
HEMATOLOGY AND ONCOLOGY
Howard M. Katzenstein, MD, Michael Briones, DO, and Benjamin K. Watkins, MD

CASE 1

Approximately 12 hours ago, you delivered a term male infant via spontaneous vaginal delivery to a 30-year-old G2P2 female whose pregnancy was complicated by poorly controlled gestational diabetes. The infant has developed respiratory distress and is noted to be irritable. On examination you note diffuse redness of the skin and tachypnea.

What is the most likely diagnosis?
A. Sepsis
B. Persistent pulmonary hypertension (PPHN)
C. Meconium aspiration
D. Polycythemia
E. Congenital heart disease

Discussion

The correct answer is **D**. Polycythemia occurs in 1% to 5% of neonates. The central venous hematocrit level peaks 6 to 12 hours after birth. Physical findings observed with polycythemia include irritability, lethargy, seizures, respiratory distress, cyanosis, plethora or ruddiness, and apnea. Hypoglycemia occurs in 12% to 40% and hypocalcemia occurs in 1% to 11% of infants with polycythemia.[1] Necrotizing enterocolitis and disseminated intravascular coagulation are rare but serious complications.

What is the diagnostic definition of polycythemia?
A. Peripheral hematocrit >70%
B. Central hematocrit >65%
C. Peripheral hematocrit >60% with signs of hyperviscosity
D. Signs of hyperviscosity regardless of hematocrit

Discussion

The correct answer is **B**. Polycythemia is defined as a central hematocrit >65%. Neonates with a hematocrit >65% are at risk for hyperviscosity syndrome. Hyperviscosity syndrome is a condition that consists of hypoglycemia, central nervous system injury, and hypocalcemia. Only 47% of infants with polycythemia have hyperviscosity and only 24% of infants with hyperviscosity have polycythemia.[1]

Which of the following is not associated with neonatal polycythemia?
A. Delayed cord clamping >3 minutes
B. Infants of diabetic mothers with poor glycemic control
C. Intrauterine growth restriction
D. Dizygotic twin pregnancy
E. Trisomy 21

Discussion

The correct answer is **D**. Delayed cord clamping for greater than 3 minutes has been associated with increased blood volume delivered to the infant which can increase as much as 30%. Polycythemia, in infants of diabetic mothers with poor glycemic control as well as infants with intrauterine growth retardation results from chronic fetal hypoxia that causes increased erythropoiesis. The incidence of polycythemia in infants of diabetic mothers is 40%. Multiple genetic disorders such as trisomy 13, trisomy 18, trisomy 21, and Beckwith–Wiedemann syndrome (BWS) are associated with polycythemia. Twin-to-twin transfusions occur only in monozygotic monochorionic twins due to placental vascular anastomoses. The incidence of twin-to-twin transfusion syndrome has been estimated to be 13% to 33%.[1]

Objectives

1. Know the common clinical signs and symptoms associated with neonatal polycythemia
2. Identify conditions and disorders associated with an increased risk of neonatal polycythemia
3. Know other associated metabolic abnormalities commonly seen in patients with neonatal plycythemia

CASE 2

A 4-day-old Caucasian male presents to clinic because "he is yellow." He was born at term via spontaneous vaginal delivery to a 32-year-old G1P1 female and is noted to have new onset jaundice. Maternal labs are blood type A+, RPR nonreactive, rubella immune, Group B Strep negative. He is bottle fed and has been taking 2 to 3 ounces every 2 to 3 hours. On examination he is diffusely jaundiced. Total bilirubin is 17.1 mg/dL. The conjugated (direct) fraction is 0.6 mg/dL.

What is the most likely cause of his jaundice?
A. Sickle cell disease
B. Hereditary spherocytosis (HS)
C. Physiological jaundice
D. ABO incompatibility
E. Biliary atresia

Discussion

The correct answer is **B**. Hereditary spherocytosis is a predominantly autosomal- dominant inherited hemolytic anemia; however, an estimated 25% of cases are due to spontaneous mutations. In the United States, the incidence of Hereditary spherocytosis is approximately 1 case in 5,000 people. It is most commonly caused by a defect in spectrin or one of the proteins involved in the attachment of spectrin to the membrane that affects the structural integrity of the cell membrane. The instability of the red cell membrane results in spheroidal and osmotically fragile cells. These cells will be rapidly eliminated from the circulation by the spleen resulting in hemolysis. Red cell trapping by the spleen can also result in significant splenomegaly. Approximately 30% to 50% of cases of Hereditary spherocytosis will present with jaundice in the first week of life. The degree of anemia can vary greatly from patient to patient, however the anemia is typically mild. Laboratory studies will show an increased MCHC and a decreased MCV due to red cell dehydration. The reticulocyte count may also be elevated depending on the degree

of anemia. Most children will remain asymptomatic and their physical examination often is benign except for a palpable spleen that occurs in 75% of cases. However, children with Hereditary spherocytosis are at increased risk for aplastic crises which often occurs following a viral infection, most commonly Parvovirus B19. Aplastic crisis may require red cell transfusion until the crisis resolves. Splenic sequestration may also occur following infection and is associated with a sudden decrease in the hemoglobin and splenic enlargement. If red cell transfusion support is required then smaller aliquots, 3 to 5 mL/kg, should be given. Once a transfusion is given the spleen will often release the sequestered red cells resulting in a higher than expected increase in the patients hemoglobin and hematocrit which is why smaller aliquots are given. Patients with HS require lifelong folic acid in order to support the increased erythropoiesis that occurs due to decreased red blood cell life span. Splenectomy is the only known Hereditary spherocytosis treatment, however it is controversial and reserved for patients with significant complications. The most sensitive test for HS is the incubated osmotic fragility. The osmotic fragility test uses different hypotonic solutions varying in salinity from 0.1% to 0.9%. The patient's blood is added to each of the different solutions and examined for hemolysis. Hereditary spherocytosis cells will lyse at higher concentrations than normal cells due to the inability of their membrane to conform to fluid shifts.[2]

What is the most common defect in HS?
A. Ankryin
B. Pyruvate kinase deficiency (PKD)
C. Spectrin
D. Glucose-6-phosphate dehydrogenase (G6PD) deficiency
E. Point mutation in the β-globin chain of hemoglobin

Discussion

The correct answer is **C**. Hereditary spherocytosis is most commonly caused by a defect in spectrin or one of the proteins involved in the attachment of spectrin to the membrane that affects the structural integrity of the cell membrane. The instability of the red cell membrane results in spheroidal and osmotically fragile cells. These cells will be rapidly eliminated from the circulation by the spleen resulting in hemolysis. Approximately 30% to 45% of Hereditary spherocytosis patients present with combined ankyrin and spectrin deficiency, 30% with isolated spectrin deficiency, and 20% with band 3 deficiency.[2] PKD is the second most common enzymatic defect of red blood cells after G6PD deficiency. Pyruvate kinase converts phosphoenolpyruvate to pyruvate which is one of the two glycolytic reactions resulting in the production of ATP in the red blood cell. PKD results in a mild hemolytic anemia that is often asymptomatic.[3] A point mutation in the β-globin chain of hemoglobin is the defect present in sickle cell anemia. This results in a substitution of valine for glutamic acid at the sixth position. The β-globin gene is located on chromosome 11.

Objectives

1. Know the genetic inheritance patterns for Hereditary Spherocytosis
2. Know the typical clinical presentation of children with Hereditary Spherocytosis
3. Identify laboratory abnormalities seen in affected patients
4. Know appropriate diagnostic test to confirm a diagnosis of Hereditary Spherocytosis

CASE 3

You recently delivered a term male infant via spontaneous vaginal delivery to a 30-year-old G2P2 female. You note prolonged bleeding at the site of a heel stick and order a CBC and coagulation studies. The platelet count is noted to be 20,000. Mother reports no history of thrombocytopenia and her platelet count is 250,000. A head ultrasound shows no evidence of intracranial hemorrhage.

Your next plan of care is
A. Observation
B. Transfuse random donor platelets
C. Transfuse maternal platelets
D. Transfuse washed maternal platelets

Discussion

The correct answer is **C**. Neonatal alloimmune thrombocytopenia (NAIT) has an estimated incidence of 1 in 1,000 to 5,000 live births in Caucasian populations. NAIT is caused by maternal immunization against fetal paternally derived platelet-specific antigens. The mother lacks a common platelet antigen, most commonly HPA-1a, and when exposed to the antigen on neonatal platelets, the mother forms neutralizing IgG. The antibodies will cross the placenta and mediate destruction of fetal and newborn platelets. Due to the ability of IgG to cross the placenta, NAIT can occur with the first pregnancy unlike hemolytic disease of the newborn which only occurs in subsequent pregnancies. Treatment for throm-

bocytopenia in the full-term newborn should occur when the platelet count is less than 30×10^9/L, due to the risk of intracranial hemorrhage that can occur in 10% to 15% of cases of NAIT; however this remains controversial and varies from provider to provider. The most appropriate treatment is washed maternal platelets because the platelets will lack the antigen the antibody is formed against. The platelets need to be washed so additional maternal antibody will not be transferred to the infant. Random donor platelets from individuals also lacking the common platelet antigen, HPA-1a, are rare but if available can be used. If washed maternal platelets and HPA-1a random donor platelets are not available then transfusion with unwashed random donor platelets should not be delayed. High-dose IVIG may also be given but it has less predictable efficacy and the increase in platelet count is not seen immediately. The dose is typically 2 g/kg given over 2 to 5 days. Spontaneous recovery typically occurs after 1 to 6 weeks, when the antibodies have disappeared. The parents should be informed that the risk and severity of hemorrhage (ante and postnatal) increases with subsequent pregnancies.[4]

What is the appropriate sequence of the location of erythropoiesis occurring in fetal development?
A. The yolk sac from 2 to 8 weeks, then the liver from 8 to 20 weeks, and the bone marrow from >20 weeks
B. The yolk sac from 2 to 20 weeks, then the liver from 20 to 36 weeks, and the bone marrow from >36 weeks
C. The yolk sac from 2 to 8 weeks, then the kidney from 8 to 20 weeks, and the bone marrow from >20 weeks
D. The yolk sac from 2 to 20 weeks, then the kidney from 20 to 36 weeks, and the bone marrow from >36 weeks

Discussion

The correct answer is **A**. Hematopoiesis in the embryo and fetus can be divided into three periods conceptually: mesoblastic, hepatic, and myeloid. All blood cells are derived from embryonic connective tissue and blood formation can first be detected by the 14th day of gestation. Isolated foci of erythropoiesis can be observed throughout the extraembryonic mesoblastic tissue in the area vasculosa of the yolk sac at 3 to 4 weeks postconception. As the gut continues to develop, erythropoiesis is taken over by the liver and spleen around 6 to 8 weeks. Between the 5th and 10th weeks, the liver will significantly increase in size with an associated increase in the total nucleated cell count. The bone marrow will begin to be responsible for erythropoiesis around week 20. Midway through the third trimester the majority of hematopoiesis occurs in the bone marrow where it will stay throughout life, however stem cells can still be found in the liver and spleen during the first few weeks of postnatal life.[5]

Objectives

1. Identify the most common antigens responsible for alloimmune thrombocytopenia
2. Know the recommended treatment for affected patients
3. Identify the sequence of normal erythropoiesis in the developing fetus

CASE 4

You recently delivered a term newborn to a G2P2 female. The mother received no prenatal care. Shortly after delivery you notice diffuse jaundice, pallor, and hepatosplenomegaly. Maternal labs are blood type O−, RPR nonreactive, rubella immune, Group B Strep negative. The newborns blood type is A+.

Which clinical or laboratory feature would be more likely associated with hemolytic disease due to ABO incompatibility versus Rh disease in the newborn?
A. Late anemia occurring between the second and the sixth week of life
B. Need for exchange transfusion
C. Anemia at birth
D. Negative or weakly positive DAT (Coombs test)
E. Hydrops fetalis

Discussion

The correct answer is **D**. All newborns born to type O mothers should have cord blood sent for typing and DAT (Coombs) testing. The cord blood will be DAT positive in only 30% of ABO-incompatible pregnancies. If positive, it is typically weakly positive. A DAT sent from the newborn is rarely positive especially after the first day of life. In Rh disease, the DAT is typically strongly positive. The majority of neonates with Rh isoimmunization will develop late anemia between the second and the sixth week of life due to the persistence of anti-D antibodies. On the other hand, ABO incompatibility typically causes anemia for a shorter duration usually only lasting 2 to 4 weeks depending on the amount of maternally transferred antibody. Anti–Rh-D antibodies cross the placenta and can result in immune hemolysis in the fetus that can ultimately result in hydrops fetalis in some patients. IgG antibodies against A or B antigens due to

ABO incompatibility do not cross the placenta, thus anemia and jaundice are not seen immediately after birth but within the first 24 hours. Approximately 50% to 70% of patients with Rh disease will require exchange transfusion due to the severity of the anemia, but less than 10% of newborns with ABO incompatibility require an exchange.[6]

Which of the follow is NOT an indication for exchange transfusion in neonates with hemolytic disease of the newborn?
A. Hemoglobin 9.2 g/dL
B. Cord bilirubin >4 mg/dL
C. Total serum bilirubin >20 mg/dL regardless of gestational age
D. Rate of bilirubin rise >0.5 mg/dL despite intensive phototherapy
E. None of the above

Discussion

The correct answer is **E**. One of the primary goals of exchange transfusion is to prevent kernicterus due to the rapidly increasing bilirubin from ongoing hemolysis. Exchange transfusion will remove circulating bilirubin and antibody-coated RBCs. A double-volume exchange will remove approximately 70% of the fetal RBCs. However, only 25% of the total bilirubin will be removed due to 75% of bilirubin being present in the extravascular state. A rebound of serum bilirubin will often occur and additional exchange transfusions may be required. Exchange transfusion is not a benign procedure and has an estimated morbidity rate of 5% and a mortality rate of 0.5%. The most common adverse effects include apnea, bradycardia, cyanosis, vasospasm, hypoglycemia, and hypocalcemia. Due to the risks associated with the procedure it should be reserved for those newborns with severe anemia and the presence of a rapidly worsening jaundice despite optimal phototherapy in the first 12 hours of life.[6]

Objectives

1. Know differences in clinical presentation between neonates with ABO hemolytic disease versus those with Rh-hemolytic disease
2. Know indications for exchange transfusions in neonates with hemolytic jaundice
3. Know potential benefits and complications associated with an exchange transfusion

CASE 5

A 6-day-old term male newborn presents with blood streaked stool. He was born at home to a G2P2 female by a midwife as was the first child. He received no postnatal care. He is currently breast feeding for 5 to 10 minutes every 3 to 4 hours. When drawing labs you notice oozing from the venipuncture site and hematoma formation; CBC is normal. The prothrombin time (PT) is 20 seconds (control 11.5 seconds) and the activated partial thromboplastin time (aPTT) is 72 seconds (control 36 seconds).

What should you give next?
A. Vitamin K
B. Fresh-frozen plasma (FFP)
C. Factor VIII
D. Platelet transfusion
E. Cryoprecipitate

Discussion

The correct answer is **A**. Vitamin K deficiency bleeding (VKDB) is a rare but potentially life-threatening condition of early infancy. Vitamin K stores at birth are low and breast fed infants are at risk as vitamin K concentrations are low in human milk. Classical VKDB occurs in the first week of life and is related to delayed or inadequate feeding. In these cases VKDB can be prevented by giving a small dose of vitamin K at birth. Late VKDB peaks at 3 to 8 weeks and often presents with intracranial hemorrhage. Late VKDB is most frequently due to malabsorption of vitamin K due to an undiagnosed cholestasis. Late VKDB is preventable with parenteral vitamin K. Without vitamin K prophylaxis, the incidence of VKDB is reported as 4 to 7 cases per 100,000 births. The treatment of nonlife-threatening bleeding due to VKDB in infants up to 6 months of age is 1 to 2 mg of intravenous or subcutaneous vitamin K. Reduced bleeding from vitamin K can be seen as soon as 20 minutes following administration. In severe bleeding or those infants requiring emergency surgery, FFP should be administered at a dose of 10 to 15 mL/kg which will have an immediate effect.[7]

Objectives

1. Understand the potential causes of Vitamin K deficiency bleeding
2. Distinguish between the clinical presentation and etiology of early VKDB and late VKDB
3. Know recommended treatment for affected patients

CASE 6

A healthy 2-day-old boy born at term undergoes circumcision prior to discharge from the hospital. Bleeding was noted at the site of circumcision 10 hours after the procedure and has increased steadily over the past 4 hours. Findings on physical examination are unremarkable except for bleeding along 2 to 3 mm of the surgical site; no petechiae or purpura are seen. The family history is negative for any known bleeding disorders. Pertinent laboratory findings include a platelet count of 350,000/μL, PT of 12 seconds (control 11.5 seconds), aPTT of 120 seconds (control 36 seconds).

Of the following, the MOST likely cause of the bleeding is
A. Disseminated intravascular coagulation
B. Factor VIII deficiency hemophilia
C. Immune thrombocytopenic purpura
D. NAIT
E. von Willebrand disease

Discussion

The correct answer is **B**. Deficiencies of factors VIII (hemophilia A) and IX (hemophilia B) comprise the spectrum of common hemophilias and bleeding disorders seen. The X-linked disorders of hemophilia A and B are similar in clinical manifestations and treatment. The clinical manifestation of factor VIII and IX deficiencies correlates with the baseline factor levels of the patient. Severe hemophiliacs have a factor level of less than 1% and are at risk for spontaneous bleeding such as hemarthrosis, hematomas, gastrointestinal bleeding, and intracranial hemorrhage. Hemophilia patients at 1% to 5% factor levels are termed moderate and tend to have less severe bleeding complications. Factor levels above 5% are considered to have a mild form of the disease and they rarely have spontaneous bleeding and bleeds that do occur are usually precipitated by trauma. von Willebrand Disease results from either a quantitative or qualitative deficiency in von Willebrand factor. It usually manifests with mucosal-type bleeding; however, some forms can have bleeding severity similar to patients with hemophilia. Hemophilia A (factor VIII deficiency) is a congenital X-linked recessive inheritance disease that results in absent or decreased circulating factor VIII activity, leading to bleeding. The incidence is 1:5,000 male births. Because it is an X-linked recessive disorder, there is usually a family history, however 30% of newly diagnosed patients will have a negative family history meaning that spontaneous mutation is the likely cause of the disease.

Hemophilia B (factor IX deficiency) is caused by a congenital deficiency or absence of factor IX. It is also an X-linked recessive disorder with an incidence of 1 in 25,000 male births and accounts for about 20% of hemophilia patients. Factors VIII and IX are important cofactors in the coagulation cascade in that both act as cofactors on the phospholipid surface of the platelets causing further activation of FX and FV, ultimately producing thrombin. Patients with a deficiency in factor VIII or IX are unable to produce enough thrombin to sustain stable clot formation. The hallmarks of hemophilia patients are prolonged bleeding along with deep tissue bleeding such as hemarthrosis and muscle hematomas. Management relies on factor replacement for bleeding complications.[8]

How does fetal hemoglobin differ from adult hemoglobin?
A. Decreased oxygen affinity
B. Is composed of two α and two γ subunits
C. Increased red blood cell life span
D. Is composed of two α subunits and two β subunits
E. Is composed of two α subunits and two δ subunits

Discussion

The correct answer is **B**. Fetal hemoglobin is composed of two α and two γ subunits compared to adult hemoglobin which contains two α and two β subunits. The γ subunit is commonly referred to as the "fetal" hemoglobin subunit. Fetal hemoglobin has an increased affinity for oxygen compared to adult hemoglobin, shifting the oxygen dissociation curve to the left. The γ subunit is what is responsible for the increased affinity. This increased affinity allows the fetus to extract oxygen from maternal oxygenated hemoglobin across the placenta. The increased affinity also results in decreased oxygen delivery to the tissues, however in the fetus this is overcome by an increased hematocrit. Other factors that shift the oxygen dissociation curve to the left include decreased temperature, decreased $PaCO_2$, decreased 2, 3-DPG, and increased pH. At birth, fetal hemoglobin comprises 50% to 95% of the infant hemoglobin. At approximately 6 months of age, the fetal hemoglobin will begin to decrease as adult hemoglobin (hemoglobin A) increases.[9]

Helpful Tip: The hemoglobin molecule is a tetramer of protein subunits:
A. Alpha subunit – α
B. Beta subunit – β
C. Gamma subunit – Υ
D. Delta subunit – δ

Objectives

1. Know the inheritance pattern for Hemophilia A, Hemophilia B and von Willebrand disease
2. Know typical clinical presentation of affected neonates
3. Understand the differences in composition between Fetal Hemoglobin compared to Adult Hemoglobin
4. Understand differences in properties and affinity between Fetal Hemoglobin and Adult Hemoglobin

CASE 7

You recently delivered a term newborn with Down syndrome who was found to have an elevated WBC count of 75,000/mm[3]. The neonate is otherwise well appearing with no signs of infection. A blood smear reveals 60% abnormal lymphocytes that appear to be peripheral blasts.

What is the most likely diagnosis?
A. Acute lymphoblastic leukemia (ALL)
B. Acute myeloid leukemia (AML)
C. Transient myeloproliferative disorder (TMD) or transient abnormal myelopoiesis (TAM)
D. Leukocyte adhesion deficiency
E. Infection

Discussion

The correct answer is **C**. Approximately 5% of neonates with Down syndrome will develop a clonal myeloproliferation characterized by peripheral leukocytosis known as transient myeloproliferative disorder (TMD) or transient abnormal myelopoiesis (TAM). TMD is indistinguishable from AML at the initial presentation. The natural history of TMD, as the name implies, is spontaneous regression within 3 to 7 months. Despite the transient nature of TMD it has been associated with 20% mortality rate. Deaths tend to occur from hepatic infiltration/hepatic fibrosis, renal failure, and DIC. Due to the transient nature of the disease, patients presenting without symptoms or significant organ involvement can be observed without treatment. Symptomatic patients or those with significant organ involvement may be treated with leukopheresis or low-dose chemotherapy. After resolution of the TMD there remains a 15% to 30% risk of developing AML or myelodysplastic syndrome (MDS) that tends to occur within 1 to 3 years of life.[3]

Objectives

1. Understand the characteristics of transient myeloproliferative disorder in patients with Down's syndrome
2. Know the natural history of treatment options for this disorder

CASE 8

The parents of this patient ask if their child will be at risk for other types of cancer in the future.

What is your most appropriate response?
A. It is unknown if patients with Down's Syndrome are at increased risk for cancers over the lifespan
B. There is not an increased risk of cancer in patients with Down's Syndrome compared to the general population
C. Patients with Down's Syndrome have an increased risk of cancer over their lifespan compared to the general population
D. Patients with Down's Syndrome should be monitored monthly for the development of cancer

Discussion

The correct answer is **C**. Children with Down's Syndrome have an increased risk of developing acute leukemia. Previous studies estimated the excess risk to be 3 to 100 fold, more recent studies estimate the risk to be 10 to 20 fold. The previous reported leukemia incidence in children with Down's Syndrome have the ratio of lymphoid to myeloid leukemias of approximately 4:1, however, current analysis of these patients now suggests that this ratio is 1:1. This shift toward a significantly greater proportion with AML likely reflects the more accurate diagnosis of acute megakaryocytic leukemia (which was often previously diagnosed as L2 ALL). It is currently unclear why Down's Syndrome predisposes children to the development of leukemia. Possible mechanisms include developmental errors with disruption of hematopoiesis, ineffective regulation of granulopoiesis, immune deficiency leading to decreased immune surveillance, abnormal cell cycle kinetics, susceptibility to viral infections, genetic predisposition to nondisjunction, increased chromosomal fragility, impaired DNA repair mechanisms, and oncogene activation. The increased risk of leukemogenesis in children with Down's Syndrome suggests that chromosome 21 may play an important role. It has been demonstrated that the extra chromosome 21 is usually of maternal origin. Genes present on chromosome 21 that may be involved include the ETS (ETS2 and ERG) gene family, interferon response genes, cystathionine-β-synthase, superoxide dismutase, and carbonyl reductase. In addition, gene mapping studies have localized the critical region for the Down's Syndrome phenotype to chromosome 21, band q22.1 to 22.2, the same region as AML-1, a gene which is commonly involved in myeloid leukemias but none have been a proven etiological factor. The megakaryocytic subtype (FAB M7) is the most common form of AML in children with Down's Syndrome. Overall, children with Down's Syndrome are estimated to have a 400-fold increase in their risk of developing megakaryocytic leukemia and the M7 subtype is very rare in non-Down patients.

An important entity in patients with Down's Syndrome, is neonates have a unique predilection to develop TMD, a rare clonal myeloproliferation characterized by peripheral leukocytosis indistinguishable at presentation from acute megakaryocytic leukemia, FAB M7, or AML with minimal differentiation, FAB M0. Its predilection for Down's Syndrome neonates coupled with its unique characteristics of a relative paucity of leukemic blasts within the marrow, variable pancytopenia, a propensity for mild to life-threatening hepatic infiltration, and typically a spontaneous regression without any intervention help to clinically distinguish this entity. Between 4% and 10% of newborn infants with DS are thought to develop TMD. Presentation can be variable from asymptomatic which spontaneous regression within 3 to 7 months of life without intervention, to massive hepatosplenomegaly with hepatic fibrosis, and respiratory failure which requires therapy. In both instances of the asymptomatic presentation and the more severe form, among those who survived there was up to a 20% to 30% risk of subsequent leukemia. Patient who have resolution of their TMD, should have CBC diff performed monthly until the age of 2 years, then every 2 to 3 months until the age of 3 years, and then every 3 months until age of 5 years, then yearly.

Objectives

1. Know risk for development of cancer in the future for neonates with Down's Syndrome
2. Understand potential causes for the increased risk of leukemia in patients with Down's Syndrome

CASE 9

The fetus of a 32-year-old G1P0 mom is noted to have a sacral mass on prenatal ultrasound. The mom is referred to you and your pediatric surgery colleagues for prenatal counseling and asks about the plan for surgical resection after the baby is born.

Which subtype(s) of sacrococcygeal teratomas (SCTs) require surgical resection of the coccyx at surgery to minimize the possibility of recurrence?
A. Altman type I—entirely outside, sometimes attached to the body only by a narrow stalk
B. Altman type II—mostly outside
C. Altman type III—mostly inside
D. Altman type IV—entirely inside; this is also known as a presacral teratoma or retrorectal teratoma
E. All of the above

Discussion

The correct answer is **E**. SCT is the most common congenital tumor and accounts for about 40% of all germ cell tumors (Fig. 14-1). The estimated incidence is 1 case per 35,000 to 40,000 live births. There is a female-to-male ratio of 4:1. SCTs are often found on screening prenatal ultrasound due to the presence of a large sacral mass. If present at birth the risk of malignancy is less than 10% but the risk increases the later the presentation. After 1 year of age the risk of malignancy increases to 75%. Anatomically, teratomas are divided into gonadal (testicular or ovarian) or extragonadal lesions. Histologically, they are classified as either mature or immature based on the presence of immature neuroectodermal elements within the tumor. Mature teratomas can contain skin, hair, fat, cartilage, bone, teeth, and other mature elements. The most common malignant component within a teratoma is a yolk sac tumor. α-fetoprotein (AFP) and B-human chorionic gonadotropin (b-HCG) are the tumor markers used in diagnosing malignant teratomas. The AFP is normally elevated in infancy until 8 to 9 months of life making the use of AFP as a marker of disease status more difficult during the first months of life however it is useful in evaluating disease response. Complete surgical excision is recommended which includes removal of the coccyx; however the sacrifice of vital organs is not indicated for benign neoplasms.[11]

Objectives

1. Know the reported incidence of sacrococcygeal teratomas
2. Identify most common germ cell elements present in these tumors
3. Identify tumor markers

CASE 10

A 3-month-old ex–38-week full-term newborn presents for routine 6-month checkup. On examination you notice bilateral undescended testes. An ultrasound confirms bilateral testes in the inguinal canal.

When is the appropriate time for surgical intervention?
A. Immediately
B. If testes do not descend by 1 year of age
C. If testes do not descend by 2 years of age
D. If testes do not descend by 5 years of age
E. If testes do not descend by 10 years of age

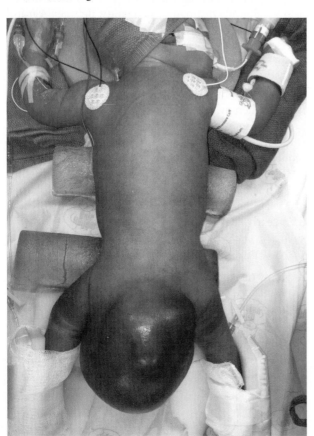

FIGURE 14-1. Neonate with saccrococcygeal teratoma. (Used with permission of Dr. Matthew Clifton, Emory University.)

Discussion

The correct answer is **B**. Three percent of full-term male newborns will have cryptorchidism at birth with the incidence decreasing as the infant ages and occurring in approximately 1% of male infants aged 6 months to 1 year. Spontaneous testicular descent after the first year of life is uncommon. Orchiopexy is advised on the undescended testicle after 6 months and before 18 months. Earlier intervention however may not prevent the subsequent development of testicular germ cell tumors. Factors that predispose to cryptorchidism include prematurity, low birth weight, small size for gestational age, twinning, and maternal exposure to estrogen during the first trimester. Males with undescended testes are 10 to 50 times more likely to develop testicular cancer and 10% of testicular cancer patients have been found to have had undescended testis. Undescended testes situated in the abdomen are more likely to result in malignancy than those in the inguinal canal. Eight percent to 22% of undescended testes occur in the abdomen; however this location is responsible for 45% of malignancies. Seminoma is the most common malignant tumor type associated with cryptorchidism. Testicular cancer usually develops in adulthood, typically in the fourth decade of life.[11]

Objectives

1. Know appropriate surgical management of cryptorchidism
2. Identify predisposing factors associated with crypotorchidism

CASE 11

A recently delivered female term newborn is found to have multiple cutaneous hemangiomas in her head, neck, and trunk.

Which internal organ would most likely also be affected?
A. Kidney
B. Brain
C. Spleen
D. Liver
E. Lung

Discussion

The correct answer is **D**. Infantile hemangiomas are common and occur in 1% to 2% of Caucasian infants at birth and 10% at 1 year of age. Hemangiomas are more frequently found in females with a ratio of 3:1. They are also more commonly found in premature infants and debatably in infants born to mothers having undergone prenatal chorionic villus sampling. Infants with multiple cutaneous hemangiomas are more likely to be associated with internal hemangiomas. The most common sites for internal hemangiomas in order of frequency are the liver, GI tract, central nervous system, eyes, and lungs. The hallmark of an infantile hemangioma is a rapid growth from birth to 6 months and then proliferation slows considerably from 6 months to a year of age. The involution phase may be rapid or prolonged. Fifty percent of infantile hemangiomas have complete involution by 5 years of age and 70% do so by the age of 7. The workup for infantile hemangioma may include MRI or ultrasound to evaluate for internal hemangiomas and to differentiate from high-flow vascular lesions such as arteriovenous malformations. The majority of infantile hemangiomas require no treatment unless there is significant vital organ compression or potential for disfigurement. Liver hemangiomas can often be life threatening due to intractable high-output cardiac failure from intralesional arteriovenous shunting, intraperitoneal hemorrhage, respiratory distress due to pulmonary congestion, and massive hepatomegaly compressing abdominal vasculature and producing abdominal compartment syndrome.[19] Treatment varies and includes topical and systemic steroids, interferon α, and vincristine.[12] β blockers (propranolol) have also recently been shown to induce involution.[13]

Objectives

1. Identify clinical variables associated with multiple cutaneous hemangiomas
2. Identify sites of involvement
3. Understand the natural history of the disease
4. Know treatment options for symptomatic infantile hemagiomas

CASE 12

A 4-week-old newborn presents to you with an 18-cm large violaceous mass on the right shoulder that developed over the past 48 hours. At birth her parents noticed fullness to the area with overlying erythema which remained stable until presentation. You suspect Kasabach–Merritt syndrome.

Which of the following is NOT associated with Kasabach–Merritt syndrome?
A. Prolonged aPTT and PT
B. Thrombocytopenia
C. Usually associated with other congenital anomalies
D. Undergoes spontaneous resolution
E. Lesions can extend into internal structures

Discussion

The correct answer is **C**. Kasabach–Merritt syndrome is the association between thrombocytopenia and a giant hemangioma of infancy. Kasabach–Merritt syndrome appears to be a complication of two rare, aggressive histo-pathologic subtypes: kaposiform hemangioendothelioma and tufted hemangioma. Most patients will present in the first few weeks of life. The lesions are typically solitary and involve the extremities, neck, or trunk. Occasionally the lesions are located internally without cutaneous findings and should be considered in an infant with unexplained thrombocytopenia. It is common to have a stable lesion that suddenly expands rapidly over a period of several weeks to months. The rapid growth is usually followed by spontaneous regression. The thrombocytopenia typically resolves as the lesion regresses. The pathogenesis of Kasabach–Merritt syndrome is not well understood, but platelets are believed to be trapped by abnormal endothelium within the hemangioma. The platelet count is typically less than 50,000/μL. Disseminated intravascular coagulopathy (DIC) also frequently occurs resulting in a prolonged aPTT and PT. Imaging studies are necessary to evaluate the extent of the lesion and determine if surgical resection is feasible. The mortality rate can be as high as 40% when associated with DIC. Initial treatment includes platelet and FFP transfusion in order to help correct the coagulopathy. Surgical intervention is often effective, but most lesions are unresectable. Vascular ligation or embolization has also been used in some patients with a large feeding vessel. Glucocorticoids, interferon α, and vincristine have also been used with some success.[14] Kasabach–Merritt syndrome has not been found to be associated with other congenital anomalies.

Objectives

1. Define clinical presentation of Kasabach-Merritt syndrome
2. Understand the natural history of this disease
3. Know associated hematologic abnormalities associated with Kasabach-Merritt syndrome
4. Know treatment options for patients with Kasabach-Merritt syndrome

CASE 13

You recently delivered a 27-week preterm newborn to a 35-year-old G2P2 female due to severe preeclampsia. Birth weight was 850 g. The family asks about the long-term risk factors associated with prematurity and low birth weight.

What malignancy has been found to be associated with being born at very low birth weight?
A. Medulloblastoma
B. Wilms tumor
C. Hepatoblastoma
D. Neuroblastoma
E. ALL

Discussion

The correct answer is **C**. Hepatoblastoma is the most common liver tumor in the pediatric age group and accounts for 65% of all liver tumors in children. The overall rate is one case per million children under the age of 15 years, which translates into approximately 100 cases per year in the United States.[15] Hepatoblastoma usually affects children younger than 3 years of age, and the median age of diagnosis is 1 year. Hepatoblastoma has been found to be associated with very low–birth-weight (VLBW) status, which is commonly defined as a birth weight less than 1,500 g. A recent study has shown that the rate of hepatoblastoma among VLBW infants was 50-fold higher than infants weighing 2,500 to 3,999 g (OR 50.6; 95% CI: 6.6–388).[16] VLBW likely is not the direct causative factor in hepatoblastoma but rather signals the involvement of correlated factors. There are current ongoing studies investigating exogenous and endogenous causes for the increase of this tumor observed in VLBW infants. There have been other proposed risk factors associated with hepatoblastoma including maternal smoking, maternal alcohol consumption, and oral contraceptive use during pregnancy but large epidemiological studies have not been done.

Objective

1. Know the risk for malignancy in children who were born premature

CASE 14

You recently delivered a 4,300-g product of a 39-week uncomplicated pregnancy to a 33-year-old G2P2 female. At delivery you notice an enlarged tongue and an omphalocele. Shortly after birth he develops severe hypoglycemia. You suspect Beckwith–Wiedemann syndrome.

What are the current recommendations for screening for malignancy?
A. Abdominal ultrasound and AFP every 3 months
B. Abdominal ultrasound and AFP every 6 months
C. Abdominal ultrasound and AFP yearly
D. Abdominal ultrasound every 6 months
E. No screening necessary

Discussion

The correct answer is **A**. Children with Beckwith-Wiedemann syndrome (BW) often present with asymmetric organomegaly, hypoglycemia, and omphaloceles. They are also at increased risk for certain malignancies including adrenal cortical carcinoma, hepatoblastoma, and Wilms tumor. BWS has been found to have abnormalities at the 11p15 gene locus. Only 15% of the cases are familial. Children with BWS should be followed with abdominal ultrasounds, AFPs, and urinalyses every 3 months. Screening with ultrasounds and urinalyses should be continued until 6 years of age while AFPs can be stopped at 3 years. WAGR is another genetic syndrome that is associated with Wilms tumor. It is also found with aniridia, genitourinary defects, and mental retardation. Patients with WAGR have cytogenetic deletions at 11p13 which includes the WT1 gene as well as PAX6. A loss of one copy of the WT1 in nephrogenic cells results in genitourinary malformations, while Wilms tumor results from acquired point mutations in the remaining WT1 allele in renal precursor cells. The loss of one allele for PAX6 leads to aniridia. Children with WAGR should also be followed every 3 months with abdominal ultrasounds and urinalysis until 6 years of age. AFP does not need to be checked as they are at no increased risk for hepatoblastoma.[17]

Objectives

1. Know the clinical presentation in a neonate with Beckwith-Wiedemann syndrome
2. Know malignancies associated with a diagnosis of Beckwith-Wiedemann syndrome
3. Know recommendations for screening for malignancy in affected children

CASE 15

A 6-month-old previously healthy full-term newborn presents to you with a week-long history of intermittent fevers up to 38.5°C and abdominal distention. On examination you note pallor and significant hepatosplenomegaly with abdominal distention. On skin examination you also note erythematous papules. Laboratory evaluation reveals hemoglobin of 7.8 g/dL, white blood cell count of 2,000 thou/uL and platelet count of 60,000 thou/uL. No blasts are seen on the peripheral smear.

What is the most likely diagnosis?
A. Neuroblastoma
B. ALL
C. Langerhans cell histiocytosis (LCH)
D. Acute myelogenous leukemia (AML)
E. Infection

Discussion

The correct answer is **C**. The etiology of LCH is unknown. It is considered to be a reactive disorder. An exaggerated activation of cytokines or loss of control of cytokine activation may be involved. An abnormal immune response to a viral infection has also been proposed. Multisystem disease is typically seen in children younger than 2 years of age. The presentation can be similar to acute leukemia with bone marrow suppression, hepatosplenomegaly, and constitutional symptoms. The cutaneous findings include erythematous papules that may ulcerate and resolve. Bony lesions are common and typically occur in older children. The skull is the most often affected bone and patients may present with painful scalp nodules. Pathological fractures may occur in weight-bearing bones. Diabetes insipidus is a common complication of LCH as lesions are often found in the skull base in the area of the pituitary. LCH has been shown to spontaneously resolve in a subset of patients, however there is another subset that has dissemination leading to end-organ dysfunction and possibly death. Involvement of the bone marrow, liver, and lungs has been found to be adverse prognostic factors. In patients with single system involvement, observation alone may be warranted as lesions often resolve spontaneously. Systemic corticosteroids in combination with oral methotrexate or intravenous vinblastine have also been shown to induce remission. Multisystem LCH requires multiagent chemotherapy and bone marrow transplantation is currently being evaluated in very high-risk patients.[18] Peripheral smear reveals no blasts making leukemia unlikely, and while neuroblastoma 4S often presents with hepatosplenomegaly in the infant, it rarely causes bone marrow suppression.

Which of the following is a true statement regarding neuroblastoma?

A. Neuroblastoma in infancy is typically associated with a worse outcome
B. Neuroblastoma in infancy always requires emergent chemotherapy due to the potential for rapid progression
C. Neuroblastoma can often be detected by analysis of urine VMA and HVA
D. Neuroblastoma surveillance is part of routine newborn screening
E. Neuroblastoma can often be detected by analysis of AFP and bHCG

Discussion

The correct answer is **C**. Neuroblastoma is the most common malignancy during the first year of life. The incidence is 9.5 cases per million children. Sixteen percent of neuroblastoma will be diagnosed in the first month of life. Forty-one percent are diagnosed in the first 3 months. Neuroblastoma 4S is a unique category of neuroblastoma and despite widespread dissemination the prognosis remains favorable. It is defined as a localized primary tumor in a patient less than 1 year of age with dissemination limited to the skin, liver, and/or <10% of bone marrow. Skin lesions are bluish, firm papules and nodules on the trunk and extremities that are often confused with rubella. Infants with stage 4S disease and favorable biological features are often treated with observation alone as these tumors have been found to spontaneously regress. In patients that require treatment due to vital organ compression, the chemotherapy is typically mild and intended to stop further progression until spontaneous resolution can occur. The overall event free survival rate is excellent at 85% to 90% and the younger the age at presentation the better the survival rate. Infants with poor outcome are typically those with extensive hepatic infiltration resulting in respiratory compromise and occasionally renal and venous obstruction. Ninety percent to 95% of patients with neuroblastoma will secrete one or both of the urinary catecholamines, homovanillic acid (HVA) or vanillylmandelic acid (VMA). In the past, routine screening for urinary VMA/HVA was done in the hopes that earlier detection would lead to increased cure rates. Routine screening resulted in a marked increase in overall incidence of neuroblastoma, however it was not found to reduce the incidence of advanced-stage patients with poor prognosis and thus it resulted in no significant change in outcome. Screening actually resulted in the over diagnosis of tumors that would have spontaneously resolved. Routine screening is no longer recommended.[19]

Objectives

1. Know clinical presentation of a child with Langerhans cell histiocytosis (LCH)
2. Identify factors associated with a poor prognosis in children with LCH
3. Know hematologic abnormalities commonly seen in children with LCH
4. Understand treatment options for patients with LCH
5. Know clinical presentation of children with neuroblastoma
6. Know factors associated with favorable and unfavorable prognosis in patients with neuroblastoma
7. Know recommendations for routine screening for neuroblastoma in the newborn

CASE 16

A male infant is born without a thumb on his right hand. Laboratory testing reveals a platelet count of 60,000 thou/uL. An x-ray of the right forearm reveals an absence of his radius.

Which of the following is the most appropriate next step?

A. Bone marrow biopsy
B. Computed tomography of head
C. Genetics consultation
D. Intravenous corticosteroid therapy
E. Intravenous immunoglobulin therapy

Discussion

The correct answer is **C**. Thrombocytopenia with absent radius (TAR) was defined as a syndrome in 1969 and further classified as the association of hypomegakaryocytes, thrombocytopenia, and abnormalities in the gastrointestinal, hematological, and cardiac system. Internationally, the frequency is 0.42 cases per 100,000 live births in Spain. No ethnic or racial predilections exist. The male to female ratio is 1:1. TAR syndrome is characterized by the absence of the radius bone in the forearm and a dramatically reduced platelet count. This syndrome may occur as a part of the 1q21.1 deletion syndrome. Due to its association with other syndromes a genetics consultation is recommended in all patients. In distinguishing TAR from other syndromes involving skeletal abnormalities of the upper extremities, the following may be of assistance: Fanconi anemia is an autosomal-recessive disorder causing bone marrow failure, skeletal defects, cutaneous pigmentation, microcephaly, and short stature.[20] Cases may present with thrombocytopenia. Upper limb abnormalities also involve the radial ray. Hypoplastic thumbs may be accompanied by radial hypoplasia but absence of the radius is associated with absence of the thumbs. Spontaneous chromosome breakage is a consistent feature of Fanconi anemia and is a reliable diagnostic test. The thumb is always present in TAR but may be hypoplastic or absent in Fanconi anemia.

Objectives

1. Know the clinical features associated with a diagnosis of Thrombocytopenia Absent Radius syndrome (TAR)
2. Identify differences in clinical features between TAR and Fanconi anemia
3. Identify other abnormalities in patients with TAR

CASE 17

A 2-day-old infant male weighing 4.9 kg presents with a left-sided abdominal mass and hematuria. While the workup for the mass is underway, his left arm becomes cold, painful, and pulseless.

The most likely diagnosis is
A. Wilms tumor
B. Neuroblastoma
C. Infantile polyarteritis
D. Paradoxical embolism
E. Kawasaki disease

Discussion

The correct answer is **D**. This case is a classic finding of renal vein thrombosis (RVT) in an infant of a diabetic mother. In neonates a RVT can proceed to embolization and cross the patent foramen ovale due to the elevated pulmonary pressure in the newborn and result in an arterial thrombus as is seen in the patient described above. RVT in neonates is the most common type of spontaneous venous thrombosis. Approximately 25% of cases are bilateral and 52% to 60% extend into the inferior vena cava. Overall survival now approaches 100%. Clinical sequelae in survivors include chronic renal impairment and hypertension. There was no difference in renal outcomes irrespective of whether the infant received no therapy, unfractionated heparin, or low–molecular-weight heparin, with 70% of affected kidneys

having irreversible renal atrophy. Approximately 20% of children have hypertension on long-term follow-up and 3% of children developed chronic renal failure.[21] Recurrent thrombosis rates appear low. Thrombophilic abnormalities did not predict recurrence or outcome; hence, their presence or absence is not useful in determining initial therapy. Because the existing direct evidence suggests no benefit, anticoagulant and thrombolytic therapy remains controversial.[22] Wilms tumor and neuroblastoma are not associated with thrombi and infantile PAN and Kawasaki disease are not associated with a left-sided abdominal mass.

Which coagulation factor or test in the neonate is different from that of a 2-year-old child?
A. Factor V
B. Factor IV
C. Thrombin time
D. Fibrinogen level
E. Platelet count

Discussion

The correct answer is **C**. The significant differences in the hemostatic system of neonates and older children or adults are (1) decreased plasma concentrations of many of the procoagulant proteins, including factors II, VII, IX, X, XI, and XII, prekallikrein, and high–molecular-weight kininogens; (2) a unique fetal glycoform of fibrinogen which is due to increased sialic acid which would be reflected in a prolonged thrombin time which is the correct answer in this case; (3) decreased plasma concentrations of the coagulation inhibitors AT III, heparin cofactor II, TFPI, protein C, and protein S, with a concomitant slower rate of thrombin inhibition; (4) a unique glycoform of plasminogen that is less efficiently converted to plasmin by tPA; (5) markedly elevated D-dimer levels until at least 3 days after birth; (6) increased plasma factor VIII and vWF concentration and elevated levels of circulating Ultralarge von Willebrand (ULvWF) multimers; and (7) modest, transient hyporesponsiveness of platelets to certain agonists such as collagen and epinephrine, but increased agglutination with low-dose ristocetin. Most of these differences resolve within the first 6 months of life. Thus factor IV, factor V, fibrinogen, and the platelet count are all similar to the child.[23]

Objectives

1. Identify clinical presentation of a neonate with renal vein thrombosis
2. Know long term sequelae of a renal vein thrombosis
3. Know recommendations for treatment options in patients with renal vein thrombosis

CASE 18

You recently delivered a 39-week full-term newborn via spontaneous vaginal delivery to a 30-year-old G1P1 male. On eye examination before being discharged home you notice leukocoria of the right eye. Ultrasound of the eye reveals a tumor suggestive of retinoblastoma. On discussion with the family the father reveals that he had an enucleation of one of his eyes at 1 year of age due to an unknown malignancy. The family asks how retinoblastoma is inherited.

What is the most likely mode of inheritance in this case?
A. Autosomal dominant
B. Autosomal recessive
C. X-linked dominant
D. X-linked recessive
E. Spontaneous mutation

Discussion

The correct answer is **A**. Retinoblastoma is the most common intraocular malignancy in children. The incidence is 1 in 18,000 live births in the United States. Retinoblastoma can be present at birth and is almost entirely restricted to early childhood with 80% of cases occurring before 4 years of age. A germline mutation is much more likely in this case considering the father's medical history however retinoblastoma also results from sporadic mutations. The inherited form is autosomal dominant with high but incomplete penetrance. The sporadic form occurs in 60% of cases. Genetic counseling should be given to the family of a child with inherited retinoblastoma. There is a 45% chance that a patient with the disease will pass it on to their offspring. Due to the incomplete penetrance there is also the chance that a sibling of the patient could develop retinoblastoma even if neither parent is affected because a germline mutation may be present but not phenotypically expressed. If genetic testing is done and an infant is known to have a germline mutation but no signs of retinoblastoma they should be screened at birth and then every 4 months until the child is 4 years of age.[23]

Which of the following is true concerning retinoblastoma?
A. Occurs from a mutation in the RB1 gene on chromosome 13
B. Increased risk of second malignancy
C. Bilateral disease is more likely to be due to a germline mutation
D. Somatic mutations are more common
E. All of the above

Discussion

The correct answer is **E**. The mutation occurs in the RB1 gene located on chromosome 13. A two-hit model has been proposed stating that as few as two stochastic mutational events are required for tumor initiation. The first hit can occur in the germline (heritable cases) or somatically in individual retinal cells (sporadic cases). In both cases, the second hit occurs somatically and leads to tumor formation. Unilateral or bilateral disease can occur. The majority of unilateral cases (85%) will be due to a sporadic mutation where as 90% with bilateral involvement will be due to germline mutations. Bilateral disease is typically diagnosed at a younger age compared to unilateral disease. Patients with the heritable disease are also at greatly increased risk for the development of second primary tumors, specifically osteosarcoma, melanoma, or brain tumors. The risk is significantly increased in areas exposed to radiation. The risk of developing osteosarcoma is highest between the ages of 10 and 20 years whereas the greatest risk for developing brain tumors occurs between the ages of 25 and 35 years.[24]

Objectives

1. Know the inheritance pattern for retinoblastoma
2. Know the typical clinical presentation of a newborn with retinoblastoma
3. Understand how the genetic mutation associated with retinoblastoma relates to disease presentation
4. Know risk for secondary malignancy in patients with a history of retinoblastoma

CASE 19

A 3,000-g baby boy is born at term to a G1P0 mother. On the second day of life he appears pale, but the physical examination is otherwise normal. Laboratory studies reveal the following: mother's blood type O, Rh negative; baby's blood type A, Rh positive; hematocrit 38%; reticulocyte count 5%.

Which of the following is the most likely cause of the anemia?
A. Fetomaternal transfusion
B. ABO incompatibility
C. Physiologic anemia of the newborn
D. Sickle cell anemia
E. RH disease of the newborn

Discussion

The correct answer is **B**. Hemolytic disease of the newborn occurs when there is transplacental passage of maternal antibody directed against fetal red cell antigens not shared by the mom. The antibodies that cross the placenta are IgG antibodies and may be against either the ABO group or against the Rh antigens. Although ABO incompatibility is more common than Rh disease, it is usually less severe. ABO "setup" occurs typically with a Group O mom and a Group A or B infant since individuals with Group O blood make naturally occurring anti-A and anti-B isohemagglutinins. It is very uncommon in incompatible infants born to Group A or B mothers, probably because the naturally occurring isohemagglutinins in these individuals are more likely IgM than IgG, and clear any fetal cells that might get into the maternal circulation, but cannot cross the placenta. Hemolytic disease of the newborn occurs more commonly with Group O moms and Group A infants, than with Group B infants, perhaps related to the density of the antigens on fetal red cells. It is rare for exchange transfusion to be required in ABO hemolytic disease of the newborn, as the combination of phototherapy (i.e., bilirubin lights) and insuring adequate hydration is usually sufficient to reduce the serum bilirubin. However, there are cases in which the maternal ABO IgG titers are so high that the serum bilirubin concentration cannot be controlled by these steps alone and exchange transfusion must be performed. When the mother is Rh− and the infant Rh+ there is also the possibility of Rh sensitization, but that does not occur in the first born child since Rh sensitization requires exposure of maternal circulation to Rh+ cells for antibodies to form. To prevent this exposure, Rh negative mothers are given anti-D immunoglobulin (RhoGam) at 28 weeks and at delivery. Doses of RhoGam should also be given after abortions, amniocentesis, or any other trauma likely to expose the mother to fetal blood cells.[6]

Objectives

1. Identify potential causes of hemolytic disease of the newborn
2. Know typical clinical presentation associated with various causes of hemolytic disease in the newborn period
3. Know indications for RhoGam administration to Rh-mothers

CASE 20

A 2-week-old African-American male is referred for evaluation and management of an abnormal FS newborn hemoglobinopathy screen. Family testing reveals that the father has HbAS, while the mother has only HbA. You repeat the infant's studies and the laboratory now reports an FSA pattern on hemoglobin electrophoresis.

The most likely diagnosis for this infant that explains these laboratory studies is

A. Nonpaternity
B. Sickle β+ thalassemia
C. Sickle β0 thalassemia
D. Sickle cell trait
E. Sickle cell anemia

Discussion

The correct answer is **B**. Overall; SCD occurs in 1 of 2,500 to 1 of 2,000 US newborns. Its incidence is highest in persons of African, Mediterranean, Middle Eastern, Indian, Caribbean, and Central and South American ancestry. The disease occurs less commonly in other ethnic groups, including individuals of Northern European descent. Accurate incidence data for many groups are unavailable. SCD is estimated to occur in 1 of 346 black infants and in 1 of 1,114 Hispanic infants in the eastern United States. The primary rationale for newborn screening and presymptomatic diagnosis is prevention of mortality from pneumococcal sepsis and splenic sequestration during infancy and childhood. Prophylactic penicillin has been shown to reduce the incidence of pneumococcal sepsis by 84% and is used in conjunction with pneumococcal conjugate and polysaccharide vaccines and urgent evaluation and treatment of febrile illness with parenteral antibiotics. Four SCD genotypes (sickle cell anemia HBSS, sickle-hemoglobin C disease HbSC, and two types of sickle β thalassemia [sickle β thalassemia+ and sickle β thalassemia 0]) account for most SCD cases in the United States. Less common forms of SCD are caused by coinheritance of hemoglobin S with other hemoglobin variants such as hemoglobin D-Punjab and hemoglobin O-Arab. In this scenario, the mother likely has β thalassemia trait and the father has sickle cell trait. Their child has sickle β thalassemia +, having inherited one abnormal hemoglobin gene from each parent. The classic newborn screening pattern in sickle β thalassemia+ is typically FSA, however, sometime the amount of hemoglobin A produced is so small that it sometime is missed. Sickle cell anemia (HBSS) also produces an FS pattern in newborn screening, however both parent should be both sickle cell trait. Sickle β thalassemia 0 would also have an FS pattern but HBA would appear later as the child get older. Sickle cell trait would have an FAS pattern.[25]

Objectives

1. Identify at risk population for Sickle Cell Disease
2. Know the various subtypes of Sickle Cell Disease and how they are diagnoses using the hemoglobin electrophoresis
3. Know rationale for routine newborn screening to identify Sickle Cell Disease

CASE 21

You recently delivered a 38-week male term newborn to a 34-year-old G2P2 African-American female. On initial examination you notice 4 or 5 hypopigmented macules to his trunk and a periungual fibroma on his left hand. You suspect the infant has tuberous sclerosis (TS).

What malignancy are they at greatest risk of developing?
A. Neurofibroma
B. Astrocytoma
C. Neuroblastoma
D. Medulloblastoma
E. Acoustic neuroma

Discussion

The correct answer is **B**. TS is an autosomal-dominant disease with variable penetrance. Spontaneous genetic mutations are actually responsible for the majority of cases and are present 75% of the time. The prevalence is 1 case in every 6,000 people. Two foci have been found for the TS complex. The TSC1 gene is located on chromosome 9q34, and the TSC2 gene is on chromosome 16q13. The TSC1 gene encodes hamartin and the TSC2 gene encodes tuberin. Hamartin and tuberin work together in the Golgi apparatus as a tumor suppressor. TS is very heterogeneous with a wide clinical spectrum that can range from severe mental retardation to being relatively asymptomatic with normal intelligence. On physical examination more than 90% of cases will have hypomelanotic macules, ash leaf spots. Visualization of the macules can be difficult in fair-skinned patients and can be enhanced by the use of a Wood ultraviolet lamp. Significant neurologic manifestation can be seen con-

sisting of seizures, cognitive impairments, and behavioral abnormalities. The brain lesion most commonly seen is a cortical tuber. Tubers are located in the convolutions of the cerebral hemispheres and can be present in the subependymal region. Tubers around the foramen of Monro may result in cerebrospinal fluid obstruction and hydrocephalus. A tuber can occasionally differentiate into a malignant subependymal giant cell astrocytoma (SEGA). SEGAs will typically present by the age of 3 or 4 years old. The major and minor criteria for diagnosing TS are listed below (Table 14-1). There is an increased risk of developing schwannomas, meningiomas, and ependymomas with neurofibromatosis type 2.[27] There is no increased risk of developing neuroblastoma or medulloblastoma in patients with TS.

Objectives

1. Know clinical features associated with Tuberous sclerosis
2. Know the genetic inheritance patterns associated with Tuberous sclerosis
3. Know diagnostic criteria for Tuberous sclerosis

CASE 22

You are taking care of a 6-day-old full-term male newborn with hyperbilirubinemia. On the third day of life he developed an indirect hyperbilirubinemia requiring phototherapy. The hyperbilirubinemia improved and the phototherapy was stopped. A male sibling also required phototherapy for indirect hyperbilirubinemia in the neonatal period and is currently a healthy 3-year old with no medical problems. You suspect G6PD deficiency.

Which of the following is true concerning G6PD deficiency?
A. Heinz bodies are seen on peripheral smear
B. Is an autosomal-dominant disorder
C. Is thought to be protective against cholera
D. Children require penicillin prophylaxis
E. All of the above

Discussion

The correct answer is **A**. G6PD deficiency is the most common human enzyme defect. It is an X-linked disorder that is present in more than 400 million people worldwide. G6PD is an enzyme that catalyzes the first reaction in the pentose phosphate pathway that results

TABLE 14-1.   **Updated Diagnostic Criteria for Tuberous Sclerosis**

Genetic Diagnosis	The identification of either a TSC1 or TSC2 pathogenic mutation in DNA from normal tissue is sufficient to make a definite diagnosis of tuberous sclerosis complex (TSC). A pathogenic mutation is defined as a mutation that clearly inactivates the function of the TSC1 or TSC2 proteins (e.g., out-of-frame indel or nonsense mutation), prevents protein synthesis (e.g., large genomic deletion), or is a missense mutation whose effect on protein function has been established by functional assessment (www.lovd.nl/TSC1, www.lovd/TSC2, and Hoogeveen-Westerveld et al., 2012 and 2013). Other TSC1 or TSC2 variants whose effect on function is less certain do not meet these criteria, and are not sufficient to make a definite diagnosis of TSC. Note that 10% to 25% of TSC patients have no mutation identified by conventional genetic
Clinical Diagnostic Criteria	
Major Features	1. Hypomelanotic macules (≥ 3, at least 5-mm diameter) 2. Angiofibromas (≥ 3) or fibrous cephalic plaque 3. Ungual fibromas (≥ 2) 4. Shagreen patch 5. Multiple retinal hamartomas 6. Cortical dysplasias* 7. Subependymal nodules 8. Subependymal giant cell astrocytoma 9. Cardiac rhabdomyoma 10. Lymphangioleiomyomatosis (LAM)[†] 11. Angiomyolipomas (≥ 2)[†]
Minor Features	1. "Confetti" skin lesions 2. Dental enamel pits (>3) 3. Intraoral fibromas (≥ 2) 4. Retinal achromic patch 5. Multiple renal cysts 6. Nonrenal hamartomas

Reproduced with permission from Northrup H, Krueger DA, on behalf of the International Tuberous Sclerosis Complex Consensus G. Tuberous Sclerosis Complex Diagnostic Criteria Update: Recommendations of the 2012 International Tuberous Sclerosis Complex Consensus Conference. *Pediatric Neurology*. 2013;49(4):243–254.

in production of NADPH. NADPH maintains glutathione in its reduced form. Reduced glutathione is a scavenger for oxidative metabolites and converts hydrogen peroxide to water. Red blood cells rely heavily on G6PD because it is the only source of NADPH required for protection against oxidative stress. Therefore, oxidative stress in patients with G6PD deficiency results in rapid response. The ingestion of fava beans has been known to result in acute hemolysis in patients with G6PD and is commonly known as favism. Fava beans contain a high level of divicine, isouramil, and convicine which increase the activity of the hexose monophosphate shunt resulting in oxidative stress. Acute hemolysis usually occurs within 24 hours after ingestion of the beans. Anemia is usually severe and can lead to acute renal failure. Blood transfusions may be required. Oxidative stress can also occur with multiple drugs, most commonly sulfonamides, and with infections. Most individuals with G6PD deficiency are asymptomatic throughout their life however neonatal jaundice is a common

presentation. The jaundice typically occurs within 1 to 4 days. It is usually responsive to phototherapy. Heinz bodies are small round inclusions that are seen within the red blood cells in patients with G6PD deficiency. Heinz bodies are irreversible precipitates of denatured hemoglobin. The exact mechanism of Heinz body formation is poorly understood but is thought to occur when there is oxidative stress in the lack of NADPH presence. When the interior thiols of the hemoglobin molecule are exposed to oxidation the hemoglobin molecule will lower its solubility. The insoluble hemochromes will then aggregate resulting in Heinz bodies.[28] Schistocytes or red blood cell fragments can also be seen on peripheral smear and are due to the splenic destruction. G6PD deficiency has been found to be associated with protection against malaria not cholera. The highest prevalence of G6PD deficiency is reported in areas with the highest rates of malaria. In vitro work has also shown that parasite growth is significantly slower in G6PD deficient red blood cells when compared to normal cells. The thought is that the increased oxidative stress that is present in G6PD deficient cells results in increased oxidative injury to the parasite.[29] Patients with G6PD deficiency do not require penicillin prophylaxis.

Objectives

1. Know the inheritance pattern for G6PD
2. Know typical clinical presentation of neonate with G6PD
3. Understand the metabolic pathways affected by G6PD

CASE 23

A 6-month-old male presents to you for decreased activity and pallor. He was born at 38 weeks' gestational age and at birth was found to have a cleft palate that has since been repaired and a triphalangeal thumb. A complete blood count (CBC) reveals a white blood cell count of 12,000 thou/uL, hemoglobin of 7 g/dL, and a platelet count of 175,000 thou/uL. The mean corpuscular volume (MCV) is 98 and the reticulocyte count is 0.5%.

What is the most likely diagnosis?
A. Fanconi anemia
B. Diamond–Blackfan anemia
C. Transient erythoblastopenia of childhood (TEC)
D. Acquired severe aplastic anemia
E. ALL

Discussion

The correct answer is **B**. Diamond–Blackfan anemia (DBA) is an autosomal-dominant disorder characterized by pure red cell aplasia, congenital anomalies, and cancer predisposition. It is caused by mutations in structural ribosomal proteins that result in erythroid failure by which the exact mechanism is poorly understood. The major diagnostic criteria include macrocytic anemia (elevated MCV) with reticulocytopenia and a normocellular bone marrow with a paucity of erythroid precursors. The neutrophil and platelet counts remain normal. Minor diagnostic criteria include an elevated erythrocyte adenosine deaminase activity (eADA), elevated fetal hemoglobin, one or more congenital anomalies described in DBA and no evidence of another inherited bone marrow failure syndrome. Congenital anomalies occur in as many as 30% to 47% of patients with DBA and include a

distinct facial appearance, genitourinary anomalies, heart defects, and a triphalangeal thumb.[30] Fifty percent of patients are diagnosed by 3 months of age, 75% by 6 months, and 92% by the first year of life. Only 10% of patients have clinically significant anemia at birth. The mainstay of treatment for DBA includes red cell transfusions, corticosteroid therapy, and hematopoietic stem cell transplant (HSCT). Approximately 80% of patients will respond to corticosteroids; however the remaining 20% will require chronic red cell transfusion therapy. HSCT is the only definitive treatment for DBA. It has been shown that patients who receive HSCT from an HLA-matched sibling before the age of 9 have significantly improved event-free survival than those older than 9 (90% vs. 70%). DBA has been found to be associated with an increased risk of developing cancer. Increased risk for leukemia, lymphoma, and solid tumors have all been reported.[31] Fanconi anemia is also an inherited bone marrow failure syndrome and is found with congenital anomalies. They can have thumb abnormalities; however they do not have triphalangeal thumbs and they typically present with pancytopenia instead of pure red cell aplasia. Transient erythroblastopenia of childhood (TEC) will also present with a pure red cell aplasia with reticulocytopenia however presents at a later age (mean 16–26 months)[32] and is not associated with congenital anomalies. As the name implies it is transient and resolves within 2 to 3 months. Severe aplastic anemia (SAA) is caused by an immune dysfunction and is associated with pancytopenia. SAA is associated with a high mortality rate and is treated with immunosuppression and hematopoietic stem cell transplantation in refractory cases.[33]

Objectives

1. Know the clinical characteristics of a patient with Diamond-Blackfan anemia
2. Know the inheritance pattern associated with a diagnosis of Diamond-Blackfan anemia
3. Know hematologic parameters seen in patients with Diamond-Blackfan anemia
4. Know treatment options for patients with Diamond-Blackfan anemia
5. Know risk for associated malignancies in affected patients

REFERENCES

1. Pappas A, Delaney Black V. Differential diagnosis and management of polycythemia. *Pediatr Clin North Am.* 2004;51(4): 1063–1086.

2. Boguslawska D, Heger E, Chorzalska A, et al. Hereditary spherocytoisis: identifications of several HS families with ankyrin and band 3 deficiency in a population of southwestern Poland. *Ann Hematol.* 2004;83:28–33.

3. Grace R, Lux S. Disorders of the red cell membrane, In: Nathan D, Oski F, eds. *Hematology of Infancy and Childhood.* 7th ed. Philadelphia, PA: WB Saunders; 2009:659–780.

4. Chakrovoty S, Roberts I. How I manage neonatal thrombocytopenia. *Br J Haematol.* 2012;156(2):155–162

5. Brugnara S, Platt O. The neontal erythrocyte and its disorders. In: Nathan D, Oski F, eds. *Hematology of Infancy and Childhood.* 7th ed. Philadelphia, PA: WB Saunders; 2009: 21–53.

6. Lily H. Immune hemolytic disease of the newborn. In: Nathan D, Oski F, eds. *Hematology of Infancy and Childhood.* 7th ed. Philadelphia, PA: WB Saunders; 2009:67–93.

7. Shearer M. Vitamin K deficiency bleeding (VKDB) in early infancy. *Blood Rev.* 2009;23(2):49–59.

8. Dunn AL, Abshire TC. Recent advances in the management of the child who has hemophilia. *Hematol Oncol Clin North Am.* 2004;18:1249–1276.

9. Bunn H, Nagel R: Hemoglobins: normal and abnormal. In: Nathan D, Oski F, eds. *Hematology of Infancy and Childhood.* 7th ed. Philadelphia, PA: WB Saunders; 2009:911–942.

10. Cooper T, Hasle H, Smith F. Acute myeloid leukemia, myeloproliferative and myelodysplastic disorders. In: Pizzo PA, Poplack DG, eds. *Principals and Practice of Pediatric Oncology.* JB Lippincott; 2011:566–600.

11. Olson T, Schneider D, Perlman E. Germ cell tumors. In: Pizzo PA, Poplack DG, eds. *Principals and Practice of Pediatric Oncology.* JB Lippincott; 2011:1045–1064.

12. Holland K, Drolet B. Infantile hemangioma. *Pediatr Clin North Am.* 2010;57(5):1069–1083.

13. Schupp C, Kleber J, Günther P, et al. Propranolol therapy in 55 infants with infantile hemangioma; dosage, duration, adverse effects, and outcome. *Pediatr Dermatol.* 2011 ;28(6): 640–644.

14. Wilson D. Acquired platelet defects. In: Nathan D, Oski F, eds. *Hematology of Infancy and Childhood.* 7th ed. Philadelphia, PA: WB Saunders; 2009:1576–1577.

15. Raney B. Hepatoblastoma in children: a review. *J Pediatr Hematol Oncol.* 1997;19(5):418–422.

16. Reynolds P, Urayama K, Von Behren J, et al. Birth Characteristics and Hepatoblastoma risk in young children. *Cancer.* 2004;100(5):1070–1076.

17. Plon S, Malkin D. Childhood cancer and heredity. In: Pizzo PA, Poplack DG, eds. *Principals and Practice of Pediatric Oncology.* JB Lippincott; 2011:17–34.

18. Mcclain K, Allen C, Hicks J. Histiocyte diseases. In: Pizzo PA, Poplack DG, eds. *Principals and Practice of Pediatric Oncology.* JB Lippincott; 2011:703–713.

19. Brodeur G, Hogarty M, Mosse Y, et al. Neuroblastoma. In: Pizzo PA, Poplack DG, eds. *Principals and Practice of Pediatric Oncology.* JB Lippincott; 2011:877–915.

20. Greenhalgh K, Howell R, Bottani A, et al. Thrombocytopenia-absent radius syndrome: a clinical genetic study. *J Med Genet.* 2002;39:876–881.

21. Shaz BH, Hillyer CD, Abrams CS, et al. *Transfusion Medicine and Hemostasis: Clinical and Laboratory Aspects.* 1st ed Elsevier; 2009.

22. Cantor A. Developmental Hemostasis: Relevance to Newborns and Infants. In: Nathan D, Oski F, eds. *Hematology of Infancy and Childhood.* 7th ed. Philadelphia, PA: WB Saunders; 2009:148–177.

23. Goodnight SH, Hathaway WE. *Disorders of Thrombosis and Hemostasis: A Clinical Guide.* New York, NY: McGraw Hill; 2001;3–19.

24. Hurwitz R, Shields C, Shields J, et al. Retinoblastoma. In: Pizzo PA, Poplack DG, eds. *Principals and Practice of Pediatric Oncology.* JB Lippincott; 2011:809–834.

25. Heeney M, Dover G. Sickle Cell Disease. In: Orkin SH, Nathan DG, Ginsbury D, Look AT, Fisher DE, Lux SE, eds. *Hematology of Infancy and Childhood.* 7th ed. Philadelphia, PA: WB Saunders; 2009:950–1014.

26. Meyers R, Aronson D, Von Schweinitz D, et al. Pediatric liver tumors. In: Pizzo PA, Poplack DG, eds. *Principals and Practice of Pediatric Oncology.* JB Lippincott; 2011:853–854.

27. Hasam R. The nervous system. In: Kliegman R, Behrman R, Jenson H, eds. *Nelson Textbook of Pediatrics.* Philadelphia, PA: Saunders; 2007:2485–2487.

28. Cappellini M, Fiorelli G. Glucose-6-phosphate dehydrogenase deficiency. *Lancet.* 2008;371(9606):64–74.

29. Miller J, Golenzer J, Spira D, et al. Plasmodium falciparum: thiol status and growth in normal and glucose-6phosphate dehydrogenase deficiency human erythrocytes. *Exp Parasitol.* 1984;57:239–247.

30. Lipton J, Ellis S. Diamond-Blackfan anemia: diagnosis, treatment, and molecular pathogenesis. *Hematol Oncol Clin North Am.* 2009;23(2):261–282.

31. Vlachos A, Muir E. How I treat Diamond-Blackfan anemia. *Blood.* 2010;116:3715–3723.

32. Prassouli A, Papadakis V, Tsakris A, et al. Classic transient erythroblastopenia of childhood with human parvovirus B19 genome detection in the blood and bone marrow. *J Pediatr Hematol Oncol.* 2005;27(6):333–336.

33. Scheinberg P, Young N. How I treat acquired aplastic anemia. *Blood.* 2012;120(6): 1185–1196.

Chapter 15
NEUROLOGY
Shannon E. G. Hamrick, MD and William A. Carey, MD

Physical Examination

CASE 1

You are asked to evaluate a 2-day-old newborn in the well-baby nursery at your hospital. During the discharge examination the general pediatrician had identified asymmetry of the pupils. He is concerned this may be a sign of serious neurologic or ophthalmologic disease, so he would like your opinion before sending the baby home. On examination you find that the right pupil measures 3 mm, while the left pupil is slightly less than 4 mm. Both are reactive to light. There is no evidence of ptosis or abnormal extraocular movement. The remainder of the neurological examination is normal.

What does this pupillary inequality most likely represent?
A. Horner's syndrome
B. An early sign of infantile botulism
C. Congenital third nerve palsy
D. Normal variation in pupil diameter
E. Optic atrophy

Discussion

The correct answer is **D**. Inequality of pupillary diameter can be a sign of significant pathology in the newborn. In order to make an accurate clinical diagnosis, it is important to consider a discrepancy of pupil size in the context of a patient's history and the results of a comprehensive neurological examination. Recall that pupillary constriction is mediated by the pupillary light reflex, in which afferent signals from the ophthalmic nerve stimulate parasympathetic efferent signals from midbrain nuclei. Pupillary dilation, on the other hand, is mediated by sympathetic efferent signals from the ipsilateral superior cervical ganglion and epinephrine in the systemic circulation.

In the case presented above, we can assume that the baby had an uneventful delivery and was well, as the pediatrician was preparing to discharge her at 2 days of age. More importantly, you identified normal pupillary size and a pupillary discrepancy of <1 mm. These findings alone would be considered normal. However, you also identified no associated abnormalities of the eye or ocular structures and the baby had no other abnormalities on the neurologic examination. Together, these facts suggest that the baby has a normal variation of pupil diameter. Horner's syndrome would have been suggested by a history of a prolonged second stage of labor, the presence of ptosis in association with a miotic pupil and evidence of ipsilateral brachial plexus injury. Congenital third nerve palsy would have been suggested by the presence of ptosis in association with a dilated pupil and lateral deviation of the affected eye. Optic atrophy occurs most commonly as a complication of extreme prematurity, hydrocephalus or hypoxic-ischemic encephalopathy, though it also occurs as a component of septo-optic dysplasia.

The finding of bilaterally fixed, dilated pupils is cause for alarm in any patient, regardless of age. In the newborn, fixed, dilated pupils are most commonly seen in the setting of brainstem injury, such as in severe, acute hypoxic-ischemic events. This neurological examination finding also is an important aspect of the brain death examination, so it is worthwhile to list here the various other causes of bilateral pupillary dilatation. Parasympatholytic drugs, such as atropine and cyclopentolate, may paralyze the pupillary constrictors such that the sympathetically innervated pupillary dilators function without a counterbalance. Severe central nervous system injuries, such as that seen with encephalitis or nonaccidental trauma, are two other causes of parasympathetic paralysis that should be considered. Excessive sympathetic stimulation, whether from exogenous or endogenous adrenergic compounds, is another possible cause of fixed, dilated pupils.

As part of your neurological examination, you assessed the baby's cranial nerves as well as her tone, movement, and primitive reflexes. You explain to the baby's mother that a comprehensive assessment is important, even though you were consulted to look specifically at her daughter's eyes.

Which of the following is a *true* statement regarding the newborn neurological examination?

A. A coordinated suck-swallow reflex involves five different cranial nerves
B. Organized sleep-wake cycles are not present until term gestation
C. Flexor muscle tone develops in a rostral-to-caudal pattern over the course of gestation
D. The tonic neck (or "fencing") reflex is the primitive reflex that develops earliest in the course of gestation
E. Cranial nerve IX mediates the motor component of the pharyngeal ("gag") reflex

Discussion

The correct answer is **A**. Comprehensive neurological examination of the newborn typically proceeds with the following assessments, in order: state of alertness, cranial nerves, motor functions, then primitive reflexes.

Specific states of alertness have been well described for healthy term newborns and are defined by eye-opening, pattern of respiration, spontaneous movements, and vocalization. With eyes closed the baby may be in quiet or active sleep, with the former characterized by regular respirations and absent movement. Irregular respiration and some degree of spontaneous movement are typical of active sleep. With eyes open the baby is considered awake, with the exact state defined by the pattern of breathing, movement and vocalization. True alertness is difficult to ascertain prior to 28 weeks of gestation, as most extremely premature babies open their eyes for only brief periods of time. Spontaneous alerting and prolonged periods of wakefulness develop around 28 weeks, and by 32 weeks a sleep-wake cycle may be identified. As term gestation approaches, babies demonstrate more activity during wakeful periods and attend to environmental stimuli.

Examination of the cranial nerves typically begins with an assessment of the pupillary reflex, which involves CN II afferents and CN III parasympathetic efferents as discussed above. Observation of the resting position of the eyes and their movements in response to lateral rotation of the head (the "doll's eye" maneuver) or during tracking permits the assessment of CN III, IV, and VI.

Cranial nerves V and VII may be assessed simultaneous by alternately touching each side of the face lightly with a somewhat sharp object (e.g., the broken edge of a tongue-depressor). In this test, the CN V mediates facial sensation and CN VII affects the grimace that would be elicited. These cranial nerves also participate in the suck-swallow reflex, along with CN IX, X, and XII. Cranial nerves V, VII, and XII participate in sucking by their control of the muscles of mastication, perioral, and buccal muscles, and tongue, respectively. Cranial nerves IX and X, which respectively mediate the sensory and motor components of the pharyngeal reflex, jointly mediate swallowing. Cranial nerves I, VIII, and IX are difficult to test clinically, especially in the intensive care nursery environment.

Motor functions may be considered in three distinct categories. Posture and tone often are assessed together, as a baby's posture reflects his or her acquisition of tone in the flexor muscles of the extremities. Passive movement of the extremities would reveal little tone in a 28-week newborn, while lower extremity flexor tone would be identified in a 32-week newborn. As the development of flexor tone proceeds in a caudal-to-rostral direction, it appears in the upper extremities by 36 weeks and is completely developed by term. Similar to the development of tone, spontaneous movement and power may be considered together and reflect the developmental progression of flexor tone. Thus at 28 weeks a newborn would tend to move an extremity without any flexion, while by 36 weeks full, alternating lower extremity flexion is seen along with some degree of upper extremity flexor movement. Finally, deep tendon reflexes may be elicited quite easily in the pectoral and brachioradialis muscles and at the knee and ankle.

Assessment of the so-called primitive reflexes is the final component of the newborn neurological examination. In term infants, the Moro reflex is characterized by abduction and extension of the arms with opening of the hands, followed by anterior flexion of the arms. In keeping with the developmental progression of flexor tone, only opening of the hands is seen at 28 weeks, while by 32 weeks the abduction-extension is present. There is a similar developmental progression of the palmar grasp, which is first present at 28 weeks and gradually becomes quite strong by term gestation. Two other primitive reflexes, the "walking" and tonic neck reflexes, do not appear until approximately 36 weeks.

As you are leaving the nursery the pediatrician asks you to clarify one aspect of your examination. To him it seemed that the baby's deep tendon reflexes were normal at the elbow, knee, and ankle—but he also noticed that the baby had a few beats of clonus when her foot was held in dorsiflexion. He asks you whether it is possible to differentiate benign clonus from pathological clonus.

Which of the following is a true statement regarding clonus and jitteriness in a newborn?

A. Jitteriness is often accompanied by diminished deep tendon reflexes
B. Jitteriness is a manifestation of neuronal irritability
C. Hypercalcemia is a common cause of jitteriness in newborns
D. Ankle clonus may be present in healthy newborns, but should disappear within the first few days of life
E. Ankle clonus lasting eight to 10 beats always is considered abnormal

Discussion

The correct answer is **B**. Jitteriness is a motor disorder that reflects neural irritability resulting from another, underlying condition. Metabolic causes, such as hypoglycemia or hypocalcemia, are commonly associated with jitteriness in the newborn, as are neurologic disorders, such as hypoxic-ischemic encephalopathy and neonatal opioid withdrawal. A jittery baby will demonstrate a generalized, coarse tremor that is exacerbated by environmental stimuli and accompanied by brisk deep tendon reflexes. Clonus, on the other hand, represents a self-reexcitation of the myotatic ("stretch") reflex. By 3 months of age this spinal reflex arc is inhibited by the corticospinal tract, but in the newborn the caudal CST is not yet fully myelinated. Thus, several beats of ankle clonus may be elicited during examination of the healthy term newborn. Conditions that impair the function of motor centers or the CST may result in clonus of the affected myotomes.

Neonatal encephalopathy is a commonly seen neurological syndrome that may present with signs of neuronal irritability, so it merits some discussion here. While often considered in the context of intrapartum hypoxia-ischemia, neonatal encephalopathy may result from a variety of prenatal and postnatal causes as well (e.g., severe placental insufficiency, congenital or perinatal infection, or metabolic disease). However, in the setting of perinatal hypoxia-ischemia there is a well-described progression of neurological signs that typify the more severe cases of encephalopathy. In the first hours of life an affected newborn will appear stuporous or comatose and display little spontaneous movement and rather reduced tone. The latter half of the first day of life may be characterized by the gradual development of jitteriness and lower brain stem dysfunction, with further involvement of brain stem nuclei over the next 2 days of life. Encephalopathic newborns may suffer from persistent hypotonia and uncoordinated, ineffective sucking and swallowing (which may relate to injury of any one of the five cranial nerves that govern this complex movement).

Objectives

1. Understand the significance and pathophysiology of neurologic abnormalities in a newborn
2. Know the function of the various cranial nerves and how to assess them in a newborn examination
3. Know normal variation in neurologic findings in a newborn

Neurodiagnostic Tests

CASE 2

You receive a call from a general pediatrician who just admitted a 33-week newborn to the intermediate special care nursery at his hospital. He appropriately performed a rule-out sepsis workup, including a lumbar puncture. Most of the test results so far are reassuring, but he would like to discuss with you the results of the cerebrospinal fluid (CSF) analysis. The fluid was characterized as mildly xanthochromic, but clear. There were 178 red blood cells/mm^3; 21 white blood cells/mm^3; the protein concentration was 137 mg/dL; and the glucose concentration was 41 mg/dL (a random blood glucose concentration was 55 mg/dL at the same time).

Which of the following conditions does the above CSF analysis most likely represent?

A. Hemorrhagic infarction
B. Bacterial meningitis
C. Congenital viral infection
D. Traumatic lumbar puncture
E. Normal CSF

Discussion

The correct answer is **E**. CSF analyses provide information about the gross physical characteristics of the CSF (turbidity and color), the total and differential cell counts, as well as CSF chemistry. Turbid fluid would be expected in the presence of high white blood cell counts or large amounts of cellular debris. Xanthochromia may reflect the breakdown of red blood cells within the CSF, though typically this represents small, clinically insignificant bleeding related to the process of delivery. Similarly, red blood cells are very commonly seen on CSF analysis in the newborn population. More than 100 RBC/mm^3 may be seen in otherwise healthy term newborns, while even higher RBC counts may be present in the CSF of well-preterm newborns.

An elevated white blood cell count, when seen in the setting of increased protein concentration and decreased glucose concentration in the CSF, may represent infection in any patient. However, each of these laboratory values must be compared to age-specific norms in order to draw appropriate clinical conclusions. Healthy term and preterm newborns may have up to 30 WBC/mm³ CSF, the majority of which may be neutrophils. CSF protein concentrations likewise are higher in newborns than in older infants and adults, with a normal range that spans approximately 50 to 150 mg/dL. Glucose concentrations tend to range between 30 to 120 mg/dL, with a higher CSF glucose:blood glucose range than that seen in adults.

Several days later the same pediatrician again contacts you about this 33-week newborn. While the baby initially demonstrated some mildly decreased tone in all the four extremities, it is now more evident that the baby is generally hypotonic and demonstrates little spontaneous movement. He would like to transfer the baby to you, but to prepare her parents he would like to know what types of testing are likely to happen once she is admitted to your intensive care nursery.

Which of the following is a true statement regarding neuroimaging in the newborn?
A. Ultrasonography cannot detect posterior fossa abnormalities
B. Ultrasonography is the most sensitive imaging modality for the detection of periventricular leukomalacia
C. Magnetic resonance imaging (MRI) is particularly helpful in detecting cerebral myelination
D. MRI is the most sensitive imaging modality for the detection of intracranial calcifications
E. Magnetic resonance spectroscopy may be used to detect metabolic abnormalities only in the setting of hypoxic-ischemic encephalopathy

Discussion

The correct answer is **C**. Ultrasonographic (US) imaging of the newborn brain is most easily accomplished via the anterior fontanelle. However, posterior fossa structures are best imaged via the posterior and mastoid fontanelles. While not as sophisticated as computed tomography (CT) or magnetic resonance imaging (MRI), US offers the advantage of bedside imaging. CT provides more detail than US in many respects and outperforms MRI in the detection of intracranial calcifications and anomalies of the skull bones. However, the benefits of this modality must be weighed against the significant radiation dose to which the neonate is exposed. MRI is the most sensitive means

by which to image the neonatal brain. In addition to the major structural anomalies detected by CT, MRI readily can identify a variety of developmental abnormalities (e.g., neuronal migration disorders), subtle structural defects (e.g., agenesis of the corpus callosum), vascular anomalies, and myelination disorders, including periventricular leukomalacia. Volumetric MRI has implications for long-term developmental prognostication. MR spectroscopy may detect a wide range of biochemical abnormalities in the brain, whether due to hypoxia-ischemia or an inborn error of metabolism.

Two days after admitting the baby to your intensive care nursery you are still unsure of the diagnosis. The neurological examination is notable for generalized hypotonia and weakness, including the facial musculature. To this point the infectious and metabolic disease workups are negative and the neuroimaging studies revealed no structural abnormalities. You are concerned that the baby may have a congenital neuromuscular disorder.

Which of the following is a true statement regarding diagnostic testing for neuromotor disorders?
A. Nerve conduction velocity is prominently decreased in spinal muscular atrophy
B. Nerve conduction velocity is prominently decreased in congenital myasthenia gravis
C. Electromyography is normal in cases of spinal muscular atrophy
D. Electromyography is normal in cases of peripheral nerve disease
E. Muscle biopsy is abnormal in cases of spinal muscular atrophy

Discussion

The correct answer is **E**. Nerve conduction velocity (NCV) is used to detect disorders of the peripheral nerves. Conduction velocity is slower in newborns than in older children and adults due to the small diameter and immature myelination of the peripheral nerves. Nevertheless, NCV may be used to diagnose disorders of myelination or, more rarely, the axon. Electromyography may be used to detect abnormalities at every level of the motor unit: anterior horn cell, peripheral nerve, neuromuscular junction, and muscle. Fibrillations at rest are seen in disorders of the anterior horn cells and peripheral nerve, whereas these are usually absent in congenital myasthenic syndromes and myopathies. Muscle biopsy likewise provides information about disorders of the entire motor unit, revealing characteristic patterns of atrophy, qualitative changes in muscle fibers, and biochemical data.

Objectives

1. Know how to interpret laboratory values of CSF
2. Understand the role of cranial sonography and MRI in the diagnostic evaluation of a newborn with abnormal neurologic findings
3. Understand the use of nerve conduction studies in the evaluation of a newborn with abnormal neurologic findings

Development of the Nervous System-1

CASE 3

A newborn has been transferred to you from a community hospital in your region to evaluate for microcephaly and dysmorphisms. On your examination, you find a male infant appropriately sized for weight and length but with a head circumference <3%. He has marked ocular hypotelorism, a flat nose, and when you examine his palate you find a cleft. He has clonic spasms with stimuli, but the remainder of his physical examination is normal.

Based on physical examination, this infant is most likely to have
A. Aqueductal stenosis
B. Fetal alcohol syndrome
C. Holoprosencephaly (HPE)
D. Wolf–Hirschhorn syndrome
E. Miller–Dieker syndrome

Discussion

The correct answer is **C**. HPE is the most common structural malformation of the forebrain and has a wide clinical spectrum depending upon the extent of hemispheric separation. It is characterized by variable degrees of craniofacial and midline anomalies. In its most severe form there is cyclopia or synophthalmia with a proboscis, and in less severe forms, such as our case, there is hypotelorism with midface hypoplasia or a single maxillary central incisor.

Aqueductal stenosis (A) presents with hydrocephalus, not microcephaly. Infants with fetal alcohol syndrome (B) often do have microcephaly with midface hypoplasia. Classically the defining feature is a smooth or long philtrum with thin upper lip. Cleft palate is a less common feature. Wolf–Hirschhorn syndrome (D) is on the differential for congenital microcephaly but these infants characteristically have hypertelorism, as well as dysplastic ears, hypotonia, seizures, and heart disease. The answer

E, Miller–Dieker, one of the lissencephaly syndromes, also has midface abnormalities but is incorrect because it has other notable findings on physical examination (classically bitemporal hollowing, heart disease, genital anomalies, and clinodactyly).

Prosencephalic development has its peak in the second and third months of gestation, and is characterized by three sequential important events: prosencephalic formation, prosencephalic cleavage, and midline prosencephalic development; disorders result from interruption or disturbances in these events. Aprosencephaly or atelencephaly is the most severe disorder, and can be distinguished from anencephaly by the intact skull and dermal covering. (Anencephaly is the failure of anterior neural tube closure.) Abnormalities in prosencephalic cleavage lead to HPE or holotelencephaly. The most severe form of HPE, alobar HPE, results in a single-sphered cerebral structure with a common ventricle with a distended posterior cyst, absence of olfactory bulbs/tracts, and hypoplasia of optic nerves. The cortical mantle often shows heterotopias (a sign of disordered neuronal migration). Less severe forms are semilobar or lobar HPE. Finally, and least severe, midline prosencephalic developmental anomalies include agenesis of the corpus callosum or agenesis or the septum pellucidum, and forms of septo-optic dysplasia.

Agenesis of the corpus callosum is frequently seen with other brain anomalies, most notably disorders of neuronal migration, due to the fact that callosal development and neuronal migration occur during the same developmental time frame. It is also frequently seen with Chiari II malformations. Agenesis of the corpus callosum without other CNS anomalies can be essentially asymptomatic. However, identification of agenesis of the corpus callosum on ultrasonography is an indication for an MRI as it is so frequently seen with migrational disorders.

Which is not a feature of Aicardi syndrome?
A. Male sex
B. Impaired cognition
C. Agenesis of the corpus callosum
D. Infantile spasms
E. Cerebrocortical heterotopias

Discussion

The correct answer is **A**. Aicardi syndrome is an example of agenesis of the corpus callosum in conjunction with a defect in neuronal migration. It is seen in *females* only and is also characterized by *chorioretinal lacunae*.

Neuronal migration, which peaks between the third and fifth months of gestation, is the process by which millions of nerve cells migrate from their site of origin (e.g., ventricular and subventricular zones) to their permanent location (e.g., cortex or deep gray nuclei). Radial glial cells serve as the escorts for migrating neurons and they enable columnar organization of the cortex; they then differentiate into astrocytes. Disorders in neuronal migration lead to abnormalities in gyral formation.

At which point in gestation does the number of cerebral gyri begin to increase most rapidly?
A. 18 to 20 weeks
B. 22 to 24 weeks
C. 26 to 28 weeks
D. 32 to 34 weeks
E. >42 weeks

Discussion

The correct answer is **C**. Between 26 and 28 weeks is the greatest increase in major gyri, though this continues throughout the third trimester and just beyond term birth, as well. Completion of neuronal migration is the inciting event: as the surface area of the outer cortical layers have exceeded that of the inner cortical layers, the mechanics of compressive pressures produce the gyri. When migration is disturbed gyral patterns are abnormal, and frequently the corpus callosum is absent or hypoplastic, as midline prosencephalic development is occurring concomitantly with migration, and callosal fibers are dependent on normal neuronal migration.

Which disorder of neuronal migration is most severe?
A. Focal cerebrocortical dysgenesis
B. Heterotopias
C. Polymicrogyrias
D. Lissencephaly and pachygyria
E. Schizencephaly

Discussion

The correct answer is **E**. In fact, the severity is depicted by the reverse order of the answers. Schizencephaly results from an agenesis of a germinative zone and thus an absence of a cerebral wall, leading to clefts. The etiology is likely multifactorial: a genetic or physical insult such as early infection or infarction. Lissencephaly (D) means "smooth brain," while pachygyria is a less severe form of lissencephaly. Pathologically it appears that migrating neurons never made it to their final destination, with heterotopic neurons in columns. Lissencephaly can be isolated or part of more complex syndromes such as Walker–Warburg or Fukuyama congenital muscular dystrophy. Many responsible genes have been identified but like schizencephaly the etiology may be multifactorial and related to a physical disruption. Polymicrogyria (C), or excessive and small gyri, falls into two broad categories: layered, which is postmigrational and caused by a destructive process, and nonlayered which is a

migrational disorder. Heterotopias (B) are collections of neurons in the subcortical white matter where they have arrested migration. Heterotopias always accompany more severe migration disorders, and are frequently seen in a multitude of genetic or metabolic disorders, but isolated collections are also found incidentally at autopsy. Only MRI is sensitive enough to detect heterotopias. Focal cerebrocortical dysgenesis (A), also called cortical dysplasia, is likely a late event resulting in a disorganized area of cortex.

With the more severe migrational disorders, cognitive and motor impairments are common, as are seizures. For the less severe disorders, topography and size determine the clinical significance (seizures being the predominant feature).

Microcephaly is an important yet nonspecific finding. The differential diagnosis for congenital (*not* postnatally acquired) microcephaly includes genetic causes: isolated microcephaly (e.g., autosomal recessive and dominant, and X-linked forms) or syndromic mirocephaly (e.g., trisomy 21, 13, 18, or contiguous gene deletions such as Wolf–Hirschhorn or 22q11, or single gene defects such as HPE or Smith–Lemli–Opitz). There are also congenitally acquired forms of microcephaly from a prenatal disruption in vascular supply (e.g., death of a monozygotic twin or stroke) or from a prenatal infection (e.g., TORCHES) or from exposure to a teratogen (e.g., alcohol, hydantoin, poorly controlled diabetes, or maternal phenylkenonuria) or from deprivation states, such as maternal hypothyroidism, malnutrition, or placental insufficiency.

Children with severe microcephaly (defined as <3 SD) who have been imaged by either CT or MRI will show an abnormality what percentage of the time?
A. 10%
B. 30%
C. 50%
D. 75%
E. 90%

Discussion

The correct answer is **D**. MRI is a higher-yield test than a CT scan, as MRI can reveal abnormalities that are difficult to visualize on CT, such as callosal malformations, migrational or myelination disorders. Because certain malformations (e.g., lissencephaly) are associated both with specific genes and with severe developmental impairment, the MRI can be helpful for diagnosis and prognosis, as well as genetic counseling. In addition, specific targeted genetic testing should be considered on the basis of the imaging results. Children with microcephaly are at risk for epilepsy, mental retardation, and cerebral palsy.

In our microcephalic infant with dysmorphic facies above, the MRI revealed semilobar HPE. The anterior (frontal) brain is fused and underdeveloped but the inter-hemispheric fissure is noted posteriorly and the posterior portion of the corpus callosum is present. The deep gray nuclei are partially separated and there is a small third ventricle and large dorsal cyst.

What is the next step in his management?
A. Genetic consult
B. 7-dehydrocholesterol level
C. Craniofacial consult
D. Urine-specific gravity
E. All of the above

Discussion

The correct answer is **E**. All of the above may be appropriate. An estimated 30% to 50% of HPE cases are due to genetic abnormalities. Approximately 25% of patients have recognizable syndromes (e.g., Smith–Lemli–Opitz [SLOS] or trisomy 13). There are established HPE genes. Other risk factors include the use of retinoids or statins (or other alterations in cholesterol biosynthesis) or alcohol during gestation or maternal diabetes.

A reasonable approach to the evaluation for HPE is to discuss the case with a geneticist and obtain a chromosomal microarray and 7-dehydro-cholesterol levels (for SLOS). If these are negative, molecular analysis for the most common genes implicated in HPE is warranted. Parental samples are also helpful in interpretation of the infant's results, and for future genetic counseling.

Abnormalities in hypothalamic function are common, most frequently diabetes insipidus (in 70%), but also inappropriate antidiuretic hormone secretion and poikilothermia. Anterior pituitary dysfunction is less common. Severity of diabetes insipidus correlates with the degree of hypothalamic non-separation.

Objectives

1. Know the embryology of the development of the human brain
2. Know the various types of neuronal migration abnormalities
3. Know the clinical characteristics and features of newborns with developmental abnormalities of brain development
4. Know the common features associated with holo-prosencephaly
5. Identify the syndromes commonly associated with abnormalities in brain development

Development of the Nervous System-2

CASE 4

You are asked to perform a prenatal consult in your hospital's perinatology clinic. The woman with whom you will meet is a healthy 25-year-old primigravida who is 20 weeks pregnant. She learned last week that her fetus is affected by myelomeningocele, so she has returned for a follow-up appointment and additional testing.

Which of the following is a true statement regarding neural tube defects?
A. Like myelomeningocele, encephalocele is an example of an open neural tube defect
B. Like myelomeningocele, encephalocele often is complicated by hydrocephalus
C. The cerebellum is the neural structure most commonly involved in encephalocele
D. Aside from hindbrain herniation, additional cerebral anomalies are rarely associated with myelomeningocele
E. A newborn with a myelomeningocele that spans L3 and L4 likely would be unable to flex the hips

Discussion

The correct answer is **B**. Encephalocele and myelomeningocele are disorders of abnormal neurulation that occur at the opposing poles of neural tube closure. Encephalocele most commonly appears as a closed neural tube encasing the occipital lobe within. Hydrocephalus and agenesis of the corpus callosum frequently accompany encephalocele. Surgery is indicated early in the neonatal period if the mass leaks CSF, but later intervention is preferred.

Myelomeningocele is an example of an open neural tube defect, most commonly occurring in the lumbar spine. Failed closure of the caudal pole of the neural tube leads to defects in the lumbar spine and dermis with protrusion of the neural placode at the affected level. The anatomic level of the spinal defect is important in determining eventual neuromotor function (see Table 15-1) and the likelihood that CSF shunting will be required. Another common anatomical finding in myelomeningocele is the presence of herniation of the hindbrain through the foramen magnum, the Chiari type II malformation. The presence of hindbrain herniation is associated with brain stem dysfunction and severe obstructive hydrocephalus. Caesarian delivery before the onset of labor may be associated with better neuromotor function than delivery after the onset of labor and postnatal repair should occur within the first few days of birth.

TABLE 15-1.   **Anatomic Level of Spinal Defect and Function**

SPINAL CORD LEVEL	MYOTOME (APPROXIMATE)
L1	Hip flexion
L2	Hip adduction
L3	Knee extension
L4	Ankle inversion/dorsiflexion
L5	Hip abduction, knee flexion, great toe extension
S1	Hip extension, ankle eversion/plantarflexion
S2	Toe flexion
S2–S4	Bladder, colon, and pelvic musculature

The fetus in this case is affected by a myelomeningocele that spans the L2 to L4 vertebrae. There is herniation of the hindbrain and ventricular dilatation, but no other congenital anomalies have been identified. The fetal karyotype is normal.

Based on the information provided above, would it be appropriate to offer this maternal–fetal dyad prenatal surgical repair of the myelomeningocele?

A. No, because there is evidence of hindbrain herniation
B. No, because there is evidence of ventricular dilatation
C. No, because prenatal surgery has not been shown to improve outcomes
D. Yes, because the maternal and fetal characteristics are favorable
E. Yes, because the fetus is still previable

Discussion

The correct answer is **D**. The *Management of Myelomeningocele Study* or "MOMS trial" compared the safety and efficacy of prenatal surgical repair of myelomeningocele to that of standard postnatal surgery. A fetus was considered eligible if the gestational age were between 19.0 and 25.9 weeks; the rostral pole of the defect were located between T1 and S1; hindbrain herniation were present; no significant anomalies unrelated to the MM were present; and the karyotype were normal. A mother was considered eligible if she were at least 18 years of age; had a body mass index <35; were not otherwise at risk for preterm delivery; and had no obstetric complications (e.g., placental abruption, prior classical caesarian section).

Compared to babies who underwent standard postnatal surgery, babies treated prenatally were less likely to die or need a CSF shunt during the first year of life (relative risk 0.7). Shunt placement rates were 40% among those treated prenatally and 82% among the postnatal surgery group. Hindbrain herniation also was less common at 12 months of age in the prenatal surgery group. Neurodevelopmental outcomes were better among babies whose MM was repaired prenatally, with composite mental development–motor function significantly improved at 30 months of age. Prenatal repair also was correlated with a higher likelihood that the neurological functional level would be higher than the anatomical level of the defect.

Adverse neonatal outcomes among babies treated prenatally were limited to prematurity (average gestational age at delivery 34 weeks vs. 37 weeks) and respiratory distress syndrome. Maternal complications included chorioamniotic membrane separation, spontaneous rupture of membranes, placental abruption, and increased likelihood of blood transfusion upon delivery.

Toward the end of the consultation, the mother asks you whether her future children will be at increased risk of myelomeningocele or hydrocephalus. She is specifically concerned with the latter, as she has read online that hydrocephalus and other causes of macrocephaly can be familial.

Which of the following is a true statement regarding congenital macrocephaly?

A. X-linked aqueductal stenosis is a common cause of congenital hydrocephalus
B. Macrencephaly results from reduced neuronal proliferation
C. Tay–Sachs disease is an example of an autosomal dominant neurodegenerative condition
D. The classic "cherry red spot" of Tay–Sachs disease reflects the fact that Tay–Sachs predominantly affects white matter
E. Neurodegenerative diseases associated with macrocephaly are rarely associated with seizures

Discussion

The correct answer is **A**. Macrocephaly, or increased head circumference, may result from a variety of developmentally distinct primary disorders. Congenital hydrocephalus most often results from abnormalities of the cerebrum or CSF circulatory system. Thus, HPE, aqueductal stenosis, myelomeningocele with associated hindbrain herniation and Dandy–Walker malformation are common causes of hydrocephalus. Less commonly, an imbalance between CSF production and resorption may result in extra-axial fluid accumulation (i.e., "communicating hydrocephalus").

Macrencephaly likely results from excessive neuronal proliferation or inadequacy of the programmed cell death that normally occurs during brain development. Autosomal dominant macrencephaly is associated with relatively preserved neurodevelopment, though the autosomal recessive variety is characterized by cognitive and motor dysfunction as well as seizures.

Macrocephaly also may be identified in the setting of inborn errors of metabolism (e.g., pyruvate carboxylase deficiency) or neurodegenerative disorders. These conditions, many of which are autosomal recessive, are characterized by the accumulation of complex molecules in either or both the gray or white matter. Gray matter–predominant diseases often present with seizures, retinal disease, and impaired cognitive development. Gangliosidoses, such as Tay–Sachs disease/GM2 gangliosidosis (hexosaminidase A deficiency), may present with these signs in association with macrocephaly. White matter–predominant diseases tend to present with severe motor deficits in association with seizures. Alexander disease (autosomal dominant, gain-of-function mutation in glial fibrillary acidic protein) and Canavan disease (N-acetylaspartoacyclase deficiency) are classic examples.

Neurocutaneous syndromes (e.g., neurofibromatosis [NF] and Sturge–Weber disease) and chromosomal anomalies (e.g., Fragile X syndrome and 47, XXY karyotype/Klinefelter syndrome) may present with macrocephaly as well.

Objectives

1. Know the various types of neural tube defects
2. Understand normal development of the neural tube
3. Know the options for surgical management of the fetus with a neural tube defect
4. Know other abnormalities commonly found in children with neural tube defects
5. Know the potential causes of macrocephaly and associated clinical syndromes

Encephalopathy

CASE 5

Baby Coleman is a 40-week-old male, born at 3,200 g to a G1P0 29-year-old female with unremarkable prenatal labs and good prenatal care. He was noted to have variable decelerations during monitoring prior to delivery. At birth he required positive pressure ventilation but by 10 minutes was breathing spontaneously with a normal heart rate. The cord gas showed a pH of 7.0 and a base deficit of –16. He was taken to a transitional unit for observation and blood work to rule out sepsis. Over the

course of the next hour he became more lethargic and hypotonic with periods of hypoventilation. His follow-up blood gas had a pH of 6.9 with an elevated CO_2 and a base deficit of –18.

This infant is most likely encephalopathic due to which of the following?
A. A urea cycle defect
B. Hypoxic-ischemic encephalopathy (HIE)
C. An organic academia
D. A congenital brain malformation
E. Meningitis

Discussion

The correct answer is **B**. The neurological syndrome that accompanies perinatal hypoxia-ischemia can be varied, but the clinical features evolve over the first hours, days, and weeks of life. In the initial few hours after birth it is common to see a depressed level of consciousness with ventilatory disturbances—the severity depends upon the severity of insult. Pupillary responses are usually intact early in the course of encephalopathy, but abnormalities in tone may be present (hypotonia more common than hypertonia). Seizures may occur and are usually subtle (ocular or oral–buccal–lingual abnormalities, "rowing"-type movements or apnea).

Although a congenital brain malformation or remote antenatal insult could present with an encephalopathic picture it should not be accompanied by either an acute acidosis or a worsening clinical neurological syndrome.

Inborn errors of metabolism, such as a urea cycle defect or an organic academia, comprise a group of disorders in which a single gene defect causes a clinically significant block in a metabolic pathway resulting either in accumulation of substrate behind the block or deficiency of the product. Inborn errors of metabolism can present with an encephalopathy. However, more typically the encephalopathy is delayed. For example, urea cycle defects (e.g., citrullinemia, ornithine transcarbamylase deficiency, and argininosuccinic aciduria), which affect the ability to detoxify nitrogen and are characterized by hyperammonemia, have an onset after 24 hours. Organic acidemias (e.g., methylmalonic or propionic acidemia, multiple carboxylase deficiency) are caused by abnormal metabolism of proteins, fats or carbohydrates and are characterized by marked metabolic acidosis with or without ketosis, often with elevated lactate and mild to moderate hyperammonemia. Common signs include vomiting, signs of encephalopathy, neutropenia, and thrombocytopenia, but generally not until an exposure to milk or an increase in catabolism has occurred. Neurological signs (e.g., seizures, obtundation) may be the predominant feature in several other inborn errors of metabolism (IEMs), as well (e.g., nonketotic hyperglycinemia, GLUT-1 deficiency, sulfite oxidase deficiency, molybdenum cofactor deficiency, peroxisomal disorders, pyridoxine responsive seizures).

Meningitis certainly can cause a clinical decompensation as described. However, given this infant's birth history, hypoxic-ischemic encephalopathy would be more likely.

The infant was intubated due to ineffective ventilation. His CXR was unremarkable and the sepsis screen was benign. At approximately 5 hours of life the infant had apnea with focal clonic movements of his right arm. An EEG revealed abnormally suppressed background activity and confirmed seizures.

What is the only proven treatment to improve outcomes following HIE?
A. Phenobarbital
B. Hypothermia, total body
C. Hypothermia, selective brain cooling
D. Mannitol
E. B and C

Discussion

The correct answer is **E**. In 2005, several randomized controlled trials showed a positive effect of hypothermia as a treatment for HIE. Both total body (i.e., cooling blanket) and selective head cooling are efficacious. Hypothermia must be initiated prior to 6 hours of life. Treatment with hypothermia reduces the risk of death or moderate to severe disability by about 25%. Neither mannitol nor phenobarbital has been proven in a prospective fashion to reduce brain injury or improve outcomes following HIE. An EEG is important to obtain as nearly half of the seizures seen in neonates with HIE are subclinical, and the presence of seizures is thought to worsen neurodevelopmental outcomes.

Baby Coleman was cooled using a cooling blanket to an esophageal temperature of 33.5°C for 72 hours. He was treated transiently with phenobarbital for his seizures, which did not recur. At 3 days of life he was extubated and breathing spontaneously. He was tolerating gavage breast milk feeds but he had a poorly coordinated suck and swallow. His upper extremities and trunk remained hypotonic. His parents are asking what they can expect for baby Coleman's future.

Which neurodiagnostic test would provide the most prognostic information for the parents?
A. Cranial ultrasound
B. Head CT
C. Brain MRI
D. EEG
E. NIRS

Discussion

The correct answer is **C**. An MRI is most sensitive at detecting the patterns of brain injury seen following term hypoxia-ischemia. The typically affected areas for term infants with HIE are the deep gray nuclei (i.e., basal ganglia and thalamus) and the posterior limb of the internal capsule (PLIC) (see Fig. 15-1). In terms of prognostication, the absence of signal in the PLIC is strongly associated with poor neurodevelopmental outcome. Injury to the basal ganglia and thalamus is strongly associated with impairment in feeding (e.g., gastrostomy tube) and communication abnormalities. A cranial ultrasound is advantageous in its simplicity, but it is less informative and much less sensitive to cortical or posterior fossa injury. A CT scan, less desirable because of radiation exposure, is also less informative on cortical and white matter injury, though will identify major injuries. EEG can be helpful for prognosis because prolonged seizures or abnormal background both portend a worse outcome. NIRS is not predictive of outcome in this setting. It is worth noting that hypothermia may delay changes in magnetic resonance diffusivity; thus the optimal time for MRI will be in the days following completion of therapy.

Baby Coleman's brain MRI revealed mild–moderate injury in his basal ganglia bilaterally. These abnormalities put him in a higher risk category for cerebral palsy.

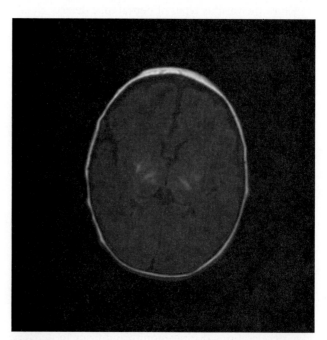

FIGURE 15-1. Axial T1-weighted MRI in a term neonate at approximately 10 days of life following perinatal hypoxic-ischemic insult, demonstrating T1 hyperintensity in ventrolateral thalami and the posterolateral putamina with loss of normal T1 hyperintensity in the posterior limb of the internal capsule. (Used with permission of Dr. Nilesh Desai, Department of Radiology, Emory University.)

For a survivor of HIE, what is the expected rate of cerebral palsy?
A. 10%
B. 25%
C. 50%
D. 75%
E. 90%

Discussion

The correct answer is **B**. In the era of hypothermia, outcomes following HIE have improved. Cooling is now accepted as standard of care. Data from the original trials would suggest that approximately 30% of babies with moderate HIE who are cooled will die or survive with moderate/severe disability. Approximately 70% of those with severe HIE who are cooled will die or survive with moderate/severe disability. Of survivors, including those with both moderate and severe HIE, approximately 25% have disabling cerebral palsy and 25-40% have a severely abnormal mental developmental index.

Objectives

1. Know the clinical features associated with hypoxic-ischemic encephalopathy in the newborn
2. Know the differential diagnosis of the newborn presenting with clinical signs of encephalopathy
3. Know the role of therapeutic hypothermia in the newborn with a diagnosis of hypoxic-ischemic encephalopathy
4. Know long-term outcome of newborns with hypoxic-ischemic encephalopathy
5. Understand the role of CNS imaging to evaluate the newborn with hypoxic-ischemic encephalopathy

Intracranial Hemorrhage and Vascular Injury-1

CASE 6

Baby boy Wilson is a full-term male infant who has been transferred to your nursery from the well-baby nursery on his first day of life due to a witnessed focal upper extremity (right arm) seizure with subsequent postictal state. His mother had been treated with magnesium for preeclampsia, but otherwise the prenatal and maternal history was benign and his delivery course was unremarkable with Apgar scores of 7 and 9. He is nonencephalopathic on examination, with a normal respiratory rate and normal oxygen saturation. While you are ruling him out for infectious or metabolic causes of seizure, you suspect that he has suffered a perinatal stroke.

Which of the following statements about newborn stroke is inaccurate?
A. The incidence of neonatal stroke is approximately that of congenital diaphragmatic hernia
B. Approximately 80% of neonatal strokes are hemorrhagic
C. The most common presenting sign is seizures, typically in a well-appearing newborn
D. The left middle cerebral artery (MCA) is the most frequently involved vessel
E. The majority of neonatal strokes are unilateral

Discussion

The incorrect statement is **B**. Approximately 80% of neonatal strokes are *ischemic*, and the remainder are due to cerebral venous sinus thrombosis (CVST) or hemorrhage. "Perinatal stroke" can refer to both ischemic and hemorrhagic cerebrovascular injury from arterial or venous pathology, from early gestation through the first 28 days of life, though some authors define it from early gestation only through the first 7 days of life. "Neonatal stroke" generally is meant to refer to cerebrovascular events from around the time of birth through 28 days of life. Neonatal *arterial* ischemic stroke (AIS) is defined as an acute, symptomatic, focal infarction in a cerebral arterial territory between birth and 28 days of life, confirmed by neuroimaging. Neonatal stroke has an incidence of approximately 1 in 2,300 live births. The presentation for both neonatal arterial and venous stroke is often seizures, most typically focal motor seizures. In fact, stroke accounts for approximately 10% of the seizures in term neonates. Many children with perinatal stroke are asymptomatic as newborns but present with early handedness or developmental delay. The MCA is the most frequently involved arterial site in newborns, left more common than right, and typically the stroke is unilateral (see Fig. 15-2).

The site of cerebral venous thrombosis is most frequently the superior sagittal sinus (or multiple sinuses). As mentioned above, the presenting sign is typically a seizure, but venous thrombosis can also lead to *intracranial hemorrhage* from venous congestion. In a review of 29 term neonates with evidence of intraventricular hemorrhage, 9 (31%) also had CVST on imaging.

The preferred diagnostic test is MRI with MR angiography or venography. Ultrasound may miss superficial an ischemic lesions and CT carries the risk of radiation and can miss venous thrombosis and early arterial stokes. Diffusion-weighted imaging can identify an infarction earlier than other MRI sequences or CT.

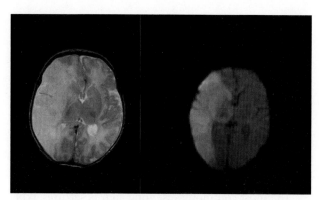

FIGURE 15-2. Axial T2-weighted MRI on the left, and diffusion weighted image on the right, of the same term neonate demonstrating right-sided middle cerebral artery distribution infarction. (Used with permission of Dr. Nilesh Desai, Department of Radiology, Emory University.)

Baby Wilson undergoes a brain MRI with diffusion-weighted imaging which reveals restricted diffusion within the left MCA-territory, suggestive of a relatively recent infarction. His parents tell you that they had no idea it was possible for a baby to have a stroke.

Which of the following statements about neonatal stroke is correct?
A. Most newborn strokes are due to maternal cocaine use
B. The baby probably has congenital heart disease, too
C. The obstetrician delivered the head incorrectly
D. Preeclampsia is the only risk factor you identify
E. Thrombophilia is not possible without a positive family history

Discussion

The only correct statement above is **D.** General etiologies for perinatal stroke are numerous and include vascular maldevelopment, vasculopathy or vasospasm (i.e., cocaine exposure, which is not the most common cause of stroke), vascular emboli or thrombus (idiopathic, or due to hypercoagulation, infection, ECMO, congenital heart disease or monochorionic twin gestation), or hypoxia-ischemia. This baby has no signs or symptoms consistent with congenital heart disease, and occlusion of neck vessels during delivery is possible but highly unlikely in an uncomplicated delivery. Much investigation has centered around risk factors: suspected *maternal* risk factors for arterial infarction include a history of infertility, chorioamnionitis, premature rupture of membranes, and preeclampsia. Suspected *neonatal* risk factors include cardiac disease, coagulation disorders, infection, trauma, drugs, and perinatal asphyxia. The contribution to stroke of thrombophilic disorders is difficult to ascertain as population-based normative data are not well estab-

lished, but estimates suggest inherited thrombophilia in 10% to 20% of newborn cases and up to 50% in childhood arterial stroke cases. It is reasonable to consider testing for the genetic polymorphisms (factor V Leiden, prothrombin gene mutation, thermolabile form of the MTHFR gene), though other thrombophilia testing is more accurate beyond the neonatal period. A placental study from the Canadian Pediatric Ischemic Stroke Registry revealed that placental pathology was evident in 10 of 12 (83%) patients with AIS or CVST, with 50% showing a placental thromboinflammatory process.

Neonatal AIS carries an extremely low recurrence rate, so withholding anticoagulation therapy is a reasonable option, unless the etiology is due to thrombophilia or some types of congenital heart disease. Thrombus propagation in CVST is not uncommon and anticoagulation therapy is more commonly used than for arterial infarcts. In a prospective study from Toronto the lack of anticoagulation predicted propagation. Complete thrombus recanalization occurred by 3 months of age in 90% of patients. No major complications were noted in preliminary studies of low–molecular-weight heparin (LMWH) for neonates with CVST, but it is also unclear whether anticoagulation is beneficial, except in a patient with a propagating thrombus. Thrombolytic agents are not currently recommended in neonates; more information about the safety and effectiveness of these agents is needed. Hemiplegia is a common clinical manifestation in affected children. Physical therapy is documented to have a beneficial effect in children with cerebral palsy though it has not been specifically evaluated in the setting of perinatal stroke. A small study suggests that constraint of the functional arm leads to increased use of the weak arm. (constraint therapy)

How would you discuss outcomes with Baby Wilson's parents? Which statement is inaccurate?
A. You can reassure them that the mortality rate for arterial stroke is <5%
B. You tell them there is a good chance for some degree of motor impairment
C. You tell them that chances are his IQ will be unaffected but that school age problems may develop
D. You tell them he will have childhood epilepsy
E. You mention that perinatal stroke is the leading cause of hemiplegic cerebral palsy

Discussion

The incorrect statement is **D.** Risk of future seizures following a neonatal arterial stroke is approximately 25%; however half of these are a single episode (and the other half develop epilepsy). The mortality rate for neonatal arterial stroke is very low (2%), while for CVST it is estimated to be approximately 5% to 20%.

Perinatal stroke is the most common etiology of hemiplegic cerebral palsy. Estimates of the incidence of cerebral palsy after perinatal arterial stroke vary widely between studies: 9% to 88%. Cognitive deficits also vary widely, 0% to 55%, and may be unapparent during toddler years and appear during school age. For a unilateral MCA stroke, the most commonly seen infarction, approximately 80% of children will have a normal IQ.

Of CVST survivors, moderate to severe neurological sequelae include neuromotor deficits (42%) and cognitive and behavioral impairments (27%). The majority of children with neonatal CVST will walk independently, usually before 2 years of age. Estimates for epilepsy beyond infancy range from 6% to 41% for neonatal CVST.

While you are reviewing Baby Wilson's MRI in the neuro reading room, one of the interns' comments on the small amount of subdural blood over his cerebral convexities.

You tell her all of the following except
A. Call neurosurgery and risk management immediately
B. This is likely an incidental finding in a recently delivered newborn
C. Traumatic subdurals can be rapidly lethal
D. Most lethal subdurals are in the posterior fossa and cause brainstem compression
E. Subarachnoid bleeding is generally well tolerated in newborns

Discussion

The best answer is **A**. It has recently been recognized by studying normal newborns with brain MRI after birth that approximately 8% to 18% will have an incidental subdural hemorrhage with no neurological symptoms.

The deep venous drainage of the cerebrum joins at the convergence of the tentorium and falx into the vein of Galen. Within the inferior margin of the falx is the inferior sagittal sinus and its confluence with the vein of Galen forms the straight sinus. This runs posteriorly to join the superior sagittal sinus and this convergence forms the transverse sinus (which proceeds inferiorly to the internal jugulars). The superficial venous drainage of the cerebrum is called the superficial bridging veins, which then empty into the superior sagittal sinus. A subdural hemorrhage results from tearing of any of these veins or sinuses.

A tear of an infratentorial large vein can extend into the posterior fossa, compress the brainstem and become lethal. These are typically large term infants who rapidly become symptomatic after birth with signs of midbrain or brainstem compression (coma, lateral deviation of eyes, unequal pupils, nuchal rigidity or bradycardia). Another traumatic and serious lesion is occipital osteodiastasis where the occipital sinuses are torn in a breech delivery, resulting again in posterior fossa hemorrhage. Superficial vein rupture causes the convexity subdural hematomas and is often accompanied by cerebral contusion. These infants can be irritable or hyperalert, or have seizures, or occasionally will have third cranial nerve dysfunction (nonreactive, dilated pupil) on the side of the hematoma. Risk factors for traumatic subdural hemorrhages include abnormal presentation (breech, foot, face or brow presentation), difficult extractions, or cephalopelvic disproportion. These lesions can also occur in nontraumatic scenarios in situations of coagulation disorders. Although a CT scan can be obtained quickly, an MRI is more sensitive in demonstrating a posterior fossa hemorrhage.

Severe, traumatic hemorrhages have a very poor prognosis with survival being the exception. If recognized promptly and drained, survival without impairment is theoretically possible. Survivors often develop hydrocephalus from CSF obstruction. Convexity subdural hematomas have a better prognosis with over 50% of affected children being normal at follow-up. Surgery is not mandatory in these cases if neurological signs are stable.

A *primary subarachnoid* hemorrhage (i.e., not due to extension from blood in subdural, intraventricular or intracerebral spaces) arises from the small vessels (leptomeningeal arteries or bridging veins) in the subarachnoid space. The leptomeningeal anastomotic channels involute with maturity, so bleeding at this site is more common with prematurity or trauma. The bleeding is typically located above the convexities or posterior fossa, and is generally well tolerated with minimal to no clinical signs. If symptomatic, the typical clinical picture is of a well baby with seizures on the second day of life. Only rarely is there significant enough hemorrhage to cause a catastrophic deterioration. Often the diagnosis of a primary subarachnoid hemorrhage is made when a lumbar puncture is done for another indication, and high RBCs and protein levels are discovered. Ultrasound is insensitive to the periphery of the brain but the diagnosis can be made by CT or MRI. No treatment is warranted in the majority of cases. Hydrocephalus resulting from impaired CSF absorption is an infrequent sequelae. The outcome of asymptomatic cases, or cases with seizures, is still excellent.

Objectives

1. Know the morbidity and mortality associated with perinatal strokes
2. Know the potential causes of a perinatal stroke in the newborn
3. Recognize the common clinical presentation of a newborn with a perinatal stroke
4. Know the long-term neurocognitive outcomes of children affected by a perinatal stroke
5. Understand the role of neuroimaging in the evaluation of a newborn with a suspected perinatal stroke

Intracranial Hemorrhage and Vascular Injury-2

CASE 7

You are caring for a 4-month-old female who had been born at 24 weeks of gestation to a mother with chorioamnionitis. Her initial clinical course was notable for early-onset *Escherichia coli* sepsis and severe hypotension for which she was prescribed several inotropes. Gratefully, a head ultrasound on day-of-life three revealed no evidence of intracranial hemorrhage and a follow-up ultrasound 3 weeks later revealed no cystic change in the periventricular white matter.

Which of the following is a true statement regarding intraventricular hemorrhage among premature newborns?

A. They most commonly originate in the choroid plexus
B. Ventricular shunting occurs in the majority of cases of grade IV IVH
C. Ventricular shunting in cases of severe IVH is associated with an increased risk of adverse neurodevelopmental outcome
D. Treatment with diuretics, such as acetazolamide, reduces the need for ventricular shunting in cases of severe IVH
E. None of the above

Discussion

The correct answer is **C**. Intraventricular hemorrhages originate in the subependymal germinal matrix, a highly vascularized region of the developing human brain. The capillaries within the germinal matrix are supported only by a thin basement membrane and, thus, are liable to rupture during periods of increased cerebral blood flow (CBF). Such fluctuations in cerebral perfusion are common among premature newborns, as their cerebral arterioles are only capable of regulating CBF over a narrow range of systemic blood pressures. This impairment of cerebrovascular autoregulation is a major contributor to IVH in the premature newborn.

Most clinical studies of intraventricular hemorrhage refer to the severity grading system proposed by Papile. On this scale, hemorrhage that is confined to the germinal matrix is classified as grade I. Bleeding that escapes into the ventricular space without distending the ventricle is classified as grade II, while that which fills and enlarges the ventricle is considered grade III. Grade IV hemorrhages at one time were thought to result from "extension" of intraventricular blood into the adjacent cerebral cortex. However, it has been demonstrated that these bleeds are in fact hemorrhagic infarctions that arise from the medullary veins of the periventricular white matter, thus they are more appropriately termed *periventricular hemorrhagic infarctions*. It is important to note that the presence of grade IV hemorrhages may coincide with lower-grade IVHs that emanate from the germinal matrix.

Intraventricular hemorrhages of grades III and IV often are considered together as "severe" forms of IVH. Among patients with severe IVH, ventricular shunting is required in substantial minority (20–30%). However, the need for ventricular shunting appears to be an independent risk for adverse neurodevelopmental outcomes. There are no clearly effective measures for preventing severe posthemorrhagic hydrocephalus among patients with severe IVH, and recent evidence suggests that once-promising diuretic regimens are of no benefit—and may, in fact, be harmful.

With the advent of improved intracranial imaging has come recognition of cerebellar injury (hemorrhage, infarction, or atrophy), especially in preterm infants. The incidence of cerebellar injury is highest in the most preterm infants. Hemorrhages are typically focal and unilateral, and often occur along with other cerebral lesions such as IVH, PVL, and parenchymal hemorrhage. Term-equivalent preterm infants with injury may show cerebellar atrophy. Neurodevelopmental impairments such as hypotonia, fine motor incoordination, and ataxia may be attributable to cerebellar injury, as cognitive, language, and behavioral abnormalities.

As part of a research study, the baby undergoes MRI of the brain at 40 weeks corrected gestational age. Her parents had been under the impression that she would be a "normal control," but the neurologist just informed them that the images revealed a significant degree of periventricular leukomalacia. They are distraught and confused.

Which of the following is a true statement regarding periventricular leukomalacia?

A. It affects only cerebral white matter, not cerebral gray matter
B. The periventricular location of cysts correlates with the end-zones of penetrating blood vessels
C. Inflammation and infection likely play little role in the pathogenesis of noncystic PVL
D. MRI is of little prognostic value in noncystic PVL
E. Motor deficits are more common than cognitive-behavioral impairments in noncystic PVL

Discussion

The correct answer is **B**. Periventricular leukomalacia is characterized by the impaired development of cerebral white matter and gray matter structures. Injury to the periventricular white matter is most prominent because this region often is subject to repeated episodes of hypoxia-ischemia in preterm newborns. Immature development of the vascular supply, limited cerebral autoregulation, and prolonged periods of bradycardia and desaturation all combine to deprive the periventricular white matter of oxygen and energy substrates. Likewise, the immature oligodendrocytes are more susceptible to hypoxia-ischemia than their more mature counterparts. Through similar biochemical and signaling mechanisms, inflammation and infection also play a role in the pathogenesis of PVL.

Cystic periventricular leukomalacia likely results from fairly acute, severe episodes of hypoxia-ischemia. Because the periventricular zone is particularly predisposed to injury, it is in this location that focal, macroscopic necrosis may occur. These large areas of necrosis eventually coalesce into fluid-filled cysts that are visible on bedside ultrasound or gross pathological examination. More commonly, however, PVL takes on a noncystic form that is characterized by diffuse, microscopic areas of glial scarring. MRI is a sensitive means by which to demonstrate the hypomyelination, reduced white matter and gray matter volumes, and abnormal fiber tract development that underlie the adverse neurodevelopmental outcomes associated with noncystic PVL (the most common of which are cognitive-behavioral deficits).

As you discuss the baby's case with her parents, you review the many factors that contribute to abnormal white matter development in premature neonates. The parents seem particularly interested in learning more about whether their daughter may have suffered from a "lack of blood and oxygen in her brain."

Which of the following is a true statement regarding cerebrovascular physiology in premature neonates?
A. Anemia substantially decreases CBF
B. Hypoglycemia substantially increases CBF
C. Hypoxia has no effect on cerebrovascular autoregulation
D. Hypercarbia has no effect on cerebrovascular autoregulation
E. The lower limit of the cerebral autoregulatory range is well below the normal systemic blood pressure

Discussion

The correct answer is **B**. The ability of the cerebral vasculature to regulate CBF is quite limited in newborns in comparison to adults. This is especially true of premature newborns, for whom the range of blood pressures over which autoregulation occurs is quite narrow. What is more, among the most premature babies the lower limit of the autoregulatory blood pressure range is essentially identical to the normal systemic blood pressure—thus, even mild hypotension may result in reduced CBF. Hypoxia, hypercarbia, and acidosis all have been shown to exacerbate impairments of cerebral autoregulation. Anemia, rapid volume infusions, and hypoglycemia all increase CBF.

Objectives

1. Know the risk of intraventricular hemorrhage in the preterm infant
2. Understand the clinical symptoms associated with an increased risk for intraventricular hemorrhage in the preterm infant
3. Know the definitions for Papile's criteria for grading intraventricular hemorrhage
4. Understand the role of neuroimaging in the preterm infant to identify intraventricular hemorrhage and/or periventricular leukomalacia
5. Know the long-term neurocognitive outcomes of preterm infants who experience intraventricular hemorrhage and/or periventricular leukomalacia

Cranial and Neurologic Trauma

CASE 8

You are called to attend the delivery of a newborn whose estimated fetal weight is in excess of 4 kg. The obstetrician indicates that the second stage of labor has been prolonged by the occiput posterior presentation of the fetal head. The obstetrician already has attempted vacuum extraction without success and now will apply forceps to facilitate delivery.

Which of the following types of cranial trauma are associated with operative vaginal delivery?
A. Facial nerve palsy
B. Skull fracture
C. Cephalohematoma
D. Subgaleal hemorrhage
E. All of the above

Discussion

The correct answer is **E**. The facial nerve is the cranial nerve most likely to be affected by birth trauma. While its occurrence is associated with operative vaginal delivery, facial nerve injury does not result directly from the application of forceps to the fetal head. In fact, it is the compression of the fetal face against the maternal sacrum that leads to compression of the nerve as it exits the stylomastoid foramen. As the facial nerve exits the stylomastoid foramen it divides into two branches: the temporofacial that innervates the zygomatic region, eye and upper face, and the cervicofacial which innervates the mandibular region and platysma muscle. Because the injury occurs so close to the foramen, typically both upper and lower facial muscles are affected. Thus, it is typical to see a wide palpebral fissure, an eye that cannot firmly close, and flat nasolabial fold on the affected side. During crying, the mouth on the ipsilateral side cannot move well so the mouth appears to pull to the opposite side, resulting in an abnormal grimace. Seventy-five percent of the time the left side is affected due to the frequency of intrauterine positioning to that side. The prognosis is excellent with the majority recovering completely within a few weeks. Artificial tears to prevent corneal injury may be warranted if eye closure is not complete.

Similar to facial nerve injury, skull fracture results from compression of the fetal head during descent, its occurrence associated with—but not necessarily caused by—application of forceps. Cephalohematoma and subgaleal hemorrhage are both associated with operative delivery. Cephalohematoma represents subperiosteal bleeding and thus may be identified as a distinct, somewhat firm fluid mass that does not cross suture lines. On the contrary, subgaleal hemorrhage fills the subaponeurotic space of the scalp and thus appears as a swelling with indefinite borders along the posterior aspect of the head.

A final perinatal nerve injury to consider in these settings is laryngeal nerve injury. Similar to the others, it results from abnormal intrauterine lie or traumatic delivery. In this case, lateral neck flexion against the right thyroid cartilage compresses the laryngeal nerve between either the hyoid bone, which catches the superior branch and results in swallowing difficulty, or the cricoid cartilage, which catches the recurrent branch and results in disturbances in vocal cord closure, causing stridor or dyspnea. Most infants will recover spontaneously by 6 to 12 months of life though supportive care (e.g., gavage feeding or tracheostomy) may be required until that time.

Following delivery of the fetal head, the obstetrician soon realizes that shoulder dystocia also has complicated the baby's delivery. Despite several maneuvers to reposition the mother, the obstetrician then attempts to deliver the baby by grasping his head and applying forceful, side-to-side traction to the baby's neck. Following delivery you note that the infant breathes quietly and regularly, with asymmetry of the pupils and limited movement of his upper extremities.

What is the most likely neuroanatomical site of injury?
A. Intracranial
B. Spinal
C. Nerve root
D. Nerve
E. Muscle

Discussion

The correct answer is **C**. Even with the lack of detail given on the baby's physical examination, a brachial plexus injury is a far more common injury seen following traumatic birth than an injury to the spinal cord (B). Injury to an individual neuron (D) or muscle (E) would not cause this constellation of findings. An intracranial injury (A) due to perinatal hypoxia-ischemia should result in more of a neurological syndrome than just muscle weakness and discordant pupils.

The brachial plexus consists of cervical nerve roots 5 to 8 and thoracic root 1. Injury results from lateral traction, which stretches the plexus away from the cervical cord. The clinical scenarios at highest risk for brachial plexus injury are ones that result in excessive traction during delivery: fetal macrosomia, abnormal presentation, dysfunctional or augmented labor, and fetal depression. In the most severe lesions the root avulses from the cord, but more commonly there is hemorrhage or edema to the nerve sheath or axon. MRI may clearly identify avulsed nerve roots, a condition that portends a poor outcome.

There are two types of brachial plexus injury: Erb's palsy, the most common (90%), which affects the fifth and sixth (sometimes seventh) nerve roots, and Klumpke's palsy, which affects the eighth cervical and first thoracic. Motor deficits are more pronounced than sensory deficits because sensory dermatomes overlap and the anterior root is more disturbed than the posterior root. Erb's palsy is responsible for the classic "waiter's tip" posture.

Which of the following is not a component of the "waiter's tip" posture?
A. Injury to C5, causing shoulder adduction
B. Injury to C5, causing external shoulder rotation
C. Injury to C5 and C6 causing elbow extension
D. Injury to C5 and C6 causing pronation
E. Injury to C6 and C7 causing wrist and finger flexion

Discussion

The correct answer is **B**. External shoulder rotation is not part of the waiter's tip, which is characterized by should adduction and internal rotation, with an extended elbow, pronated arm, and flexed wrist and fingers. These positions are preserved by the loss of their counterpart to weakness (i.e., injury to C5 causes weak shoulder abduction and external rotation, so adduction and internal rotation occur). Other deficits seen include an incomplete Moro and an absent biceps reflex. The grasp reflex should be preserved. Approximately 5% of Erb's palsy cases will extend to cervical roots 3 and 4, which supply the phrenic nerve and affect the ipsilateral diaphragm. Klumpke's palsy is technically a weakness of the distal extremity only, though often used to describe a complete brachial plexus injury (both proximal and distal). With the distal injury there would be a loss of palmar grasp, and the wrist and fingers would be extended. Due to T1 damage there would be miosis and ptosis (Horner's syndrome), such as seen in the case above.

The diagnosis of brachial plexus injury is made by clinical examination, though EMG can be used as an adjunct test. In the case of severe injury, MRI can also be used as an adjunct by demonstrating pseudomeningoceles, which suggest avulsion of roots. In cases with concomitant respiratory symptoms, chest ultrasound or fluoroscopy can aid in diagnosing diaphragmatic paralysis. The classic finding is an elevated hemidiaphragm (ipsilateral) and "seesaw" movements with respiration.

In cases of nerve root avulsion, the likelihood of spontaneous recovery of function is very low. More commonly the pathological lesion, as above, is hemorrhage or edema to the nerve sheath or axon and resolution with full function is expected. Onset of recovery by the first few weeks of life is a good prognostic sign. Management is aimed at the prevention of contractures: immobilization of the limb across the upper abdomen with passive range of motion exercises at each affected joint is appropriate. In severe cases, surgical exploration may be appropriate, and although rare, has generally led to improved motor and sensory outcomes.

Spinal cord injury during delivery is much more uncommon and much more devastating. It is excessive traction or torsion that produces the spinal cord injury that can occur during delivery, in contrast to the compression injuries that characterize spinal cord injury later in life. Hyperextension of fetal head is a very high-risk position. Breech delivery can cause injury to the lower cervical or upper thoracic area cord, whereas cephalic delivery (especially by mid-forceps) can cause injury to the upper and mid cervical cord. The acute pathological lesion seen is hemorrhage—both epidural and intraspinal—or edema, laceration, or even transsections. It is rare to see actual fractures of the vertebrae, which are very cartilaginous at this stage of development; the cord itself is less elastic than the vertebrae.

The clinical picture of an infant with an acute, midcervical spinal cord injury includes all of the following except
A. Hyperreflexia of the lower extremities
B. Areflexia of lower extremities
C. Flaccid weakness of lower extremities
D. Respiratory failure
E. Distended bladder

Discussion

The correct answer is **A**. Hyperreflexia occurs in the chronic phase of spinal cord injury, not the acute phase. Clinically an infant with a lower cervical or upper thoracic spinal cord injury will acutely manifest flaccid weakness with areflexia of lower extremities, a defined sensory level around the lower neck or upper trunk, diaphragmatic breathing, distended bladder, and atonic anus. If the upper extremities are involved it may represent concomitant brachial plexus injury (or if only the distal hand is affected it may represent anterior horn cell injury). Occasionally Horner's syndrome is appreciated from injury to the exiting root at T1, destined for the sympathetic ganglia. An infant who has mid or upper cervical injury will show these findings but also respiratory failure with need for mechanical ventilation, as diaphragmatic innervation occurs from cervical segments 3, 4, and 5. Unfortunately, hypoxic-ischemic encephalopathy is also a frequent co-occurrence. This initial clinical presentation (also called "spinal shock") will eventually develop into a more chronic picture of hyperreflexia and spasticity, with "triple flexion" at hips, knees, and ankles.

Clinical cases of cord damage that do not include a compatible birth history should be differentiated from a spinal mass, a dysraphic state, an abscess or an infarction (such as due to a vascular catheter) by imaging of the cord with MRI. This is critical as some may be surgically remediable. Aside from this, surgical intervention for spinal cord injury is rarely indicated except in the rare case of a major epidural hemorrhage contributing to the cord trauma. The role of steroids in the acute management of a spinal cord injury is not proven, but efficacy if started within 8 hours of injury has been extrapolated from adult spinal cord patients. Outcome prediction in the neonatal period is difficult but the absence of spontaneous respirations beyond a day of life is suggestive of long-term mechanical ventilation with severe motor disability.

Objectives

1. Know the clinical signs of the various types of brachial plexus injuries in the newborn
2. Know the location of neurologic injury for the various types of brachial plexus injury in the newborn

3. Know the clinical signs and symptoms of a spinal cord injury in the newborn
4. Distinguish between a caput, cephalohematoma, and a subgaleal hemorrhage
5. Know the clinical signs and symptoms associated with Horner's syndrome

Seizures

CASE 9

You receive a call from a general pediatrician who is evaluating an hour-old newborn with apparent seizure activity. After indicating that the baby will need to be transported to the intensive care nursery, you ask him to characterize the seizure activity. He reports that the baby seems to have "jerky movements" of the neck, right arm, and left leg. These episodes occur at random, during which time the baby seems to be awake and alert.

Which type of seizure is the pediatrician most likely describing?
A. Focal clonic
B. Multifocal clonic
C. Myoclonic
D. Tonic
E. Subtle

Discussion

The correct answer is **C**. Neonatal seizures are typically classified according to their clinical manifestation. *Clonic* seizures are characterized by low-frequency, rhythmic jerking movements that may affect the bulbar, axial, or appendicular structures. Newborns with clonic seizures may remain conscious during seizure episodes and there may be no obvious postictal state. Among all categories of seizures, clonic seizures are most likely to be manifest as electroencephalographic abnormalities. Clonic seizures may be further categorized as focal or multifocal in nature. *Focal clonic* seizures affect structures on just one side of the body and often result from localized cerebral abnormalities (e.g., stroke). In contrast, *multifocal clonic* seizures involve both sides of the body, with jerking movements occurring either at random or in a pattern that reflects neuroanatomical progression of the seizures (i.e., a Jacksonian march). Multifocal seizures often are caused by more generalized cerebral disease.

Myoclonic seizures are distinguished from clonic seizures by the high-frequency jerking movements seen in myoclonus and the tendency for myoclonus to affect the flexor muscles of the upper extremities. Myoclonic seizures are rarely correlated with abnormalities on electroencephalography (EEG), whether focal, multifocal, or generalized. *Tonic* seizures most commonly are generalized and manifest as tonic extension of the upper and lower extremities, though tonic flexion of the upper extremities may be present. *Subtle* seizures are distinct from the other types of seizures in that they are characterized by neither clonic nor tonic movements. Instead, subtle seizures manifest as more complex movements (e.g., chewing or "bicycling"), ocular phenomena (e.g., deviation of the eyes), or autonomic changes. Subtle seizures most commonly occur in premature newborns and are inconsistently correlated with electroencephalographic findings.

Upon arrival to the intensive care nursery the newborn is found to have normal vital signs. He appears well developed and does not seem to have any obvious congenital anomalies. However, the neurological examination is notable for frequent, repetitive jerking movements of the upper and lower extremities. You indicate to the baby's father that a number of tests will be performed, including an electroencephalogram.

Which of the following is a true statement regarding EEG in neonates?
A. Electrical seizures may be seen on EEG in the absence of clinical seizures
B. EEG provides diagnostic and prognostic information only if performed during a seizure episode
C. Prolonged EEG monitoring is necessary to capture a complete seizure episode, as neonatal seizures tend to be long lasting
D. Multifocal electrical seizures are difficult to distinguish from normal, transient electrical discharges
E. The burst-suppression pattern is difficult to distinguish from the pattern seen during sleep

Discussion

The correct answer is **A**. The presence of electrical seizures in the absence of clinical seizures is termed electroclinical dissociation. This phenomenon is most likely to occur in premature newborns or in term newborns who have received antiepileptic medications. Electroclinical dissociation most likely results from a developmental difference in chloride transport between cerebrocortical neurons and those from lower levels of the motor system. In response to gamma-aminobutyric acid (GABA) or GABA agonists (i.e., most antiepileptic drugs), neonatal cortical neurons export chloride and consequently depolarize. Maturation of chloride transport in the brainstem and spinal cord results in no such excitation.

Thus, activation of GABA receptors could facilitate electrical discharge within a cortical seizure focus, while at the same time preventing the conduction of that impulse through the rest of the motor system.

EEG provides diagnostic and prognostic information both during and between seizure episodes. Neonatal seizures tend to be brief, with most lasting less than 1 to 2 minutes. Seizures most often appear as single or multiple foci of spike wave discharges. These localized, rhythmic discharges tend to spread to adjacent cortical areas before fading into a voltage-depressed state. Thus, seizures may be readily distinguished from transient neuronal discharges, which are randomly located, arrhythmic, do not spread, and are not followed by reduced voltage.

Between seizures, the interictal (or "background") EEG may provide important diagnostic and prognostic information. Underlying diagnosis aside, a normal electrical background usually is associated with good neurodevelopmental outcomes. Abnormalities on the background EEG may range from subtle voltage asymmetries to more worrisome findings such as discontinuous activity or markedly reduced voltage. Of particular concern is the burst-suppression pattern, which is characterized by long periods of low or absent voltage that are interrupted by synchronous bursts of high-voltage spikes. Burst-suppression is commonly seen in states of severe, bilateral cortical disease and portends a poor outcome. Burst-suppression may be distinguished from the neonatal sleep state in that sleep is characterized by more regular, brief periods of low voltage between bursts and normalization of the EEG pattern with stimulation.

While this question was meant to review the role of EEG in the diagnosis and management of neonatal seizures, it is important to point out that EEG is just one part of a more comprehensive approach to the neonate with seizures. As shown in Table 15-2, the etiologies of neonatal seizures are numerous and diverse. However, it is possible to identify the categorical cause of most neonatal seizures by taking into account the maternal medical and obstetric histories, the newborn physical and neurological examinations and the results of just a few additional tests. A *serum electrolyte panel* may identify common metabolic causes, such as hypoglycemia or hypocalcemia, while an *ammonium level* may reveal more complex metabolic disease. *Blood, urine, and CSF* should be sent for total and differential cell counts, chemistries, and culture. It is important to remember that for many neonates with meningitis only the CSF will yield a positive bacterial culture. *Neuroimaging* may reveal disorders of cerebrocortical and cerebrovascular development or stroke. Given the rapidity of CT and bedside ultrasound techniques, either may be used safely early in the diagnostic process. MRI offers superior imaging of cerebral anatomy and may reveal abnormalities invisible on CT (e.g., heterotopias)

TABLE 15-2. Etiology of Neonatal Seizures

CATEGORICAL ETIOLOGY OF SEIZURES	EXAMPLES
Developmental defects	Lissencephaly
	Polymicrogyria
	Gray matter heterotopia
Epilepsies	Benign familial neonatal seizures
	Myoclonic encephalopathy
Hemorrhage/vascular	Subdural hemorrhage
	Subarachnoid hemorrhage
	Intraventricular hemorrhage
Hypoxic-ischemic encephalopathy	
Infection	Bacterial meningoencephalitis
	Viral encephalitis (HSV, CMV)
Metabolic	Hypoglycemia
	Hypocalcemia
	Hyponatremia
	Nonketotic hyperglycinemia
	Hyperammonemia
	Aminoacidopathies
	Organic acidopathies
	Pyridoxine dependency
Toxic	Neonatal abstinence syndrome
	Systemic infusion of local anesthetic

as well as no risk from radiation, but the availability of MRI and the time required for the procedure may be barriers to its use in the acute setting. Finally, it is important to note that the incidence of neonatal abstinence syndrome may present with seizures. *Meconium screening* is indicated to identify whether a newborn was exposed in utero to medications or drugs associated with neonatal withdrawal (e.g., opioids).

The baby now has been in your care for the past 5 hours. During this time you have identified no signs of metabolic disease, infection, or neuroanatomical abnormalities. You report to the baby's parents that the EEG still shows generalized bursts of seizures bilaterally, despite that fact that he has received 40 mg/kg of each phenobarbital and fosphenytoin.

What should be your next diagnostic or therapeutic step?

A. Administer sodium benzoate, sodium phenylacetate, and arginine IV
B. Administer pyridoxine IV
C. Initiate a third antiepileptic drug
D. Initiate therapeutic hypothermia
E. Broaden your antibiotic coverage

Discussion

The correct answer is **B**. Pyridoxine dependency is an uncommon cause of neonatal seizures, but one that must be considered when standard antiepileptic medications fail to work. This disorder results from defects in glutamic acid decarboxylase, the enzyme that converts glutamate (an excitatory neurotransmitter) to GABA (an inhibitory neurotransmitter). The resulting imbalance of excitatory and inhibitory neurotransmitters result in generalized seizure activity and excitotoxic neural injury. Underlying most cases of pyridoxine dependency is the impaired binding of activated pyridoxine to the active site of glutamic acid decarboxylase. Because this defect is present throughout fetal development, myoclonic seizures may begin in utero and cerebrocortical abnormalities may be present at birth. In the setting of recalcitrant seizures, it is appropriate to administer 50 to 100 mg of pyridoxine intravenously while performing continuous EEG. The diagnosis of pyridoxine dependency would be suggested by the resolution of electrical seizures within minutes of the pyridoxine infusion (though in some cases resolution occurs after a few hours). Adjunctive diagnostic tests include the detection of low levels of GABA and elevated levels of glutamate in the CSF, elevated pipecolic acid in the plasma and aminoadipic semialdehyde levels in urine.

Sodium benzoate, sodium phenylacetate, and arginine often are prescribed together to treat the hyperammonemia that results from various defects in the urea cycle. While these conditions may cause seizures in neonates, the initial metabolic tests in this case were negative. Empirically adding a third antiepileptic drug or expanding antibiotic coverage may be indicated in some settings. However, in this case the seizure pattern and recalcitrance was suggestive of pyridoxine dependency and there was no laboratory evidence of infection. Finally, therapeutic hypothermia is indicated only as a treatment of neonatal hypoxic-ischemic encephalopathy. Neither the clinical history nor the laboratory findings are suggestive of HIE.

Objectives

1. Know the potential etiologies of seizures in the newborn
2. Know the various types of seizures commonly seen in the newborn
3. Understand the role of EEG in the evaluation and management of a newborn with seizures
4. Know the potential treatment options for the newborn with seizures
5. Understand the role of neuroimaging in the newborn with seizures

Infections

CASE 10

Baby Brown is a 7-day-old female infant who was born precipitously at 38 weeks of gestation to a 32-year-old G3 with excellent prenatal care. Her prenatal labs were unremarkable except that she was GBS+ with incomplete intrapartum antibiotic therapy due to the quick delivery. Baby girl Brown received ampicillin and gentamicin, and at 48 hours her blood culture was negative and she was discharged home with her parents. On her seventh day of life she was noted to have poor feeding, irritability, and fever. In the emergency room she has a seizure. As part of her workup the emergency room physician performs a lumbar puncture, which shows many polymorphonuclear (PMN) leukocytes, an elevated protein level, and a low glucose value. The Gram stain and culture are pending.

In the era of intrapartum Group B Streptococcus (GBS) screening and prophylaxis, which organism is most likely responsible for baby girl Brown's meningitis?
A. *Escherichia coli*
B. *Enterococcus spp.*
C. *Listeria monocytogenes*
D. *Staphylococcus aureus*
E. GBS

Discussion

The correct answer is **E**. GBS, Even though screening and antibiotic prophylaxis has markedly reduced GBS infection rates, it is still the most common cause of neonatal meningitis. Like sepsis, there are distinguishing characteristics and consequences to early- versus late-onset meningitis. Early-onset meningitis is more common in the preterm infant, occurs within the first 48 hours of life due to vertical transmission, typically has a history of maternal peripartum infection, and has a clinical presentation of sepsis and a high mortality rate. Late-onset meningitis occurs typically after a week of life and is more common in term infants—the transmission can be vertical or from postnatally acquired organisms. The presentation of late-onset sepsis often resembles that of the case presented above, and the mortality rate is relatively low. There is much overlap in the bacterial pathogens between early-onset sepsis with meningitis and late-onset sepsis with meningitis, though distinctions can be made: GBS is still the most common organism in both early-onset and late-onset, with *E. coli* the second most common. A French series from 2011 reports that *E. coli* is the most common in preterm infants, whereas a study from the NICHD Neonatal Research Network in 2004 on VLBW infants reports that gram-positive organisms were most frequently seen in late-onset meningitis when in conjunction with sepsis, whereas *enterococcus* was most common for preterm infants with meningitis only. Meningitis is more common in premature infants than in full-term infants, due to the higher rate of bacteremia, indwelling catheters and immature immunity. Certainly, preterm infants with a history of intraventricular hemorrhage and resultant hydrocephalus, who have indwelling ventricular drainage devices, are at risk for meningitis from both gram-positive and enteric organisms.

Acutely the predominant cells seen in CSF sampling are PMN leukocytes, but after a few weeks the proportion shifts to a mononuclear (histiocyte and macrophage) predominance with very low lymphocytes. Interestingly, the classic CSF findings for acute infection (elevated WBC with PMN predominance, elevated protein, and low glucose relative to blood glucose) are most pronounced for late-onset meningitis as compared to early-onset, and for gram-negative organisms compared to GBS.

Seizures are present in 50% of neonatal meningitis cases. Other clinical features that may be present include a bulging anterior fontanel, cranial nerve palsies (especially seventh, third and sixth), and extensor rigidity.

The pathogenesis is hematogenous spread of bacteria into the choroid plexus and entrance into the ventricles.

Which of the following statements regarding the neuropathology of bacterial meningitis is false?
A. 30% to 50% of cases will be accompanied by cerebral infarction
B. Vasculitis is present in the majority of cases
C. Cystic encephalomalacia results most commonly from abscesses
D. 50% of affected patients will develop hydrocephalus
E. Subdural empyema is a rare occurrence in neonates

Discussion

The correct answer is **C**. Cystic encephalomalacia and porencephaly likely represent destruction from infarctions rather than abscesses, which are rare with the most common types of meningitis. The organisms most likely to produce true abscesses, though, are *Citrobacter, Serratia marcescens, Proteus, Pseudomonas,* and *Enterobacter* (*L. monocytogenes* classically produces microabscesses). Cerebral infarction is also a frequent complication, seen in 30% to 50% in autopsy series, most typically venous hemorrhagic infarctions, though arterial occlusion from vasculitis and thrombosis can occur. Vasculitis, both

arterial and venous, is a natural extension of the inflammation in the arachnoid space and ventricles.

The ventriculitis seen with bacterial meningitis can be very exudative and ultimately produce obstructions to CSF flow, causing hydrocephalus. This obstruction is usually at the aqueduct or fourth ventricle or within the subarachnoid space, and is estimated to occur in 50% of cases, based on autopsy data. Cerebral atrophy can also appear as ventricular dilation on cranial ultrasound. Subdural effusions and empyema are rare occurrences in newborns, although they become more common later in infancy.

In our case above, ampicillin and gentamicin were started immediately. The Gram stain showed gram-positive cocci. Meningitis complicates approximately 15% of early-onset GBS sepsis but 57% of late-onset GBS sepsis. Of infants with GBS meningitis, 20% will have a negative blood culture.

Initial antibiotic coverage should be chosen to eradicate both common gram-positive and gram-negative organisms until the culture results can refine the treatment. Ampicillin is generally chosen to cover GBS and *L. monocytogenes* and an aminoglycoside or third-generation cephalosporin are chosen to cover gram negatives, depending upon local susceptibility patterns. Synergy between the combination of ampicillin and aminoglycoside is beneficial for many common organisms. The duration of therapy depends upon the response to therapy: repeated CSF samples are necessary to prove eradication of the organisms.

Gram-negative organisms, which may take longer to treat in part due to difficulty in attaining appropriate CSF concentrations of aminoglycosides and getting the antibiotic to the precise site of infection, are treated for 2 weeks beyond the first negative CSF culture, or a total of 3 weeks. Gram-positive organisms treated with ampicillin (which penetrates the CSF more easily) could be treated for 2 weeks following eradication by CSF sample, though practically speaking a 3-week treatment for all types of meningitis is prudent. Neither intrathecal nor intraventricular antibiotic administration improves outcomes, though there are select cases where ventriculostomy and intraventricular instillation of antibiotics is indicated.

What should be your next diagnostic or therapeutic step?
A. Mannitol to decrease her elevated intracranial pressure
B. Dexamethasone to reduce intracranial pressure and prevent deafness
C. Continuous blood pressure monitoring
D. Phenobarbital for seizure prophylaxis
E. Vasopressin for fluid management

Discussion

The correct answer is **C**. The management of neonatal bacterial meningitis is supportive, along with antibiotics. Attention to systemic hypotension is critical, as diminished CBF in a setting of injury (with increased intracranial pressure and impaired autoregulation) can exacerbate ischemia. Likewise ventilation parameters must be optimized, and coagulation studies must be followed closely. Although cerebral edema is common, the pressure release effect of the fontanels is protective; however tonsillar herniation in the newborn has been reported. Although corticosteroids are used in conjunction with antibiotics for treatment of *Haemophilus influenza* meningitis in older infants, this has not been proven to be beneficial in newborns with other infectious agents. Likewise, hyperosmolar solutions such as mannitol to decrease intracranial pressure have not been studied for efficacy in the human newborn with bacterial meningitis. Acute hydrocephalus may rarely warrant a ventriculostomy, which may also be utilized for antibiotic administration. Clinicians should have a high suspicion for seizures, which may occur early or late in the disease, but prophylaxis with an antiepileptic is not proven to be of benefit. Routine electrolytes and urinary measurements should be assessed for inappropriate antidiuretic hormone secretion (which would be made worse by vasopressin).

Further management following the acute stabilization should include cranial imaging, to detect complications such as ventricular enlargement, infarction, cystic encephalomalacia, and cortical atrophy. As discussed before, MRI is most sensitive and does not carry the risk of radiation that CT scans do. Bedside ultrasound can be very useful for serial studies during the phase of ventricular enlargement.

Baby girl Brown's parents ask you about her prognosis. Which of the following statements regarding mortality and morbidity is *false*?
A. The mortality rate from meningitis is much lower for gram-positive organisms than for gram negatives or fungal infections
B. Mortality of GBS meningitis is dropping and now <15%
C. 50% of survivors of GBS have some neurological sequelae
D. 90% of survivors of gram-negative meningitis have significant neurological sequelae
E. There is a 20% chance that baby girl Brown will be deaf

Discussion

The false statement is **D**. The outcome of survivors of gram-negative meningitis is similar to that of GBS for term infants, though more ominous for preterm infants.

It is worth noting that disseminated fungal infections can lead to fungal meningitis, classically with diffuse microabscesses. This is most common in low–birth-weight newborns with indwelling catheters, especially in those on

TABLE 15-3. **Infections**

PRE- OR PERINATAL INTRACRANIAL INFECTION	CLASSIC NEUROPATHOLOGY AND SEQUELAE
Cytomegalovirus	Meningoencephalitis, *periventricular calcifications*, microcephaly, migrational disorders, chorioretinitis, progressive hearing loss, neurodevelopmental disability, seizures
Enteroviruses	"Aseptic" meningitis or meningoencephalitis, seizures
Herpes simplex virus	Meningoencephalitis with necrosis, cerebral edema, cystic encephalomalacia, seizures, neurodevelopmental disability
Human immunodeficiency virus	Meningoencephalitis, cerebral atrophy, basal ganglia and white matter calcifications, vasculopathy, CNS lymphoma or opportunistic infections possible, progressive and static encephalopathies, neurodevelopmental disability
Lymphocytic choriomeningitis	Hydrocephalus, chorioretinitis, cerebral calcifications, neurodevelopmental disability
Rubella	Meningoencephalitis, microcephaly, impaired myelination, vasculopathy, chorioretinitis, cataracts, neurodevelopmental disability, deafness
Syphilis	Meningitis, hydrocephalus, infarction, optic and auditory nerve atrophy, seizures, cranial nerve palsies
Toxoplasmosis	*Granulomatous* meningoencephalitis, *diffuse cerebral calcifications*, periaqueductal inflammation, hydrocephalus, microcephaly, chorioretinitis, neurodevelopmental disability, seizures, blindness, deafness
Varicella	Meningoencephalitis, myelitis of anterior horn cells and dorsal root ganglionitis, denervation atrophy, seizures, neurodevelopmental disability

total parenteral nutrition and receiving multiple broad-spectrum antibiotics. The presentation is often more insidious than a bacterial meningitis, with a similar outcome. In addition to amphotericin B, 5-fluorocytosine is added for CSF penetration.

Pre- or perinatal infections of the CNS by "TORCH" pathogens—viruses such as herpes simplex (HSV), varicella virus, cytomegalovirus (CMV) or human immunodeficiency virus (HIV), a protozoan (*Toxoplasma gondii*) or a spirochete (*Treponema pallidum*), as well as non-TORCH viruses like enterovirus or lymphocytic choriomeningitis all can cause neurological consequences, though many of them are asymptomatic in the neonatal period. These infections are covered in detail in the chapter on infectious diseases; only the classic neuropathology for each is listed in Table 15-3.

Objectives

1. Know the pathogens that typically cause meningitis in the newborn
2. Know the clinical signs and symptoms of newborns with meningitis
3. Know the long-term prognosis in children with a history of neonatal meningitis
4. Understand the treatment and management strategies in patients with neonatal meningitis

Neonatal Abstinence and Withdrawal Syndromes

CASE 11

You have been called to the well-baby nursery to assess a 1-day-old term newborn who seems "jittery" according to his nurse. The nurse tells you that the baby is slightly small for gestational age and that so far he has fed poorly. He also has not slept much and has been inconsolable over the past few hours. You are suspicious that this newborn is showing signs of opioid withdrawal.

Which of the following is not a clinical feature of neonatal opioid withdrawal?
A. Fever
B. Increased muscle tone
C. High-pitched crying
D. Depressed deep tendon reflexes
E. Diarrhea

Discussion

The correct answer is **D**. Neonatal opioid withdrawal most commonly presents with signs of neurologic and gastrointestinal dysfunction, reflecting the organ systems in which most opioid receptors are located. Neurologic features are characterized by excitability, such as tremors, hyperactive deep tendon and primitive reflexes, increased muscle tone, autonomic signs and, in severe cases, seizures. Gastrointestinal signs may include constant, uncoordinated sucking, poor feeding, and diarrhea, all of which may result in poor weight gain and dehydration.

After examining the newborn and considering the nurse's observations, you indicate to her that the newborn is most likely suffering from neonatal abstinence syndrome. She expresses some surprise at this diagnosis, as "you don't see that kind of thing around here."

Which of the following is a true statement regarding the epidemiology of neonatal abstinence syndrome and/or maternal drug use in the United States?
A. Opioids are the illicit drugs most commonly used by pregnant women
B. Clinically important neonatal withdrawal most commonly results from in utero benzodiazepine exposure
C. Among women in the first trimester of pregnancy, the rate of heavy alcohol use exceeds the rate of tobacco use
D. The rate of neonatal abstinence syndrome has declined over the past decade
E. Compared with nonpregnant women of the same age, pregnant women 15 to 17 years of age are more likely to use tobacco and illicit drugs

Discussion

The correct answer is **E**. While the rates of smoking and illicit drug use among pregnant women are lower than those among nonpregnant women across most age groups, the opposite is true among women 15 to 17 years of age, of whom 20% smoke and 15% use illicit drugs. Among all women in the first trimester of pregnancy, tobacco use (15%) is more common than heavy alcohol use (12%). Marijuana is the illicit drug most commonly used by pregnant women. Unfortunately, the rate of neonatal abstinence syndrome has increased substantially over the past decade and now may affect 0.3% of newborns each year. Among all in utero drug exposures, opioids result in the most clinically important neonatal withdrawal syndrome.

You inform the newborn's mother that her baby is showing classic signs of opioid withdrawal. Having heard that her baby is unwell, the mother reveals that she receives treatment in a methadone maintenance program, a fact that she did not disclose to her obstetrician. You thank her for her willingness to share that information and then proceed to describe how you will manage her baby's opiate withdrawal in the intensive care nursery.

Which of the following is a correct statement regarding the pharmacologic management of neonatal opioid withdrawal?

A. Benzodiazepines are effective as second-line therapy
B. Opioids are contraindicated as they increase the likelihood of narcotic addiction in later life
C. Early initiation of pharmacologic therapy improves the long-term developmental outcomes of affected patients
D. Clonidine may be effective as a primary or adjunctive therapy
E. Paregoric is one of the safest means by which to administer morphine

Discussion

The correct answer is **D**. In a randomized, double-blind, placebo-controlled trial, adjunctive clonidine reduced the duration of pharmacologic treatment for neonatal narcotic abstinence syndrome with no untoward effects. While it is unknown whether postnatal opioid exposure improves long-term outcomes or increases the risk of adverse behavioral outcomes, opioids are the recommended first-line therapy for neonatal opioid withdrawal. Benzodiazepines are not effective in the treatment of neonatal opioid withdrawal and paregoric is unsafe because it contains a variety of opioids and several toxic ingredients. In fact, along with clonidine, morphine and methadone are the only medications for which treatment regimens have been specified by American Academy of Pediatrics' Committee on Drugs and Committee on Fetus and Newborn.

Objectives

1. Understand the epidemiology of neonatal abstinence syndrome in the United States
2. Know the clinical signs and symptoms of neonatal abstinence syndrome
3. Know the options for pharmacologic management of neonatal withdrawal syndrome

Hypotonia

CASE 12

Baby Johnson is a 2-week old, ex–36-week gestation male infant whose delivery was induced due to severe

polyhydramnios. He has been in your intensive care nursery since birth due to hypotonia with arthrogryposis. On examination you find an infant who is supported by continuous positive airway pressure and receives nasogastric feedings. His examination is notable for generalized weakness that includes the face, with a thin chest and legs, talipes equinovarus, and depressed tendon reflexes.

Before reading the text below, which of the following diagnoses is most likely? The denouement will be given at the end of the review

A. Zellweger (cerebrohepatorenal) syndrome
B. Werdnig–Hoffman disease
C. A peripheral hypomyelination disorder
D. Congenital myasthenia
E. Congenital myotonic dystrophy

Discussion

The correct answer is **A**. Neonatal hypotonia has a very broad differential diagnosis. A structured approach to the evaluation is to march down the possible anatomical sites of the motor system, from the most central (i.e., cerebrum) to the most distal components (i.e., muscle). Most of the central causes can be distinguished by other signs (e.g., encephalopathy, seizures) and preserved tendon reflexes (which eventually become hyperactive). Serum CPK, CSF protein, EMG, nerve conduction velocities, nerve, and muscle biopsies are all normal. Causes of neonatal encephalopathy include hypoxia-ischemia, intracranial hemorrhage or infection, metabolic disorders, trauma, and also endocrine (e.g., hypothyroidism). Developmental disorders, such as neuronal migration abnormalities may cause hypotonia, as can other cerebral causes primarily distinguished by neonatal hypotonia such as Zellweger (cerebrohepatorenal syndrome), oculocerebrorenal syndrome of Lowe and Prader–Willi syndrome.

Prader–Willi syndrome is characterized by profound neonatal hypotonia, weakness, and all of the following except

A. Almond-shaped eyes and a dolichocephalic head
B. Poor weight gain as a neonate, followed by future obesity
C. Diminished deep tendon reflexes
D. Hydronephrosis
E. Hypogonadism

Discussion

The correct answer is **D**. The feature that is not classically seen with Prader–Willi syndrome is hydronephrosis. Prader–Willi syndrome can be diagnosed by FISH for the chromosome 15 deletion in 70% of patients. The other

30% have uniparental disomy; therefore they have a normal FISH study, but an abnormal DNA methylation test.

Spinal cord injury or dysraphism can result in hypotonia and weakness and are discussed comprehensively in **Cranial and Neurologic Trauma (Case 8)**.

Disorders of the lower motor neuron are the most common cause of *severe* neonatal hypotonia with weakness, and the hallmark disease is SMA Type 1, also known as Werdnig–Hoffman disease. Another rare cause is Pompe disease or glycogen storage disease, Type 2.

The clinical features of type 1 SMA include profound hypotonia, weakness, and all of the following except
A. A large, fasciculating tongue
B. Preserved facial motility
C. Normal sensory function
D. Areflexia
E. Preserved sphincter function

Discussion

The incorrect feature is **A**. A large fasciculating tongue is characteristic of Pompe disease, due to the accumulation of glycogen. In Pompe disease, glycogen deposits in anterior horn cells as well as skeletal muscle, the heart, liver, and brain. Type 1 SMA is the hereditary (autosomal recessive), infantile form of anterior horn cell degeneration. It is clinically apparent at birth in 35% of cases, often with report of decreased fetal movement in the third trimester. The hypotonia and weakness is typically more prominent than distal weakness, and lower extremities may be more affected than upper extremities. Infants with SMA are areflexic (D). Because the cranial nerve nuclei are less involved initially, facial motility is preserved (B). Tongue fasciculations may be noted, and the tongue appears small and atrophic. Sensory function is normal (C) and sphincter function is present (E), two findings that help distinguish SMA type 1 from spinal cord or peripheral nerve disease. The areflexia and absence of facial weakness helps differentiate SMA from a primary muscle disorder. Infants who present at birth and have respiratory failure will often die by 4 months of life. The diagnosis can be made by examining chromosome 5q13; muscle biopsy will also show changes of denervation such as panfascicular atrophy. Serum CPK and CSF protein are normal. Management is supportive: frequent oropharyngeal suctioning, tube feedings, monitoring for respiratory infections or failure.

The next anatomical site in the motor system is the peripheral nerve, felt to be a relatively rare cause of neonatal hypotonia. The largest group of congenital peripheral nerve disorders is a heterogeneous group, all with failure of proper myelination (known as chronic motor-sensory hypomyelination polyneuropathy). These infants present with severe weakness and hypotonia at birth and a minority will have arthrygryposis multiplex congenita. There is muscular atrophy with weak to absent tendon reflexes. Muscles innervated by cranial nerves are variably spared, but sensation is impaired (helping to distinguish from Type 1 SMA). Approximately 40% of affected infants die.

The diagnostic tests would show which of the following results in cases of congenital peripheral nerve hypomyelination?
A. Elevated CPK
B. Normal CSF protein
C. Normal NCV
D. Normal muscle biopsy
E. Onion-bulb formation on nerve biopsy

Discussion

The correct answer is **E**. The diagnosis is definitively made by a peripheral nerve biopsy; classic features are hypomyelination and potentially "onion-bulb" formation (due to Schwann cell reactive proliferation). An NCV will be reduced and a muscle biopsy usually shows evidence of denervation, though often there is relative preservation of muscle cells. CPK is normal but CSF protein is elevated. Management consists of trying to optimize the motor function that is present: preventing contractures, scoliosis, and pulmonary infections.

Disorders at the level of the neuromuscular junction infrequently manifest in the newborn period, but are important to consider as they are some of the few treatable causes of neonatal hypotonia. Neonatal neuromuscular junction disorders include congenital myasthenia, transient myasthenia, hypermagnesemia, rare effects of aminoglycosides, and infantile botulism.

What distinguishes congenital from transient neonatal myasthenia?
A. Cranial nerve involvement
B. Genetic versus immune process
C. Response to neostigmine
D. Electrophysiological testing
E. Survival

Discussion

The correct answer is **B**. Transient neonatal myasthenia gravis, due to passive antibody transfer from myasthenic mothers (antibody decreases available acetylcholine receptors postsynaptically), has an onset within the first 24 hours of life but often after a few hours of normalcy. Once the clinical syndrome begins it evolves rapidly, with disturbances of cranial nerve musculature, weakness in sucking and swallowing, respiratory difficulty (30% require ventilation), general hypotonia and weakness, but normal tendon reflexes. Ptosis or other oculomotor abnormalities are uncommon with transient myasthenia, another distinguishing factor from congenital myasthenia. The diagnosis is made by response to an anticholinesterase, commonly neostigmine (beneficial effect seen for 1 to 3 hours—edrophonium has a shorter onset but shorter duration). Serum CPK, CSF protein, EMG, nerve conduction, and muscle biopsy would all be normal. Electrophysiological testing with repetitive nerve stimulation will show decrements in the amplitude of the motor unit potential. Only 10% to 20% of infants born to myasthenic mothers will manifest the transient syndrome. Management is supportive (potentially requiring tube feeds and ventilation), avoidance of aminoglycosides (see subsequent paragraph), and treatment with anticholinesterase agents. The role of exchange transfusion has not been proven beneficial, but may transiently improve symptoms.

Congenital myasthenia is due to a genetic defect of the neuromuscular junction rather than an immune-mediated process. The onset is usually a few weeks of life, with a milder presentation than the transient phenomenon: less feeding difficulties, less pronounced weakness, or hypotonia. However, early ocular involvement is common. Diagnostic test results are the same, as is management, though an additional agent to increase acetylcholine release (3,4 Diaminopyridine) is often added.

Hypermagnesemia, from maternal eclampsia treatment with IV magnesium sulfate, may result in a transient paralysis with hypoventilation, apnea, weakness and hypotonia, and hypo- or areflexia. Smooth muscle is also affected, potentially causing an ileus or meconium plus syndrome. Serum magnesium levels usually exceed 4.5 mEq/L in symptomatic neonates. Hypermagnesemia results in impaired release of acetylcholine from the presynaptic nerve ending. Calcium administration may have a beneficial effect though not supported by clinical trials. Most affected infants will recover by 3 days of life.

Aminoglycosides, especially when used in high doses, can impair release of acetylcholine from the presynaptic nerve ending. Calcium administration may have a beneficial effect, as may neostigmine, but the management is generally supportive. Aminoglycosides should be avoided in any known myasthenic syndrome.

Infant botulism typically presents between 2 weeks and 6 months of age (and in newborns is **not** related to infected honey ingestion, but rather contact with soil and dust leading to an intestinal infection by *Clostridium botulinum*). The clinical features aside from weakness and hypotonia include impaired suck and swallow, facial diplegia, and constipation. A descending and symmetrical paralysis progresses. Interestingly, there is loss of pupillary response to light, which is helpful in distinguishing this diagnosis from congenital myasthenia. Serum CPK, CSF

protein, nerve conduction, and muscle biopsy would all be normal. EMG shows a characteristic tetanic facilitation; additionally isolation of *C. botulinum* from the stool is diagnostic. Management is again supportive (tube feedings and mechanical ventilation are required in a majority of cases), with avoidance of aminoglycosides. Treatment with human botulism immune globulin shortens duration of mechanical ventilation, tube feedings, and hospital stay. With appropriate management the condition is completely survivable.

Finally, hypotonia can be due to a primary muscle disorder, another heterogeneous group of disorders. In general, they are characterized by proximal weakness, often with facial involvement, depressed tendon reflexes, and no fasciculations or sensory abnormalities. CSF protein is normal. Serum CPK is elevated (although in the slowly progressive disorders or congenital myotonic dystrophy this may not be the case in the neonatal period). An EMG study is consistent with myopathic changes, and muscle biopsy is diagnostic (general myopathy with disproportionate distribution or size of muscle fibers, or particular features such as central cores, rod bodies, myotubular fibers, abnormal mitochondria, or lipid or glycogen accumulation).

The most common muscle disorder causing hypotonia is congenital myotonic dystrophy, an inherited muscle disease that is distinct from adult-onset myotonic dystrophy. It can present prenatally, with polyhydramnios, and is apparent in the newborn within hours to days of life.

Which of the following is not a feature of congenital myotonic dystrophy?
A. Uniparental disomy
B. Poor suck and swallow
C. Intolerance of gastric feeds
D. Ventricular dilation
E. Mental retardation

Discussion

The incorrect choice is **A**. Uniparental disomy is not a mode of inheritance for this disorder. Transmission (autosomal dominant) is through an affected mother, although the mother may have a mild disease of which she is unaware. Congenital myotonic dystrophy shows genetic anticipation, due to trinucleotide repeats at chromosome 19q13.3. Myotonia can be elicited from the mother (a clenched fist tightly that cannot immediately open on command). The clinical presentation of myotonic dystrophy is characterized by hypotonia, muscular atrophy, facial diplegia ("tent"-shaped upper lip), and respiratory and feeding issues. Smooth muscle is also affected and a portion of the feeding difficulties may be from poor intestinal motility. In addition, there is usually arthrogryposis of the lower extremities. EMG can detect electrical myotonia, though this can be difficult to elicit in newborns. Cranial imaging often reveals ventricular dilation for unclear reasons. The basis for the low IQ often seen in affected children is also unclear. Muscle biopsy reveals essentially an arrest in muscle maturation. Management is supportive for feeding and ventilation, as well as treatment of the joint deformities. Prolonged ventilation as a newborn is associated with a mortality rate of 25%. Of survivors, nearly 100% have some degree of mental retardation.

Congenital muscular dystrophy is a group of progressive disorders of the muscle, typically autosomal recessive in inheritance, that can be either "pure" (muscle only) or have CNS involvement (white matter abnormalities, Fukuyama, Muscle-eye-brain, and Walker–Warburg). In general they may show improvement during late infancy and early childhood but ultimately all are progressive with a reduced life expectancy.

Other myopathic disorders are rare but classified on the basis of their distinct histology: central core disease, nemaline myopathy, myotubular myopathy, and congenital fiber type disproportion. In addition to hypotonia and weakness there may be postural deformities such as developmental dislocation of the hip, pectus excavatum, pes cavus, and eventually kyphoscoliosis and lumbar lordosis. Mitochondrial myopathies include carnitine deficiency and cytochrome-c oxidase deficiency; metabolic myopathies include disorders of glycogen or lipid metabolism.

Arthrogryposis multiplex congenita is a congenital syndrome characterized by limited movement with fixed positions of multiple joints, caused by a fetal disturbance in the motor system, of many possible etiologies. The more distal joints are most commonly affected, for example talipes equinovarus or flexion deformities of the wrist. The affected muscles appeared atrophied and tendon reflexes are depressed or absent, or difficult to obtain due to the joint contractures. Approximately 50% of patients exhibit other organ system anomalies, but rather than representing a true disturbance in development they are typically explainable by the disturbance in fetal movement (i.e., micrognathia and impaired facial/masticatory movements).

Which of the following is not explained by a disturbance in intrauterine movement?
A. High-arched palate
B. Pulmonary hypoplasia
C. Clinodactyly
D. Congenital heart disease
E. Retrognathia

Discussion

The correct answer is **D**. Congenital heart disease is assumed to be an associated anomaly rather than pathogenically explained by diminished fetal movement. A high-arched palate (A) is presumed to occur from impaired tongue movement and micrognathia, while retrognathia (E) may occur from impaired masticatory movements. Pulmonary hypoplasia (B) is presumed to occur from impaired breathing movements and clinodactyly (C) from impaired finger movements. Other notable findings in addition to the joint contractures may be polyhydramnios from impaired swallowing, and a short umbilical cord from infrequent movement.

Which site in the motor system is the most frequent cause of arthrogryposis multiplex congenita?
A. Cerebrum/brain stem
B. Anterior horn cells
C. Peripheral nerve/root
D. Neuromuscular junction
E. Muscle

Discussion

The correct answer is **B**. The pathogenesis can occur at any level of the motor system from cerebrum to muscle (or even as a result of mechanical intrauterine obstruction), but the most common site of disease is probably the anterior horn cell, followed by "central" causes. Cerebral (A) causes include developmental dysgenesis such as the neuronal migrational disorders or hydrocephalus, or ischemic or infectious causes of injury early in gestation. Microcephaly, pontocerebellar hypoplasia, and fetal alcohol syndrome are also notable central causes. Anterior horn cell disorders include dysgenesis, destruction, or degeneration (i.e., similar to Werdnig–Hoffman). Interestingly, classic Werdnig–Hoffman (chromosome 5-linked) newborns infrequently exhibit contractures despite the severity of the intrauterine muscular weakness; this may be due to the uniformity of anterior horn cell involvement. Neural tube defects are common causes of fixed congenital contractures, and many patients with Mobius syndrome are afflicted. Peripheral neuropathies (C) (i.e., hypomyelinative) and neuromuscular junction disorders (D) (i.e., congenital myasthenia or infant of myasthenic mother) are rare but possible etiologies of arthrogryposis. The more common muscle disorders (E) that can be responsible for arthrogryposis are congenital muscular dystrophy, congenital myotonic dystrophy, and myotubular myopathy. Myopathies due to glycogen storage or mitochondrial disorders also have been known to cause arthrogryposis. Marfan's syndrome or other causes of connective tissue disorders are rare causes of arthrogryposis multiplex congenita. Intrauterine obstructions such as amniotic bands or uterine anomalies can result in diminished fetal movement and the arthrogryposis complex.

The evaluation of arthrogryposis multiplex congenita needs to consider each level of the motor system. Imaging of the CNS is necessary as approximately 10% to 30% of cases are exclusively central in origin, especially the severe cases. Assessment of the neuromuscular unit may include serum CPK, EMG, nerve conduction velocities, and muscle biopsy. CSF examination or nerve biopsy may be warranted.

Management is aimed at improving joint or muscle function. Treatment consists of passive stretching exercises and serial casting, with surgical release of the tendons and ligaments of the joint in the case of enduring deformities.

The outcome depends upon the etiology of arthrogryposis. Central causes have an unfavorable outcome. As mentioned above, congenital myasthenia is treatable. In cases where the muscle appears well formed (on biopsy) there may be a good prognosis for muscle function, though certain myopathies (severe congenital muscular dystrophy) have a very poor prognosis.

Back to Baby Johnson: you decide to classify him based on your review of the above material. You determine that he has no features of an encephalopathy. His tendon reflexes are depressed, but present, excluding an anterior horn cell disease where they'd be absent, and making the neuromuscular junction an unlikely site (where they'd be normal). His face is weak, excluding a peripheral nerve disorder. His sensation is intact, also excluding a peripheral nerve disorder.

Before ordering any ancillary test, now which of these choices is highest on your differential?
A. Zellweger (cerebrohepatorenal) syndrome
B. Werdnig–Hoffman disease
C. A peripheral hypomyelination disorder
D. Congenital myasthenia
E. Congenital myotonic dystrophy

Discussion

The correct answer is **E**. Baby Johnson was diagnosed with congenital myotonic dystrophy. His muscle biopsy showed small round muscle fibers that had an immature appearance and incomplete differentiation into distinct fiber types. Upon meeting the mother you detect that she has developmental delay and the classic myotonic grip. You plan a family meeting to discuss the baby's worrisome prognosis.

Objectives

1. Know the differential diagnosis of congenital hypotonia

2. Know the clinical features of common causes of congenital hypotonia
3. Understand the genetic inheritance pattern of common causes of congenital hypotonia
4. Know the appropriate diagnostic evaluation for newborns with congenital hypotonia
5. Know the causes of arthrogryposis multiplex congenita and the appropriate diagnostic evaluation
6. Know the clinical features associated with a diagnosis of myotonic dystrophy

Vascular Malformations

CASE 13

Which statement about vein of Galen aneurysmal malformations is false?
A. Vein of Galen aneurysmal malformations make up the majority of newborn intracranial vascular malformations
B. The phrase vein of Galen malformation is a misnomer
C. The most common feeding artery is the posterior choroidal artery
D. A cranial bruit and diminished carotid pulses are characteristic
E. The likelihood of neurologically intact survival is improving

Discussion

The incorrect answer is **D**. A cranial bruit and *increased* carotid pulses are characteristic of vein of Galen aneurysmal malformations (vein of Galen aneurysmal malformation, see Fig. 15-3), which make up the majority of newborn intracranial vascular malformations. Interestingly, anatomical studies show that the dilated vein is actually a remnant of a transitory venous structure (the median prosencephalic vein of Markowski) that drains the choroid plexus and is the precursor to the actual vein of Galen (situated within the roof of the third ventricle). The aneurysmal venous dilation is typically fed by the posterior choroidal artery, occasionally the anterior, middle or posterior cerebral artery or rarely the anterior choroidal artery. When sizable, a vein of Galen aneurysmal malformation leads to an extracardiac left-to-right shunt with decreased cerebrovascular resistance and increased venous return to the heart, leading to high

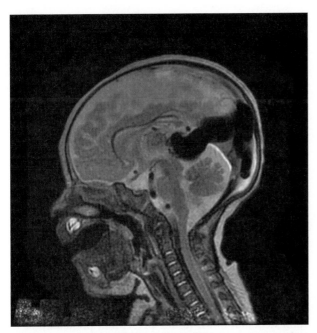

FIGURE 15-3. Sagittal T2-weighted MRI in a neonate revealing vein of Galen malformation. (Used with permission of Dr. Nilesh Desai, Department of Radiology, Emory University.)

Neurocutaneous Syndromes and Intracranial Neoplasms

CASE 14

A pediatric resident rounding in the newborn nursery notes that a term, male infant has a head circumference >95%. Just as you are discussing the difference between macrocephaly (large head) and macrencephaly (enlargement of extracerebral spaces or excessive intracranial tissue proliferation), a nurse informs you that she thinks the baby is seizing. You tell the intern that the combination of macrencephaly and seizures is concerning for neurocutaneous syndromes or congenital brain tumors.

Which of the following is a common defining feature of the neurocutaneous syndromes?
A. Noncommunicating hydrocephalus
B. Cellular hyperproliferation
C. Glaucoma
D. Supratentorial pathology
E. Cerebral calcifications

Discussion

The correct answer is **B.** In Neurofibromatosis (NF), there is hyperproliferation of glia, predominantly astrocytes. Loss of the neurofibromatosis protein via abnormalities of the Ras pathway leads to the overproliferation that causes tumors. In Sturge–Weber there is hyperproliferation of blood vessels in the leptomeninges. In tuberous sclerosis (TS) the hyperproliferation involves both glia and neurons. Similar to neurofibromatosis the genetic defects responsible for tuberous sclerosis result in loss of tumor suppressive mechanisms. Hydrocephalus (A) is possible if a tumor obstructs CSF flow but it is not a common defining feature. Glaucoma (C) is a feature of Sturge–Weber. The tubers, hamartomas, and other types of overproliferation are not exclusive to the supratentorium (D). Supratentorial predominance is a feature of neonatal brain tumors, which make them distinct from brain tumors at later infancy and beyond. Cerebral calcifications (E) are frequently seen in Sturge–Weber after the first 6 months of life.

In neurofibromatosis 1 (autosomal dominant inheritance, though many are spontaneous new mutations), the macrencephaly from the excessive proliferation of glia generally is not present right at birth. In newborns, an estimated 40% with neurofibromatosis will exhibit the classic café-au-lait spots (>6 that are >5 mm). Seizures

output heart failure in the neonate. Cardiac ischemia can occur from coronary artery steal during diastole. Intracranially, it also leads to ischemia from steal, hemorrhage and/or thrombosis, and mass effect with hydrocephalus. Cranial Doppler study of the vein and arterial feeders can make the diagnosis, and MRI with MR angiography can better define the feeding vessels, as well as concurrent injury. Conventional angiography is the definitive defining tool, especially in preparation for intervention. Successful intervention is challenging, especially in the setting of heart failure and coagulopathy, and in many cases cerebral injury has already occurred. Treatment approaches include arterial embolization or venous coil placement. Historically the prognosis was grim with no benefit to treatment, but more recent series suggest an improvement in outcome, with one series reporting 66% intact survival in 16 newborns treated with transarterial deposition of n-butyl cyanoacrylate. Non-Vein of Galen ateriovenous malformations often present with intracranial hemorrhage, sometimes seizures or congestive heart failure.

Objective

1. Know the clinical signs of symptoms associated with CNS vascular malformations

can be another presenting feature of the disease in the newborn period.

Characteristic features of Sturge–Weber (sporadic) include the facial port-wine stain, glaucoma and seizures; cerebral calcifications often appear after 6 months. Bilateral disease is associated with worse developmental outcomes than unilateral disease.

In tuberous sclerosis (autosomal dominant, though many are spontaneous new mutations) a depigmented ash leaf–shaped macule is classic in the newborn period, and cardiac rhabdomyomas may be seen early, as well. The classic neuropathologies that may cause seizures or infantile spasms include subependymal and cortical–subcortical tubers, and white matter heterotopias.

Unilateral macrencephaly is defined by enlargement of one hemisphere with localized abnormal cell proliferation (both neuronal and glial) and irregular migration and cortical organization. Seizures occur during the neonatal period and neurodevelopment is severely impaired. Linear nevus sebaceous syndrome is associated with hemimegalencephaly, as well as facial hemihypertrophy, due to lipomatous-hamartomatous lesions.

Chromosomal disorders that can be associated with macrencephaly include Fragile X, Klinefelter syndrome, Sotos syndrome, Weaver syndrome, Proteus syndrome, and Simpson–Golabi–Behmel syndrome, among others.

This infant is examined closely and noted to have a depigmented ash leaf macule. He undergoes a diagnostic MRI, because this is the most sensitive neuroimaging modality to detect the manifestations of hyperproliferation (i.e., tubers, vascular anomalies, heterotopias) in cases of macrencephaly. The MRI reveals a cortical tuber. The family is informed of the presumptive diagnosis of tuberous sclerosisand they request confirmatory testing.

Which of the following neurocutaneous syndromes have genetic testing available?
A. Tuberous sclerosis
B. Neurofibromatosis 1
C. Sturge–Weber
D. A and B
E. B and C

Discussion

The correct answer is **D**. Both tuberous sclerosis and neurofibromatosis 1 can be diagnosed through genetic testing. Tuberous sclerosis can be diagnosed by genetic mutational analysis of TSC1 or TSC2 genes. Of note, patients with a TSC2 mutation are more likely than those with a TSC1 mutation to present with infantile spasms, developmental delay, or angiofibromas. However, in approximately 15% of clinical cases genetic mutations are not identified. Clinical genetic testing can also confirm the

presence of a mutation in the neurofibromatosis 1 gene. Prenatal testing for the neurofibromatosis 1 mutation is also possible using amniocentesis or chorionic villus sampling. There is no etiologic genetic defect known for Sturge–Weber syndrome.

Each of the more common neurocutaneous syndromes is associated with a higher risk of neurodevelopmental impairment than the general population. Patients with both tuberous sclerosis and neurofibromatosis 1 are frequently diagnosed with epilepsy, intellectual impairment, behavioral issues and a higher rate of autism spectrum disorders. Likewise, Sturge–Weber patients often have epilepsy and cognitive impairments, as well as complications such as hemiparesis and visual field deficits.

Brain tumors presenting at birth are very rare, with a biological behavior that is distinct from those presenting in older infancy and childhood. A supratentorial location is common, in contradistinction to brain tumors seen after 2 months of life. Teratomas are the most common neonatal brain tumor presenting prenatally or at birth, and neuroepithelial tumors are the most common presenting in the first 2 months of life. Perinatal teratomas are particularly large and the site of origin is often ventricular. The more common neuroepithelial tumors include medulloblastoma, astrocytoma, choroid plexus tumors and various ependymomas. Less commonly seen are oligodendroglioma and glioblastoma. Mesenchymal craniopharyngiomas are seen, and infrequently sarcomas, hemangioblastomas, fibromas, and meningiomas have been described. Also reported are unusual tumors derived from midline remnant of the notochord.

Neonatal brain tumors can present dramatically as in the cases of macrocrania with cranial-pelvic disproportion and dystocia, or with massive hydrocephalus, intracranial hemorrhage, or with seizures or other neurological signs.

Which of the following neonatal brain tumors have the best prognosis?
A. Teratoma
B. Medulloblastoma
C. Low-grade astrocytoma
D. Ganglioglioma
E. Choroid plexus papilloma

Discussion

The correct answer is **E**. When present in neonates, choroid plexus papillomas, are generally considered curable. Teratomas have a mortality rate >90%, and newborn medulloblastomas have a mortality rate >80%. Among newborn brain tumor survivors, a majority will have IQ scores consistent with mental retardation. Management depends on the histology but generally includes surgery, often plus chemotherapy, and, as a last resort due to severe adverse neurological effects in infants, radiation therapy.

Objectives

1. Identify the clinical features associated with neurocutaneous syndromes
2. Know the genetic inheritance pattern of the various types of neurocutaneous syndromes
3. Know the recommended diagnostic evaluation of CNS vascular abnormalities and neurocutaneous syndromes in the newborn

REFERENCES

1. Adams-Chapman I, Hansen NI, Stoll BJ, et al. Neurodevelopmental outcome of extremely low birth weight infants with posthemorrhagic hydrocephalus requiring shunt insertion. *Pediatrics.* 2008;121:e1167–e1177.
2. Adzick NS, Thom EA, Spong CY, et al. A randomized trial of prenatal versus postnatal repair of myelomeningocele. *N Engl J Med.* 2011;364:993–1004.
3. Agthe AG, Kim GR, Mathias KB, et al. Clonidine as an adjunct therapy to opioids for neonatal abstinence syndrome: a randomized, controlled trial. *Pediatrics.* 2009;123(5):e849–e856.
4. Anand P, Birch R. Restoration of sensory function and lack of long-term chronic pain syndromes after brachial plexus injury in human neonates. *Brain.* 2002;125:113–122.
5. Ansong AK, Smith PB, Benjamin DK, et al. Group B streptococcal meningitis: cerebrospinal fluid parameters in the era of intrapartum antibiotic prophylaxis. *Early Hum Dev.* 2009;S5–S7.
6. Armstrong-Wells J, Johnston SC, Wu YW, et al. Prevalence and predictors of perinatal hemorrhagic stroke: results from the kaiser pediatric stroke study. *Pediatrics.* 2009;123:823–828.
7. Arnon SS, Schechter R, Maslanka SE, et al. Human botulism immune globulin for the treatment of infant botulism. *N Engl J Med.* 2006;354:462–471.
8. Ashwal S, Michelson D, Plawner L, et al. Practice parameter: Evaluation of the child with microcephaly (an evidence-based review): report of the Quality Standards Subcommittee of the American Academy of Neurology and the Practice Committee of the Child Neurology Society. *Neurology.* 2009;73:887–897.
9. Barkovich AJ. *Pediatric Neuroimaging.* 4th ed. Philadelphia, PA: Lippincott Williams & Wilkins; 2005.
10. Bednarek N, Mathur A, Inder T, et al. Impact of therapeutic hypothermia on MRI diffusion changes in neonatal encephalopathy. *Neurology.* 2012;78:1420–1427.
11. Berenstein A, Fifi JT, Niimi Y, et al. Vein of Galen malformations in neonates: new management paradigms for improving outcomes. *Neurosurgery.* 2012;70:1207–1213.
12. Berfelo FJ, Kersbergen KJ, van Ommen CH, et al. Neonatal cerebral sinovenous thrombosis from symptom to outcome. *Stroke.* 2010;41:1382–1388.
13. Biran V, Verney C, Ferriero DM. Perinatal cerebellar injury in human and animal models. *Neurol Res Int.* 2012;2012:858929.
14. Bracken MB, Shepard MJ, Collins WF, et al. A randomized, controlled trial of methylprednisolone or naloxone in the treatment of acute spinal-cord injury. Results of the second national acute spinal cord injury study. *N Engl J Med.* 1990;322:1405–1411.
15. Bruner JP, Tulipan N, Reed G, et al. Intrauterine repair of spina bifida: preoperative predictors of shunt-dependent hydrocephalus. *Am J Obstet Gynecol.* 2004;190:1305–1312.
16. Buser JR, Maire J, Riddle A, et al. Arrested preoligodendrocyte maturation contributes to myelination failure in premature infants. *Ann Neurol.* 2012;71:93–109.
17. Campbell C, Sherlock R, Jacob P, et al. Congenital myotonic dystrophy: assisted ventilation duration and outcome. *Pediatrics.* 2004;113:811–816.
18. Chau V, Poskitt KJ, Sargent MA, et al. Comparison of computer tomography and magnetic resonance imaging scans on the third day of life in term newborns with encephalopathy. *Pediatrics.* 123:319–326.
19. Comi AM. Presentation, diagnosis, pathophysiology, and treatment of the neurological features of Sturge-Weber syndrome. *Neurologist.* 2011;17:179–184.
20. Elbers J, Viero S, MacGregor D, et al. Placental pathology in neonatal stroke. *Pediatrics.* 2011;127:e722–e729.
21. Garges HP, Moody MA, Cotton CM, et al. Neonatal meningitis: what is the correlation among cerebrospinal fluid cultures, blood cultures, and cerebrospinal fluid parameters? *Pediatrics.* 2006;117:1094–1100.
22. Gaschignard J, Levy C, Romain O, et al. Neonatal bacterial meningitis: 444 Cases in 7 years. *Pediatr Infect Dis J.* 2011;30:212–217.
23. Glass HC, Glidden D, Jeremy RJ, et al. Clinical neonatal seizures are independently associated with outcome in infants at risk for hypoxic-ischemic brain injury. *J Pediatr.* 2009;318–323.
24. Gluckman PD, Wyatt JS, Azzopardi D, et al. Selective head cooling with mild systemic hypothermia after neonatal encephalopathy: multicentre randomised trial. *Lancet.* 2005;365:663–670.
25. Hahn JS, Hahn SM, Kammann H, et al. Endocrine disorders associated with holoprosencephaly. *J Pediatr Endocrinol Metab.* 2005;18:935–941.
26. Harteman JC, Groenendaal F, Kwee A, et al. Risk factors for perinatal arterial ischaemic stroke in full-term infants: a case-control study. *Arch Dis Child Fetal Neonatal Ed.* 2012;97:F411–F416.
27. Hudak ML, Tan RC; COMMITTEE ON DRUGS; COMMITTEE ON FETUS AND NEWBORN, AAP Committee on Drugs, et al. Neonatal drug withdrawal. *Pediatrics.* 2012;129:e540–e560.
28. Isaacs H Jr. I. Perinatal brain tumors: a review of 250 cases. *Pediatr Neurol.* 2002;27:249–261.
29. Kirton A, Armstrong-Wells J, Chang T, et al. Symptomatic neonatal arterial ischemic stroke: the international pediatric stroke study. *Pediatrics.* 2011;128:e1402–e1410.
30. Lee J, Croen LA, Backstrand KH, et al. Maternal and infant characteristics associated with perinatal arterial stroke in the infant. *JAMA.* 2005;293:723–729.
31. Leventer RJ, Guerrini R, Dobyns WB. Malformations of cortical development and epilepsy. *Dialogues Clin Neurosci.* 2008;10:47–62.
32. Libster R, Edwards KM, Levent F, et al. Long-term outcomes of group B streptococcal meningitis. *Pediatrics.* 2012;130:e8–e15.
33. Looney CB, Smith JK, Merck LH, et al. Intracranial hemorrhage in asymptomatic neonates: prevalence on MR images and relationship to obstetric and neonatal risk factors. *Radiology.* 2007;242:535–541.

34. Martinez-Biarge M, Diez-Sebastian J, Kapellou O, et al. Predicting motor outcome and death in term hypoxic-ischemic encephalopathy. *Neurology*. 2011;76:2055–2061.

35. Martinez-Biarge M, Diez-Sebastian J, Wusthoff CJ, et al. Feeding and communication impairments in infants with central grey matter lesions following perinatal hypoxic-ischaemic injury. *Eur J Paediatr Neurol*. 2012;16:688–696.

36. Mills JF, Dargaville PA, Coleman LT, et al. Upper cervical spinal cord injury in neonates: the use of magnetic resonance imaging. *J Pediatr*. 2001;138:105–108.

37. Moharir MD, Shroff M, Pontigon AM, et al. A prospective outcome study of neonatal cerebral sinovenous thrombosis. *J Child Neurol*. 2011;26:1137–1144.

38. Nakagawa TA, Ashwal S, Mathur M, et al. Clinical report – Guidelines for the determination of brain death in infants and children: an update of the 1987 task force recommendations. *Pediatrics*. 2011;128:e720–e740.

39. O'Leary H, Gregas MC, Limperopoulos C, et al. Elevated cerebral pressure passivity is associated with prematurity-related intracranial hemorrhage. *Pediatrics*. 2009;124:302–309.

40. Patrick SW, Schumacher RE, Benneyworth BD, et al. Neonatal abstinence syndrome and associated health care expenditures: United States, 2000–2009. *JAMA*. 2012;307:1934–1940.

41. Pineda-Alvarez DE, Dubourg C, David V, et al. Current recommendations for the molecular evaluation of newly diagnosed holoprosencephaly patients. *Am J Med Genet C Semin Med Genet*. 2010;154C:93–101.

42. Qaddoumi I, Carey SS, Conklin H, et al. Characterization, treatment, and outcome of intracranial neoplasms in the first 120 days of life. *J Child Neurol*. 2011;26:988–994.

43. Ricci D, Mercuri E, Barnett A, et al. Cognitive outcome at early school age in term-born children with perinatally acquired middle cerebral artery territory infarction. *Stroke*. 2008;39:403–410.

44. Rintoul NE, Sutton LN, Hubbard AM, et al. A new look at myelomeningoceles: functional level, vertebral level, shunting, and the implications for fetal intervention. *Pediatrics*. 2002;109:409–413.

45. Roach ES, Golomb MR, Adams R, et al; American Heart Association Stroke Council; Council on Cardiovascular Disease in the Young. Management of stroke in infants and children: a scientific statement from a Special Writing Group of the American Heart Association Stroke Council and the Council on Cardiovascular Disease in the Young. *Stroke*. 2008;39:2644–2691.

46. Rutherford MA, Pennock JM, Counsell SJ, et al. Abnormal magnetic resonance signal in the internal capsule predicts poor neurodevelopmental outcome in infants with hypoxic-ischemic encephalopathy. *Pediatrics*. 1998;102:323–328.

47. Shah DK, Mackay MT, Lavery S, et al. Accuracy of bedside electroencephalographic monitoring in comparison with simultaneous continuous conventional electroencephalography for seizure detection in term infants. *Pediatrics*. 2008;121:1146–1154.

48. Shah PS. Hypothermia: a systematic review and meta-analysis of clinical trials. *Semin Fetal Neonatal Med*. 2010;15:238–246.

49. Shah SS, Ohlsson A, Shah VS. Intraventricular antibiotics for bacterial meningitis in neonates. *Cochrane Database Syst Rev*. 2012;7:CD004496.

50. Shankaran S, Laptook AR, Ehrenkranz RA, et al. Whole-body hypothermia for neonates with hypoxic-ischemic encephalopathy. *N Engl J Med*. 2005;353:1574–1584.

51. Staley BA, Vail EA, Thiele EA. Tuberous sclerosis complex: diagnostic challenges, presenting symptoms, and commonly missed signs. *Pediatrics*. 2011;127:e117–e125.

52. Stoll BJ, Hansen N, Fanaroff AA, et al. To tap or not to tap: high likelihood of meningitis without sepsis among very low birth weight infants. *Pediatrics*. 2004;113:1181–1186.

53. Tekgul H, Gauvreau K, Soul J et al. The current etiologic profile and neurodevelopmental outcome of seizures in term newborn infants. *Pediatrics*. 2006;117:1270–1280.

54. Tsuji M, Saul JP, du Plessis A, et al. Cerebral intravascular oxygenation correlates with mean arterial pressure in critically ill premature infants. *Pediatrics*. 2000;106:625–632.

55. Volpe JJ. *Neurology of the Newborn*. 5th ed. Philadelphia, PA: W.B. Saunders; 2008.

56. Westmacott R, MacGregor D, Askalan R, et al. Late emergence of cognitive deficits after unilateral neonatal stroke. *Stroke*. 2009;40:2012–2019.

57. Whitby EH, Griffiths PD, Rutter S, et al. Frequency and natural history of subdural haemorrhages in babies and relation to obstetric factors. *Lancet*. 2004;363:846–851.

58. Wu YW, Hamrick SE, Miller SP, et al. Intraventricular hemorrhage in term neonates caused by sinovenous thrombosis. *Ann Neurol*. 2003;54:123–126.

59. Wusthoff CJ, Kessler SK, Vossough A, et al. Risk of later seizure after perinatal arterial ischemic stroke: a prospective cohort study. *Pediatrics*. 2011;127:e1550–e1557.

Chapter 16

DEVELOPMENT AND BEHAVIOR

Ira Adams-Chapman, MD, MPH

CASE 1

Baby Girl Johnson is born at 25 weeks with a birth weight of 750 g. The pregnancy was complicated by preterm labor and concerns of chorioamnionitis.

During your prenatal consult with the parents, they ask you if their baby will develop like a normal child.

A. You explain to the parents that the development of the premature brain is not affected by premature birth
B. You explain to the parents that the risk for a normal developmental outcome varies based on the gestational age at birth but that risk is modified on the basis of complications that may occur after birth that we are unable to predict
C. You explain to the parents that birth weight is a much stronger predictor of neurodevelopmental outcome than gestational age
D. You explain to the parents that the majority of babies born at 25 weeks' gestational age do not have any long-term neurodevelopmental problems
E. You explain to the parents that most prematurely born children have learning disabilities and require special education services in school

Discussion

The correct answer is **B**. Preterm birth is an important risk factor for abnormal neurodevelopmental outcome. Except for pregnancies affected by intrauterine growth restriction, birth weight and gestational age generally trend together and frequently demonstrate similar risk for abnormal outcome. Both gestational age and birth weight are inversely related to the risk for abnormal neurodevelopmental outcome in preterm infants. The most appropriate response to the parents is to state that both birth weight and gestational age are important risk factors for long-term developmental outcome. However, other complications associated with prematurity including late-onset infection, intraventricular hemorrhage (IVH), and necrotizing enterocolitis further increase the risk of poor outcome.

Baby Girl Johnson has respiratory distress syndrome and requires intubation and mechanical ventilation after birth. She is treated with surfactant but remains ventilated over the next 6 weeks and is successfully extubated to noninvasive ventilatory support with CPAP at 31 weeks PCA. By 36 weeks PCA she had weaned to a nasal cannula at 1 LPM with an FIO_2 of 0.30. She is unable to wean from oxygen during the hospitalization and is discharged home on supplemental oxygen therapy at 50 cc/min with FIO_2 1.0.

The parents ask if being discharged home on oxygen is a risk for worse neurodevelopmental outcome.

What is the most accurate response?

A. All preterm infants discharged home on oxygen therapy will have abnormal neurodevelopmental outcome
B. You explain to the parents that their child has severe chronic lung disease and will have abnormal neurodevelopmental outcome
C. You explain to the parent that their child has mild chronic lung disease which has been associated with an increased risk for abnormal neurodevelopmental outcome in some studies
D. The supplemental oxygen will protect the developing brain from hypoxia which will decrease the risk for abnormal neurodevelopmental outcome
E. Children with chronic lung disease tend to have stronger muscles in the chest and trunk

Discussion

The correct answer is **C**. Chronic lung disease is defined as the need for supplemental oxygen at 36 weeks post-conceptual age (PCA). This has long been associated with an increased risk for abnormal long-term developmental outcome among preterm infants. This relationship is complex and multifactorial, including therapies historically used in the management of chronic lung disease in this population, including postnatal steroids. The severity of the lung disease likely affects the risk the abnormal outcome but has been difficult to quantify in clinical trials which have primarily focused on the need for supplemental oxygen at 36 weeks PCA as the study endpoint.

Walsh et al.[1] have proposed a physiologic definition for bronchopulmonary dysplasia based on the need for supplemental oxygen but also accounts for the amount of respiratory support required at 36 weeks PCA.

Many preterm infants have truncal weakness in the months following hospital discharge. This is not always more pronounced among those with chronic lung disease. However, children with ongoing respiratory symptoms will typically have increased work of breathing with activity and exercise which often makes it difficult for them to master many of the early gross motor skills which require strength in the trunk, including rolling, sitting, and crawling.

Mr. Johnson recalls that his daughter received a 5-day course of steroids to facilitate weaning off the ventilator at 4 weeks of age. He asks how this therapy could potentially impact her long-term outcome.

Select the most appropriate response.
A. The use of postnatal steroids is preterm infants is never recommended
B. The use of postnatal steroids has been shown to decrease the incidence of chronic lung disease
C. Postnatal steroids have been shown to facilitate weaning from the ventilator but have not been shown to modify the incidence of chronic lung disease
D. Postnatal steroid use in preterm infants has been associated with an increased risk for motor and cognitive impairment in some studies but data are limited and inconclusive
E. Both C and D

Discussion

The correct answer is **E**. Postnatal steroids administered within the first week of life to prevent chronic lung disease have been associated with an increased risk of spontaneous bowel perforation and growth impairment, therefore its use is not recommended in the extremely premature infant during the first week of life for this purpose.[2] Later administration of steroids after 7 days has been shown to facilitate weaning from the ventilator and also to decrease the risk of chronic lung disease but did not affect mortality at hospital discharge. Also, of greater concern is that neurodevelopmental outcome studies have shown that postnatal steroid use may be associated with an increased risk of cognitive and motor impairment, including cerebral palsy. The AAP does not recommend the routine use of postnatal steroids in preterm infant and recommended that providers inform parents of the risks and potential benefits.[3] Some researchers believe that the potential benefit outweighs the risk in a subgroup of patients with severe chronic lung disease. Clinical trials are ongoing to further evaluate its use in select populations.

CASE 2

Baby Boy Brown was born at 25 weeks' gestation and weighed 750 g. At 1 week of age he developed increased apnea and bradycardia requiring increased ventilator support and hypotension which prompted a sepsis evaluation. The blood culture was positive for Klebsiella pneumoniae. He was treated with a 14-day course of antibiotics and a repeat blood culture was negative.

The mother is concerned that the baby has an infection and wants to know if there are any long-term problems that could occur related to this infection.

What is the most appropriate response?
A. Late-onset sepsis has been associated with an increased risk for abnormal cognitive and motor outcomes in early childhood
B. The baby will not have any long-term problems secondary to this infection since he improved so quickly once the antibiotics were started
C. Preterm infants with a late-onset infection are at higher risk for subsequent infections while in the neonatal intensive care unit (NICU)
D. We are very concerned about Baby Boy Brown because the majority of preterm infants born at his size and birth weight do not develop infections while hospitalized
E. The risk for having long-term developmental problems varies based on the organism causing the infection

Discussion

The correct answer is **A**. The majority of preterm infants will have at least one late-onset infection during their initial hospitalization.[4] Stoll et al. from the NICHD Neonatal Research Network reported that 67% of extremely low-birth infants had at least one late-onset infection prior to hospital discharge. The most common pathogen causing late-onset infection in preterm infants is coagulase-negative Staphylococcus (CoNS). Clinically, neonates tend to have more severe clinical symptoms when they are infected with gram-negative organisms. The risk of death is higher in infants with both gram-negative and fungal infections. The risk for neurodevelopmental impairment (NDI) does not vary by pathogen, except that those with gram-negative infections are more likely to have hearing impairment compared to those with CoNS infection. In an analysis of outcome of extremely preterm infants being screened for sepsis, those with fungal infections were more likely to die and survivors had worse neurodevelopmental outcomes than uninfected preterm infants.[5] These risks are highest among those <750 g birth weight. Various quality improvement strategies have been shown to decrease the risk of nosocomial infections, including judicious care of central lines, minimizing catheter days, compliance with hand-washing guidelines, and antibiotic stewardship. Having one late-onset infection does not automatically increase the risk of the infant developing yet another infection.

Mrs. Brown asks if any additional tests will be needed as a result of this infection.

Which additional tests would be appropriate to order for Baby Boy Brown?
A. Blood culture
B. Lumbar puncture
C. Hearing evaluation
D. MRI of the brain
E. A, B, and C

Discussion

The correct answer is **E**. Late-onset infection in a preterm infant should be considered a serious complication. Appropriate follow-up care ensures that the infants receive the appropriate duration of antibiotic therapy and also guides the decision making for further evaluation. A repeat blood culture should be obtained to ensure that the bacteremia has resolved. Although there is a lot of variability in clinical practice, available data suggest that a lumbar puncture should be performed in preterm infants with documented bacteremia.[6] Hearing evaluations are a routine part of newborn care; however, it is particularly important in an infant with a documented history of gram-negative sepsis because they have a higher risk for hearing impairment. Early detection is important to improve long-term outcomes. There are growing concerns that preterm infants with infection are at increased risk for cytokine-mediated central nervous system injury to the developing white matter.[7,8] Researchers speculate that this may be responsible for the apparent increased

risk for NDI in preterm children with a history of infection. However, at this time, the decision to perform additional neuroimaging varies based on the clinical scenario but would not be routinely recommended in all infants.

Objectives

1. Understand risk factors for neurodevelopmental impairment in preterm infants
2. Understand how neonatal comorbidities contribute to the risk of abnormal neurodevelopmental outcome
3. Understand how postnatal steroid use modifies the risk for abnormal neurodevelopmental outcome

CASE 3

Mrs. Morgan stops visit by the NICU to thank the doctors and nurses for the wonderful care they provided for her 28-week preterm twins. The twins have been discharged home and are back for follow-up medical appointment. The twins recently celebrated their first birthday last week.

Mrs. Morgan is concerned that the twins are not yet rolling over from prone to supine. She asks if she should be concerned.

Select the best option for how you should counsel this mother.
A. The twins are 12 months chronological age but only 9 months adjusted age. Not rolling over at 9 months of age is considered normal and she should not be concerned
B. The twins are 12 months of age and this is not considered normal for a 12-month-old child. She should contact her pediatrician immediately
C. Most premature infants have trouble mastering their motor milestones. This should not be a concern and she should wait until the children are at least 16 months old before bringing this concern to the attention of the pediatrician
D. The twins are 12 months chronological age but 9 months adjusted age. Most children are able to roll over by 6 months of age. You should recommend that she contact her pediatrician or your high-risk infant follow-up program
E. The twins should be referred to a neurologist for further evaluation

Discussion

The correct answer is **D**. Understanding the patterns of normal gross motor develop is important to all parents. Providers should provide appropriate anticipatory guidance so that parents understand expected developmental progression based on the child's age. Children born extremely prematurely should master appropriate developmental milestones based on their "adjusted" or "corrected" age rather than their chronological age. If milestones are not appropriate for the "corrected age," a referral should be made to early intervention services, particularly in an at-risk prematurely born child. In this vignette, the twins have delay in the emergence of gross motor skills. It would not be appropriate to delay referral for further evaluation until 16 months of age. The appropriate referral resource for these twins will vary based on the resources available in your local area. In some regions, these children are followed by a pediatric neurologist while in other areas they are followed in a high-risk infant follow-up program or other center or community-based programs.

It is an accepted clinical practice to adjust for prematurity for at least the first 2 years of life. There are limited data to support this practice among contemporary cohorts. In 1983, Siegel[9] attempted to determine if age-adjusted or unadjusted comparisons of neurodevelopmental outcome was a better predictor of outcome at 3 to 5 years of age by performing serial developmental assessments on two simultaneous cohorts of term and a preterm cohort infants. The data were inconsistent across different time points. In a systematic review of available data on this issue, Wilson and Cradock[10] concluded that accepted clinical practice is to adjust until 2 years of age. Some feel that age-adjusted comparisons are more predictive of motor performance rather than cognitive performance. Furthermore, most of the available data present outcomes from cohorts from several decades prior and may not reflect current outcomes. Further study is needed in this area.

The twins are enrolled in an early intervention program and begin receiving weekly physical therapy. They make nice progress over the next several months.

Mrs. Morgan asks if it is likely that the twins will continue to have developmental problems or learning disabilities as they approach school age.

The most appropriate response to Mrs. Morgan would be which of the following?
A. It is difficult to predict if the twins will continue to have problems in other areas of their development. Close observation is recommended
B. Children who have problems meeting their early motor development will also have problems with language and cognitive function
C. Early gross motor developmental delay is a strong predictor for a later diagnosis of cerebral palsy

D. Preterm twins are more likely to have developmental delays compared to singleton preterm infants
E. Based on the fact that they have early gross motor delays, it is highly likely that they will also have cognitive delays and learning disabilities

Discussion

The correct answer is **A**. Predicting the developmental trajectory of prematurely born infants can be very difficult. It is important to help parents understand that preterm brain injury is often localized and results in focal deficits. Some children will have delays in all areas of their development, while others will have isolated deficits in one domain. Close developmental follow-up is recommended for preterm infants, particularly those who exhibit early signs of gross motor delay.

In a longitudinal cohort study of LBW infants <33 weeks' gestation compared to a control reference group, the Etude Epidemiologique sur les Petits Ages Gestationnels (EPIPAGE) Study Group evaluated neurodevelopmental outcomes up to 8 years of age.[11] At age 8, they found that a significant percentage of children continued to have neurocognitive and motor delays and 42% of those 24 to 28 weeks and 31% of those 29 to 32 weeks continued to require special healthcare resources. Overall, the risk for abnormal outcome was inversely related to gestational age. Abnormalities on cranial ultrasound were the most important predictor of cerebral palsy at age 5. Cerebral palsy was observed in 9% of this cohort.[12]

Helpful Hint: The five domains for developmental assessment are gross motor, fine motor, cognitive, language, and social skills. It is important to perform a thorough evaluation using a developmental screening tool that will address potential issues in each domain. Age-appropriate developmental assessments should be utilized.

After the parents leave, the residents ask you if there are differences in how to provide perinatal counseling to parents expecting preterm ELBW singleton infants compared to those expected preterm ELBW twin or higher-order multiple gestations.

What is the most appropriate response to the residents?
A. There are no reported differences in risk of morbidity or mortality for singletons compared to twins or triplets
B. Twins tend to have a higher risk of inpatient mortality but similar risk of neurodevelopmental outcome among survivors
C. Twins tend to have a higher risk of inpatient mortality and a higher risk of adverse neurodevelopmental outcome among survivors

D. The pregnancy history, including the type of twinning, does not impact the risk of death or neurodevelopmental outcome for twin pregnancies
E. Monoamniotic–monochorionic twins have a lower risk of adverse pregnancy and developmental outcome than diamniotic–dichorionic twins

Discussion

The correct answer is **C**. Overall, twins have a higher risk of death and adverse neurodevelopmental outcomes compared to singletons. This statement is true for twins born at full term and those born premature. One of the most important explanations for the higher risk of complications in twin gestations relates the increased risk of preterm delivery.

In several large population cohorts studies which include normal birth weight and term infants, twins have a higher risk of both neonatal and fetal death particularly when one twin dies in utero. Similarly, the prevalence of cerebral palsy ranges from 4 to 7.4 times higher in twins compared to singletons.[13–15] If one twin ties in utero, the survivors had a 10-fold increased risk of developing CP.[15]

The increased prevalence of CP in twins is strongly correlated to the increased risk of preterm birth; therefore, it is important to identify exactly which variables are independent predictors of twin outcomes. Scher et al. reported that the risk of death was actually lower in twins whose BW was <2500 g but higher among larger birth weight and more mature twins compared to singletons.

Few studies have reported neurodevelopmental outcome assessments on preterm multiple gestation survivors. Wadhawan et al.[16] from the NICHD NRN evaluated neurodevelopmental outcomes of ELBW from multiple gestation pregnancies and compared their outcomes to singleton ELBW infants. Twin ELBW infants had a higher rate of severe IVH compared to both singletons and higher-order multiple gestation pregnancies. Triplets had a higher risk for the composite outcome of death or NDI compared to singletons (adjusted OR: 1.7 [95% CI: 1.29–2.24]). There was a trend toward worse outcomes in twin pregnancies but this did not reach statistical significance (adjusted OR 1.27 [95% CI: 0.95–1.71]).[16] Very preterm infants evaluated in the EPIPAGE study were evaluated at 5 years of age. In unadjusted outcomes, twins had higher rates of in-hospital mortality; however, no differences were seen in rates or cerebral palsy or developmental performance at 5 years of age.[17] In adjusted analyses, twins had slightly lower scores on the Mental Processing Composite Scale compared to singletons.

Neurodevelopmental outcome on children affected by twin-to-twin transfusion syndrome (TTTS) have limited generalizability because they are small, include newborns from various gestational ages, and represent select population. However, available data suggest that when there is death of a co-twin, the risk for developmental impairment is higher in monochorionic twins compared to dichorionic twins. In a systematic review by Ong et al., 267 twin pregnancies with a fetal demise of one twin, the surviving twin was more likely to have a neurologic abnormality in monochorionic compared to dichorionic twins.[13,18]

On the basis of the population-based registry data, normal birth weight and term twins have a higher risk of cerebral palsy compared to singleton peers. The relative risk for CP for twin ≥2,500 g ranges from 3.3 to 5.5.[13] After adjustment for gestational age and birth weight, reports of differences in the risk of cerebral palsy among low–birth-weight infants have been inconsistent. In terms of cognitive impairment, outcomes again have been somewhat variable. Some have shown no difference in cognitive performance. The study by Wadhawan et al.[16] evaluated outcomes at 2 years of age using the Bayley Scales of Infant Development (BSID)-IIR, found that twins were more likely to have a Mental Developmental Index <70 compared to singleton ELBW infants but these differences were not seen after adjustment for other neonatal morbidities.

Which of the following options best characterizes risk for adverse neurologic outcome and CNS injury in twin pregnancies complicated by twin-to-twin transfusion?

Select the best answer.
A. The type of twinning does not affect the risk for CNS injury
B. The smaller twin (donor twin) is at greater risk for CNS injury
C. The larger twin (recipient twin) is at greater risk for CNS injury
D. Both twins have equal risk of CNS injury
E. Intracranial hemorrhage and/or stroke is an infrequent complication in pregnancies affected by twin-to-twin transfusion

Discussion

The correct answer is **C**. Twin-to-twin transfusion results in the shunting of blood from the donor twin (typically smaller twin and anemic) to the recipient twin (typically larger twin and polycythemia). This volume overload in the recipient twin is associated with an increased risk for intracranial hemorrhage in the larger infant. Due to this increased risk for CNS injury, this infant would similarly have an increased risk of abnormal developmental outcome.

Objectives

1. Know the risk for CNS injury and abnormal developmental outcome in high-risk pregnancies, including twin gestations
2. Understand the unique risks associated with twin-to-twin transfusion syndrome
3. Know the complications associated with twin-to-twin transfusion syndrome

CASE 4

The pediatric residents have just started their rotation in the NICU. During patient care rounds the resident reports that Baby Jones had a cranial ultrasound on yesterday and he is reported to have a Grade 3 IVH on the right side. They ask you to explain the differences in the Papile grading system for IVH.

Which image below best characterizes a Grade 3 IVH based on Papille Criteria?
See images:
A. Figure 16-1
B. Figure 16-2
C. Figure 16-3
D. Figure 16-4
E. Figure 16-5

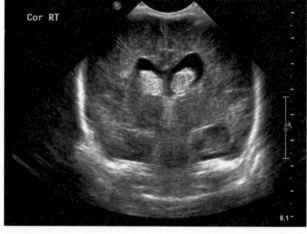

FIGURE 16-2. Used with permission of Dr. Ira Adams Chapman.

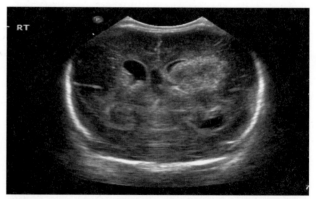

FIGURE 16-3. Used with permission of Dr. Ira Adams Chapman.

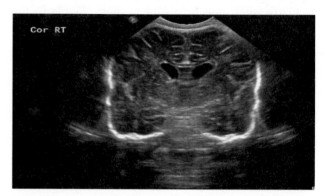

FIGURE 16-4. Used with permission of Dr. Ira Adams Chapman.

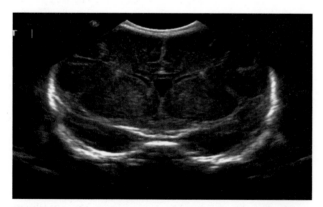

FIGURE 16-1. Used with permission of Dr. Ira Adams Chapman.

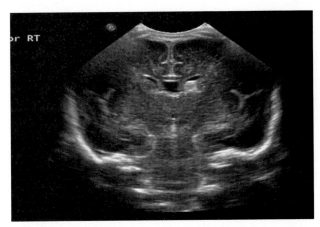

FIGURE 16-5.   Used with permission of Dr. Ira Adams Chapman.

Discussion

The correct answer is **B**. In 1978 Papile et al.[19] developed the most commonly used grading system to describe differences in IVH in preterm infants based on cranial ultrasound findings. This system distinguishes between the location of blood and the degree of ventricular dilatation. The grading system is as follows:

Grade 1 IVH	Subependymal hemorrhage
Grade 2 IVH	Blood extending into the ventricular system
Grade 3 IVH	Blood extending into the ventricular system AND ventricular dilatation
Grade 4 IVH	Parenchymal hemorrhage

This system allows for some consistency for classifying ultrasound findings. The system is limited by the fact that the degree of ventricular dilatation is subjective and there can be significant variability in the amount of involvement within a grading stage. This system also does not have a classification for the patient with isolated ventricular dilatation but no IVH.

In general, rates of IVH have decreased over time. In 2010, Stoll et al.[20] reported outcomes of 9,575 low–birthweight infants and found that 10% had Grade 1 IVH, 6% had Grade 2 IVH, 7% had Grade 3 IVH, and 9% had Grade 4 IVH. Isolated ventriculomegaly was reported in 2% and PVL was present in 4%.

Figure 16-1 represents a normal cranial ultrasound.

Figure 16-2 represents bilateral Grade 3 IVHs.

Figure 16-3 represents bilateral nonspecific ventriculomegaly. You will note the lack of hemorrhage in the ventricles even though both ventricles are enlarged.

Figure 16-4 represents a Grade 4 IVH on the left. This image represents the classic appearance of periventricular hemorrhagic infarction with the fan-shaped distribution near the ventricular angle. Pathologically, these lesions are frequently associated with secondary hemorrhage into the periventricular white matter surrounding this region. The echogenic material fills the ventricle and is also present in the parenchymal space. Though frequently associated with severe IVH, it is no longer felt that a Grade 4 hemorrhage is an extension of a Grade 3 hemorrhage. In contrast, these lesions most likely result secondary to hemorrhage venous infarction.

Figure 16-5 represents a Grade 1 IVH.

The resident asks you to explain how this ultrasound finding will modify the risk for abnormal neurodevelopmental outcome for Baby Jones.

Select the best answer.
A. Increasing severity of IVH increases the risk for abnormal neurodevelopmental outcome
B. Increasing severity of IVH does not increase the risk of abnormal neurodevelopmental outcome
C. Early timing of the hemorrhage is correlated with an increased risk of abnormal neurodevelopmental outcome
D. All children with Grade 3 IVH develop cerebral palsy
E. Intracranial hemorrhage does not affect the risk of cerebral palsy or abnormal neurodevelopmental outcome

Discussion

The correct answer is **A**. In general, increasing severity of IVH is associated with an increased risk of IVH. However, it is important to remember that even low grades of IVH such as Grade 1 and 2 have been associated with an increased risk of motor and cognitive impairment.[21,22]

O'Shea et al.[23] reported 24-month developmental outcomes of 949 children born ≤28 weeks' gestation who had at least one cranial ultrasound performed within 2 weeks of life. Developmental evaluations were performed using the BSID-IIR. They found that 41% of children with IVH also had white matter damage. They found that only those children with both IVH and WMI had an increased risk of adverse developmental outcome. Of note, the rate of WMI in this study using solely cranial ultrasounds for diagnosis was higher than rates reported in other studies.

Klebermass-Schrehof et al.[24] reported an increased risk of IVH in preterm children. This risk was similar at all gestational ages for those with severe Grades 3 and 4 IVH. For those with Grades 1 and 2 IVH the risk was inversely related to gestational age.

Increasing severity of IVH is correlated with an increased risk for adverse neurodevelopmental outcome. Adams-Chapman et al.[25] evaluated developmental outcomes at 2 years of age using the BSID-IIR and noted an incremental decrease in performance on cognitive and motor performance and an increased risk of cerebral palsy with increasing severity of IVH. Those children with a Grade 3 or 4 IVH who required shunt insertion had the highest overall risk of poor outcome. However, 14% of children in this cohort with severe Grade 3 or 4 IVH and shunt insertion had normal developmental outcome at 2 years of age. Further studies are needed to see how these results correlate with school-age outcomes in these high-risk infants.

Posthemorrhagic ventricular dilatation in the absence of parenchymal lesions may have a better prognosis. In a review of a cohort of 32 preterm infants with PHH requiring neurosurgical intervention evaluated at 5 years of age, 59.4% had no NDI. Rates of cerebral palsy and cognitive impairment were similar when compared to control preterms with no ICH.[26]

The resident asks you to explain the significance of isolated ventricular dilatation and how that may impact the long-term developmental outcome of this patient.

A. Patients with isolated ventriculomegaly should be referred emergently to pediatric neurosurgery for evaluation of a shunt insertion
B. Isolated ventriculomegaly is most likely of no clinical consequence to affected patients
C. Isolated ventriculomegaly is only important when seen with an associated IVH
D. Isolated ventriculomegaly is rarely reported in preterm infants
E. Isolated ventriculomegaly in children born preterm has been associated with an increased risk of NDI

Discussion

The correct answer is **E**. Increasingly, preterm infants have been noted to have isolated ventricular dilatation without evidence of hemorrhage. Anatomically, this region of the brain is where the periventricular white matter resides. There are limited data reporting neurodevelopmental outcomes of affected infants. The ELGAN Study group reported neurodevelopmental outcomes at 2 years of age of extremely preterm children and found that those with ventriculomegaly had an increased risk of cerebral palsy at follow-up.[27] MRI data will likely help researchers better understand the significance of these findings in the future.

The resident continues to inquire about the predictive value of the cranial ultrasound. You have discussed the predictive value of an abnormal study (i.e., IVH or isolated ventriculomegaly) but the resident asks what the predictive value of a normal cranial ultrasound is.

What is the most appropriate response?

A. Most premature infants with a normal cranial ultrasound will have a normal developmental outcome
B. A normal cranial ultrasound is a poor predictor of developmental outcome
C. When combined with other neuroimaging studies, the positive predictive value of a normal cranial ultrasound increases
D. Abnormalities on cranial ultrasound are equally sensitive as they are specific for long-term neurodevelopmental outcome
E. A and C

Discussion

The correct answer is **E**. Cranial ultrasounds remain the primary mode of CNS imaging in the critically ill preterm newborn. These studies are portable, reproducible, and do not result in additional radiation exposure to the newborn. The value of being able to obtain cranial sonograms such not be minimized. Although severely abnormal findings on a cranial ultrasound are strongly correlated with neurodevelopmental outcome, they are not an absolute predictor. Rather, an abnormal cranial ultrasound findings is a variable that must be evaluated in the context of all risk factors associated with neurodevelopmental outcome, including gestational age, chronic lung disease, late-onset infections, meningitis, sensory impairment, necrotizing enterocolitis, and nutrition.

Neuroimaging with MRI has helped researchers better understand the normal development of the preterm brain. This information is further enhanced by animal data demonstrating the maturation-dependent vulnerability of the oligodendrocytes in the preterm brain. These circumstances help explain the increased risk for injury to the developing white matter in preterm infants and may represent some of the apparent gaps in prediction using traditional modeling based on known risk factors. In general, the extent of diffuse white matter abnormalities is underestimated by traditional cranial sonography.

In an analysis of MRI findings and neurodevelopmental performance at 2 years of age, Woodward et al.[28] reported that approximately 21% of the preterm infants had white matter abnormalities on MRI. Overall, 17% of this cohort had severe NDI at follow-up and these white matter abnormalities were strongly associated with an increased risk of cognitive delay (odds ratio, 3.6; 95% CI, 1.5–8.7), motor delay (odds ratio, 10.3; 95% CI, 3.5–30.8), cerebral palsy (odds ratio, 9.6; 95% CI, 3.2–28.3), and neurosensory impairment (odds ratio, 4.2; 95% CI, 1.6–11.3).

In 2012, Woodward et al.[29] compared neurodevelopmental outcome of preterm born children at 4 and 6 years to term controls. All subjects have a near-term MRI and neurocognitive evaluations at follow-up. They found no differences in outcome between preterm and term infants who both had a normal MRI. In contrast, preterm infants with moderate/severe white matter abnormalities were more likely to have abnormalities in cognitive performance, motor functioning, and executive function. In general, all preterms were three times more likely to have abnormalities in executive functioning at both 4 and 6 years of age.

Although it is clear that MRI is a more sensitive and specific predictor of CNS injury in the preterm population, neither cranial sonography nor MRI is an absolute predictor of neurodevelopmental outcome. Studies are ongoing to determine how to best incorporate the use of these imaging modalities into routine neonatal care.

O'shea et al.[23] from the the Extremely Low Gestational Age Newborn (ELGAN) Study Group reported that intracranial hemorrhage alone was not predictive of motor or developmental impairment at 2 years of age. Instead, evidence of white matter abnormality on cranial ultrasound was a much stronger and independent predictor. Similar findings were reported by Hintz et al.[30] from the NICHD Neonatal Research Network who reported results from early and late cranial ultrasounds, near-term MRI, and neurodevelopmental outcomes at 2 years of age. Although all cranial ultrasound abnormalities were associated with an increased risk of abnormal neurodevelopmental outcome at 2 years of age, on multivariate analysis, early cranial ultrasound findings within the first week of life were not independently predictive of outcome. These authors found that the late (near term) neuroimaging studies (late cranial ultrasound or near-term MRI) were independent predictors of outcome. This study also highlighted the importance of cerebellar lesions on neurodevelopmental outcome. The yield for detecting these cerebellar lesions is much higher using MRI for neuroimaging compared to ultrasound, even when mastoid windows are used to enhance visualization.

Baby Girl Axel was born at 26 weeks' gestation and weighted 900 g at birth. She developed necrotizing enterocolitis at 2 weeks of age and had a surgical resection of her terminal ileum. Her cranial ultrasounds immediately after delivery showed evidence of a Grade 2 IVH. She became clinically ill during the episode of NEC including bacteremia with *Escherichia coli*, hypotension, and disseminated intravascular coagulopathy. A repeat cranial ultrasound showed bilateral Grade 3 IVH. She has

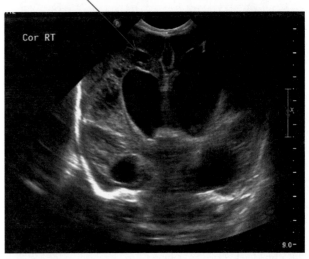

Multiple cystic echolucencies consistent with diagnosis of PVL in addition to bilateral PHH

FIGURE 16-6.   Used with permission of Dr. Ira Adams Chapman.

serial ultrasounds over the next several weeks and was noted to develop both posthemorrhagic hydrocephalus and cystic changes in the periventricular white matter. See Figure 16-6.

How would you best explain these findings to Baby Axel's parents? Are there risk factors from her history that would have allowed you to predict this outcome?

A. You explain to her parents that these findings are not of any concern and that her neurodevelopmental outcome will most likely be normal

B. You explain to her parents that these findings are abnormal but PVL is typically not associated with abnormal neurodevelopmental outcome in preterm infants

C. You explain to the parents that these findings are abnormal and frequently associated with long-term cognitive and motor difficulties

D. You explain to her parents that these findings are abnormal and always associated with severe spastic quadriplegia and cognitive impairment

Discussion

The correct answer is **C**. The findings in this cranial ultrasound represent significant bilateral ventricular dilatation and multiple isolated cystic changes in the periventricular area. As previously discussed, MRI is a more sensitive imaging modality to detect white matter

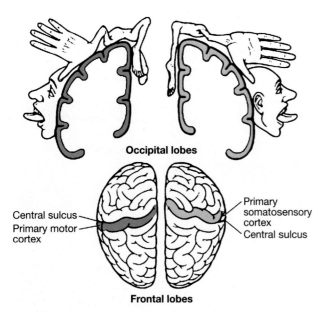

Occipital lobes

Central sulcus
Primary motor
cortex

Primary
somatosensory
cortex
Central sulcus

Frontal lobes

FIGURE 16-7. Reproduced with permission from the Merck Manual: Professional Version, edited by Robert Porter. Copyright 2015 by Merck Sharp & Dohme Corp., a subsidiary of Merck & Co., Inc., Kenilworth, NJ. Available at http://www.merckmanuals.com/professional/. Accessed 5-12-15.

injury; however, in some patients clearly defined cystic changes can be seen with routine cranial sonography. Injury to the white matter has been associated with an increased risk for cerebral palsy and cognitive impairment, both in early childhood and at school age. The geographic locations outlined from the homunculus remind us that there is a pathophysiologic correlate to site of injury and clinical outcomes (Fig. 16-7).

Basic science research has also helped neonatologist better understand that the developing white matter is uniquely vulnerable to cytotoxic injury which is frequently associated with sepsis and inflammatory conditions, including necrotizing enterocolitis. The developing oligodendroglia has been shown to be vulnerable to hypoperfusion and cytokine-mediated injury. Elevated levels of inflammatory mediators have been associated with an increased risk of white matter abnormalities on MRI and abnormal developmental performance at 2 years of age.[27,28,31,32]

Objectives

1. Know how to identify the types of intraventricular hemorrhage
2. Know the significance of isolated parenchymal hemorrhage without intraventricular hemorrhage
3. Know the significance of isolated ventriculomegaly
4. Understand how the risk for adverse neurologic outcome varies based on abnormalities on neuroimaging

5. Understand the limitations of cranial ultrasounds to predict long-term developmental outcomes

CASE 5

Your neighbor delivered a male infant at 34 weeks' gestation after a pregnancy complicated by preterm labor and suspected chorioamnionitis. He was discharged home after a 2-week stay in the NICU step down unit due to immature feeding but was successfully breast-feeding at discharge. The little boy is now 3 years of age and is still not walking independently and only has 10 words in his vocabulary.

His parents ask for your advice because they know that you are a neonatologist. They were told at discharge that their baby should be fine but they are concerned that his developmental progress is delayed.

What is the best advice that you can give these parents?
A. You should advise the parents not to worry because the child's developmental progress is within expected norms
B. You should advise the parents to request further evaluation for their child's development because his developmental progress is delayed for his age
C. You should advise the parents that all preterm infants have developmental delays but typically "catch up" by school age
D. You should advise the parents to immediately take the child to the emergency room and demand an MRI of the brain

Discussion

The correct answer is **B**. Understanding normal child development is critically important, even for the late preterm infant. Recent data suggest that late preterm infants are at higher risk for developmental problems in early childhood and at school age than previously thought.[33–36] There are critical windows in normal brain development that continue until the final weeks of gestation. Any disruption in this process can result in an increased risk of injury to the developing brain. Cortical brain volumes increase by 50% during the last 6 weeks of gestation.[34] Brain maturation and synaptogenesis are also occurring in this time period. As outlined in Figure 16-8 there are significant changes in both brain volume and organization that continue throughout gestation.[37] Kugelman and Colin[34] summarized neurodevelopmental outcome data available for late preterm infants (see Table 16-1). Late preterm infants are at increased risk for cerebral palsy, decreased school performance and

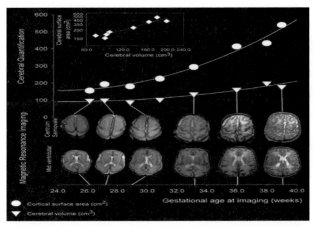

FIGURE 16-8. Reproduced with permission from Kapellou O, Counsell SJ, Kennea N, et al. Abnormal cortical development after premature birth shown by altered allometric scaling of brain growth. *PLoS Med.* 2006;3(8):e265.

attention, and behavioral issues compared to term controls. Interpretation of current data is limited by the lack of systematic neuroimaging and follow-up of late preterm cohorts therefore reported outcomes may be biased toward those with abnormal outcomes. Additional studies are needed in this area.

Baby Girl Bryan was born at 27 weeks' gestation and had a birth weight of 550 g. After hospital discharge she is referred to your High-Risk Infant Follow-Up Program for an evaluation and returns today for an assessment at 18 months adjusted age.

What type of assessment should be performed at the visit today?
A. A comprehensive physical examination
B. A parent interview
C. A developmental screen
D. A screen for autism
E. All of the above

Discussion

The correct answer is **E**. Children with suspected developmental delay should be referred for further evaluation as soon as possible. There is federal legislation in the United States in the Individuals with Disabilities Education Act (IDEA) Part C which mandates that all children less than 3 years of age with significant developmental delay in one or more domains should receive early intervention services in their natural environment. Although this provision is federally mandated,

TABLE 16-1. Long-Term Neurodevelopmental Outcome of Late Preterm Infants

REFERENCE	STUDY DESIGN	PARTICIPANTS	MAIN OUTCOMES
Chyi et al.[38]	Retrospective	767 LP/13 671 term	Increased risk for below-average reading competence at all grade levels, increased need for individualized education programs at early school ages, and increased need of special education
Gray et al.[39]	Prospective	260 LP/General population	Increased rate of behavior problems at age 8 years
Huddy et al.[40]	Retrospective	83 LP	Increased rate of hyperactivity, behavioral, or emotional problems
Woythaler et al.[41]	Prospective	1200 LP/6300 term	Increased risk of mental or physical developmental delay at age 24 months
Morse et al.[42]	Retrospective	7152 LP/152 661 term	Increased risk for developmental delay or school-related problems through age 5 years
Lipkind et al.[43]	Retrospective	13 207 LP/199 599 term	Increased need for special education and lower adjusted math and English scores at school age. Linear association between GA and test scores through 39 weeks' gestation
Quigley et al.[44]	Retrospective	537 LP/6159 term	Increased risk for poorer educational achievement at age 5 years
Talge et al.[45]	Retrospective	168 LP/168 term	Increased risk for behavioral problems and lower IQ at age 6 years
Odd et al.[46]	Prospective	741 (32–36 weeks)/13 102 term	Despite an increased risk for special educational needs, there was little evidence of a reduction in IQ, memory, or attention measures at school age
Gurka et al.[47]	Prospective	53 LP/1245 term	No difference regarding cognition, achievement, behavior, and socioemotional development throughout childhood

Reproduced with permission from Kugelman A, Colin AA. Late preterm infants: near term but still in a critical developmental time period. *Pediatrics.* 2013;132(4):741–751.

TABLE 16-2. **Developmental Screening Tools**

DEVELOPMENTAL SCREENING TOOL	AGE RANGE	ADMINISTRATION	ITEMS	ADVANTAGES/DISADVANTAGES
Ages and Stages Questionnaire (ASQ Third Edition)	4–60 months	10–15 minutes Parent report English/Spanish/French	30	• 0.70–0.90 sensitivity; 0.76–0.9 specificity • Easy to score • Normed in 2008 on diverse ethnic and SES background • Risk categorization in five domains to indicate need for further screening
Battelle Developmental Inventory Screening Tool (BDI-ST)	1–95 months	10–15 min <3 years old 20–30 minutes >3 years old Some special training required	100	• Sensitivity 0.72–0.94; specificity 0.72–0.93 • Normed in 2,500 children based on demographic from census • Scores in five domains • Provides pass/fail score and age equivalents • Designed for use by various providers
Child Developmental Inventory (CDI)	18 months–6 years	30–50 minutes	300	• 0.80–1.00 sensitivity; 0.94–0.96 specificity • Parent Questionnaire to evaluate social, self-help, language, and general developmental skills • Provides developmental quotients and age equivalents • Normative sample included 568 children from MN from working-class families and 43 high-risk children
Denver Developmental Screening Tests	2 weeks–6 years	10–20 minutes No special training required	125	• 0.56–0.83 sensitivity; 0.43–0.80 specificity • Normed on 2,096 term children from Colorado from diverse SES profile • Risk categorization classifies children as normal, suspect, or delayed
Bayley Scales of Infant Development Screener (BINS)	3–24 months	15–25 minutes to administer Special training required	11–13	• 0.75–0.86 sensitivity; 0.75–0.86 specificity • Normed on 1,700 children matching demographic from 2000 census • Risk categorization grading children as low, moderate, or high risk in each of four domains
Bayley Scales of Infant Development-III Revision	1–42 months	50–90 minutes to administer Special training required	Varies depending on age and ceiling	• Five domains evaluated are cognitive, gross motor, fine motor, receptive language, and expressive language • Age equivalents available • Some concern that scores higher in current version of BSID compared to previous versions but strongly correlated with other instruments
Parent's Evaluation of Developmental Status (PEDS)	0–8 years	5–10 minutes to administer and score No special training required	10	• 0.74–0.79 sensitivity; 0.70–0.80 specificity overall but lower sensitivity and specificity in preterm populations • Questions designed as a high-level screen for developmental delay • Limited utility in high-risk population • Normed on population of 771 children from diverse ethnic and SES backgrounds • More detailed instrument to confirm abnormal findings • Risk categorization as low, medium, or high risk
Modified Checklist for Autism in Toddlers (MCHAT)	16–30 months	5–10 minutes	23–29	• Sensitivity 0.85–0.97; specificity 0.93–0.99 • Easy to use parent questionnaire • May over identify children with language delay and developmental delay • Risk categorization to determine need for further evaluation • Standardized and validated instrument

Adapted with permission from Council on Children With Disabilities, et al. Identifying infants and young children with developmental disorders in the medical home: an algorithm for developmental surveillance and screening. *Pediatrics.* 2006;118(1):405–420.

this is operationalized by each state. Eligibility criteria, scope of available services, and the delivery of those specific services vary widely by state. It is important for providers to be aware of their local environment and appropriately refer patients for rehabilitation and therapy services.

There are a variety of commonly used developmental assessment tools. A comprehensive evaluation should be performed to assess the major domains of his overall developmental status, including his cognitive skills, expressive and receptive language skills, fine motor skills, gross motor skills, and social development.

The BSID-IIIR is a frequently used developmental assessment tool in the United States because it evaluates each of the above areas. The instrument has been normed to a mean score of 100 with a Standard Deviation ±15 points. Two standard deviations below the mean are considered abnormal. In addition, the child is assigned an age-equivalent score in each domain evaluated. Historically, researchers were concerned that early speech and language delays, which are common in the ELBW population, falsely lowered developmental outcome scores in this population and thereby overestimated rates of NDI in preterm children. An advantage of the 2005 revision of the BSID is that the child receives a separate subscale score for expressive and receptive language rather than these items being collapsed into the cognitive items. Unfortunately, new concerns have surfaced because researchers have reported significantly higher overall scores using the BSID-III in similar populations compared to the second edition. These differences cannot be fully explained by differences in the population raising the concern that the new version of the BSID may be underestimating impairment in the preterm population.[5, 48] Additional research is needed in this area and studies are ongoing to compare performance on the BSID-III in early childhood and then at school age to determine which measure is more predictive.

In addition to screening high-risk infants, the American Academy of Pediatrics recommends routine developmental screening for all children at the well-child visit at 9, 12, and 30 months of age. In addition, a screen for signs of autism is recommended at the 18-month well-child visit.

There are a variety of developmental screening instruments that can be used for both the general population and high-risk populations as outlined in Table 16-2. A more expanded version of available developmental assessment tools has been published by the AAP.[49]

Some of the advantages and disadvantages of each tool are outlined. More specific neurocognitive assessments can be performed by providers with specialized training in both the administration and interpretation of the results, including the frequently used Stanford–Binet Intelligence Scale and Wechsler Preschool and Primary

Scale of Intelligence Scale (WPPSI). The WPPSI can be administered to children ages 2 years and 6 months to 7 years. The Stanford–Binet can be administered to children 2 years of age or greater.

Objectives

1. Understand the risk for CNS injury among late preterm infants
2. Understand limitations of current data available regarding neurodevelopmental outcome of late preterm infants
3. Recognize available standardized developmental screening tools used to evaluate term and preterm children

CASE 6

You have new residents in the High-Risk Infant Follow-Up Clinic today. They are trying to master the neurologic examination and have questions about immature reflexes and when they should disappear.

Currently you are evaluating a former 28-week infant who is now 9 months adjusted age.

Which immature reflexes should be present?
A. Moro reflex
B. Atonic neck reflex (ATNR)
C. Grasp reflex
D. All of the above
E. None of the above

Discussion

The correct answer is **E**. Similar to gross motor milestones, you should expect that immature reflexes should resolve at the expected time for the child's adjusted age. Both the Moro reflex and the atonic neck reflex (ATNR) typically resolve by 4 to 6 months of age. The Grasp reflex typically resolves by 6 months of age. Persistence of immature reflexes can be an indicator of neurologic injury and must be evaluated in the context of the rest of the neurologic examination (Table 16-3).

The students ask what are the other important components of the neurologic examination. You explain that you must also evaluate for abnormalities in tone, posture, symmetry, and also the deep tendon reflexes. On your examination of this infant, you note that the child

TABLE 16-3. **Primitive Reflexes**

REFLEX	APPEARANCE	DISAPPEARANCE
Moro	Birth	4 months
Hand grasp	Birth	3 months
Crossed adductor	Birth	7 months
Toe grasp	Birth	8–15 months
ATNR	2 weeks	6 months
Head righting	4–6 months	Persists voluntarily
Protective equilibrium	4–6 months	Persists voluntarily
Parachute	8–9 months	Persists voluntarily

has stiffness and increased tone in the right upper extremity and right lower extremity. When the child is trying to reach for a toy in the midline, you notice that he reaches with the left hand faster than the right. Deep tendon reflexes are brisk in both the right upper and lower extremity and there is sustained clonus in the right ankle.

Which of the following diagnoses are these findings most consistent with?
A. Normal neurologic examination for a child of this age
B. Spastic quadriplegia
C. Spastic diplegia
D. Hypotonia
E. Spastic hemiplegia

Discussion

The correct answer is **E.** These findings are consistent with an examination of a child with spastic hemiplegia involving the right hand, right upper extremity, and right lower extremity. The child has abnormalities of tone and function involving the right side of the body. The examination of a child with spastic quadriplegia would show involvement in all four extremities. Spastic diplegia is the most common form of cerebral palsy which classically shows involvement in both lower extremities.

The residents ask you how soon you can make a diagnosis of cerebral palsy.
A. At birth
B. 6 months of age
C. 12 months of age
D. 24 months of age
E. Variable

Discussion

The correct answer is **E.** By definition, cerebral palsy is a nonprogressive neurologic disorder associated with a central nervous system injury that is affecting posture, tone, and function. The appropriate time for the clinician to make this diagnosis varies depending on the clinical scenario. Some infants have devastating neurologic injury with significantly compromised function immediately after birth. More commonly, abnormalities of tone and posture manifest over time. Many preterm infants have transient early minor abnormalities in their neurologic examination therefore many are hesitant to make a diagnosis prior to 12 months of age in the child who is more mildly affected.

The overall prevalence of cerebral palsy is approximately 1 to 2 cases per 1,000 live births, with an increased prevalence among low–birth-weight infants. Cerebral palsy is a clinical diagnosis. The international working group defined cerebral palsy as "a group of permanent disorders of the development of movement and posture, causing activity limitation, that are attributed to nonprogressive disturbances that occurred in the developing fetal or infant brain."[50] It is important to counsel parents that even though the injury is nonprogressive, from a clinical perspective, the clinical manifestations and functional implications change significantly over time. The current guidelines do not indicate a level of functional impairment required for a diagnosis of cerebral palsy; however, the majority of clinical trials in neonatology exclude children with mild impairment and only include children with moderate-to-severe impairment of gross motor function as the outcome measure. The Gross Motor Functional Classification Score (GMFCS) developed by Palisano et al.[51] is often used as a standardized measure of functional skills in children with a diagnosis of cerebral palsy (see Table 16-4). Classification of type of CP is generally based on the predominant tone abnormality which includes spastic, ataxia, or dyskinetic which may be dystonia or athetosis.[52] Some children have involvement of the upper extremities more so than the lower extremities while other have findings localized to one side. The inter-rater reliability has been questioned using the above criteria. An alternative classification system has been proposed by the Surveillance for Cerebral Palsy in Europe (SCPE)[53] collaborative which includes the following categories: unilateral spastic CP, bilateral spastic CP, dystonic CP, choreoathetoid CP, and ataxia (Fig. 16-9).

Himpens et al.[54] reported in a meta-analysis that the prevalence of CP decreases with increasing gestational age beginning at 27 weeks: 14.6% at 22 to 27 weeks' gestation, 6.2% at 28 to 31 weeks, 0.7% at 32 to 36 weeks, and 0.1% in term infants. Spastic CP is more common in

TABLE 16-4.   Age-Specific Age Band of the Gross Motor Function Classification System Levels I to V

	BEFORE SECOND BIRTHDAY	BETWEEN THE SECOND AND THE FOURTH BIRTHDAY
Level I	Infants move in and out of sitting and floor sit with both hands free to manipulate objects. Infants crawl on hands and knees, pull to stand, and take steps holding on to furniture. Infants walk between 18 months and 2 years of age without the need for any assistive mobility device.	Children floor sit with both hands free to manipulate objects. Movements in and out floor sit are performed without adult assistance. Children walk as the preferred method of mobility without the need for any assistive mobility device.
Level II	Infants maintain floor sitting but may need to use their hands for support to maintain balance. Infants creep on their stomach or crawl on hands and knees. Infants may pull to stand and take steps holding on to furniture.	Children floor sit may have difficulty with balance when both hands are free to manipulate objects. Movements in and out of sitting are performed without adult assistance. Children pull to stand on a stable surface. Children crawl on hands and knees with a reciprocal pattern, cruise holding onto furniture, and walk using an assistive mobility device as preferred method of mobility.
Level III	Infants maintain floor sitting when the low back is supported. Infants roll and creep forward on their stomachs.	Children maintain floor sitting often by 'W-sitting' (sitting between flexed and internally rotated hips and knees) and may require adult assistance to assume sitting. Children creep on their stomach or crawl on hands and knees (often without reciprocal leg movements) as their primary methods of self-mobility. Children may pull to stand on a stable surface and cruise short distances. Children may walk short distances indoors using and assistive mobility device and adult assistance for steering and turning.
Level IV	Infants have head control but trunk support is required for floor sitting. Infants can roll to supine and may roll to prone.	Children floor sit when placed, but are unable to maintain alignment and balance without use of their hands for support. Children frequently require adaptive equipment for sitting and standing. Self-mobility for short distances (within a room) is achieved through rolling, creeping on stomach, or crawling on hands and knees without reciprocal leg movement.
Level V	Physical impairments limit voluntary control of movement. Infants are unable to maintain antigravity head and trunk postures in prone and sitting. Infants require adult assistance to roll.	Physical impairments restrict voluntary control of movement and the ability to maintain antigravity head and trunk postures. All areas of motor function are limited. Functional limitations in sitting and standing are not fully compensated for through the use of adaptive equipment and assistive technology. At Level V, children have no means of independent mobility and are transported. Some children achieve self-mobility using a power wheelchair with extensive adaptations.

Reproduced with permission from Gorter JW, Ketelaar M, Rosenbaum P, et al. Use of the GMFCS in infants with CP: the need for reclassification at age 2 years or older. *Dev Med Child Neurol.* 2009;51(1):46–52.

preterm infants while nonspastic forms of CP are more common among term infants. In this particular study, severity of CP was not associated with gestational age even though the absolute risk for CP is significantly higher with lower gestational age.

Objectives

1. Identify abnormal neurologic examination findings
2. Identify age appropriate developmetnal milestones
3. Understand the significance of transient abnormalities on neurological examination in preterm
4. Know the classification systems for a diagnosis of cerebral palsy
5. Know the risk factors for and prevalence rates of cerebral palsy

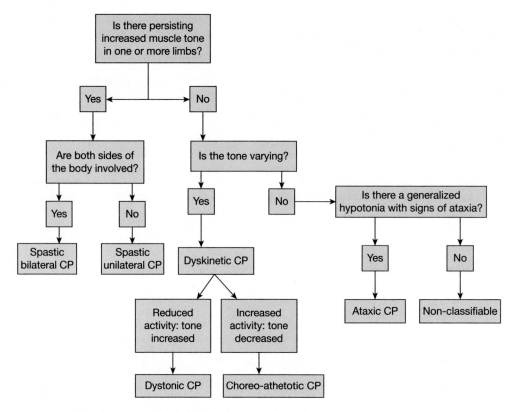

FIGURE 16-9.   SCPE hierarchical classification of cerebral palsy.

CASE 7

You are preparing to discharge Baby Girl Martin from the NICU after a 3-month hospitalization. She was born at 28 weeks' gestation and had two late-onset infections with CoNS and Klebsiella. She had a spontaneous intestinal perforation on day of life 2 managed with a penrose drain, bowel rest, and a 7-day course of antibiotic therapy. She has demonstrated consistent upward growth in her weight, height, and head circumference. She has retinopathy of prematurity and received Avastin injections. Her cranial ultrasounds showed bilateral Grade 2 IVHs.

Which of the following would you recommend at hospital discharge?
A. High-risk infant follow-up program and/or early intervention
B. Ophthalmology
C. Gastroenterology
D. A and B
E. All of the above

Discussion

The correct answer is **D**. Recommendations for follow-up care after discharge is heavily influenced by the availability of pediatric subspecialists in your local area and local practice patterns. The best answer for this question is choice "D." Baby Girl Martin should be followed in a high-risk infant follow-up program and/or early intervention because she has multiple risk factors that increase her risk for long-term developmental difficulties, including multiple late-onset infections and IVH. It is imperative that she have close follow-up with a pediatric ophthalmologist to ensure that the retinae continue to develop appropriately. The need for Avastin injections indicates that her ROP was severe. Many infants with spontaneous intestinal perforations do not require ongoing evaluations with the gastroenterologist, particularly if she has demonstrated consistent weight gain during the hospitalization and has not had any feeding difficulties. The parents and primary care provider should be on the alert for any feeding-related difficulties.

Baby Girl Martin had an abnormal ABR the day prior to discharge. The mother asks you to explain exactly what this means and what needs to be done next.

Select the most appropriate response to Mrs. Martin.

A. It is recommended that all newborns have a hearing evaluation prior to hospital discharge and all abnormal screening evaluations must be evaluated further

B. We decided to perform a hearing evaluation on your daughter only because she had a history of IVH

C. Complications during her hospitalization do not affect the risk for late-onset hearing loss

D. You daughter is deaf in one ear and is immediately being referred to ENT for evaluation for hearing aids

Discussion

The correct answer is **A**. Routine hearing screening prior to hospital discharge or within the first 2 weeks of life is recommended by the American Academy of Pediatrics in an effort to ensure early identification by 6 months of age of all children with early hearing loss. It is recommended that all newborns have an OAE and an automated auditory brain response evaluation prior to hospital discharge. If the baby does not pass the first attempt, the test should be repeated prior to discharge. If the child refers again, the patient should be referred for a follow-up audiological evaluation after hospital discharge (Fig. 16-10). Choice C is incorrect because we know that medical risk factors definitely increase the risk for late-onset hearing loss. Therefore, even for children who pass the initial screening evaluation prior to hospital discharge, a follow-up evaluation is recommended no later than 24 to 30 months of age for all newborns who have a history of medical complications known to be associated with hearing loss including NICU hospitalization greater than 5 days, ECMO, and infectious complications. Furthermore, any child demonstrating language delays in early childhood should be referred for a repeat hearing evaluation.

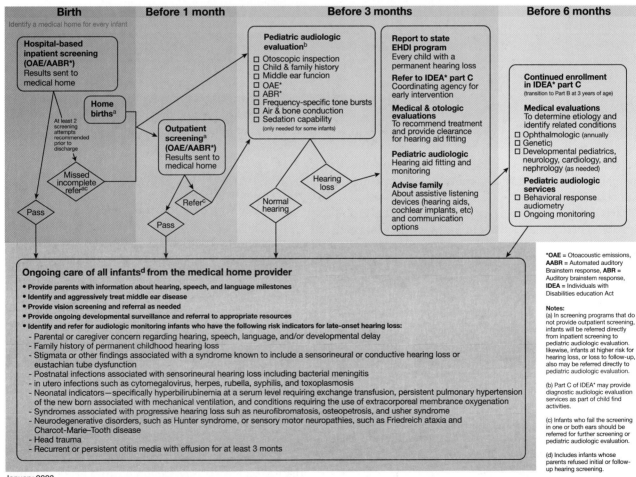

Universal newborn hearing screening, diagnosis, and intervention
Guidelines for pediatric medical home providers

FIGURE 16-10. Reproduced with permission of American Academy of Pediatrics, Joint Committee on Infant Hearing. Year 2007 position statement: Principles and guidelines for early hearing detection and intervention programs. *Pediatrics.* 2007;120(4):898–921.

CASE 8

A 23-week female infant was delivered by emergency C-section last night to a 25-year-old G1P0 mom after a placental abruption. Her birth weight was 500 g. The baby is intubated and receiving mechanical ventilator support. The father immediately went to the internet to find out more information about premature babies and what he should expect. The following morning he confides in you that he is overwhelmed by all of the information on the internet and asks you to explain the difference between the terms impairment, disability, and handicap.

Which of the following best explains the difference between these terms?

A. Impairment refers to any physical or psychological loss or limitation in structure or function
B. Disability refers to the inability or limitation to perform expected activities as a result of impairment
C. A person can have an impairment which is not disabling
D. Handicap refers to the inability of a person to take advantage of opportunities or the environment as other people
E. All of the above are true

Discussion

The correct answer is **E**. The World Health Organization has defined these three terms.

Impairment is defined as any loss or abnormality of psychological, physiological, or anatomical structure or function.

Disability is defined as any restriction or lack of the ability to perform an activity in the manner considered normal human functioning.

Handicap is defined as a disadvantage that limits or prevents an individual from fulfillment of a normal role or activity.

Mrs. Morrison delivered a term male infant at 39 weeks' gestation who had a birth weight of 2,950 g. Prenatal ultrasound showed abnormalities consistent with a diagnosis of hypoplastic left heart syndrome. The newborn was hypoxic at birth and admitted to your NICU. His echocardiogram confirmed these finding.

The mom asks you to help her understand if her child will be considered impaired, disabled, or handicapped.

What is your most appropriate response?

A. The child will most likely be impaired
B. The child will most likely be disabled
C. The child will most likely be handicapped
D. The child will most likely be impaired and disabled but may not be considered handicapped
E. The child will most likely be impaired, disabled, and handicapped

Discussion

The correct answer is **D**. Based on the definitions above outlined by the WHO one can differentiate between these different levels of abnormal function. The term "impairment" primarily refers to abnormalities in structure or function. The child in this scenario has a diagnosis of HLHS with single ventricle physiology which would be considered a physical impairment. Most children with single ventricle physiology will have mild hypoxemia and exercise intolerance. This would be considered a disability because the structural abnormality in the heart will affect the ability to perform tasks which are physically demanding. The definition of handicap refers to the ability to perform activities relative to your peer group. Based on the information provided in the vignette, one is unable to determine how baby Morrison will function relative to his peer group.

The newborn has surgery on DOL 3 and does well. Two weeks later he is ready for discharge from the hospital. He is being discharged home with supplemental gavage feedings.

The mother asks if they should monitor for neurologic problems after discharge.

A. Children with cyanotic heart disease do not have an inherent increased risk for developmental delay, therefore, no additional monitoring is required
B. Children with cyanotic heart disease will have abnormal developmental outcome due to the chronic hypoxemia
C. Children with cyanotic heart disease are not at increased risk for developmental problems if the corrective or palliative surgery is performed within the first week of life
D. Children with cyanotic heart disease are at increased risk for developmental problems after discharge due to multiple factors including the abnormal cardiac anatomy and abnormal CNS blood flow

Discussion

The correct answer is **D**. Children with a history of complex congenital heart disease have an increased risk for developmental difficulties in early childhood. Gaynor and colleagues reported outcomes from a multi-center cohort study of 1770 children requiring surgery for CHD between 1996-2009.[55] The Bayley Scales of Infant Development-IIR was used for the assessments and these were performed at a mean age of 14.5 ± 3.7 months. They reported that those with CHD had a psychomotor developmental index ≥2 SD below the population mean in 36.8% of children and a mental developmental index ≥2 SD below the population mean in 15.3% of children. Independent predictors of motor outcomes included: genetic/extracardiac anomalies, low birth weight and white race. Similarly, independent predictors for cognitive outcomes were low birth weight, lower maternal education and the prescence of genetic/extracardiac anomalies.

Neuroimaging data has shown that many children with CHD have evidence of abnormal brain developmental prior to surgery, including decreased brain volumes, abnormal metabolism and delayed cortical maturation and folding.[56-60] Up to 20% of affected children have evidence of white matter injury on MRI prior to surgery.[16] Furthermore, Beca showed that CNS abnormalities present at birth predicted 2 year outcomes among those with CHD.[61]

The resident does not want to offend the parents by using insensitive terminology but also wants to be sure that the information is accurately presented.

He asks what is the most appropriate terminology to use when discussing outcomes of children with severe developmental issues.

A. You tell the resident that you should tell the parents that the child will have severe mental retardation in the future

B. You tell the resident that you should tell the parents that most children outgrown their developmental problems before the age of 3

C. You tell the resident to tell the parent that we have no idea which children will have learning difficulties solely based on problems experienced in the NICU

D. You tell the resident to tell the parent that based on the information available to us at this time, we would expect that he will have a higher risk for intellectual disability

Discussion

The correct answer is **D**. The term mental retardation has been used for decades to describe children and adults with motor and mental impairment. This term was used indiscriminately to various types of people and also used in a derogatory manner. Rosa's Law was passed in 2010 which requires that the term "mental retardation" be removed from all federal legislation and be replaced with the term "intellectual disability" in federal health, education, and labor policy.

It is important that parents of extreme preterm born children understand that the risk for developmental difficulties occurs over a continuum. During the first few years of life, much of the emphasis is on achievement of gross motor milestones. Of equal importance, is the emergence of language and cognitive milestones that occurs somewhat later. Approximately 30% to 45% of extremely prematurely born children will require special support between preschool and kindergarten, with the highest rates being among the most immature.

More data are emerging on the longer term neurodevelopmental outcome of preterm children at school age and young adulthood.

In 2009, the Victorian Infant Study Group published developmental outcomes of a cohort of preterm children born between 22 and 27 weeks' gestational age to term controls at 8 years of age.[62] They found that the preterm cohort had an increased risk of disability compared to term controls (59% vs. 13%; $p < 0.05$) which included 19% in the preterm group compared to 3% of controls with moderate/severe disability. Similarly, these preterm children had higher rates of both CP and intellectual difficulties at 8 years.

Larroque et al.[11] highlighted the school difficulty that many very preterm children experience by reporting neurodevelopmental outcomes at 8 years of age from a cohort of preterm children born between 22 and 32 weeks' gestation compared to term controls in France. Parents reported that 5% were enrolled in special needs classrooms, 18% had repeated a grade in a regular mainstream classroom. Furthermore, even though the majority were in mainstream classrooms, 15% of them required special educational support in the classroom. Behavior problems were twice as common among the very preterm cohort. Others have reported lower developmental quotients even among those free of severe motor disability.[63] A Norwegian cohort of extremely low–birth-weight children (BW <1,000 g) and born between 22 and 27 weeks' gestation were evaluated at 5 years of age with the Weschlers Preschool and Primary Scale of Intelligence-Revised and the Movement ABC.[64] Moderate-to-severe disability was more common among those born <25 weeks' gestational age. IQ scores were positively correlated with gestational age, maternal education, and preeclampsia. Higher movement ABC scores were associated with gestational age, antenatal steroids, and female gender.

Objectives

1. Know recommendations for high risk infant follow-up
2. Know eligibility criteria for early intervention services

3. Know recommendations for routine follow-up audiology screening for high risk children
4. Distinguish between the terms impairment, handicap and disability
5. Understand the risk for CNS injury in newborns with surgical congenital heart disease
6. Know data regarding school age neurodevelopmental outcomes of prematurely born children

CASE 9

Baby Boy Wilson was born at 40 weeks' gestation and had a birth weight of 3,570 g. He was born to a G10P9009 mom after an uncomplicated pregnancy. One hour before birth mom developed acute onset of vaginal bleeding and was rushed to the hospital. At presentation, fetal bradycardia was noted and an emergent cesarean delivery was performed. The uterus had ruptured and the baby was free floating in the abdomen. The NICU team initiated resuscitation which included intubation, chest compressions, epinephrine, and a fluid bolus. Apgar scores were 1, 1, 1, 3, and 4 at 1, 5, 10, 15, and 20 minutes, respectively. After admission to the NICU a neurologic examination was performed which was consistent with moderate–severe encephalopathy. Whole body cooling was started.

The father asks you to describe the most likely outcome for his son if he survives the hospitalization. What is the most accurate response to this parent?
A. Hypothermia has been shown to be an effective therapy to decrease neonatal death in newborns with clinical evidence of hypoxic ischemic encephalopathy
B. Inadvertent hyperthermia has been associated with worse outcome among neonates with HIE
C. Neonates with HIE who survive have similar neurodevelopmental outcomes to survivors who did not receive hypothermia at 2 years of age
D. All of the above

Discussion

The correct answer is **D**. Numerous clinical trial evaluating the efficacy and safety of either selective head hypothermia or whole body hypothermia in term born neonates have been performed in the United States and Europe. The summary of these various clinical trials is represented in a 2013 meta-analysis of 11 randomized controlled clinical trials which included over 1,500 infant with moderate/severe encephalopathy and a clinical history consistent with intrapartum asphyxia.[65]

Hypothermia was associated with a significant reduction in the composite outcome of death *or* severe neurologic disability at 18 months among survivors. Many investigators were concerned that the decreased mortality seen at 18 months would be offset by an increase in late deaths among survivors.

As a representative example of published clinical trials, the outcome data for the NICHD Neonatal Research Network Hypothermia randomized controlled trial at 18 months and 6 to 7 years of age is outlined below.

NICHD NRN 18-Month Hypothermia Data: There was not a statistically significant difference in each individual component of the primary outcome at 18 months; however, the composite outcome of death or moderate/severe disability was statistically lower among those receiving hypothermia compared to controls at 18 months of age.[66]

Outcomes of NICHD Hypothermia Clinical Trial at 18 Months:

	HYPOTHERMIA $N = 102$	CONTROL $N = 106$	RR (95% CI)
Death	24%	37%	RR = 0.68 95% CI 0.44–1.05, p = ns
CP	19%	30%	RR = 0.68 95% CI 0.38–1.22, p = ns
Death or moderate/ severe disability	44%	62%	RR = 0.72 95% CI 0.54–0.95, $p < 0.05$

NICHD NRN 6- to 7-year ND Outcome Data: In the NICHD Neonatal Research Network clinical trial Shankaran, et al reported outcomes at 6 to 7 years of age from their cohort of 208 children.[67] There were an equal number of deaths in both the hypothermia group and the control group between the 18-month and 6- year visit. Overall, at 6 years the mortality rate was 28% in the hypothermia group compared to 44% in the control group, RR 0.66 (95% CI 0.45–0.97). Death or severe disability was 41% versus 60% ($P = 0.03$), death or IQ less than 55 was 41% versus 60% ($P = 0.03$), and death or CP 41% versus 60% ($P = 0.02$) in the hypothermia and control groups, respectively. Survivors were less likely to have cerebral palsy or IQ less than 70. At 6 to 7 years of age, overall there were fewer deaths among children who received hypothermia. Among survivors, the likelihood of having IQ scores <70 were similar between the two groups. The composite outcome of death *or* IQ <70 was significantly lower among those who received hypothermia.

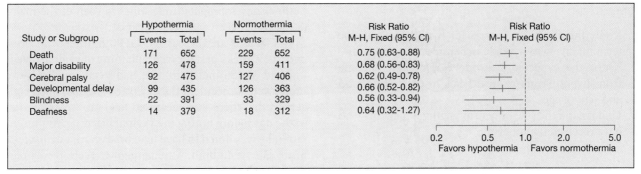

FIGURE 16-11.   Reproduced with permission from Tagin MA, Woolcott CG, Vincer MJ, et al. Hypothermia for neonatal hypoxic ischemic encephalopathy: An updated systematic review and meta-analysis. *Arch Pediatr Adolesc Med.* 2012;166(6):558–566.

Outcomes of NICHD Hypothermia Trial at 6-7 Years:

	HYPOTHERMIA (N = 97)	CONTROL (N = 93)	RELATIVE RISK (95% CI, p)
Death/ IQ <70	47%	62%	RR 0.78 95% CI 0.61–1.01, p = 0.06
Death	28%	44%	RR 0.66 95% CI 0.45–0.97, p = 0.04
Death or severe disability	41%	60%	0.03

Tagin, et al. performed a meta-analysis of the evaluate the efficacy of hypothermia to improve neurodevelopmental outcomes for each component of primary outcome of death or neurodevelopmental impairment are outlined in Figure 16.11.[68]

In general, the benefit of hypothermia is greatest for those with moderate encephalopathy. Other interventions such as MRI neuroimaging, cytokines levels, and EEG findings may also be helpful in predicting outcomes but none are completely predictive. A combination of clinical examination and ancillary testing data are most useful to predict outcome. Close neurodevelopmental follow-up is recommended for children with a history of moderate/severe HIE who undergo hypothermia.

The eligibility criteria for most clinical trials in the US and Europe have included the following:

Clinical Criteria		
Gestational age	≥36 weeks	
Admission	≤ 6 hours of age	
Labor and delivery	History of significant perinatal event	
Laboratory findings	pH ≤ 7.0 or Base deficit ≥16 mmol/L	
Clinical Exam	**Moderate Encephalopathy**	**Severe Encephalopathy**
Level of consciousness	Lethargic	Stupor or coma
Spontaneous Activity	Decreased activity	No activity
Posture	Distal flexion or complete extension	Decerebrate
Tone	Hypotonia	Flaccid
Primitive Reflexes	Weak suck or incomplete Moro	Absent suck and Moro
Autonomic Instability	Constricted pupils Bradycardia Inconsistent respiratory effort or periodic breathing	Deviated, dilated or unresponsive pupils Variable heart rate Apnea

Objectives

1. Know the eligibility criteria for hypothermia in the term infants with hypoxic ischemic encephalopathy
2. Know the expected neurodevelopmental outcome from hypothermia clinical trials in early childhood and school age
3. Understand the role of neuroimaging in patients who have received hypothermia

CASE 10

Baby Boy Wilson survives his NICU stay and is discharged home on seizure medications and nasogastric feedings. His discharge neurologic examination was abnormal. He has a weak gag reflex, severe head lag, and hypotonia. The baby is enrolled in your High-Risk Developmental Follow-Up Clinic and presents for the first evaluation at 4 months of age.

Baby Boy Wilson is rolling over from prone to supine. He is able to bring his hands to the midline to grasp a toy but is not yet transferring. He prop sits with support. He focuses visually on your face and is able to track a bright toy continuously across the midline.

What is your assessment of Baby Boy Wilson's developmental status at this time?

A. His developmental skills are within normal limits for his age therefore he should be discharged from ongoing evaluations in the follow-up clinic
B. His developmental skills are within normal limits for his age but he remains at risk for developmental issues based on his NICU complications and he should return for additional evaluations
C. You assure the parents that if his development is normal at 1 year of age, it is likely that he will never have any developmental issues
D. You refer Baby Boy Wilson to a neurologist because you are concerned about his gross motor developmental delays

Discussion

The correct answer is **B**. Understanding the progress of normal motor development is critically important in the assessment of the high-risk neonate. Parents should understand anticipated developmental milestones so that the child can receive the appropriate intervention as early as possible. Newborns with a history of HIE have a significant risk for abnormal long-term developmental outcomes and should be monitored carefully. Table 16-5

outlines developmental milestones in each of the major domains between ages 0 to 5 years.

Ms. Tate is an 18-year-old G1P0 mother who presents at 39 weeks' gestation complaining of vaginal bleeding and abdominal pain. She had been involved in a motor vehicle accident the day prior and had been concerned that there was decreased fetal movement earlier in the day before noting the vaginal bleeding. At presentation he was noted to have fetal bradycardia with a fetal heart rate of 40 bpm. An emergent C-section was performed. The infant was depressed at birth and required vigorous resuscitation including intubation, chest compressions, and two doses of epinephrine. Apgar scores were 1, 1, 3, 3 and 4 at 1, 5, 10, 15, and 20 minutes, respectively.

Ms. Tate brings little baby Joseph Tate back for a visit after they are discharged home when he is 9 months of age. Mom reports that he is able to hold his head up briefly when placed on his tummy and he is able to roll from his back to his side. He brings his hands together in the midline. He is not yet able to sit without full support. He will focus on objects with his eyes and will grasp a toy with his hands and he is able to bring his hands together in the midline.

She is concerned about his developmental status and asks your opinion. She asks you to estimate the approximate age-equivalent level of functioning.

What is the most appropriate response to Ms. Tate?

A. Normal
B. 2 months
C. 4 months
D. 6 months

Discussion

The correct answer is **C**. Ms. Tate sends you a letter to thank you for your wonderful NICU care when Joseph celebrates his second birthday! She updates you on his status and tells you that he is sitting independently, crawls on hands and knees, pulls to stand, and is cruising. He is not yet able to walk independently. He babbles constantly and says "mama" and "dada" to everyone he meets. He reaches for objects but has difficulty manipulating objects and uses the entire hand to pick up small objects.

What is his current age-equivalent level of functioning based on her report?

A. Normal
B. 6 months
C. 9 months
D. 12 months

TABLE 16-5: Developmental Milestones

	GROSS MOTOR/PHYSICAL	COGNITIVE	LANGUAGE/ COMMUNICATION	SOCIAL/EMOTIONAL	REASONS FOR CONCERN
2 Mo	Begins to hold head up Begins to weight bear on hands in prone position	Pays attention to faces Becomes bored if not active and engaged	Turns head to sounds Coos and vocalizes	Begins to smile Begins to self soothe	Does not respond to loud noises Does not watch things as they move Poor head control
4 Mo	Holds head up steady Bears weight on feet in supported standing May roll over from prone to supine position Reaching for objects and able to hold and grasp toy Brings hands to mouth Pushes up on arms in prone position	Recognizes familiar people from a distance Able to grab a toy with one hand Responds to affection Uses hands and eyes together Tracks across the midline to follow toy	Begins to babble Babbles with expression Cries in different ways to express anger, fatigue, and hunger	Smiles spontaneously, especially at people Enjoys playing with people Copies some movements and facial expressions	Does not hold head up Does not smile at people Difficulty tracking objects or faces Does not bear weight on feet in supported standing
6 Mo	Rolls over in both directions Begins to sit without support In standing, starts to bounce Begins to crawl (may crawl backward before going forward)	Looks around at things nearby Brings objects to mouth Tries to get things that are out of reach Begins to pass things from one hand to the other	Responds to sounds by making sounds Strings vowels together when babbling ("ah," "eh," "oh") and likes taking turns with parent while making sounds Responds to name Uses consonant sounds (jabbering with "m," "b")	Knows familiar faces Enjoys playing with others, especially caregivers Enjoys seeing self in mirror	Does not attempt to get objects that are out of reach No affection for caregivers Not rolling Not responding to sounds around him
9 Mo	Stands with support Beginning to cruise Sits without support Transitions from sitting to crawling Pulls to stands Crawls	Looks for hidden toy Plays peek-a-boo Moves objects smoothly from one hand to another Picks up small objects with tips of fingers (fine pincer grasp)	Understands "no" Makes variety of different sounds including "mama" and "dada" Copies sounds and gestures of others Uses fingers to point	Stranger anxiety Has preferred toys and objects Has preferred people	Unable to sit without support Unable to bear weight on feet in supported standing Does not respond to noises or name
12 Mo	Gets into sitting position without help May stand alone Cruises May take a few steps with hands held	Finds hidden toys easily Explores using toys in different ways, banging, hitting Looks at correct picture when you name object Places objects into and removes them from box Follows simple commands	Responds to simple verbal requests Uses simple gestures, such as waving or shaking head Says "mama" and "dada" and expression such as "uh-oh" Tries to repeat words	Shy or nervous with strangers Engages adults for play Repeats sounds or actions to get attention Puts out arms or legs to help with getting dressed Plays games like "peek-a-goo" or "pat-a-cake"	Unable to crawl Unable to stand and weight bear on feet with support Does not point or gesture Does not search for objects when you hide them

Age	Movement/Physical	Cognitive	Language/Communication	Social/Emotional	Act Early
18 Mo	Walks alone May walk up steps or run Pulls small toy while walking Learns to undress Drinks from cup and uses spoon	Pretend play Understands what common objects are used for Points to one body part Scribbles Follows simple commands	Says several single words Shakes head "no" appropriately Points to indicate that he wants something	Likes to hand people toys to play with them Shows affection to familiar people Points to indicate something is interesting Will play alone but prefers parent to be close	Not learning new words Does not point Loses skills he once had Not concerned when caregiver leaves the room
24 Mo	Stands on tiptoes Runs Kicks a ball Walks upstairs holding rail Throws ball	Begins to sort shapes and colors Completes sentences and rhymes in familiar books Builds tower of 4 or more blocks Names items in a picture book	Points to things or pictures when named Knows names of familiar people and objects Says sentences in 2–4 words Points to things in a book	Copies others, especially adults Gets excited when with other children Shows more independence Plays alongside other children	Does not copy actions or words Does not follow simple commands Unable to walk steady Unable to use 2 word phrases
36 Mo	Climbs well Rides tricycle Runs easily Walks up and down stairs alternating feet	Can operate toys with buttons, levers, and moving parts Plays make believe with dolls, animals, and people Does puzzles with 3 or 4 pieces Copies a circle with crayon Turns pages of book Build tower with 6 cubes	Follows instructions with 2–3 steps Understands words like "in," "on," and "under" Says words like "I," "me," "we," and "you" and some plurals (cars, dogs, cats) Speech understandable to strangers Holds conversations with 2–3 sentences	Copies adults and friends Takes turn in games Shows empathy to friends Understands the idea of "mine" and "his" or "hers" Separates easily from parents Dresses and undresses self	Unable to speak in sentences Speech not understood by strangers Does not enjoy playing with other children Does not understand simple instructions
48 Mo	Hops and stands on one foot Catches a bouncing ball	Names colors and shapes Understands "same" and "different" Draws a person with 2–4 body parts Uses scissors	Knows basic rules or grammar including "he" and "she" Sings familiar songs from memory Tells stories Can tell first and last name	Enjoys doing new things Plays cooperatively with other children Enjoys talking about what they like and enjoy	No interest in interactive play or make believe Can't retell a story Unable to follow 3 step commands Speaks unclearly

Data from Centers for Disease Control and Prevention.

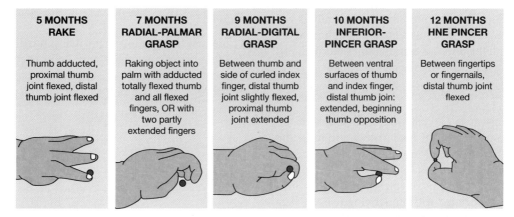

| 5 MONTHS RAKE | 7 MONTHS RADIAL-PALMAR GRASP | 9 MONTHS RADIAL-DIGITAL GRASP | 10 MONTHS INFERIOR-PINCER GRASP | 12 MONTHS HNE PINCER GRASP |

FIGURE 16-12.   Reproduced with permission from McIntire S, Nowalk A, Ziteli B. *Zitelli and Davis' Atlas of Pediatric Physical Diagnosis*. 6 th ed. Philadelphia, PA: Saunders/Elsevier; 2012.

Discussion

The correct answer is **C**. There is a range of normal functioning at all developmental levels; however, there are general guidelines describing the typical age that children will achieve certain motor milestones. Often, all milestones are similar across the various domains but preterm infants are known to have focal brain injury which often results in isolated delays in one domain but not others.

Based on the gross motor milestones reported in the vignette, the child's gross motor skills are at approximately 9- to 10-month level. Children often begin to babble and will repeat "mama" and "dada" indiscriminately at this age. By 12 months of age, many children are walking independently and refer to parental figures specifically as "mama" or "dada". The fine motor skills described in this vignette are suspect and weak in quality. The fine pincer grasp typically develops between 9 and 12 months of age and is characterized by opposition of the tip of them and the index finger when picking up small objects (Fig. 16-12). By 9 to 12 months of age you will notice that children start to point at objects and will isolate the index finger in order to do so. The development of more complex fine motor skills progresses over

time as outlined in Figure 16-13. As preterm infants approach school age it is important to monitor fine motor skills and visual spatial discrimination because both have been identified as an area of weakness for these children at school age.

Objective

1. Identify normal developmental milestones in each of the five domains from ages 0 to 5 years

CASE 11

Baby Girl Benson was born at 29 weeks' gestation to a 32-year-old G1P0 mom. The pregnancy was complicated by premature rupture of membranes 1 week prior to the delivery. The delivery was uncomplicated. Baby Girl Benson had mild respiratory distress syndrome and remained on NCPAP for 2 weeks. She had no other NICU complications other than immature feeding patterns.

Baby Girl Benson presents for her first visit in the High-Risk Infant Follow-Up Clinic at 5 months of age. Parents are very concerned that the right side of her head is flat and her head appears misshapen. They are concerned that there is a problem with the way that her brain is growing. On your physical examination you note that her neurological examination is normal.

How should you counsel the parents of Baby Girl Benson?
A. The shape of the head is a reflection of brain growth
B. You are very concerned and recommend an emergent consult with the neurosurgical team to evaluate for surgery

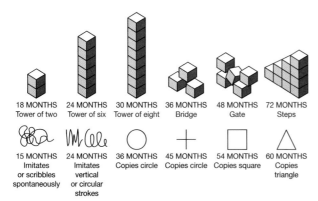

FIGURE 16-13.   Reproduced with permission from McIntire S, Nowalk A, Ziteli B. *Zitelli and Davis' Atlas of Pediatric Physical Diagnosis*. 6th ed. Philadelphia, PA: Saunders/Elsevier; 2012.

C. This condition is very common and typically is not related to any type of underlying brain abnormality

D. Even though the physical examination is normal, you are very concerned about the plagiocephaly

Discussion

The correct answer is **C**. Positional deformities of the skull are not uncommon in high-risk children. In the absence of other abnormal examination findings suggesting premature closure of the fontanelle or lack of integrity of the cranium, this is typically an isolated finding that is not associated with underlying disease. Parents should be reassured that the shape of the head is not a reflection of brain function. Plagiocephaly can result in facial asymmetry and cosmetic concerns. The infant should be carefully examined for any evidence of synostosis. In contrast, abnormal closure of the various sutures results in craniosynostosis. This can be an isolated abnormality or associated with a syndrome. Children diagnoses with craniosynostosis should have a thorough physical examination and neurologic exam. In the figure below, various types of craniosynostosis and associated syndromes are presented (Fig. 16-14).[69]

Objectives

1. Identify the location of normal suture lines
2. Identify plagiocephaly and its impact on development and function
3. Identify the various forms of craniosynostosis and associated syndromes

CASE 12

Mrs. Sanders delivers a preterm infant at 28 weeks' gestation whose birth weight is 1,250 g. The mother has not breastfed any of her other children and is not particularly interested in trying to breastfed this baby.

What is your recommendation to the mother regarding the advantages of providing breast milk for her baby?

A. There are no advantages to the preterm infant by providing breast milk; therefore, the decision to breastfed should purely be based on parental preference

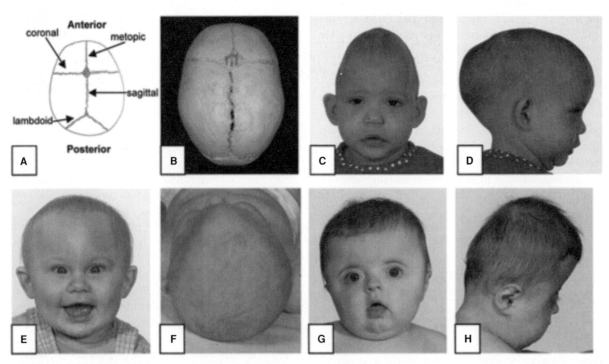

FIGURE 16-14. Diagnostic features of craniosynostosis. (**A**) Schematic diagram showing positions of the major cranial sutures. (**B**) CT scan (vertex view of skull) showing major sutures; anterior is at top. (**C, D**) Sagittal synostosis: note long, narrow head. (**E, F**) Metopic synostosis: note hypotelorism and triangular profile of forehead. (**G, H**) Bicoronal synostosis: broad, flattened head.

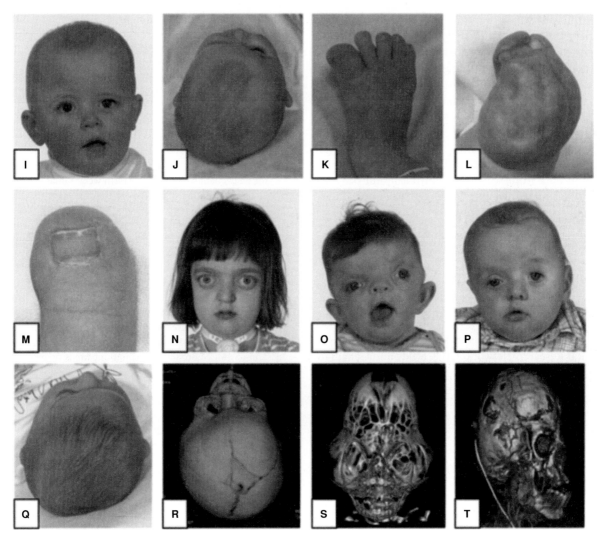

FIGURE 16-14. (*Continued*) (**I, J**) Right unicoronal synostosis: note flattened brow and anterior position of ear on affected side, deviation of nasal tip, and prominent brow on unaffected side. (**K–M**), Congenital anomalies of feet or hands characteristic of Pfeiffer syndrome (**K**), Apert syndrome (**L**) and craniofrontonasal syndrome (**M**). (**N**) Crouzonoid facial appearance. (**O**) Severe hypertelorism, grooved nasal tip, and left unicoronal synostosis in craniofrontonasal syndrome. (**P**) Ptosis and left unicoronal synostosis in Saethre–Chotzen syndrome. (**Q**) Positional plagiocephaly: prominence on right anteriorly and left posteriorly, with right ear anterior and parallelogram shape to skull. (**R**) CT reconstruction showing left unicoronal synostosis. (**S**) CT reconstruction showing cloverleaf skull. (**T**) CT venogram showing abnormal venous drainage in multisuture syndromic craniosynostosis. See text for further details. (Reproduced with permission from Johnson D, Wilkie AO. Craniosynostosis. *Eur J Hum Genet.* 2011;19(4):369–376.)

B. Preterm infant formula provides the same nutritional intake as breast milk

C. The advantages to breast-feeding are only seen during the first 2 months after birth

D. Breast milk is the preferred form of nutrition for preterm infants and is associated with both short-term and long-term benefits

Discussion

The correct answer is **D**. All mothers who deliver preterm infants are encouraged to provide breast milk for their infant based on data showing improving feeding tolerance, less necrotizing enterocolitis, and a decreased risk of infection. Very preterm infants enrolled in EPIPAGE and the LIFT trial were evaluated at ages 2 and 5 years of age.[70] Breast-feeding rates at discharge were low; however, breast-feeding at discharge was associated with improved developmental performance and improved head growth. Paradoxically, breastfed children had lower weights at hospital discharge compared to formula-fed infants.

Vohr et al. from the NICHD Neonatal Research Network evaluated the impact of breast milk during hospitalization on neurodevelopmental outcome status at

2 years of age. Every 10 mL/kg intake of breast milk was associated with an incremental increase in both motor and cognitive scores on the BSID-IIR.[71] These benefits persisted at 30 months adjusted age.[72] Similarly, Anderson et al.[73] showed improvement in cognitive performance for preterm infants who were breastfed.

In 2012 the American Academy of Pediatrics Section on Breastfeeding[74] issued a statement that all infants should be exclusively breastfed for the first 6 months of life using their mother's milk. This recommendation was based on data from studies in both term and preterm populations showing improvement in cognitive functioning for those receiving breast milk for at least 3 months.[75] Furthermore, the AAP recommended that human donor milk be provided for preterm infants whose mothers are unable to provide an adequate supply of breast milk. Currently, there is a paucity of data regarding the long-term benefits of donor milk in preterm infants. Two clinical trials are ongoing to determine if the use of human and/or donor milk result in improved neurocognitive performance in early childhood (NICHD Neonatal Research Network MILK Study and Canadian DoMINO Study).

Objectives

1. Understand the benefits of breast milk for the preterm infant
2. Know the potential short-term and long-term impacts of breast milk on feeding tolerance and growth for the preterm infant
3. Understand the impact of breast milk feeding on long-term neurocognitive outcome

REFERENCES

1. Walsh MC, Yao Q, Gettner P, et al. Impact of a physiologic definition on bronchopulmonary dysplasia rates. *Pediatrics*. 2004;114(5):1305–1311.
2. Stark AR, Carlo WA, Tyson JE, et al. Adverse effects of early dexamethasone treatment in extremely-low-birth-weight infants. *N Engl J Med*. 2001;344(2):95–101.
3. Committee on Fetus and Newborn. Postnatal corticosteroids to treat or prevent chronic lung disease in preterm infants. *Pediatrics*. 2002;109(2):330–338.
4. Stoll BJ, Hansen NI, Adams-Chapman I, et al. Neurodevelopmental and growth impairment among extremely low-birth-weight infants with neonatal infection. *JAMA*. 2004;292(19):2357–2365.
5. Adams-Chapman I, Bann CM, Das A, et al. Neurodevelopmental outcome of extremely low birth weight infants with Candida infection. *J Pediatr*. 2013;163(4):961–967.e3.
6. Stoll BJ, Hansen N, Fanaroff AA, et al. To tap or not to tap: High likelihood of meningitis without sepsis among very low birth weight infants. *Pediatrics*. 2004;113(5):1181–1186.
7. Back SA, Luo NL, Borenstein NS, et al. Late oligodendrocyte progenitors coincide with the developmental window of vulnerability for human perinatal white matter injury. *J Neurosci*. 2001;21(4):1302–1312.
8. Rezaie P, Dean A. Periventricular leukomalacia, inflammation and white matter lesions within the developing nervous system. *Neuropathology*. 2002;22(3):106–132.
9. Siegel LS. Correction for prematurity and its consequences for the assessment of the very low birth weight infant. *Child Dev*. 1983;54(5):1176–1188.
10. Wilson SL, Cradock MM. Review: Accounting for prematurity in developmental assessment and the use of age-adjusted scores. *J Pediatr Psychol*. 2004;29(8):641–649.
11. Larroque B, Ancel PY, Marchand-Martin L, et al. Special care and school difficulties in 8-year-old very preterm children: The Epipage cohort study. *PLoS One*. 2011;6(7):e21361.
12. Beaino G, Khoshnood B, Kaminski M, et al. Predictors of cerebral palsy in very preterm infants: The EPIPAGE prospective population-based cohort study. *Dev Med Child Neurol*. 2010;52(6):e119–e125.
13. Lorenz JM. Neurodevelopmental outcomes of twins. *Semin Perinatol*. 2012;36(3):201–212.
14. Bonellie SR, Currie D, Chalmers J. Comparison of risk factors for cerebral palsy in twins and singletons. *Dev Med Child Neurol*. 2005;47(9):587–591.
15. Scher AI, Petterson B, Blair E, et al. The risk of mortality or cerebral palsy in twins: A collaborative population-based study. *Pediatr Res*. 2002;52(5):671–681.
16. Wadhawan R, Oh W, Vohr BR, et al. Neurodevelopmental outcomes of triplets or higher-order extremely low birth weight infants. *Pediatrics*. 2011;127(3):e654–e660.
17. Bodeau-Livinec F, Zeitlin J, Blondel B, et al. Do very preterm twins and singletons differ in their neurodevelopment at 5 years of age? *Arch Dis Child Fetal Neonatal Ed*. 2013;98(6):F480–F487.
18. Ong SS, Zamora J, Khan KS, et al. Prognosis for the co-twin following single-twin death: A systematic review. *BJOG*. 2006;113(9):992–998.
19. Papile LA, Burstein J, Burstein R, et al. Incidence and evolution of subependymal and intraventricular hemorrhage: A study of infants with birth weights less than 1,500 gm. *J Pediatr*. 1978;92(4):529–534.
20. Stoll BJ, Hansen NI, Bell EF, et al. Neonatal outcomes of extremely preterm infants from the NICHD neonatal research network. *Pediatrics*. 2010;126(3):443–456.
21. Bolisetty S, Dhawan A, Abdel-Latif M, et al. Intraventricular hemorrhage and neurodevelopmental outcomes in extreme preterm infants. *Pediatrics*. 2014;133(1):55–62.
22. Patra K, Wilson-Costello D, Taylor HG, et al. Grades I-II intraventricular hemorrhage in extremely low birth weight infants: Effects on neurodevelopment. *J Pediatr*. 2006;149(2):169–173.
23. O'Shea TM, Allred EN, Kuban KC, et al. Intraventricular hemorrhage and developmental outcomes at 24 months of age in extremely preterm infants. *J Child Neurol*. 2012;27(1):22–29.
24. Klebermass-Schrehof K, Czaba C, Olischar M, et al. Impact of low-grade intraventricular hemorrhage on long-term

neurodevelopmental outcome in preterm infants. *Childs Nerv Sys.* 2012;28(12):2085–2092.

25. Adams-Chapman I, Hansen NI, Stoll BJ, et al. Neurodevelopmental outcome of extremely low birth weight infants with posthemorrhagic hydrocephalus requiring shunt insertion. *Pediatrics.* 2008;121(5):e1167–e1177.

26. Brouwer AJ, van Stam C, Uniken Venema M, et al. Cognitive and neurological outcome at the age of 5–8 years of preterm infants with post-hemorrhagic ventricular dilatation requiring neurosurgical intervention. *Neonatology.* 2012;101(3):210–216.

27. Kuban KC, Allred EN, O'Shea TM, et al. Cranial ultrasound lesions in the NICU predict cerebral palsy at age 2 years in children born at extremely low gestational age. *J Child Neurol.* 2009;24(1):63–72.

28. Woodward LJ, Anderson PJ, Austin NC, et al. Neonatal MRI to predict neurodevelopmental outcomes in preterm infants. *N Engl J Med.* 2006;355(7):685–694.

29. Woodward LJ, Clark CA, Bora S, et al. Neonatal white matter abnormalities an important predictor of neurocognitive outcome for very preterm children. *PLoS One.* 2012;7(12):e51879.

30. Hintz SR, Barnes PD, Bulas D, et al. Neuroimaging and neurodevelopmental outcome in extremely preterm infants. *Pediatrics.* 2015;135(1):e32–e42.

31. Kuban KC, O'Shea TM, Allred EN, et al. The breadth and type of systemic inflammation and the risk of adverse neurological outcomes in extremely low gestation newborns. *Pediatr Neurol.* 2015;52(1):42–48.

32. Back SA, Rosenberg PA. Pathophysiology of glia in perinatal white matter injury. *Glia.* 2014;62(11):1790–1815.

33. de Jong M, Verhoeven M, van Baar AL. School outcome, cognitive functioning, and behaviour problems in moderate and late preterm children and adults: A review. *Semin Fetal Neonatal Med.* 2012;17(3):163–169.

34. Kugelman A, Colin AA. Late preterm infants: Near term but still in a critical developmental time period. *Pediatrics.* 2013;132(4):741–751.

35. Adams-Chapman I. Neurodevelopmental outcome of the late preterm infant. *Clin Perinatol.* 2006;33(4):947–964; abstract xi.

36. Baron IS, Litman FR, Ahronovich MD, et al. Late preterm birth: A review of medical and neuropsychological childhood outcomes. *Neuropsychol Rev.* 2012;22(4):438–450.

37. Kapellou O, Counsell SJ, Kennea N, et al Abnormal cortical development after premature birth shown by altered allometric scaling of brain growth. *PLoS Med.* 2006;3(8):e265.

38. Chyi LJ, Lee HC, Hintz SR, et al. School outcomes of late preterm infants: Special needs and challenges for infants born at 32 to 36 weeks gestation. *J Pediatr.* 2008;153(1):25–31.

39. Gray RF, Indurkhya A, McCormick MC. Prevalence, stability, and predictors of clinically significant behavior problems in low birth weight children at 3, 5, and 8 years of age. *Pediatrics.* 2004;114(3):736–743.

40. Huddy CL, Johnson A, Hope PL. Educational and behavioural problems in babies of 32-35 weeks gestation. *Arch Dis Child Fetal Neonatal Ed.* 2001;85(1):F23–F28.

41. Woythaler MA, McCormick MC, Smith VC. Late preterm infants have worse 24-month neurodevelopmental outcomes than term infants. *Pediatrics.* 2011;127(3):2009–3598.

42. Morse SB, Zheng H, Tang Y, et al. Early school-age outcomes of late preterm infants. *Pediatrics.* 2009;123(4):e622–e629.

43. Lipkind HS, Slopen ME, Pfeiffer MR, et al. School-age outcomes of late preterm infants in New York City. *Am J Obstet Gynecol.* 2012;206(3):e1–e6.

44. Quigley MA, Poulsen G, Boyle E, et al. Early term and late preterm birth are associated with poorer school performance at age 5 years: A cohort study. *Arch Dis Child Fetal Neonatal Ed.* 2012;97(3):F167–F173.

45. Talge NM, Holzman C, Wang J, et al. Late-preterm birth and its association with cognitive and socioemotional outcomes at 6 years of age. *Pediatrics.* 2010;126(6):1124–1131.

46. Odd DE, Emond A, Whitelaw A. Long-term cognitive outcomes of infants born moderately and late preterm. *Dev Med Child Neurol.* 2012;54(8):704–709.

47. Gurka MJ, LoCasale-Crouch J, Blackman JA. Long-term cognition, achievement, socioemotional, and behavioral development of healthy late-preterm infants. *Arch Pediatr Adolesc Med.* 2010;164(6):525–532.

48. Anderson PJ, De Luca CR, Hutchinson E, et al. Underestimation of developmental delay by the new Bayley-III Scale. *Arch Pediatr Adolesc Med.* 164(4):352–356.

49. Council on Children With Disabilities, Section on Developmental Behavioral Pediatrics, Bright Futures Steering Committee, et al. Identifying infants and young children with developmental disorders in the medical home: An algorithm for developmental surveillance and screening. *Pediatrics.* 2006;118(1):405–420.

50. Rosenbaum P, Paneth N, Leviton A, et al. A report: The definition and classification of cerebral palsy April 2006. *Dev Med Child Neurol Suppl.* 2007;109:8–14.

51. Palisano R, Rosenbaum P, Walter S, et al. Development and reliability of a system to classify gross motor function in children with cerebral palsy. *Dev Med Child Neurol.* 1997;39(4):214–223.

52. O'Shea TM. Diagnosis, treatment, and prevention of cerebral palsy. *Clin Obstet Gynecol.* 2008;51(4):816–828.

53. Surveillance of Cerebral Palsy in Europe (SCPE). Surveillance of cerebral palsy in Europe: A collaboration of cerebral palsy surveys and registers. Surveillance of Cerebral Palsy in Europe (SCPE). *Dev Med Child Neurol.* 2000;42(12):816–824.

54. Himpens E, Van den Broeck C, Oostra A, et al. Prevalence, type, distribution, and severity of cerebral palsy in relation to gestational age: A meta-analytic review. *Dev Med Child Neurol.* 2008;50(5):334–340.

55. Gaynor JW, Stopp C, Wypij D, et al. Neurodevelopmental outcomes after cardiac surgery in infancy. *Pediatrics.* 2015;135(5):816–825.

56. Andropoulos DB, Hunter JV, Nelson DP, et al. Brain immaturity is associated with brain injury before and after neonatal cardiac surgery with high-flow bypass and cerebral oxygenation monitoring. *J Thorac Cardiovasc Surg.* 2010;139(3):543–556.

57. Licht, DJ, MD, Shera DM, Clancy RR, et al. Brain maturation is delayed in infants with complex congenital heart defects. *J Thorac Cardiovasc Surg.* 2009;137(3):529–536;discussion 536–537.

58. Limperopoulos C, Tworetzky W, McElhinney DB, et al. Brain volume and metabolism in fetuses with congenital heart

disease: Evaluation with quantitative magnetic resonance imaging and spectroscopy. *Circulation.* 2010;121(1):26–33.

59. Miller SP, Ferriero DM, Leonard C, et al. Early brain injury in premature newborns detected with magnetic resonance imaging is associated with adverse early neurodevelopmental outcome. *J Pediatr.* 2005;147(5):609–616.

60. Licht, DJ, Wang J, Silvestre DW, et al. Preoperative cerebral blood flow is diminished in neonates with severe congenital heart defects. *J Thorac Cardiovasc Surg.* 2004;128(6):841–849.

61. Beca, J, Gunn JK, Coleman L, et al. New white matter brain injury after infant heart surgery is associated with diagnostic group and the use of circulatory arrest. *Circulation.* 2013; 127(9):971–979.

62. Roberts G, Anderson PJ, De Luca C, et al. Changes in neurodevelopmental outcome at age eight in geographic cohorts of children born at 22–27 weeks' gestational age during the 1990 s. *Arch Dis Child Fetal Neonatal Ed.* 2010;95(2):F90–F94.

63. Charkaluk ML, Truffert P, Fily A, et al Neurodevelopment of children born very preterm and free of severe disabilities: The Nord-Pas de Calais Epipage cohort study. *Acta Paediatr.* 2010;99(5):684–689.

64. Leversen KT, Sommerfelt K, Elgen IB, et al. Prediction of outcome at 5 years from assessments at 2 years among extremely preterm children: A Norwegian national cohort study. *Acta Paediatr.* 2012;101(3):264–270.

65. Jacobs SE, Berg M, Hunt R, et al. Cooling for newborns with hypoxic ischaemic encephalopathy. *Cochrane Database Syst Rev.* 2013;1:CD003311.

66. Shankaran S, Pappas A, McDonald SA, et al. Childhood outcomes after hypothermia for neonatal encephalopathy. *N Engl J Med.* 2012;366(22):2085–2092.

67. Shankaran S, Laptook AR, Ehrenkranz RA, et al. Whole-body hypothermia for neonates with hypoxic–ischemic encephalopathy. *N Engl J Med.* 2005;353(15):1574–1584.

68. Tagin MA, Woolcott CG, Vincer MJ, et al. Hypothermia for neonatal hypoxic ischemic encephalopathy: An updated systematic review and meta-analysis. *Arch Pediatr Adolesc Med.* 2012;166(6):558–566.

69. Johnson D, Wilkie AO. Craniosynostosis. *Eur J Hum Genet.* 2011;19(4):369–376.

70. Rozé JC, Darmaun D, Boquien CY, et al. The apparent breast-feeding paradox in very preterm infants: Relationship between breast feeding, early weight gain and neurodevelopment based on results from two cohorts, EPIPAGE and LIFT. *BMJ Open.* 2012;2(2):e000834.

71. Vohr BR, Poindexter BB, Dusick AM, et al Beneficial effects of breast milk in the neonatal intensive care unit on the developmental outcome of extremely low birth weight infants at 18 months of age. *Pediatrics.* 2006;118(1):e115–e123.

72. Vohr BR, Poindexter BB, Dusick AM, et al. Persistent beneficial effects of breast milk ingested in the neonatal intensive care unit on outcomes of extremely low birth weight infants at 30 months of age. *Pediatrics.* 2007;120(4): e953–e959.

73. Anderson JW, Johnstone BM, Remley DT, et al. Breast-feeding and cognitive development: A meta-analysis. *Am J Clin Nutr.* 1999;70(4):525–535.

74. Section on Breastfeeding. Breastfeeding and the use of human milk. *Pediatrics.* 2012;129(3):e827–e841.

75. Kramer MS, Chalmers B, Hodnett ED, et al. Promotion of Breastfeeding Intervention Trial (PROBIT): A randomized trial in the Republic of Belarus. *JAMA.* 2001;285(4):413–420.

Chapter 17
PEDIATRIC SURGERY
Sarah J. Hill, MD and Matthew S. Clifton, MD, FACS, FAAP

CASE 1

You are called to the delivery room to evaluate an infant who was delivered 2 minutes ago and is having respiratory distress. The patient's mother is 17 years old and did not receive prenatal care. On your examination, the neonate is hypotonic and apneic despite nursing attempts of nasal suctioning and stimulation. You immediately intubate the baby and initiate transport to the NICU. Once you reach the ICU, a chest film is ordered (Fig. 17-1) and an ABG is sent with the following results:

ABG: pH 6.8, pCO_2 130, pO_2 18

Given the scenario and imaging above, which of the following is true about the suspected diagnosis?
A. Identifying the presence of an arterial blood vessel to the lesion prior to surgical repair is critical
B. iNO and milrinone are sometimes used to improve the hemodynamics of children with this diagnosis
C. The diagnosis could not have been made prenatally as it is most likely a result of birth trauma
D. The pathology is more commonly found on the right side

Discussion

The correct answer is **B**. This clinical scenario and image most likely represents a congenital diaphragmatic hernia (CDH). The embryogenesis of the diaphragm occurs between weeks 9 and 12. The majority (80%) of CDHs are found on the left side. Two main issues – pulmonary hypertension and pulmonary hypoplasia – affect neonates with CDH to varying degrees and determine outcome. Treatment of pulmonary hypertension is aimed at improving inotropy and decreasing the pulmonary vascular

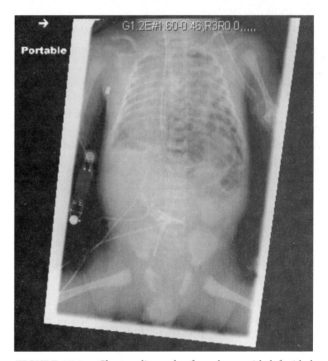

FIGURE 17-1. Chest radiograph of newborn with left-sided congenital diaphragmatic hernia.

resistance. This is accomplished with administration of vasoactive medications including inhaled nitric oxide and milrinone. Limited data are available regarding the short or long term benefits of these medications in patients with CDH.

The presence of a systemic blood vessel in a cystic lung malformation implies that the lesion is a sequestration. Given the baby's significant respiratory distress and radiographic findings, this diagnosis is less likely. Meconium aspiration could cause the respiratory distress that is presented here, however the x-ray findings do not correspond with that diagnosis.

The baby is started on iNO and transitioned to a high-frequency oscillator ventilator. Despite this, the baby has persistent respiratory failure. Discussion is held with the team regarding the possibility of transitioning the infant to ECMO.

Which of the following patients would be the most appropriate candidate for ECMO cannulation?
A. 2.8-kg, 36-week EGA infant with a grade I intraventricular hemorrhage and persistent respiratory distress. Echocardiogram shows significant pulmonary hypertension without structural cardiac abnormality. The infant is receiving mechanical ventilation on the high-frequency oscillator with mean airway pressure of 25, amplitude 30, and F_IO_2 100%. Follow-up ABG after maximal ventilator support: pH 7.32, pCO_2 34, pO_2 35
B. 1.8-kg, 31-week EGA infant with a grade I intraventricular hemorrhage and persistent respiratory distress. Follow-up ABG after maximal ventilator support: pH 7.32, pCO_2 34, pO_2 155
C. 2.6-kg, 38-week EGA infant with a no evidence of intraventricular hemorrhage and persistent respiratory distress. Echocardiogram shows total anomalous pulmonary venous return with mild to moderate pulmonary hypertension. Follow-up ABG after maximal ventilator support: pH 7.02, pCO_2 93, pO_2 40
D. 2.3-kg, 36-week EGA infant with a grade III intraventricular hemorrhage and persistent respiratory distress. Follow-up ABG after maximal ventilator support: pH 7.32, pCO_2 34, pO_2 155

Discussion

The correct answer is **A**. ECMO is often considered in appropriate neonates who have refractory respiratory distress secondary to a CDH. One consideration for determining necessity for ECMO is the oxygenation index (OI), which is calculated as follows:

$$O.I. = \frac{F_IO_2 * MAP}{P_aO_2}$$

where MAP = mean airway pressure.

Center-specific criteria exist to determine patient suitability for ECMO, but in general an OI in the range of 35 to 40 despite maximal medical therapy warrants consideration for this intervention. The following *exclusion* criteria should generally be utilized when evaluating a patient for ECMO:

i. Irreversible lung disease
ii. Birth weight <2 kg
iii. Gestational age <34 weeks
iv. Major (grade II or greater) intracranial hemorrhage
v. Lethal congenital anomalies (including uncorrectable cardiac anomalies)

Which of the following is true regarding surgical intervention for congenital diaphragmatic hernia?
A. Patients should be emergently taken to surgery for definitive treatment, on or off ECMO
B. Patients should have a chest tube for several days after surgery to ensure the lung remains fully expanded
C. Because of the high incidence of gastroesophageal reflux disease, surgeons will frequently recommend fundoplication at the time of definitive treatment
D. Regardless of the size of the defect, surgical recommendations include the use of a synthetic patch to reinforce the repair
E. None of the above

Discussion

The correct answer is **E**. The timing of CDH repair has been debated over the last decade, with recent studies showing improved survival benefit by delaying repair of the diaphragm until after the pulmonary hypertension is significantly improved and the infant has been decannulated (if ECMO was necessary). Tube thoracostomy in the postoperative setting for CDH is rare. Forcibly expanding the lung in a patient with pulmonary hypoplasia can cause barotrauma in an already compromised lung. An expected obligate pneumothorax exists after diaphragm repair; this fills initially with serous fluid, but over time the lung grows and expands to fill the space in most children. It is true that many neonates with a CDH will have symptomatic gastroesophageal reflux, however many of these patients can be treated medically. Antireflux surgery at the time of CDH repair will be unnecessary in a number of infants. Synthetic (Gore-tex®) or biologic patches (SIS®) are often required in the setting of a large diaphragmatic defect. The goal is to accomplish a tension-free repair, as excess tension has been cited as an underlying cause for recurrent herniation after repair. If a tension-free primary repair can be accomplished, no patch is necessary.

CASE 2

You are called to evaluate a 2-day-old male neonate in the well-baby nursery. The baby is the product of a 38-week gestation pregnancy that was complicated by polyhydramnios. Per nursing reports, the baby coughed and had a small amount of nonbilious emesis when the mother attempted to breast feed the child. On your examination, he is a normal appearing, term infant in no apparent distress. You note a faint holosystolic murmur, but the remainder of your examination is nonrevealing.

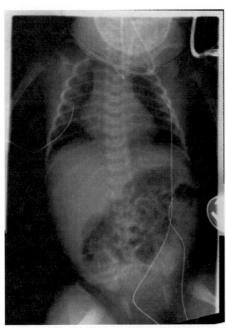

FIGURE 17-2. Chest/abdomen radiograph of newborn with esophageal atresia and a distal tracheoesophageal fistula. Note the radiopaque tube terminating in the proximal pouch. Gas in the intestinal tract indicates a fistula between the airway and distal esophagus.

Given this history, what would *not* be on your differential diagnosis?
A. Annular pancreas
B. Duodenal atresia
C. Esophageal atresia
D. Ileal atresia

Discussion

The correct answer is **D**. The clinical scenario described appears to represent a proximal bowel obstruction. It is highly unlikely that an ileal atresia would cause non-bilious emesis. The remaining three answers (annular pancreas, duodenal atresia and esophageal atresia) are all proximal obstructions that can result in nonbilious emesis.

As part of your initial work-up, you place a soft orogastric tube and obtain a chest/abdomen x-ray. See Figure 17-2.

Which of the following tests or procedures would *not* be appropriate during the further work-up of this child?
A. Echocardiogram
B. MRI of chest
C. Renal ultrasound
D. A "gap-o-gram"
E. Prone positioning of the infant

Discussion

The correct answer is **B**. The chest x-ray confirms the suspected diagnosis, esophageal atresia (EA). The tube terminates in the proximal esophageal pouch. Air in the intestinal tract indicates the presence of a distal tracheoesophageal fistula (TEF). Several classification systems for EA exist; the most commonly used is the Gross classification. According to this schema, patients are described as: Type A (pure EA, no TEF), Type B (proximal TEF, distal EA), Type C (proximal EA, distal TEF), Type D (proximal and distal TEF), and Type E (H-type fistula, with patent esophagus and coexistent TEF). The majority of patients are accounted for by Type C (85%) and Type A (10%) anatomy. The TEF in Type C patients is typically located at the carina, making it impossible to pass an endotracheal tube past the fistula, a common mistake/misperception by anesthesiology teams. See Figure 17-3.

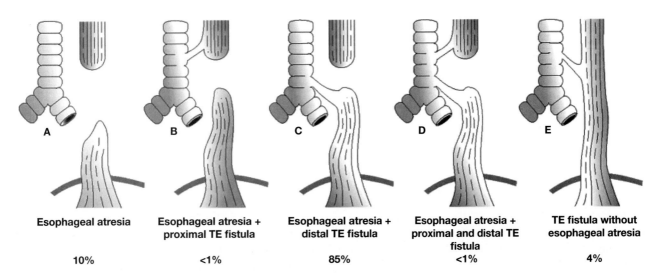

A	B	C	D	E
Esophageal atresia	**Esophageal atresia + proximal TE fistula**	**Esophageal atresia + distal TE fistula**	**Esophageal atresia + proximal and distal TE fistula**	**TE fistula without esophageal atresia**
10%	<1%	85%	<1%	4%

FIGURE 17-3. Diagram of various types of tracheoesophageal fistulas.

As a part of the VACTERL association, appropriate work-up would include an echocardiogram and renal ultrasound, as these anomalies should be identified prior to surgical intervention. Vertebral anomalies are not immediately life-threatening, thus further work-up to evaluate for abnormalities is not warranted at this time.

A "gap-o-gram" or "gag-o-gram" can be performed by gently placing a rigid tube with radiopaque markings into the esophageal pouch while applying gentle pressure on the tube during an x-ray of the chest and abdomen. This allows the surgeon to estimate the gap between the esophageal pouch and the distal esophagus. Films can be taken in the AP or lateral position to accurately estimate length. In the instance of a long-gap atresia, a delay in anastomosis may be necessary to allow time to increase the proximal pouch length. If a distal TEF is present in these patients, they should still be taken to the operating room in the first 1 to 2 days of life for ligation of the fistula.

Prone positioning of neonates with EA and distal TEF can lessen reflux and minimize soilage of the lungs from gastric fluid until fistula ligation can be performed.

After the work-up is complete, the baby is taken to the operating room for surgical repair. On postoperative day 5, the nurse notes that there is a small amount of frothy, clear fluid draining from the chest tube.

What is the most likely explanation for this finding?
A. A missed ileal atresia
B. Aspiration pneumonia
C. A leak of the esophageal anastomosis
D. A missed tracheoesophageal fistula
E. Injury to the thoracic duct resulting in chylothorax

Discussion

The correct answer is **C**. Drainage of saliva from the chest tube after an esophageal atresia repair is worrisome for an anastomotic leak. This can be confirmed by a contrast esophagram. A missed ileal atresia would present with high-volume bilious output from the orogastric tube. Aspiration pneumonia would present with increased secretions from the endotracheal tube rather than the chest tube. A second, missed tracheoesophageal fistula would be more likely to present with coughing and sputtering during oral feeding. This would escape detection in the early postoperative period while the baby remains NPO. Chylothorax is typically suspected when a high-volume effusion persists; it can be clear or cloudy in nature. The diagnosis can be confirmed by a differential cell count showing >80% lymphocytes or a triglyceride content >100 mg/dL.

CASE 3

As the staff physician for the nursery, you are presented with a 3.7-kg, 1-hour-old girl in no apparent distress. According to the mother, she had an ultrasound at 21 weeks gestation that showed a lesion in her lung. The baby is clinically asymptomatic; however, a chest x-ray demonstrates a large cystic lesion on the left.

At this point your differential diagnosis includes all of the following, *except*?
A. Congenital lobar emphysema
B. Pulmonary sequestration
C. CCAM/CPAM
D. Congenital diaphragmatic hernia
E. A large pneumothorax

Discussion

The correct answer is **E**. With the exception of a pneumothorax, each answer listed can present as a cystic pulmonary lesion on chest radiograph. Congenital lobar emphysema is thought to result from a focal cartilaginous deficiency leading to airway collapse with expiration. This causes air trapping, leading to emphysematous distention which may appear cystic on chest radiograph. Pulmonary sequestrations are portions of pulmonary tissue without direct connection to the bronchial tree. Sequestrations have an anomalous systemic blood supply and can be intralobar or extralobar depending on their position relative to the visceral pleural membrane. A congenital cystic adenomatoid malformation (CCAM) or congenital pulmonary airway malformation (CPAM) is often identified in prenatal screening but asymptomatic at birth. Although CCAM/CPAMs typically receive their blood supply from the pulmonary vessels, there are case reports of hybrid lesions which retain features of both CCAM/CPAM and sequestration. Small bowel in the thoracic space as seen with a congenital diaphragmatic hernia can be mistaken for a cystic pulmonary lesion. Most patients with CDH that are not diagnosed prenatally are discovered after delivery because of tachypnea. The degree of associated lung hypoplasia is not always predicted by the size of the diaphragm defect. A small number of patients are relatively asymptomatic, likely due to a mild degree of pulmonary hypoplasia. It would be unlikely for the child to be completely asymptomatic, but an UGI study would demonstrate filling of the intestine cephalad to the diaphragm, confirming the diagnosis.

Which of the following is the most appropriate next step?
A. CT angiogram
B. Abdominal ultrasound

C. Emergent tube thoracostomy

D. Intubation

E. Pulmonary function testing

Discussion

The correct answer is **A**. In this stable patient, an emergent chest tube or intubation is not necessary. Rather, this patient likely has a sequestration or CCAM/CPAM, which should be appropriately evaluated prior to intervention. A CT angiogram is typically performed in order to distinguish between these two diagnoses. Knowledge of a systemic vascular supply is critical for preoperative planning. Sequestration vessels typically arise from the abdominal aorta. If improperly controlled when a thoracic approach is used, there is a risk of the vessel retracting into the abdomen, leading to significant hemorrhage and potentially death.

Which of the following is not correctly paired with the appropriate timing for planned surgical intervention?

A. CCAM: delay operative intervention until >3 to 6 months of age

B. CDH: delay operative intervention until pulmonary hypertension improved

C. Sequestration: delay operative intervention until >3 to 6 months of age

D. Congenital pulmonary emphysema: delay operative intervention until >3 to 6 months of age

E. Pneumothorax: immediate tube thoracostomy

Discussion

The correct answer is **D**. There should not be a delay in surgical intervention for congenital lobar emphysema once the diagnosis is made. Failure to intervene early can lead to overdistension of the affected segment as the abnormal cartilage creates a "ball-valve" effect. This can cause mediastinal shift and cardiovascular collapse if left unchecked. Both CCAM/CPAMs and sequestrations can be performed once the child has grown at home for several months. They typically require lobectomy, and can be approached via an open thoracotomy or minimally invasive thoracoscopic technique.

True or False: Neonates with a prenatally diagnosed cystic pulmonary lesion who have a postnatal chest x-ray that does not demonstrate a lesion can be followed by serial clinical examinations and require no additional imaging.

A. True

B. False

Discussion

The correct answer is **B**. The absence of findings on a chest x-ray does not indicate the absence of a congenital lung lesion. CT angiogram of the chest is used to characterize any lesion that was noted prenatally. The current recommendation includes surgical resection of asymptomatic lesions, primarily because of the risk for recurrent pulmonary infections in the abnormal lung segment. Additionally, there is a risk of malignant degeneration. Pleuropulmonary blastoma and bronchoalveolar carcinoma have been reported in patients with known CCAMs/CPAMs.

CASE 4

You are asked to evaluate an ex-35-week premature male infant who is now 2 weeks old with new onset bilious emesis. The hospital chart indicates that the neonate required high flow oxygen for the first 24 hours of life and subsequently weaned to room air. He passed meconium within the first 24 hours of life and has been fed via a nasogastric tube without difficulty for the last 12 days. The nursing staff reports that the patient is slated for discharge in the morning. On your examination, the baby has a soft, round abdomen that is nontender. Laboratory values are unremarkable. An abdominal film is obtained (Fig. 17-4).

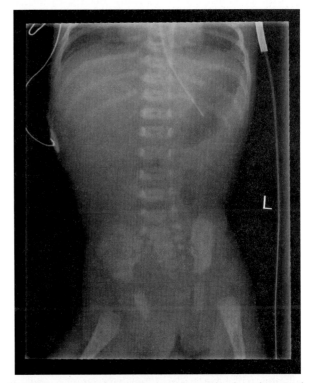

FIGURE 17-4. Chest/abdomen radiograph of newborn with malrotation. Note the paucity of distal gas. The presence of any gas beyond a "double bubble" with concomitant bilious emesis should raise suspicion for malrotation and midgut volvulus.

Given this history and radiograph, which of the following diagnoses is the most likely?
A. Hirschsprung disease
B. Malrotation with midgut volvulus
C. Ileal atresia
D. Pyloric stenosis
E. Meconium ileus

Discussion

The correct answer is **B**. Malrotation with midgut volvulus is a surgical emergency that classically presents with bilious emesis. As this is a proximal obstruction, patients will not typically manifest abdominal distension. Between 50% and 75% of patients with malrotation will become symptomatic during the first month of life. Hirschsprung disease is manifested by aganglionosis of the intestine, typically affecting distal colon (most commonly rectosigmoid), and usually presents with failure to pass meconium in the first 24 hours of life. A radiograph of a patient with Hirschsprung disease typically shows multiple dilated loops of intestine as a result of the functional distal obstruction. Congenital obstructions such as ileal atresia would likely present earlier in the patient's life, but would similarly demonstrate multiple dilated loops of intestine on abdominal x-ray. By definition, pyloric stenosis patients will present with nonbilious emesis. This typically occurs in infants between 2 and 8 weeks of life. Meconium ileus can present in a healthy appearing infant with a distended abdomen and a paucity of distal gas, but these babies will have difficulty with passage of meconium during the first 48 hours of life.

What is the most appropriate next test for this patient?
A. Barium enema
B. Suction rectal biopsy
C. Upper gastrointestinal contrast study
D. Abdominal CT scan
E. Doppler ultrasound to evaluate orientation of superior mesenteric vessels

Discussion

The correct answer is **C**. The gold standard for evaluation of intestinal malrotation is an upper gastrointestinal series whereby the duodenum is visualized to pass into the retroperitoneum, cross the midline, and the duodenal–jejunal junction (the ligament of Treitz) is noted at the level of the gastric antrum on the patient's left side. The contrast on an UGI in the setting of malrotation and volvulus will have a "corkscrew" appearance, and the intestine will not cross midline (Fig. 17-5). Despite a stable appearing patient, this study should be performed emergently. Delays in diagnosis and operative correction

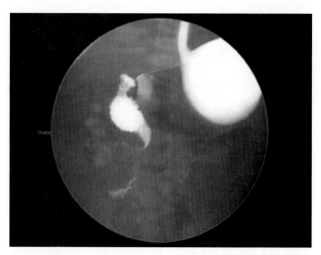

FIGURE 17-5. Upper GI contrast study of a patient with malrotation and midgut volvulus. The contrast has the typical "corkscrew" pattern that is pathognomonic for this problem.

can lead to total intestinal necrosis with potentially devastating outcomes. Ultrasound and CT scan can also be used to diagnose intestinal malrotation, as the position of the superior mesenteric artery relative to the superior mesenteric vein may be notably switched. However, these imaging modalities have neither the sensitivity nor specificity to accurately diagnose midgut volvulus.

Which of the following is true?
A. Patients with malrotation rarely have associated congenital anomalies
B. Normal intestinal rotation and fixation occurs between gestational weeks 15 to 20
C. Operative treatment for midgut volvulus typically includes a clockwise detorsion of the small bowel and a Ladd procedure
D. Recurrent volvulus is a potential complication following surgical treatment of malrotation

Discussion

The correct answer is D. Patients with malrotation have an increased risk of recurrent volvulus compared to the general population. Additional congenital anomalies are seen in half of patients with malrotation. The most frequent associated malformations are intestinal atresias or cardiac anomalies. The frequency of atresias is likely related to an intestinal ischemic event during incomplete rotation. Intestinal rotation occurs in the first trimester, between gestational weeks 5 and 10. During this time, the intestines herniate out of the peritoneal cavity into the umbilical cord. As the intestines return into the abdominal cavity at week 10, the cecocolic limb rotates a total of 270 degrees counterclockwise around the SMA. The final step in this process is fixation of the cecum and the duodenojejunal junction to the posterior abdominal wall. Because of this complex rotation, patients with volvulus typically require counterclockwise detorsion, followed by lysis of adhesions between the duodenum and the cecum (the so-called "Ladd bands"). This detorsion and mesenteric broadening allows for return of blood flow to the intestine and decreases the likelihood of a recurrent volvulus. Because the cecum will ultimately lie on the left side of the abdomen, an appendectomy is also routinely performed at the time of surgery so as to prevent confusion if abdominal pain occurs in the future.

CASE 5

You are called to evaluate an ex-28-week premature infant that is now 3 weeks old. The neonate has been tolerating enteric feeds which have been steadily advanced for the past 2 weeks with regular bowel movements. The nurse notes that the infant has started having occasional episodes of bradycardia and high gastric residuals. On your examination the baby's abdomen is protuberant with slight erythematous discoloration. You request an abdominal film, shown in Figure 17-6.

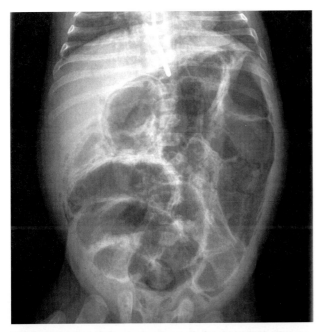

FIGURE 17-6. Abdominal radiograph demonstrating pneumatosis intestinalis.

What is the suspected diagnosis?
A. Malrotation
B. Ileal atresia
C. Necrotizing enterocolitis
D. Pyloric stenosis
E. Meconium ileus

Discussion

The correct answer is **C**. This clinical scenario is typical of necrotizing enterocolitis (NEC). Early signs of NEC are nonspecific and include physiologic abnormalities (temperature instability, bradycardia, hypotension) and feeding intolerance. The biggest risk factor for the development of NEC is related to prematurity—90% of cases occur in preterm infants, typically around 31 to 32 weeks corrected gestational age.

Which of the following is an absolute indication for operative intervention in this situation?
A. Pneumoperitoneum
B. Portal venous gas
C. Worsening metabolic acidosis
D. Pneumatosis intestinalis
E. Paracentesis yielding clear, yellow fluid

Discussion

The correct answer is **A**. Pneumoperitoneum is an absolute indication for surgical intervention. The remaining answers are relative indications for surgical consideration; alone, they do not necessitate an operative exploration.

You take the baby to the operating room and perform a laparotomy where you find that the distal 1/3 of the small bowel and the cecum are necrotic. You perform a resection with a diverting ostomy and mucous fistula.

Which of the following long-term issues is *not* a concern for this patient?
A. Rapid transit of intestinal contents and the need for long-term parenteral nutrition
B. Chronic pancreatitis
C. Vitamin A deficiency
D. Development of pernicious anemia
E. Neurodevelopmental delay

Discussion

The correct answer is **B**. There does not appear to be any increased risk for pancreatitis in patients with a history of small bowel resection for NEC. With the loss of a significant portion of their small bowel, there is an increased risk for rapid transit of intestinal contents. The preservation of the ileocecal valve and the percentage of remaining small bowel compared to the age-adjusted length of residual bowel are both independent predictors of infants who will fail at weaning parenteral nutrition. In this situation, refeeding of the proximal ostomy output into the mucous fistula may be considered to allow for increased resorption of fluid, electrolytes, and nutrients.

The terminal ileum is important for absorption of intrinsic factor (released by the parietal cells of the stomach) and vitamin B_{12}. After a significant portion of distal small bowel is resected, the patient can develop pernicious anemia. Without the distal small bowel, resorption of fat-soluble vitamins (vitamins A, D, E, and K) can be limited as well. Deficiencies of these vitamins can lead to altered vision, osteomalacia, myopathies, and bleeding dyscrasias.

Children with surgical NEC have a significantly higher rate of neurodevelopmental delay compared to similar gestational age premature infants who have a history of medical NEC or no NEC. This may be a result of severe physiologic stress that occurs during a critical period of development. It is unclear whether infants managed with laparotomy or peritoneal drainage will have a difference in neurodevelopmental outcomes. Research studies are ongoing to investigate this question.

CASE 6

A newborn baby boy is transferred to your NICU for evaluation. He was diagnosed prenatally with trisomy 21 via amniocentesis. Prenatal ultrasound detected a congenital heart defect and was also notable for polyhydramnios and a distended, fluid-filled stomach. He had several episodes of nonbilious emesis at the referring hospital after an initial feeding attempt and his abdominal radiograph is shown here (Fig. 17-7).

Which of the following statements is true?
A. Nonbilious emesis only occurs when an obstruction is proximal to the pylorus
B. The patient has a 40% to 50% likelihood of a concomitant distal atresia
C. Most patients with duodenal atresia present with nonbilious emesis
D. Additional air in the intestinal tract distal to the "double bubble" warrants an UGI to distinguish between malrotation and duodenal web
E. Echocardiogram should be deferred until after the intestinal obstruction is surgically repaired

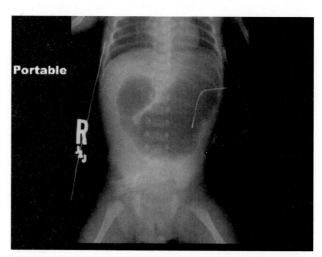

FIGURE 17-7. Abdominal radiograph in an infant with duodenal atresia showing characteristic finding of a "double bubble."

Discussion

The correct answer is **D**. The majority of patients with duodenal atresia (85%) have an obstruction distal to the ampulla of Vater, which results in bilious emesis. Duodenal atresia is thought to occur as a result of failed recanalization of the duodenum during early fetal development. The migration of the dorsal and ventral anlage of the pancreas occurs at the same time, which is felt to be the reason for an association with annular pancreas. An annular pancreas should never be divided, since important ductal structures will be injured in the process. Jejunoileal atresias occur as a result of vascular occlusion—they can occur in the same patient, though it is uncommon. Though restoration of intestinal continuity is important, knowledge of any underlying cardiac dysfunction is critical before commencing with a general anesthetic.

Air located distally in the intestinal tract in the setting of a "double bubble" has several possible diagnoses: duodenal web (which frequently have small holes in the web, allowing passage of gas distally), duodenal stenosis, and malrotation with midgut volvulus. Because malrotation with midgut volvulus is a possibility, stable infants with these radiographic findings should either have an UGI to clarify the diagnosis, or proceed directly to the operating room.

An echocardiogram performed on this patient demonstrates a balanced atrioventricular canal. The infant remains hemodynamically stable. Which of the following statements about surgical repair of this defect is true?
A. Intestinal malrotation that is coexistent with duodenal atresia should be addressed with a future operation, after intestinal continuity is restored

B. A duodenal web should be treated by complete web excision and transverse closure of the duodenotomy

C. Tapering duodenoplasty and gastrostomy tube should be performed in all patients with duodenal atresia and trisomy 21

D. Postoperative bilious output from a nasogastric tube is indicative of early postoperative anastomotic stricture

E. Laparoscopic repair with duodenoduodenostomy can be performed safely in this setting

Discussion

The correct answer is **E**. Intestinal malrotation can occur in conjunction with duodenal atresia, and if so should be addressed with a Ladd procedure at the same time at the atresia repair. The distal common bile duct and ampulla of Vater will frequently be contained within the substance of a duodenal web. Consequently, only the lateral portion of the web should be excised if this is the approach taken to address the problem. Complete web excision may lead to injury to the distal common bile duct.

The proximal portion of the duodenum in this setting is quite dilated and thick walled, and oftentimes the pylorus has become incompetent because of a long-standing distal obstruction. Nasogastric output is commonly bilious for the first several weeks after repair because of pyloric incompetence, and does not indicate a stricture. Tapering duodenoplasty is typically reserved for those infants in whom a repair proves inadequate and there is chronic atony of the proximal duodenal segment. Neither tapering nor gastrostomy tube are universally indicated for this patient population, though they are sometimes necessary. Laparoscopic repair of duodenal atresia has been described extensively, and can be performed safely, even in patients with congenital heart disease. However, this is best reserved for hospitals that have expertise in the anesthetic management of neonatal cardiac disease and surgeons trained in advanced, minimally invasive surgery.

CASE 7

You are called by a referring NICU to give advice on management for a newborn that is 36 hours old. The baby boy was born at term to Caucasian parents. Apgar's were 7 and 9. He has fed poorly since birth, has voided, but has not yet passed meconium. On physical examination the infant is well appearing. The abdomen is distended but soft and nontender, with no discoloration. There is a patent anus.

Which of the following is *not* in the differential diagnosis?

A. Hirschsprung disease
B. Malrotation with midgut volvulus
C. Meconium ileus
D. Congenital small left colon
E. Distal ileal atresia

Discussion

The correct answer is **B**. All of the other choices represent distal intestinal obstructions, which will characteristically result in a distended abdomen. Malrotation with midgut volvulus results in an obstruction at the second portion of the duodenum; consequently, the obstruction is proximal and infants are not distended. Distension can occur if the entire midgut becomes necrotic. However, the baby would likely have a discolored abdomen and be profoundly ill appearing.

An abdominal x-ray is done which demonstrates multiple dilated loops of small bowel with calcifications in the right lower quadrant.

What is the next step in management?

A. Water-soluble contrast enema
B. Sweat test
C. Send genetic testing for $\Delta F508$
D. Surgical consultation for laparotomy
E. GI consultation for colonoscopy

Discussion

The correct answer is **A**. This patient has findings consistent with meconium ileus. In this disease process, the terminal ileum becomes obstructed with dense, inspissated meconium, causing an intestinal obstruction. In newborns, the presentation is classified as either simple (limited to intestinal obstruction) or complicated (obstruction with an additional component of volvulus, intestinal necrosis and perforation, and/or meconium peritonitis). Since the child is otherwise well appearing and has a benign examination, the next step is to clear the obstruction.

A water-soluble contrast enema using 25% to 50% solution of Gastrografin (meglumine diatrizoate, Bristol-Meyers Squibb, Princeton, NJ) can be diagnostic and therapeutic. Gastrografin is hyperosmolar, causing fluid to shift into the intestinal lumen and soften the meconium. Appropriate fluid resuscitation is critical to ensure the infant does not become dehydrated as a result. A successful enema should reflux into the dilated small bowel. These enemas can be repeated at 6- to 24-hour intervals (as long as no sign of peritonitis occurs), and usually result in passage of meconium within 24 to 48 hours. Complications can include failure to reflux into the dilated intestine and perforation. After the meconium has been evacuated, gastrointestinal secretions can be maintained in a liquid form by administering 5 to 10 mL of a 10% *N*-acetylcysteine solution every 6 hours.

The most common genetic mutation causing cystic fibrosis is ΔF508, located on chromosome 7 in the *CFTR (cystic fibrosis transmembrane regulator)* gene. Sweat chloride testing for cystic fibrosis is not always diagnostic in the first few weeks of life. Laparotomy is reserved for complicated meconium ileus, or simple cases that fail to resolve within 48 hours of Gastrografin enema. Colonoscopy is never indicated as a first step in evaluating a stable newborn with a distal small bowel obstruction.

A water-soluble contrast enema demonstrates a very small caliber colon in its entirety. There is no reflux of contrast into the ileum.

Which of the following statements is *not* true?
A. Surgical management options include laparotomy with Bishop–Koop anastomosis, T-tube placement, or ileostomy and mucous fistula
B. The site of obstruction is the terminal ileum
C. The site of obstruction is the hepatic flexure of the colon
D. Pneumoperitoneum and extravasation of contrast after enema is an indication for laparotomy

Discussion

The correct answer is **C**. The site of obstruction in meconium ileus is the terminal ileum, not the colon. Complicated meconium ileus and perforation after Gastrografin enema are clear indications for surgical exploration. Once a laparotomy is performed, the goal is complete evacuation of the meconium, with ongoing enteral access to prevent recurrence. In a Bishop–Koop enterostomy, the meconium-filled segment of ileum is resected, the distal end brought up to the skin an enterocutaneous fistula, and the proximal end anastomosed to the sidewall of the distal limb (Fig. 17-8). This allows tube access to the distal limb for ongoing postoperative irrigation. Further, as long as a distal obstruction is prevented, intestinal contents will pass into the downstream limb and result in limited output from the stoma. Alternatively, a T tube can be placed intraoperatively through the sidewall of the intestine. It is used to maintain access to the intestine after evacuation of all meconium, and allows postoperative irrigation of the intestine without a stoma. Diversion with an ileostomy and mucous fistula accomplishes similar goals to the Bishop–Koop reconstruction—decompression of the obstruction with ongoing access to the distal limb to prevent ongoing obstruction.

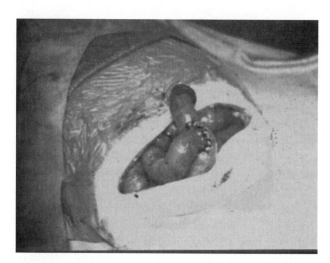

FIGURE 17-8. Bishop–Koop enterostomy.

CASE 8

A baby girl delivers at 38 weeks to a 26-year-old G1P0 mother who had good prenatal care and no abnormalities noted on prenatal ultrasound. The physical examination is normal with the exception of the perineum, which is pictured here (Fig. 17-9).

What is the diagnosis?
A. Imperforate anus with perineal fistula
A. Cloaca
B. Rectovaginal fistula
C. Neonatal Crohn disease
D. Fistula-in-ano

Discussion

The correct answer is **A**. The baby has an absent anus and fistulous connection of the rectum to the perineum in an

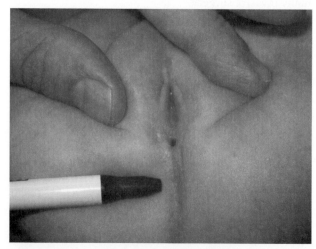

FIGURE 17-9. Photo of newborn girl with fistulous connection of rectum to the perineum.

aberrant location. Cloacal malformations are found in girls and are defined by having a single common channel into which the bladder, vagina, and rectum all converge. Rectovaginal fistulas are exceedingly rare in newborns, and would involve a fistulous connection of the rectum to the vagina deep to the hymenal membrane. Crohn disease typically peaks in the second or third decade of life though it can present at any age, even in the first months of life. Fistula-in-ano is a complication of perirectal abscess formation and is never present in a newborn.

Which of the following statements is true?
A. This baby has a fistula between the rectum and urinary tract that should be divided as soon as possible to stop soilage
B. The baby should be placed prone with the hips elevated for 24 hours. A lateral film should be done to assess the proximity of the rectum to the perineum
C. A sigmoid colostomy and mucous fistula should be performed in the next 24 hours
D. The baby should be repaired within the next day as a single procedure with a posterior sagittal anorectoplasty
E. Central IV access should be obtained and TPN initiated

Discussion

The correct answer is **D**. Anorectal malformations are approached initially based on the presence of an obvious fistula. If no fistula is visible on the perineum, the baby should be placed prone with the hips elevated to allow air in the rectum to rise and reach its most superficial point. Air that nearly reaches the perineum signifies a "low" fistula; however, if air does not reach a point near the perineum, it is difficult to draw conclusions about the nature of the fistula. It could signify a "high" fistula or a "low" fistula with meconium preventing the air from reaching its most distal point.

In the large majority of cases, the presence of a connection to the perineum means that there is no connection to the genitourinary tract more proximally. A colostomy is typically performed when a staged repair is planned for imperforate anus—these are typically the "high" lesions. This baby should be able to begin feeds immediately after the anoplasty. There is no indication to begin hyperalimentation.

CASE 9

A small, community based NICU calls for advice regarding a full-term baby boy that delivered to a G2P1 mother overnight. The baby has an absent anus. Initially, he voided clear urine. About an hour ago, he passed dark black urine. He has had mild grunting and has a harsh, holosystolic murmur on auscultation. He has started nursing and has not vomited.

Which of the following statements is true?
A. This baby has a fistula between the rectum and urinary tract that should be divided sometime during the first week of life to stop soilage
B. The baby should be placed prone with the hips elevated for 24 hours. A lateral film should be done to assess the proximity of the rectum to the perineum
C. A sigmoid colostomy and mucous fistula should be performed in the next 24 hours
D. The baby should be repaired immediately with a posterior sagittal anorectoplasty
E. Central IV access should be obtained and TPN initiated

Discussion

The correct answer is **C**. The decision to perform a colostomy should be made no longer than 24 hours after birth to stop soilage of the urinary tract and prevent perforation of the colon. Since the baby has clearly passed meconium in the urine, it can be assumed that a fistulous connection exists between the rectum and the urinary tract. These are classified as "high" lesions, and require a staged repair. Staged repair entails a sigmoid colostomy and mucous fistula initially. This prevents ongoing soilage of the urinary tract, and provides access to the distal rectum via the mucous fistula. Before performing a definitive pull-through reconstruction, a high-pressure colostogram is performed (with water soluble contrast) which details the exact location of the fistula, facilitates operative planning, and will give an anticipated level of fecal continence long term. Once a colostomy has been performed, the infant can be started on enteral nutrition.

Standard operative approaches for reconstruction after colostomy include PSARP (posterior sagittal anorectoplasty) and laparoscopic pull-through. A newly described modification of the laparoscopic approach utilizes intraoperative magnetic resonance imaging to guide the position of the rectum as it is pulled through the pelvic muscle complex.

What other work-up should be included prior to surgery?
A. Renal ultrasound
B. Echocardiogram
C. Spine MRI
D. Spine ultrasound
E. UGI with SBFT

Discussion

The correct answer is **B**. Of the items listed, the echocardiogram is the most essential before subjecting the child to an anesthetic. Renal and spine ultrasounds can be performed either before or after surgery—neither will affect the decision to perform a colostomy. However, knowing that information preoperatively may allow bundling of procedures under one anesthetic, if necessary.

Renal ultrasound is a critical part of the standard evaluation of patients with anorectal malformations. The likelihood of an infant having an associated urologic anomaly is directly correlated with level of the malformation—the higher the malformation, the more likely an associated urologic anomaly. These range from 20% of patients with perineal fistulas to 90% in the setting of cloacas (female) or rectobladder neck fistulas (male).

Since 25% of patients with anorectal malformations have an associated tethered cord, spine ultrasound is an important part of the neonatal evaluation. Spine MRI can be done as a follow-up to ultrasound if further delineation of the anatomy is necessary. Pelvic radiographs (anterior and lateral views of the sacrum) are important in defining the prognostic outcome in terms of future bowel control. Additionally, they can alert the physician to the presence of a presacral mass, a condition known as Currarino syndrome (defined as triad of sacral anomaly, anorectal malformation, and presacral mass, oftentimes a teratoma or myelomeningocele).

If the child is showing no clinical signs of intestinal obstruction (feeding intolerance, bilious emesis, abdominal distension), then there is no indication to study the patency of the GI tract.

CASE 10

You are a pediatrician called to round on a 2-day-old baby boy in the well-baby nursery that has still not passed meconium. The child was born at 39 weeks via Cesarian with no complications. He has been fed well but is quite distended (Fig. 17-10). The family has two older children who are healthy, but cannot recall if they passed meconium immediately after birth.

Which of the following is *not* included in the differential diagnosis?
A. Meconium ileus
B. Imperforate anus
C. Malrotation
D. Ileal atresia
E. Hirschsprung disease

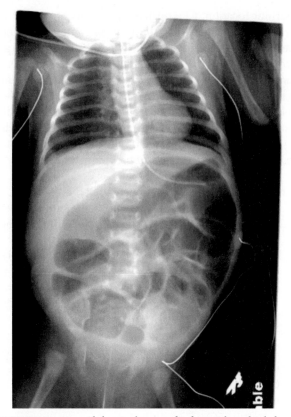

FIGURE 17-10. Abdominal x-ray of infant with multiple loops of dilated intestine.

Discussion

The correct answer is **C**. All of the listed items can result in delayed passage of meconium. However, malrotation by itself is not obstructive. Furthermore, if the malrotation resulted in midgut volvulus, the site of obstruction is the second portion of the duodenum. Midgut volvulus is a proximal obstruction but does not typically result in distension unless the entire midgut has infarcted and become edematous.

Which of the following is considered the gold standard for diagnosing Hirschsprung disease?
A. Suction rectal biopsy
B. Contrast enema
C. Ultrasound of the abdomen
D. Rectal examination showing empty rectal vault
E. UGI

Discussion

The correct answer is **A**. Hirschsprung disease is one of a host of diseases to be considered in the evaluation of a newborn with distal intestinal obstruction. During early gestation, the enteric nervous system develops as neural crest cells migrate into the gastrointestinal tract in an aboral direction. The ganglion cells are located in the submucosal (Meissner) and intramuscular (Auerbach) plexus, and function to control intestinal relaxation and peristalsis. For reasons that are unclear, this migration is halted during development in some babies. This ultimately leaves a variable length of distal bowel without ganglion, and therefore, the inability to relax. The result is a contracted, spastic distal segment of intestine with a transition to proximally dilated intestine in the region where ganglion cells are present.

Diagnosis begins with a complete history and physical examination. Particular attention should be directed to a history of failure to pass meconium within 48 hours of childbirth, chromosomal abnormalities (increased prevalence in trisomy 21), and a history of explosive stools after suppository administration. On physical examination, these children can range from lethargic to active. If enterocolitis is developing, the abdomen may be quite distended. Digital examination will reveal a tight, spastic rectum and often yields an explosive, foul smelling stool (this can potentially be lifesaving, and is an absolutely essential component of the examination). A contrast enema should be performed as part of the initial work-up; it may or may not demonstrate a distally contracted segment with transition to proximally dilated bowel. Patients may demonstrate an inverted rectosigmoid ratio (the diameter of the rectum is smaller than that of the sigmoid colon), further evidence of distal aganglionic bowel (Fig. 17-11A and B). Definitive diagnosis is achieved with a rectal biopsy—this can be done at the bedside in newborns using a suction biopsy device. Under the microscope, key features are an absence of

ganglion cells and hypertrophied nerve trunks; confirmation with acetylcholinesterase staining (demonstrating hypertrophied nerve trunks) is performed at some centers.

A suction rectal biopsy is done which demonstrates absence of ganglion cells in the submucosal and intramuscular layers of intestine. There are hypertrophic nerve trunks present that stain densely positive for acetylcholinesterase. The baby is taken to the operating room by the surgeons.

Which of the following is *not* an appropriate surgical option for this child?
A. Soave pull-through
B. Swenson pull-through
C. Duhamel pull-through
D. Leveling colostomy
E. Sigmoid colectomy with primary anastomosis

Discussion

The correct answer is **E**. About 85% of patient with Hirschsprung's have disease limited to the rectosigmoid colon region. Soave, Swenson, and Duhamel reconstructions are all reasonable choices. Reasons to divert with a stoma include total colon Hirschsprung disease, ongoing enterocolitis, and significant size mismatch between the proximal and distal ends. In this setting, the colon is biopsied at the region of transition from dilated to spastic. The "level" at which ganglion cells are identified in the dilated region of colon is brought out as a stoma (hence the term, "leveling colostomy"), with the distal

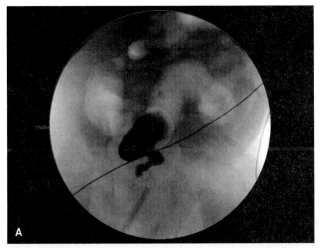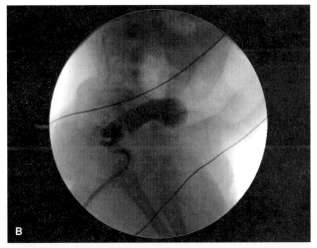

FIGURE 17-11.   A and B: Contrast enema, AP and lateral view demonstrating a narrow, spastic rectum with more dilated, air-filled sigmoid and more proximal colon.

end matured as a mucous fistula. Removing the sigmoid colon and performing a primary anastomosis would retain the distal spastic rectum and place the anastomosis at risk for rupture because of the functional obstruction located distally.

After surgery, the child does well and is discharged after a 2-week convalescence in the NICU. After 2 weeks, the family returns with the child because of feeding intolerance. He has become very distended, and has witnessed bright green emesis.

Which of the following is *not* the next step in management?
A. Rectal examination
B. UGI
C. IV metronidazole
D. IVF resuscitation
E. Rectal irrigations

Discussion

The correct answer is **B**. This patient is distended, manifesting signs of postoperative enterocolitis. It is unlikely to be the first presentation of malrotation and midgut volvulus given the history. Interestingly, and for unclear reasons, children who have undergone an operation for Hirschsprung disease remain at risk for enterocolitis. Treatment is usually nonoperative—bowel rest, fluid resuscitation, and metronidazole. Anastomotic stricture can be dealt with by rectal dilations, and tends to improve after the incision line remodels and stools solidify. The rectum is typically irrigated every 6 hours with warm normal saline at a volume of 10 mL/kg. It is important to differentiate this from an enema in that with irrigations, the saline is flushed into the rectum *and withdrawn*.

CASE 11

A baby is transferred to your NICU for further evaluation after delivering with an unclear abdominal wall defect. The mother had no access to prenatal care, and labored for over 30 hours because of the infant's size. On examination, the baby boy has low-set ears, a loud cardiac murmur, and a large membrane covered abdominal wall defect that is 10 cm in diameter. There appears to be liver and intestine herniated up into the fragile sac enclosing the viscera (Fig. 17-12). The penis appears normal but the testes are nonpalpable.

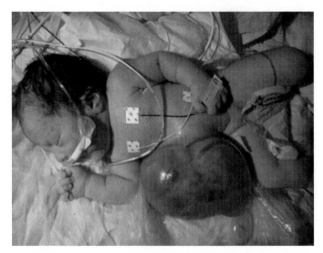

FIGURE 17-12.   Omphalocele. Note the membrane-covered abdominal wall defect encasing the abdominal viscera.

After stabilization and establishing adequate IV access, which of the following is *not* indicated?
A. Renal ultrasound
B. Cardiac ultrasound
C. Chromosome analysis
D. Testicular ultrasound
E. Cranial ultrasound

Discussion

The correct answer is **D**. Omphalocele is frequently associated with a number of other congenital anomalies, most notably chromosomal, cardiac, and renal. Testicular ultrasound is not indicated, even if they are nonpalpable at the time of delivery. Orchiopexy for cryptorchid testes is typically not performed until 12 to 18 months of life.

Which of the following is *not* an appropriate management strategy?
A. Painting the membrane with dilute povidone-iodine until it forms an eschar
B. Painting the membrane with silver sulfadiazine until it forms an eschar
C. Immediate removal of the membrane in the operating room with surgical closure of the defect
D. Placement of the viscera in a silo if the membrane ruptures
E. Delayed repair of the ventral hernia after the child has cardiac disease addressed and the viscera are covered by skin

Discussion

The correct answer is **C**. The presence of an omphalocele is not a surgical emergency in and of itself. If the defect is small enough to permit primary closure, this can be done in the neonatal period, but not until after the child has been found to be free of life-threatening congenital anomalies. Various methods have been adopted to stabilize the omphalocele membrane, including iodine solutions and silver sulfadiazine. If the membrane ruptures, silo coverage allows gradual reduction while minimizing evaporative and thermal losses.

CASE 12

You are asked to evaluate a premature infant who delivered at home to a 16-year-old mother with no prenatal care. She admits to smoking about 10 cigarettes a day, and has had several alcoholic beverages a week. On physical examination, the child appears to have an abdominal wall defect with herniation of the contents. The intestine is firm and matted, covered with meconium though there is no obvious perforation (Fig. 17-13).

What is the next step in management?
A. Echocardiogram
B. Renal ultrasound
C. Placement of occlusive bag around infant from the axillae down
D. Painting the wound with povidone-iodine or silver sulfadiazine
E. Amputation of the extruded intestine with diverting stomas

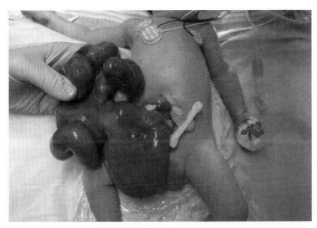

FIGURE 17-13. Gastroschisis. Note that the abdominal wall defect is located to the right of the umbilicus. The intestine is matted and foreshortened.

Discussion

The correct answer is **C**. Coverage of the abdominal wall defect by placing the inferior half of the child in a plastic bag minimizes thermal and evaporative losses. Cardiac and renal anomalies are uncommon in babies with gastroschisis and therefore are not evaluated in the absence of clinical findings to suggest a problem. Painting the intestine is not indicated, as it may cause further inflammatory damage. The intestine is frequently thickened and foreshortened/contracted. However, its appearance often improves after it has been replaced in the abdomen for several weeks. It is important to maintain as much intestinal length as possible. Typically no resections or diverting stoma operations are performed unless it is absolutely necessary (i.e., ongoing soilage from a clear perforation).

What additional work-up needs to be completed before repairing the abdominal wall?
A. Echocardiogram
B. Renal ultrasound
C. Testicular ultrasound
D. Central venous access
E. None of the above

Discussion

The correct answer is **E**. If the abdominal wall defect can be closed primarily in the perinatal time period, it should be done. Cardiac and renal ultrasounds are not necessary prior to closure if the infant does not show any signs of congenital anomaly and is stable from a cardiorespiratory perspective. The infant will need central venous access for parenteral nutrition; however, this can occur after the abdominal wall closure. If the defect is not amenable to immediate closure, a silo is placed (again, before central venous access is obtained).

Which of the following statements is *incorrect* when counseling the family?
A. The baby should have been delivered via Cesarian to prevent intestinal injury
B. Once the intestine is reduced inside, it often takes between 2 and 4 weeks or longer until enteral nutrition can be instituted
C. Even though the baby passed meconium, it is still possible for the child to have an intestinal atresia/stenosis
D. Chromosomal abnormalities are uncommon in these babies
E. This problem seems to occur more commonly in babies with mothers of low maternal age with a poorer socioeconomic status

Discussion

The correct answer is **A**. Gastroschisis typically affects mothers on the younger end of childbearing age spectrum, in poorer socioeconomic groups. The infants typically deliver several weeks before full term. There is no data to support a decision to deliver via Cesarian. The degree of inflammation seen grossly in the intestine does not have a direct correlation with the length of ileus—seemingly normal intestine may take over 4 weeks to tolerate enteral nutrition, while matted, foreshortened intestine may accept feeds earlier. The intestinal villi continue to turn over in utero, and therefore a proximal atresia can be present in an infant who has passed meconium.

REFERENCES

1. Noori S, Friedlich P, Wong P, et al. Cardiovascular effects of sildenafil in neonates and infants with congenital diaphragmatic hernia and pulmonary hypertension. *Neonatology*. 2007;91:92–100.
2. Patel N. Use of milrinone to treat cardiac dysfunction in infants with pulmonary hypertension secondary to congenital diaphragmatic hernia: A review of six patients. *Neonatology*. 2012;102:130.
3. Bahrami KR, Van Meurs KP. ECMO for neonatal respiratory failure. *Semin Perinatol*. 2005;29:15–23.
4. Bryner BS, West BT, Hirschl RB, et al; Congenital Diaphragmatic Hernia Study Group. Congenital diaphragmatic hernia requiring extracorporeal membrane oxygenation: Does timing of repair matter? *J Pediatr Surg*. 2009;44:1165–1171; discussion 1171–1162.
5. Holcomb GW, Rothenberg SS, Bax KM, et al. Thoracoscopic repair of esophageal atresia and tracheoesophageal fistula: A multi-institutional analysis. *Ann Surg*. 2005;242(3):422–428.
6. Keckler SJ, St. Peter SD, Valusek PA, et al. VACTERL anomalies in patients with esophageal atresia: An updated delineation of the spectrum and review of the literature. *Pediatr Surg Int*. 2007;23:309–319.
7. Krosnar S, Baxter A. Thoracoscopic repair of esophageal atresia with tracheoesophageal fistula: Anesthetic and intensive care management of a series of eight neonates. *Paediatr Anaesth*. 2005;15(7):541–546.
8. Spitz L, Kiely E, Brereton RJ. Esophageal atresia: Five year experience with 148 cases. *J Pediatr Surg*. 1987;22:103–108.
9. Adzick NS, Harrison MR, Crombleholme TM, et al. Fetal lung lesions: Management and outcome. *Am J Obstet Gynecol*. 1998;179:884–889.
10. Albanese CT, Rothenberg SS. Experience with 144 consecutive pediatric thoracoscopic lobectomies. *J Laparoendosc Adv Surg Tech A*. 2007;17(3):339–341.
11. Eber E. Antenatal diagnosis of congenital thoracic malformations: Early surgery, late surgery, or no surgery? *Semin Respir Crit Care Med*. 2007;28:355–366.
12. Ford EG, Senac MO Jr, Srikanth MS, et al. Malrotation of the intestine in children. *Ann Surg*. 1992;215:172–178.
13. Messineo A, MacMillan JH, Palder SB, et al. Clinical factors affecting mortality in children with malrotation of the intestine. *J Pediatr Surg*. 1992;27:1343.
14. Fraser JD, Aguayo P, Sharp SW, et al. The role of laparoscopy in the management of malrotation. *J Surg Res*. 2009;156:80.
15. Blakely ML, Tyson JE, Lally KP, et al. Laparotomy versus peritoneal drainage for necrotizing enterocolitis or isolated intestinal perforation in extremely low birth weight infants: Outcomes through 18 months adjusted age. *Pediatrics*. 2006;117:e680–e687.
16. Cass DL, Brandt ML, Patel DL, et al. Peritoneal drainage as definitive treatment for neonates with isolated intestinal perforation. *J Pediatr Surg*. 2000;35:1531–1536.
17. Grosfeld JL, Molinari F, Chaet M, et al. Gastrointestinal perforation and peritonitis in infants and children: Experience with 179 cases over ten years. *Surgery*. 1996;120:650–655.
18. Kennedy J, Holt CL, Ricketts RR. The significance of portal venous gas in necrotizing enterocolitis. *Am Surg*. 1987;53(4):231–234.
19. Moss RL, Reed RA, Barnhart DC, et al. Laparotomy versus peritoneal drainage for necrotizing enterocolitis and perforation. *N Engl J Med*. 2006;354:2225–2234.
20. Ricketts RR. The role of paracentesis in the management of infants with necrotizing enterocolitis. *Am Surg*. 1986;52(2):61–65.
21. Dalla Vecchia LK, Grosfeld JL, West KW, et al. Intestinal atresia and stenosis: A 25-year experience with 277 cases. *Arch Surg*. 1998;133:490–496.
22. Georgeson KE, Robertson DJ. Minimally invasive surgery in the neonate: Review of current evidence. *Semin Perinatol*. 2004;28(3):212–220.
23. Kimura K, Mukohara N, Nishijima E, et al. Diamond-shaped anastomosis for duodenal atresia: An experience with 44 patients over 15 years. *J Pediatr Surg*. 1990;25:977–979.
24. Rothenberg SS. Laparoscopic duodenoduodenostomy for duodenal obstruction in infants and children. *J Pediatr Surg*. 2002;37:1088–1089.
25. Hill SJ, Koontz CS, Lagness SM, et al. Laparoscopic versus open repair of congenital duodenal obstruction in infants. *J Laparoendosc Adv Surg Tech A*. 2011;21:961–963.
26. DelPin CA, Czyrko C, Ziegler MM, et al. Management and survival of meconium ileus, a 30-year review. *Ann Surg*. 1992;215:179–185.
27. Noblett H. Treatment of uncomplicated meconium ileus by Gastrografin enema: A preliminary report. *J Pediatr Surg*. 1969;4:190–197.
28. deVries PA, Pena A. Posterior sagittal anorectoplasty. *J Pediatr Surg*. 1982;17(5):638–643.
29. Georgeson KE, Inge TH, Albanese CT. Laparoscopically assisted anorectal pull-through for high imperforate anus—a new technique. *J Pediatr Surg*. 2000;35(6):927–930.
30. Rintala RJ, Pakarinen MP. Imperforate anus: Long- and short-term outcome. *Semin Pediatr Surg*. 2008;17:79.
31. Raschbaum GR, Bleacher JC, Grattan-Smith JD, et al. Magnetic resonance imaging-guided laparoscopic-assisted anorectoplasty for imperforate anus. *J Pediatr Surg*. 2010;45(1):220–223.
32. Georgeson KE, Robertson DJ. Laparoscopic-assisted approaches for the definitive surgery for Hirschsprung's disease. *Semin Pediatr Surg*. 2004;13(4):256–262.

33. Minford JL, Ram A, Turnock RR, et al. Comparison of functional outcomes of Duhamel and transanal Endorectal colo-anal anastomosis for Hirschsprung's disease. *J Pediatr Surg.* 2004;39:161–165.

34. Skaba R. Historic milestones of Hirschsprung's disease (commemorating the 90th anniversary of Professor Harald Hirschsprung's death). *J Pediatr Surg.* 2007;42: 249–251.

35. How HY, Harris BJ, Pietrantoni M, et al. Is vaginal delivery preferable to elective cesarean delivery in fetuses with a known ventral wall defect? *Am J Obstet Gynecol.* 2000;182: 1527–1534.

36. Nuchtern JG, Baxter R, Hatch EI Jr. Nonoperative initial management versus silon chimney for treatment of giant omphalocele. *J Pediatr Surg.* 1995;30:771–776.

37. Minkes RK, Langer JC, Massiotti MV, et al. Routine insertion of a silastic spring-loaded silo for infants with gastroschisis. *J Pediatr Surg.* 2000;35:843–846.

38. Sydorak RM, Nijagal A, Sbragia L, et al. Gastroschisis: Small hole, big cost. *J Pediatr Surg.* 2002;37(12):1669–1672.

Chapter 18
ETHICS
Helen O. Williams, MD

CASE 1

Ms. Jones is a 35-year-old pregnant woman with bipolar depression who presents to labor and delivery at term with vaginal bleeding. The obstetrical team is concerned about a possible placental abruption and they recommend an immediate caesarian section as the fetus is showing signs of distress. Ms. Jones refuses the caesarian and states her intention to have a normal vaginal delivery. Her husband is in agreement with the obstetricians. You are the neonatologist on call and you have been asked to speak with Ms. Jones and make recommendations to the obstetrical team.

Which one of the following is the *most* appropriate next step in Ms. Jones' case?
A. Since the fetus is in distress, an immediate caesarian should be performed and Ms. Jones' consent is not required in this emergency setting
B. A complete discussion with Ms. Jones concerning the risks of the abruption should be undertaken. If she continues to refuse caesarian section her wishes should be respected
C. Since the father of the fetus is in agreement with the obstetricians, an immediate caesarian should be performed even without Ms. Jones' consent
D. A court order should be immediately sought to allow for a caesarian section against Ms. Jones' request
E. In light of Ms. Jones bipolar depression, she is not competent to make medical decisions and the caesarian can be performed without her consent

Discussion

The correct answer is **B**. Questions concerning maternal–fetal rights remain highly controversial and ethically challenging. To frame the debate in ethical language, the main concern is that respect for maternal autonomy conflicts with the best interest of the fetus (beneficence). These questions arise in instances when pregnant women are noncompliant with medical care, use illegal substances, abuse alcohol or otherwise engage in behaviors which may be considered to be detrimental to the fetus. Although attempts have been made to criminally prosecute for these behaviors, the courts have typically decided with the pregnant woman. The rationale being that her autonomy is considered the controlling ethical principle. The fetus is typically not considered a person for purposes of assigning moral standing or legal protection.

In this scenario, the best approach would be to engage Ms. Jones in a fully informative discussion, but ultimately her decision should be respected. An informed consent discussion requires complete disclosure of potential benefits and burdens of the proposed interventions. Preconditions for informed consent include legal competence to make decisions and voluntariness or a lack of coercion.[1] There is nothing in the vignette to suggest that Ms. Jones lacks decision making capacity. The appraisal of a psychiatrist should be sought if there is concern that Ms. Jones' bipolar depression impacts on her ability to make decisions.

Helpful Tip: Bioethical Principles

The four principles of biomedical ethics are:[1]

- Beneficence—the duty to help patients whenever possible—doing good
- Nonmaleficence—The obligation to avoid harm
- Respect for autonomy—The patients' right to self-determination (or their surrogates right to make decision on their behalf)
- Justice—The fair allocation of medical resources

Helpful Tip: Competence and Capacity

- Decision making capacity—The ability to understand information and use that information to make an informed decision
- Competence—A characteristic that a person is judged to possess or not to possess. Competence is a legal concept. Children are not considered competent decision makers under the law and therefore a surrogate is needed to make decisions on their behalf

CASE 2

Mrs. West presents to labor and delivery at 21 5/7 weeks gestation in preterm labor. She is a 33-year-old Gravida 3 woman with no living children. You are asked to speak with Mrs. West about her fetus. The obstetricians inform you that they expect she will deliver soon and by her last ultrasound 10 days ago, the estimated fetal weight is 390 g. Mrs. West and her husband Dr. West (an adult cardiologist) request a full resuscitation for their infant. You hear that they are well educated and they have stated willingness to care for him regardless of disability.

Of the following, the approach that is *best* supported by ethical principles is to:

A. Discuss outcomes at 22 weeks with the West's and inform them that it is not standard-of-care to offer resuscitation. Attend the delivery to assess the baby and provide palliative care. If he appears more mature, attempt resuscitation

B. Inform the West's that a respiratory only resuscitation will be attempted for their baby but it is likely he will be too small to intubate

C. Plan on a full resuscitation with intubation, chest compressions, and epinephrine as needed

D. Discuss outcomes at 22 weeks with the West's and inform them that it is not standard-of-care to offer resuscitation. However, since the infant's father is a physician and this is a very "wanted" baby you will make an exception in their case

E. Advise your obstetrical colleagues that 22 weeks is previable and a neonatal consult is not indicated in this case

Discussion

The correct answer is **A**. The Neonatal Resuscitation Program (NRP) recommends a model of shared decision making between physicians and patients, in cases of uncertain viability. However, if a case is considered to be futile that is, "*gestation, birth weight, and/or congenital anomalies are associated with almost certain early death, or unacceptably high morbidity is likely among the rare survivors,*" the American Academy of Pediatrics affirms that resuscitation is not indicated, but exceptions to comply with parental requests may be reasonable.[2] In 1983, The President's Commission for the Study of Ethical Problems in Medicine, created a framework for

Physician's assessment of treatment options	Parents prefer to accept care	Parents prefer to forego care
Clearly beneficial E.g. Treating a duodenal atresia in an infant with trisomy 21.	Provide Treatment– *Mandatory*	Provide treatment during the review process with an Ethics Consultation or second opinion from another neonatologist/perinatologist
Ambiguous/ Uncertain E.g. Resuscitating an infant at 23 weeks	Provide Treatment– *Optional*	Forego treatment
Futile E.g. Resuscitating an infant with anencephaly	Provide treatment unless provider declines to do so because ongoing care is *Unreasonable*	Forego treatment

FIGURE 18-1. Parental decision making. (Adapted with permission from Deciding to forego life-sustaining treatment: a report on the ethical, medical, and legal issues in treatment decisions. Washington, DC: U.S. Government Printing Office; 1983.)

understanding ethical decision making in cases of uncertain outcome, the so-called *gray-zone*.[3] This framework is useful for determining which treatments are optional, obligatory, or futile (Fig. 18-1).

Jason West III was born weighing 580 g with some respiratory effort, some tone, and a heart rate >100. It is your opinion that his gestational age is at least 23 weeks. He is intermittently apneic and needs positive-pressure ventilation. You intubate him and he is admitted to the NICU for continued care. His Apgar scores were 4 and 7 at 5 and 10 minutes, respectively. Your residents are concerned about Jason's prognosis.

Of the following, the *most* accurate statement predicting Jason's prognosis on day of life one is:
A. Since Jason did well in the delivery room and only required respiratory support, his prognosis is good
B. His *SNAP* score (score of neonatal acute physiology) will best predict his prognosis
C. Our ability to assess short-term survival is poor but his prognosis is best predicted by his birth weight using population-specific data
D. His prognosis is best predicted by his Apgar scores and since his 5 minute score was 7, his prognosis is good
E. The best estimate of survival is the clinical intuition of an experienced neonatal practitioner

Discussion

The correct answer is **C**. Neonatal mortality is defined as death before 28 days of age. Predicting the outcome of neonates born near the limits of viability is an important aspect of prenatal counseling, and essential to the process of obtaining informed consent for resuscitation. For this reason, neonatal investigators have sought to refine our prognostic accuracy for these smallest "gray-zone" babies. Despite our best efforts at predicting outcomes, the data show that we have great difficulty making accurate predictions of both short- and long-term survival. However, birth weight remains the most powerful prognostic measure with bigger babies generally doing better than smaller neonates.[4]

The SNAP score is less than 50% accurate as a predictor of death. Therefore it is not generally considered useful in making decisions for the individual baby. Rather, the SNAP score is a useful epidemiological measure for studying large populations of neonates.[4] Predictions of survival based on clinician experience have also been shown to be frequently incorrect. Response to resuscitation or Apgar score should not be used as independent measures to predict survival. As Meadow's illustrated, our ability to predict survival improves as we

observe the response of the baby to a trial of therapy. By 4 days of life, birth weight–specific mortality disappears as a relevant predictor of survival.[5] In these first few days of life, infants often "declare themselves" by responding positively to treatment or by worsening despite intensive care.

Of the 100,000 babies born last year in a certain population, 200 died in the first week of life, 450 died in the first 28 days of life, and a total of 650 babies died in the first year of life. The neonatal mortality rate is:
A. 6.5/1,000 live births
B. 4.5/1,000 live births
C. 45/1,000 live births
D. 11/1,000 live births
E. Not answerable with the data given

The correct answer is **B**.

Helpful Tip:

Perinatal mortality—The Centers for Disease Control (CDC) uses two definitions for perinatal mortality:

1. Infant deaths under age 7 days and fetal deaths at 28 weeks of gestation or more
2. Infant deaths under age 28 days and fetal deaths at 20 weeks or more

Neonatal mortality—Infant death before 28 days of age.

Early neonatal mortality—infant death that occurs in <7 days of birth.

Late neonatal mortality—a death from 7 to <28 days of age.

Neonatal mortality rate (NMR)—the number of neonatal deaths during a year, divided by the number of live births during the same year, expressed per 1,000 live births.

Postneonatal mortality—Infant death occurring between 28 and 365 days of age.

Infant mortality—Infant death is defined as a live birth that results in death within the first year of life (<365 days).

Infant mortality rate (IMR)—number of infant deaths during a year, divided by the number of live births reported during the same year, expressed per 1,000 live births.

CASE 3

Ms. Smith presents for her repeat caesarian section at 39 weeks' gestation. Her infant was prenatally diagnosed with hypoplastic left heart syndrome. During the pregnancy, Ms. Smith and her partner met with neonatology, cardiology, and cardiothoracic surgery. They also did extensive research on their own. They inform you that they have decided not to seek surgical treatment for their daughter's hypoplastic left heart and have made plans to take her home with pediatric hospice.

Of the following, the *most* ethically appropriate approach is to:

A. Discuss at length with the parents the benefits of surgery in hypoplastic left heart. Honor their wishes if you are unable to change their mind

B. Override the wishes of the parents and aggressively treat the infant to comply with the Baby Doe regulations

C. Override the wishes of the parents as outcomes for children with hypoplastic left heart syndrome have improved sufficiently to make treatment obligatory

D. Confirm with the parents their understanding of the condition and support their plans for palliative care

E. Refer the parents to social services for medical neglect

Discussion

The correct answer is **D**. In pediatrics parents are typically the surrogate decision makers for their child. Parental authority is deemed ethically appropriate since parents are most likely to make decisions in the best interest of their child. Furthermore, the parents along with their child will be most impacted by the decisions they make. There are few instances where parental authority to decline medical interventions is overridden. The American Academy of Pediatrics advocates for a child's right to effective treatment likely to prevent serious harm, suffering, or death, even over parental objection.[6] For example, this principle of unacceptable harm is frequently evoked to allow the courts to authorize life-saving blood transfusion against parental wishes.

Healthcare providers may perceive a technological imperative to provide therapy that may prolong life. However, in cases where significant uncertainty remains about outcome, or in cases when the treatment itself is highly burdensome, it remains ethically appropriate to support the wishes of the parents to withhold or withdraw therapy. This is particularly true of therapies that can be viewed as death prolonging rather than lifesaving or life prolonging. Such therapies often carry a high burden of pain or disability for the patient with little possibility of restoration to a good quality of life.

Withholding and withdrawing life-sustaining therapy are considered ethically equivalent. Indeed most neonatal deaths can be attributed to either withholding or withdrawing therapy. Therapy may be withheld in the form of an order not to resuscitate (DNR) or to allow natural death (AND). DNR and AND orders require the consent of the parent. When a life-limiting diagnosis is known prior to birth, parents may choose to immediately opt for a palliative care approach. It is important to emphasize that care is never withdrawn. Rather there is a change of treatment emphasis from curative/restorative therapies to palliative care. Palliative care is a holistic approach to the care of a patient with a life-limiting illness that addresses pain prevention and treatment as well as other physical, psychological, and spiritual factors that may impact care.

The Baby Doe regulations remain in effect and ban the withholding of life-saving treatment for all children except those who are permanently comatose, near death, or for whom treatment would be inhumane because it would be futile or virtually futile. Baby Doe was born in 1982 with trisomy 21 and a tracheoesophageal fistula. Her parents chose not to seek treatment for her TEF citing concerns about quality of life. While the case was working its way to the Supreme Court, Baby Doe died as a result of withdrawal of artificial nutrition and hydration. The case gave rise to federal legislation which has since been revised in the form of the Child Abuse Prevention and Treatment Act (CAPTA). The penalty for ignoring these regulations is loss of federal child protection funds to the state. Parents, individual practitioners, and hospitals are not penalized directly by this federal legislation. The Baby Doe regulations are criticized for not recognizing the "best interest of the child" or parental authority in making decisions to limit treatment on behalf of their children. To date, no state has carried out an action against anyone in violation of these regulations.[7,8]

CASE 4

A 2-day-old former 27-week infant dies in your nursery from severe respiratory distress syndrome. Your residents are concerned about how best to support the grieving parents.

All of the following may facilitate normal grieving *except*:

A. Providing tangible evidence of the loss in the form of pictures or footprints
B. Using the term "pass-away" and avoiding the word "death"
C. Encouraging the family to express their feelings with the staff and each other
D. Saying "I am sorry for your loss"
E. Making a referral for grief counseling outside the NICU

Discussion

The correct answer is **B**. The death of a child is always a tragedy and parents need considerable support from healthcare providers as they grieve. The best way to provide this support has been studied but mostly through observation. As previously noted, the majority of NICU deaths occur following the withholding or withdrawing (WH/WD) of life-sustaining therapy. The decision to WH/WD therapy is ideally made collaboratively by parents and health care providers. This shared-decision making respects patient autonomy by supporting parental authority to make decisions on behalf of their child. However, it is also important for treating physicians to give clear recommendations to the family as to the course they consider most beneficent. A recommendation for treatment is essential to the process of informed consent but it also allows the burden of WH/WD treatment and the guilt that may ensue from these decisions to not fall exclusively on the parents.

Family centered care should be emphasized in end-of-life situations.[9] Many NICUs have palliative care or end-of-life protocols to support bereaved families. These typically include relaxed visitor restrictions, designated quiet spaces, memory boxes, photography and psychosocial and spiritual support through social work and chaplaincy. Parents may benefit greatly from holding their infant, or participating in the bathing and dressing of the baby. All healthcare providers should be aware of the Kübler-Ross stages of grieving which include denial, anger, bargaining, depression, and eventually acceptance.[10] A parent may be in the anger phase of grief around the time of their child's death and it is important that providers engage in empathic listening rather than discouraging or belittling these emotions. It is imperative to directly use the words "death," "dying," and "dead" in conversations with parents instead of the various euphemistic terms for dying such as "passing away," "going to heaven," etc. Some of these terms are laden with religious context which may or may not reflect the belief system of the family. Finally, statements that attempt to discount the family's grief are entirely without benefit and should be avoided. Platitudes such as "it was for the best," "things will get better with time," or "you can have other children" are of no benefit and may be damaging to the grieving parent.

You speak with the family about an autopsy. All of the following are true concerning autopsy *except*:

A. A change of diagnosis rarely follows autopsy examination
B. Autopsy rates in the United States are declining
C. A full autopsy remains the best method of investigating perinatal death
D. Autopsy examinations may help with counseling for future pregnancies and the process of grieving
E. It is the right of every family to be afforded the opportunity to consent to a postmortem examination

Discussion

The correct answer is **A**. Perinatal autopsy rates in the United States are declining. There is concern that neonatal practitioners do not fully appreciate the value of a postmortem evaluation. Autopsy remains the gold standard for investigating the cause of perinatal death.[11,12] The benefits of autopsy include: more accurate ascertainment of the causes of death, more accurate vital statistics, identifying conditions of interest to family members, educating healthcare providers regarding pathological findings, and local quality assurance.[13] There may be discordance between the clinical diagnosis and the autopsy diagnosis leading to a change in the listed cause of death. Autopsy promotes beneficence for the family by allowing for an accurate diagnosis and possibly counseling for future pregnancies. By forgoing autopsy there may be potential harms to society (inaccurate disease surveillance, e.g., as deaths are miscategorized) which becomes an ethical issue of justice. It is important to seek consent for autopsy and share this information with the family.

Quick Quiz:

The most common cause of neonatal death according to the CDC is:

A. Bacterial sepsis of newborn
B. Birth asphyxia
C. Congenital malformations
D. Disorders of short gestation
E. Sudden infant death syndrome

Discussion

The correct answer is **C**. Disorders of short gestation follow behind birth defects as a leading cause of neonatal morbidity.

CASE 5

The mother of a feeding and growing 26-week infant in your NICU recently discovered a family history of Huntington disease in a great uncle. She is concerned that the baby may develop the disease and would like to have him tested.

The *most* ethically appropriate next step would be to:
A. Test the infant as the outcome would affect neonatal decision making
B. Counsel mother against testing the infant since the disease does not have onset of symptoms until adulthood
C. Send an oligonucleotide array on the infant to screen for genetic disease
D. Recommend the testing as an outpatient and let the primary care pediatrician who has a relationship with the family make the decision
E. Recommend that the patient's mother be tested for Huntington disease

Discussion

The correct answer is **B**. Advances in genetic testing have allowed many diseases to be diagnosed prior to the presence of symptoms.[14] Of particular concern in pediatrics is the testing of asymptomatic children for adult onset diseases. Many such diseases are not presently amenable to treatment or preventative measures leaving little benefit to the child in obtaining the label of the diagnosis. Such genetic testing should only be performed in competent adults who have given informed consent. In addition, many genetic markers only predict a predisposition to disease but the timing and severity of disease is still uncertain. In this scenario it would be most beneficial to refer this family to genetics, so they can be properly counseled about the risk and benefits of testing for Huntington disease in the adult family members. In an asymptomatic, nondysmorphic infant there is no indication to send an oligonucleotide array.

CASE 6

A neonatal fellow is working on a project to improve admission temperatures in very–low-birth weight (VLBW) babies. She uses the plan-do-study-act approach to quality improvement and finds that three simple delivery room interventions improve the admission temperature of VLBW infants to your nursery. Her data is so compelling that she decides to write up the project for publication.

Of the following, the main characteristic *distinguishing* research from quality improvement is that research:
A. Requires a consent form
B. Allows results to be published
C. Focuses on implementation of knowledge
D. Seeks to develop new knowledge
E. Uses patient data

Discussion

The correct answer is **D**. In recent years there has been increasing emphasis placed on quality improvement (QI). Indeed, Part 4 of the American Board of Pediatrics' maintenance of certification (MOC) program now requires physicians to complete a QI project. Quality improvement differs from research in its ultimate goal. QI focuses on the implementation of current medical knowledge to improve medical care to patients. Quality improvement initiatives improve patient care by refining the use of proven therapies and identifying areas of overuse and underuse of treatments. On the other hand, research seeks to develop new knowledge by building on current evidence. Some research projects, such as database reviews, do not require a consent form. The need for consent is determined by review from the institutional review board (IRB). Both endeavors can produce useful information which may be suitable for publication.

Benchmarking is a tool that is often used to improve quality. In benchmarking, data is collected from several participating institutions. This data then undergoes an external audit with the goal of determining which strategies are most effective at improving perinatal outcomes. For example, a unit with a particularly low rate of NEC may be noted to have much higher rates of breastfeeding than the other institutions. This information would be shared with participating units and efforts could be made to raise breastfeeding rates at the units with higher rates of NEC.

REFERENCES

1. Beauchamp TL, Childress JF. *Principles of Biomedical Ethics.* 6th ed. New York, NY: Oxford University Press; 2009:xiii, 417.
2. American Heart Association and American Academy of Pediatrics. *Textbook of Neonatal Resuscitation.* 6th ed. Dallas, TX: Amer Academy of Pediatrics; 2011: xiii, 328.

3. United States President's Commission for the Study of Ethical Problems in Medicine and Biomedical and Behavioral Research. *Deciding to Forego Life-Sustaining Treatment : A Report on the Ethical, Medical, and Legal Issues in Treatment Decisions*. Washington, DC: President's Commission for the Study of Ethical Problems in Medicine and Biomedical and Behavioral Research; 1983: For sale by the Supt. of Docs., U.S. G.P.O. 554.

4. Lantos JD, Meadow W. *Neonatal Bioethics: The Moral Challenges of Medical Innovation*. Baltimore, MD: Johns Hopkins University Press; 2006: 177.

5. Meadow W, Reimshisel T, Lantos J. Birth weight-specific mortality for extremely low birth weight infants vanishes by four days of life: epidemiology and ethics in the neonatal intensive care unit. *Pediatrics*. 1996;97(5):636–643.

6. Religious objections to medical care. American Academy of Pediatrics Committee on Bioethics. *Pediatrics*. 1997;99(2):279–281.

7. Pence GE. *Medical Ethics: Accounts of Ground-Breaking Cases*. 6th ed. New York, NY: McGraw-Hill; 2011.

8. Robertson JA. Extreme prematurity and parental rights after Baby Doe. *Hastings Cent Rep*. 2004;34(4):32–39.

9. Harris L, Douma C. End-of-life Care in the NICU: A family-centered approach. *NeoReviews*. 2010;11:e194–e199.

10. Kübler-Ross E. *On Death and Dying*. 1st Scribner Classics ed. New York, NY: Scribner Classics; 1997:286.

11. Faye-Petersen OM, Guinn DA, Wenstrom KD. Value of perinatal autopsy. *Obstet Gynecol*; 1999;94(6):915–920.

12. Hickey L, Murphy A, Devaney D, et al. The value of neonatal autopsy. *Neonatology*. 2012;101(1):68–73.

13. Shojania KG, Burton EC. The vanishing nonforensic autopsy. *N Engl J Med*. 2008;358(9):873–875.

14. Jonsen AR, Siegler M, Winslade WJ. *Clinical Ethics: A Practical Approach to Ethical Decisions in Clinical Medicine*. 6th ed. New York, NY: McGraw Hill Professional; 2010: vi, 227.

Chapter 19

CORE KNOWLEDGE IN SCHOLARLY ACTIVITIES

José Nilo G. Binongo, PhD, Vijaya Kancherla, PhD, and Michael R. Kramer, PhD

CASE 1

A previous case-control study reported a relationship between administering magnesium sulfate to women at high risk for early preterm delivery and occurrence of cerebral palsy in their children. A randomized, double-blind clinical trial was conducted on 2,241 women at imminent risk for preterm delivery; 1,096 were assigned to receive magnesium sulfate, and 1,145 were assigned to receive the placebo.[1]

What is the strength of this clinical trial compared to the previously conducted case-control study?
A. A clinical trial usually requires a fewer number of participants than a case-control study
B. In a clinical trial, participants typically choose the type of intervention and this usually results in higher participant recruitment rates. Participant recruitment is more difficult in case-control studies
C. A clinical trial provides stronger evidence for a causal link between treatment and outcome; the case-control study could only hope to show an association
D. Statistical power of a clinical trial is generally higher than that of a case-control study
E. All of the above

Discussion

The correct answer is **C**. Randomized placebo-controlled, double-blind clinical trials provide the strongest evidence to demonstrate the efficacy of an intervention. Other study designs, such as cohort and retrospective studies, are prone to bias and confounding.

Why were eligible women randomly allocated into the magnesium sulfate group and placebo group?
A. To encourage participant compliance to the treatment
B. To remove potential researcher bias in participant assignment
C. To make the groups comparable with respect to known and unknown prognostic factors
D. To ensure that tests of hypothesis will have correct significance levels
E. B, C, and D

Discussion

The correct answer is **E**. With comparable groups at baseline, it is possible to establish a causal link between intervention and outcome. Although randomization does not guarantee identical groups, it minimizes the chance that systematic factors unrelated to the treatment differentially affect the outcome.

This study was described as double blind. What is the primary purpose of double blinding?
A. To reduce sample sizes
B. To increase chance of obtaining a significant finding
C. To minimize investigator and participant bias
D. To decrease variability of the outcome
E. All of the above

Discussion

The correct answer is **C**. The decisions of unblinded investigators are prone to bias; so is the treatment response of unblinded participants. Bias may result in different values of the outcome between intervention and control groups. Because the goal in a clinical trial is to make a definitive statement regarding the efficacy of the intervention, both investigator and participant bias should be minimized.

The primary outcome of the study was the composite of stillbirth or infant death by 1 year or moderate or severe cerebral palsy at or beyond 2 years. As part of the study design, the researchers determined an adequate sample size for the study. They estimated that the primary outcome would occur in 14% of the placebo group. Using a significance level of 0.05 and a power of at least 80%, an equally divided sample of 2,000 was deemed sufficient to detect a 30% reduction in the primary outcome in the intervention group. Assuming a 10% rate of participants' loss to follow-up, the researchers decided a target sample size of 2,200.

What was the null hypothesis of the study?
A. The average time from last menstrual period to the occurrence of stillbirth or infant death or moderate or severe cerebral palsy is different for the intervention and placebo groups
B. The number of pregnancies resulting in stillbirth or infant death or moderate or severe cerebral palsy is different for the intervention and placebo groups
C. The number of pregnancies resulting in stillbirth or infant death or moderate or severe cerebral palsy is the same in both the intervention and placebo groups
D. The proportion of pregnancies resulting in the composite of stillbirth or infant death or moderate or severe cerebral palsy is different for the intervention and placebo groups
E. The proportion of pregnancies resulting in the composite of stillbirth or infant death or moderate or severe cerebral palsy is the same in both intervention and placebo groups

Discussion

The correct answer is **E**. The null hypothesis is the hypothesis of no treatment effect. Because the primary outcome is a categorical variable, the null hypothesis is stated in terms of equal proportions (or risks) of stillbirth or infant death in both intervention and placebo groups. When comparing proportions, the chi-square test may be appropriate.

The primary outcome does not have to be a categorical variable; it may well be an ordinal or continuous numeric variable, such as change from baseline in birth weight. In this case, the null hypothesis is stated in terms of equal mean (or median) change in weight in both intervention and control groups, and the t-test may be appropriate. When more than two groups are compared, analysis of variance (ANOVA) and subsequent multiple comparison procedures may be considered.

If researchers succeed in invalidating the null hypothesis, then
A. They increase the sample size of the study
B. They increase the statistical power of the study
C. They lower the level of significance of the hypothesis test
D. They accept the alternative hypothesis
E. They fail to reject the alternative hypothesis

Discussion

The correct answer is **D**. The alternative hypothesis is the hypothesis that replaces the null hypothesis when the latter is invalidated. In this particular study, the alternative hypothesis is that magnesium sulfate has a significant effect on the composite outcome of stillbirth and death. To invalidate the null hypothesis requires compelling evidence; the weight of the evidence is couched in terms of the p-value, which is the probability of obtaining a difference in the outcome as extreme as or more extreme than what the researchers observed, assuming the truth of the null hypothesis. Very small value p-values lead to the rejection of the null hypothesis, and hence the acceptance of the alternative hypothesis.

In this particular study, the researchers decided that the maximum probability of rejecting the null hypothesis, assuming the null hypothesis was true, was
A. 0.10
B. 0.20
C. 0.80
D. 0.05
E. 0.95

Discussion

The correct answer is **D**. Prudent researchers care about errors. Two types of errors are possible when conducting a test of hypothesis. Type I error is made when researchers reject the null hypothesis, when in fact the null hypothesis is true. In the context of a superiority clinical trial, a type I error is made when researchers report a significant difference in clinical outcome between treated and placebo groups when actually there is no difference. Type II error is made when the researchers fail to reject the null hypothesis, when in fact the null hypothesis is false. Again, in the context of a clinical trial, a type II error is made when researchers fail to detect a significant difference between groups when in fact the intervention is effective. Type I error is considered the more serious error. To guard against type I error, researchers set the significance level before conducting the test of hypothesis. The significance level is denoted by alpha (α). In this example, the researchers reported

$\alpha = 0.05$. In other words, there was a 5% chance that the researchers would report a nonsignificant finding as significant.

Power was reported to be at least 80%. This refers to

A. The chance of declaring incorrectly that magnesium sulfate reduces the risk of moderate or severe cerebral palsy or death (because, in fact, it does not)
B. The chance of declaring correctly that magnesium sulfate reduces the risk of moderate or severe cerebral palsy or death (because, in fact, it does)
C. The chance of declaring incorrectly that magnesium sulfate does not reduce the risk of moderate or severe cerebral palsy or death (because, in fact, it does)
D. The chance of declaring correctly that magnesium sulfate does not reduce the risk of moderate or severe cerebral palsy or death (because, in fact, it does)
E. The chance that the null hypothesis is true

Discussion

The correct answer is **B**. Power is defined as the probability of rejecting the null hypothesis when it is false. In an interventional study, if a study has 80% power, there is 80% chance of declaring an effective intervention to be effective. Power is the complement of the probability of making a type II error. The probability of making a type II error is denoted by beta (β); hence, power is estimated as $1 - \beta$. Increasing statistical power also means decreasing the probability of a type II error. With 80% power, there is a 20% chance of making a type II error.

Suppose the researchers wished to detect a 40% reduction in the primary outcome (as opposed to 30%). How would this affect the sample size?

A. A larger sample will be needed
B. A smaller sample will be needed
C. The sample size will not be affected
D. The sample size will increase by 10%
E. The sample size will decrease by 10%

Discussion

The correct answer is **B**. Holding everything else constant, if the researchers wish to detect a larger effect size, a smaller sample is needed. It is easier to detect a large difference in the outcome than a small one. Deciding an appropriate effect size can be difficult, especially for clinical outcomes that have not been well studied. However, determining the amount of change in the outcome that is of clinical interest is important in calculating the sample size.

The researchers wrote that for all analyses of the primary outcome, their unit of analysis was the pregnancy. What is consistent with this statement?

A. Cases of twin pregnancy are excluded from the analysis
B. In a twin pregnancy, if both twins had moderate or severe cerebral palsy or both twins died, only one event is recorded
C. In a twin pregnancy, if both twins had moderate or severe cerebral palsy or both twins died, two events are recorded
D. A and B
E. A and C

Discussion

The correct answer is **B**. Determining the unit of analysis is important in every study. In many clinical studies, the unit of analysis is an individual. In this example, however, the unit of analysis is the pregnancy. Hence, in the case of a twin pregnancy, where both twins had the event of interest, one rather than two events is recorded.

Classify this study as a specific phase of a clinical trial

A. Phase I
B. Phase II
C. Phase III
D. Phase IV

Discussion

The correct answer is **C**. Drug intervention trials involve several phases. In phase I, researchers determine how well the proposed drug is tolerated by a small number of subjects. In phase II, researchers administer the drug to a larger group of individuals to evaluate efficacy and safety, and to determine if the intervention warrants further testing in phase III. In phase III, the primary goal is to test for treatment effect by comparing the trial drug with a standard therapy or other competitive therapies, and to monitor side effects. Phase IV studies, which are performed after the drug has been marketed for this indication, aim to assess efficacy in various populations and identify any side effects associated with long-term exposure to the drug.

Intention-to-treat (ITT) analysis has widely become the preferred analysis strategy for clinical trial findings. Suppose a pregnant woman (X) was randomly assigned to the magnesium sulfate group, but for some reason was administered the placebo during the study.

What does ITT analysis require?
A. That the woman X be removed from the study
B. That the treatment assignment of the woman X be recorded as placebo
C. That the treatment assignment of the woman X be recorded as magnesium sulfate
D. That another randomly selected woman in the placebo group be given magnesium sulfate
E. That the treatment assignment of the woman X be recorded as a missing value

Discussion

The correct answer is **C**. The strength of clinical trials lies in the researchers' ability to infer a causal connection between treatment and outcome. Such a connection is difficult to demonstrate using other study designs. Establishing cause-and-effect is made possible by randomization. To fully realize the benefits of randomization, all subjects that have been randomized must be included in the analysis. That also means subjects must be analyzed according to the treatment they were originally assigned, regardless of what occurred during the study.

When the researchers reported their findings, they started with a summary of baseline characteristics of the mothers

TABLE 19-1.   Selected Characteristics of the Mothers

CHARACTERISTIC	CONTROL GROUP (N = 1,145)	INTERVENTION GROUP (N = 1,096)
Gestational age at randomization: mean weeks ± SD	28.2 ± 2.4	28.3 ± 2.5
Prepregnancy body mass index (kg/m²) mean ± SD	26.4 ± 6.9	26.0 ± 6.7
Maternal racial/ethnic group (number [%])		
Black	495 (43.2)	483 (44.1)
White	418 (36.5)	404 (36.9)
Hispanic	206 (18.0)	184 (16.8)
Other	26 (2.3)	25 (2.3)
Time since rupture (hours)		
Median	24.4	25.2
Interquartile range	10.8–62.9	10.7–61.1

SD, standard deviation.
Adapted with permission from Rouse DJ, Hirtz DG, Thom E, et al. A randomized, controlled trial of magnesium sulfate for the prevention of cerebral palsy. *N Engl J Med.* 2008;359(9):895–905.

in both intervention and placebo groups. Table 19-1 shows some of the variables the researchers provided.

In Table 19-1, quantitative characteristics are summarized as mean ± standard deviation (SD), except for time since premature rupture of membrane, which was summarized as median and interquartile range (IQR). What does this suggest regarding time since premature rupture of membrane?
A. It had values generally lower than expected
B. It had values generally higher than expected
C. It had a skewed distribution
D. It had several missing values
E. It was considered by the researchers as the most important baseline characteristic

Discussion

The correct answer is **C**. Numeric variables are typically summarized by reporting their average and variability. The average is calculated using mean or median. The mean is popular among researchers because in calculating the mean, every single observation is taken into account. However, this can also be a disadvantage because the mean is sensitive to outliers (i.e., observations with very large or very small values). In the presence of outliers, it may be best to report the median, which is the 50th percentile. The median is resistant to extremely high or low values. Half of the observations fall below (or above) the median. If we have the entire population and the population distribution is symmetric, then the mean and the median are same. But in a right-skewed or left-skewed distribution, marked by outliers on one side of the distribution, the mean and the median are not equal.

To measure variability, researchers calculate the range, which is the difference between the maximum and the minimum values of the variable being considered. Because the range is susceptible to outliers, researchers often report the range of the middle 50% of the distribution, by removing the top 25% and the bottom 25%. The range of the middle 50% is called the IQR. When there are no outliers in the data, researchers usually report the SD as a measure of variability. The SD can be interpreted as the average difference between the observations and their average.

In this example, the median and the IQR were used to describe the distribution of time since premature rupture of membrane. This reflects the researchers' belief that the distribution is asymmetric or that outliers exist.

In Table 19-1, qualitative characteristics are summarized as counts and corresponding percentages are shown inside parentheses.

When is it essential to report the percentages?
A. When the sample sizes of the groups are different
B. When the variability of the outcome is different between groups

C. When the sample sizes are small

D. When a study design uses an intervention

Discussion

The correct answer is **A**. Categorical variables are summarized by reporting counts and percentages. It is not adequate to report that the intervention group had 483 black mothers and the control group had 495. Suppose the intervention group had a sample size of 500 and the control group had 1,000. Then we would know that there is a greater proportion of black mothers in the intervention group than in the control group. It is important to report the percentages to facilitate comparison between groups without having to grab a calculator.

The mean maternal age in the intervention group was 26.1 years (SD = 6.3) and the mean maternal age in the placebo group was 25.9 years (SD = 6.2). What does SD = 6.3 years describe?

A. The difference between the oldest and youngest mother in the sample is 6.3 years

B. The range of the middle 50% of maternal ages is 6.3 years

C. More than 50% of the mothers differ from the overall sample mean age by 6.3 years

D. The average difference between individual maternal ages in the sample and the overall sample mean maternal age is 6.3 years

E. The average difference between maternal ages in the sample and the overall sample median maternal age is 6.3 years

Discussion

The correct answer is **D**. As described previously, SD is a measure of variability (or dispersion). SD is calculated by taking the difference between each observation (x) and the overall sample mean ($\bar{x}$). Some of the differences (or

deviations) will be positive, some negative. In order for the positive and negative deviations not to cancel each other, we square each deviation $(x - \bar{x})^2$. To find the average squared deviation, we add the squared differences and divide the resulting sum by 1 less than the sample size (Equation 1). As a final step in calculating the SD, we take the square root of the average squared difference to get back the original unit of measurement (Equation 1).

$$SD = \sqrt{\frac{\sum(x - \bar{x})^2}{n-1}}$$ Equation 1

Suppose it is known that maternal age (years) in the patient population is normally distributed, with a mean = 26 and SD = 6. What are the chances of observing a mother less than 20-years old?

A. Improbable

B. Probable

C. Highly likely

Discussion

The correct answer is **B**. When a variable is normally distributed, it is said to follow the 68–95–99.7 Empirical Rule (Fig. 19-1). This means that 68% of the observations lie within 1 SD of the mean, 95% of the observations lie within 2 SDs of the mean, and 99.7% of the observations lie within 3 SDs of the mean. In this example, 68% of maternal ages lie between 20 years (i.e., 26 − 6) and 32 years (i.e., 26 + 6). In other words, there is about 16% chance that a mother in this population is older than 32 years and also 16% that a mother in this population is younger than 20 years. In Figure 19-1, 16% is derived from the sum of 13.59% and 2.28%.

The primary composite outcome of moderate or severe cerebral palsy or death was observed in 118 of

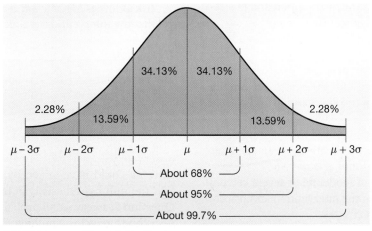

FIGURE 19-1. Normal distribution curves.

the 1,041 pregnancies in the treatment group and 128 of the 1,095 pregnancies in the placebo group. The sample relative risk was reported to be 0.97 (95% confidence interval [CI]: 0.77 − 1.23).

Interpret the sample relative risk
A. Taking magnesium sulfate is estimated to decrease the risk of moderate or severe cerebral palsy or death by 95%
B. Taking magnesium sulfate is estimated to reduce the risk of moderate or severe cerebral palsy or death by 97%
C. Taking magnesium sulfate is estimated to reduce the risk of moderate or severe cerebral palsy or death by 3%
D. Taking magnesium sulfate is estimated to increase the risk of moderate or severe cerebral palsy or death by 97%
E. Taking magnesium sulfate is estimated to increase the risk of moderate or severe cerebral palsy or death by 3%

Discussion

The correct answer is **C**. The relative risk is also called the risk ratio, which is the ratio of the risk of the event of interest (in this case, moderate or severe cerebral palsy or death), between the intervention and control groups. A relative risk of 1 means the two groups have equal risk. Because the sample relative risk comparing the risk of the event in the intervention and the control groups is less than 1, we know that the intervention group had a lower risk. In this study, intervention reduced the risk by 3%. Whether this reduction in risk is statistically significant can be determined either by constructing a confidence interval (CI) or performing a test of hypothesis.

What does the 95% CI for the true risk suggest?
A. The difference in risk of moderate or severe cerebral palsy or death between the intervention and placebo groups is significant at $\alpha = 0.10$
B. There is no significant difference in risk of moderate or severe cerebral palsy or death between the intervention and placebo groups at $\alpha = 0.05$
C. The difference in risk of moderate or severe cerebral palsy or death between the intervention and placebo groups is significant at $\alpha = 0.05$
D. There is no significant difference in risk of moderate or severe cerebral palsy or death between the intervention and placebo groups at $\alpha = 0.95$
E. The difference in risk of moderate or severe cerebral palsy or death between the intervention and placebo groups is significant at $\alpha = 0.95$

Discussion

The correct answer is **B**. The use of sample data to describe a characteristic of a population is called **statistical inference**. Statistical inference is performed either by constructing a CI or performing a test of hypothesis. Typically in clinical research 95% CIs are used. In this example, the 95% confidence for the true relative risk was calculated to be (0.77 − 1.23). We are 95% confident because we used a procedure that generates a CI that contains the true relative risk 95% of the time.

CIs and tests of hypothesis are related. If researchers construct a 95% CI for the population risk which contains 1 (the null value or value of the null hypothesis), then they fail to reject the null hypothesis that says the population relative risk is 1 at $\alpha = 0.05$. (Note that the 95% confidence level and the 5% significance level add to 100%.) Because the 95% CI that was calculated on the basis of the sample relative risk of 0.97 contains 1, we find no compelling evidence to believe that the relative risk is significantly different from 1. In other words, the difference between the risks of the two groups is not statistically significant at $\alpha = 0.05$.

If the researchers prefer a test of hypothesis, they typically perform a chi-square test. The chi-square test is used to compare event rates between two or more groups. As explained in Case 1, Question 5, when a test of hypothesis is performed, a p-value is reported.

The researchers report that for the primary research question, the p-value was 0.08. Interpret
A. The probability that the difference between the two risks is 8%
B. The difference between the two risks is at most 8% assuming the intervention is not effective
C. The probability of observing a reduction in relative risk that is at least 3% on the assumption that the intervention is not effective is 8%
D. The probability of observing a reduction in relative risk as low as 3% or lower than 3% on the assumption that the intervention is effective is 8%

Discussion

The correct answer is **C**. While it is tempting to interpret the p-value as the probability that the null hypothesis is true, this is not accurate. P-values are constructed under the assumption that the null hypothesis **IS** true; they therefore communicate the probability that the observed values (risks, means, etc.) or values more extreme could have arisen by chance alone assuming that the null hypothesis is in fact true. As explained in Question 5, a very small probability lends weight to the decision to reject the null hypothesis, while a moderate or large p-value suggests that the data are reasonably consistent with the null hypothesis.

The researchers also reported a variety of neonatal outcomes according to treatment group. Mean birth weight (g), for example, was found to be 1,410 (SD = 567) for the magnesium sulfate group and 1,424 (SD = 577) for the placebo group.

What statistical test may be used to compare the birth weights of the two groups?
A. Two-sample t-test
B. Chi-square test
C. Sign test
D. Wilcoxon signed–rank test

Discussion

The correct answer is **A**. The **chi-square test** is used when comparing two or more proportions. The sign test and Wilcoxon signed–rank test are nonparametric tests used to assess the significance of the difference between paired observations. Because the groups being considered are independent, these two nonparametric tests are inappropriate. The two-sample t-test, on the other hand, is used when comparing two means from independent groups. As such, the t-test requires that the outcome be numeric, not categorical. For small samples, the assumption is that the outcome has a normal distribution. A graph of the distribution (histogram or box plot) can be drawn to check a major departure from the normality assumption, which could result in an incorrect p-value and thus a misleading conclusion.

Question 4 also states that when more than two means are compared, **ANOVA** and **multiple comparison** procedures may be considered. The pooled t-test (which assumes that the variability of the outcome is the same in all groups) is actually a special case of ANOVA when the number of groups is 2. If there are 3 (or more) groups, a researcher may want to perform multiple t-tests to compare A versus B, A versus C, and B versus C. This practice, however, is discouraged, as conducting multiple t-tests increases the chance of finding at least one significant test result when no real population differences among the means exist. Researchers instead resort to using ANOVA, which replaces multiple t-tests with a single F-test of the assumption that the group population means are all equal. Because only one test is performed, the problem of conducting multiple tests is avoided. When a significant result is obtained, multiple comparison procedures that control the overall α level are performed subsequently.

What nonparametric test may be considered in comparing the birth weights of the two groups?
A. Sign test
B. Wilcoxon signed–rank test
C. Mann–Whitney test

Discussion

The correct answer is **B**. The t-test is an example of a parametric test because the form of the distribution of the outcome is assumed to be known (i.e., normal distribution). For small samples, the t-test is to be avoided if there is reason to believe that numeric outcome is not normally distributed, or if there are outliers in the data. Researchers resort to nonparametric tests, which make fewer assumptions about the shape of the distribution. These tests are particularly suitable for outcomes that are not measured but are ranked in order of magnitude, such as responses on a Likert scale. The nonparametric analog of the two-sample t-test is the Mann–Whitney test. For a nonparametric analog of the one-sample t-test or the paired t-test, use the sign test or the Wilcoxon signed–rank test.

CASE 2

There is incomplete knowledge of the positive and possibly negative effects of administration of gastric acid secretion inhibitors among neonates. A multicenter study was conducted to examine the relationship between ranitidine (a commonly prescribed gastric acid secretion inhibitor) treatment and unfavorable outcomes in prematurely delivered newborns.[2] Eligible infants were identified from participating neonatal intensive care units (NICU) and enrolled into two study groups: those who had been prescribed (exposed to) ranitidine treatment and those unexposed. Follow-up was conducted prospectively to observe if infants exposed to ranitidine treatment were at a greater risk for outcomes such as infections, necrotizing enterocolitis (NEC), mortality, and increased duration of hospital stay.

What type of epidemiological study design was used in this case?
A. Case-control study
B. Prospective cohort study
C. Retrospective cohort study
D. Randomized control trial

Discussion

The correct answer is **B**. A cohort is a subset of individuals identified from a defined population. This subset is categorized into two or more groups based on their observed exposure to selected factors, and followed forward in time to examine the incidence (see glossary) of a disease or other selected outcomes comparing the exposed and unexposed groups. **Cohort studies** are observational in nature and are ideally suited to relatively common outcomes. When follow-up is lengthy, or when larger sample sizes are needed in order to detect rarer outcomes, cohort studies can be expensive and time consuming. A cohort can be enrolled and followed forward in time (prospective) or be identified using historical records or administrative data (retrospective). Prospective and retrospective refer to the timing of the cohort in relation to the conduct of the study; in all cohort studies the exposure categorization is measured *before* the measured occurrence of disease, unlike a case-control study. Cohort studies can establish temporal relationship between the exposure and outcome. A cohort design is similar to randomized control trial, where the subjects are selected on the basis of exposure status; however the latter is an experimental design, where subjects are randomized to receive or not receive the exposure. See Table 19-2 for the description of various epidemiological study designs.

Of the 91 infants exposed to ranitidine, 34 contracted an infection (37.4%). Of the 183 unexposed infants, 18 contracted an infection (9.8%). The odds ratio of contracting an infection among the ranitidine exposed group compared to the unexposed group was 5.5 (95% CI 2.9–10.4).

TABLE 19-2. **Study Designs**

STUDY DESIGN	DESIGN	APPLICATIONS	STUDY TYPES	STRENGTHS	LIMITATIONS
Surveys	Observational	Prevalence estimation Study association between exposure and outcome	Cross-sectional Case series Case studies Case–case Case-crossover	Representative of the population Standardized methods of data collection Reliability in data collection Cost-effective Quick and efficient Repeatable	Cannot establish temporality Cannot make causal inferences Not recommended for rare exposures or outcomes
Case-control studies	Observational	Association between one or more exposures and outcomes	Case-control	Inexpensive and quick Moderate number of study subjects Multiple exposures can be evaluated Good for rare disease	Retrospective nature Recall bias Selection bias Control selection limitations
Cohort studies	Observational	Association between an exposure and one or more outcomes	Prospective cohort Retrospective cohort	Temporal assessment of risk Multiple outcomes can be evaluated Measures of risk–relative risk Exposure measurement bias minimal Exposure is evaluated prior to outcome	Expensive and time consuming Large study sample Attrition of participants overtime
Interventions	Experimental	Association between and intervention and an outcome in controlled intervention To evaluate the effectiveness of new therapies	Randomized control trials	Randomization controls confounding Double-blind methods minimize bias	Expensive and time consuming Ethical limitations

How were the outcomes measured in the study?

A. Cumulative incidence (risk)
B. Prevalence
C. Attack Rate
D. Cannot be calculated from the given data

Discussion

The correct answer is **A. Cumulative incidence or risk** is defined as the number of infants who acquired a new infection (e.g., in the ranitidine-exposed group) divided by the total number of infants at risk for infection (e.g., in the ranitidine-exposed group) in the study. **Prevalence** is defined as the number of infants with existing infections at a given time in the ranitidine exposed group divided by total number of infants in the ranitidine exposed group during the study period.

What measure of association was used to quantify the relationship between ranitidine exposure and infection?

A. Odds ratio
B. Risk ratio (relative risk)
C. Risk difference
D. None of the above

Discussion

The correct answer is **A**. An **odds ratio (OR)** is a measure of association between an exposure variable (e.g., risk factor) and an outcome variable (e.g., disease) (see glossary for definition of odds). OR is calculated as a ratio of the odds of a disease outcome in group A (e.g., the exposed) versus the odds of disease outcome in group B (e.g., the unexposed). An estimated OR = 1 suggests that the exposure is not associated with disease because the odds of disease are equal in the two groups; OR >1 suggests the exposure is associated with higher odds of disease in group A (e.g., those exposed in above example) compared to group B (those unexposed); OR <1 suggests the exposure is associated with lower odds of disease in group A versus group B. An odds ratio is generally estimated in case-control studies, but it can also be estimated in cross-sectional and cohort studies. The **risk ratio** is calculated as the ratio of risk of a disease among the exposed group to the risk of disease among the unexposed group. Risk ratio is estimated in cohort studies and clinical trials. When an outcome or disease is rare, the estimates for relative risk and odds ratio approximate each other, whereas, when the outcome is more common (e.g., >10%), the odds ratio will tend to exaggerate the risk ratio. Both odds ratio and risk ratios are relative measures of association. Alternately, **risk difference** is an absolute measure of association. Risk difference is measured as the difference between two risk estimates and calculated by subtracting the risk of disease in an unexposed group from a risk of disease in the exposed group. Risk difference can be estimated in cohort studies and clinical trials and allows estimation of absolute number of additional cases with a disease among the exposed group compared to unexposed group.

The team of researchers who were involved in the data collection was blinded to study aims and not involved in the direct care or clinical management of infants enrolled in the study. The final study cohort excluded infants with other critical conditions, malformations, or sepsis. All clinical diagnoses were confirmed by laboratory tests and medical chart review by expert clinicians. Infants were included in the study only if they met a preset length of hospital stay. All statistical analyses were performed by blinding the statistician to patient group assignment.

The measures described above by the study team during data collection and analysis ensures what aspects of the study?

A. Validity
B. Reliability
C. Accuracy
D. Precision

Discussion

The correct answer is **A. Validity** is a process of establishing if a study method is robust. A study is valid based on the degree to which an inference drawn from a study is strong, representative of the study sample, and the target population. There are several types of validity that need to be considered in epidemiological studies (refer to glossary). **Reliability** is defined as the degree to which results can be replicated by using the same measuring instrument (refer to glossary). **Accuracy** is the degree to which a measurement or an estimate reflects the true value of the attribute that is being measured. **Precision** is the degree to which the same value will be achieved with repeated executions of sampling or execution of a study. General studies with larger sample sizes will have greater statistical precision, but larger sample sizes will never correct for threats to validity including systematic bias.

Multivariate analysis using binary logistic regression was conducted to examine whether a selected group of characteristics (e.g., gestational age, birth weight, Apgar score, Critical Risk Index for Babies score, intraventricular hemorrhage, persistent ductus arteriosus, central vascular access, or mechanical ventilation) affected the prescription of ranitidine in the infants. These factors were also examined in association with the risk of outcome.

How was confounding due to other factors assessed during the analysis?

A. By examining if a selected group of characteristics were associated with ranitidine prescription (exposure) only

B. By examining if a selected group of characteristics were associated with both ranitidine prescription (exposure) and to the risk of infection (outcome) and not an intermediate step between the exposure and outcome

C. By examining a selected group of characteristics served as intermediary between the ranitidine prescription (exposure) and subsequent infection (outcome)

D. None of the above

Discussion

The correct answer is **B. Internal validity** of a study is established when the study groups are selected and compared in a manner where groups classified by exposure are equivalent to one another aside from exposure status and possibly random sampling error. Systematic errors during the conduct of a study introduce bias in study findings. There are several types of systematic biases including confounding, selection, and information bias which pose threats to study validity. These biases can occur at various stages of a study (refer to glossary). **Confounding** is present when an extraneous variable or factor is unbalanced (unequally distributed) in the exposure groups and predicts or is associated with a difference in the outcome. Because the extraneous variable is associated with exposure and also leads to differences in the outcomes, the unwary investigator could incorrectly attribute an outcome difference to the causal effects of the exposure when in fact the association is confounded by the extraneous variable. For instance if extremes of gestational age are likely determinants of whether an infant receives ranitidine and extremes of gestational age are also independently risk factors for incidence of infection, then gestational age could confound the true association between ranitidine exposure and infant infection. There are different ways to minimize the ill-effects of confounding bias. Randomization of study participants to assigned exposure groups is the best way to reduce confounding from both known and unknown factors. If the confounder is a known and established factor, and has been accurately measured in the study, stratification or statistical adjustment helps to minimize the impact of confounding.

What type of statistical model was used to evaluate the association between ranitidine exposure and health outcomes in preterm infants?

A. Linear regression

B. Proportional hazards

C. Logistic regression

D. Poisson regression

Discussion

The correct answer is **C. Logistic regression** is a multivariable model used to test the association between a binary or dichotomous outcome (e.g., diseased versus not diseased) and one or more continuous or categorical exposures (e.g., age, sex, smoking status, and number of cigarettes smoked per day). In a logistic regression model, the outcome variable is the logit of the disease probability (e.g., $\ln\left(\dfrac{p}{1-p}\right)$ where ln is the natural log and p is the probability of disease) and can be considered to have a linear relationship with the exposure variables in the model. The odds ratio produced from the logistic regression can be interpreted as the relative change in the odds of the outcome for each 1-unit change in the exposure. Alternately, a **linear regression** model is used to test an association between a continuous outcome (e.g., a body mass index) and one or more continuous exposures (e.g., number of minutes of exercise per day). Multiple linear or logistic regression models are useful to examine the association between an outcome and exposure, controlling for multiple other variables included in the model. Alternately, **proportional hazards model** is commonly used in survival analysis where the time-to-event is the outcome and the hazard rate is assumed to be multiplicative and constant over time. **Poisson regression** is an analytic model of choice when the outcome variable is measured as a count, exhibiting a Poisson distribution. The exposure variables in the above described models can be continuous or categorical. All of the statistical models discussed above are commonly used in epidemiological analysis.

The study concluded that ranitidine should be administered with care in preterm infants because of an increased risk of severe infections, NEC, and fatal outcome. The authors recommend that more studies are needed to further examine these effects and develop possible prophylaxis to prevent unfavorable outcomes.

How can a pediatrician who is deciding whether or not to prescribe ranitidine to an infant apply the above study findings?

A. Limit prescription of ranitidine to all infants in the clinic
B. Limit prescription of ranitidine to preterm infants
C. Limit prescription of ranitidine to children
D. Limit prescription of ranitidine and wait for confirmation of the association in future studies

Discussion

The correct answer is **B**. The study is generalizable to preterm infants with selected characteristics and receiving care in neonatal intensive care units. Infants were selected consecutively from the hospital, thus reducing selection bias. **Generalizability** (a form of external validity), is the degree to which study findings can be validly extrapolated to other populations. In the current study, findings are generalizable to preterm infants being treated in intensive care settings. Findings may not be generalizable to term infants, or to non-NICU admitted infants. Another threat to external validity is **selection bias** which could occur if, for instance, clinicians referred only the sickest patients to be enrolled in the study. In this case the selection bias makes the study population not only nonrepresentative of the larger population of newborns, but not even representative of the population of preterm, NICU-admitted newborns. Some large studies are designed using secondary data sources such as administrative billing data from insurance cohorts or Medicaid. Such data are generalizable to the source population that avail these services, such as employees of a specific organization or lower income groups, respectively.

CASE 3

Mothers of infants admitted to the NICU at Loma Linda University Children's Hospital, who had a history of tobacco use within 1 year of pregnancy but who were not currently smoking, were randomized into one of two groups.[3] Twenty-four mothers in the intervention group were given weekly encouragement to remain smoke free and enhanced support for maternal–infant bonding. Moreover, they were asked to frequently hold their babies skin-to-skin. Thirty mothers in the control group received only weekly encouragement to remain smoke free and routine breastfeeding support. The primary outcome was time to smoking relapse.[3]

Fifty-four mothers were observed for a period of 8 weeks postpartum. In comparing the time to smoking relapse between the intervention and control groups, why is the t-test inappropriate?

A. Because the t-test is only used for continuous outcomes
B. Because the t-test is only used in prospective cohort studies
C. Because some mothers did not resume smoking by the end of the 8th week postpartum
D. Because the total sample size was not large enough
E. Because the intervention did not involve the use of a drug

Discussion

The correct answer is **C**. Mothers who did not resume smoking at 8 weeks postpartum do not have a value for time to smoking relapse. Because all that is known about their time to relapse is that it is more than 8 weeks, the t-test, which compares two group means, cannot be used.

Researchers may prefer to compare the proportion of mothers who resumed smoking at 8 weeks postpartum between the two groups and then apply the chi-square test. What is a limitation of this approach?

A. The proposed approach works best for case-control studies, not for interventional studies where the number of cases and the number of controls are not decided at baseline
B. The approach assumes that the dichotomous outcome (relapse or no relapse) is available for all subjects. Subjects who are lost to follow-up or drop out of the study are excluded from the analysis. Available partial information from these subjects is not utilized
C. A mother who resumes smoking at week 1 may be quite different from a mother who resumes smoking at week 7. However, the proposed approach ignores this difference
D. Even if the relapse rates of the two groups at 8 weeks are almost identical, the relapse rates can be very different at various times prior to the end of the study. The proposed approach does not take into account what occurred in previous weeks
E. B, C, and D

Discussion

The correct answer is **E**. In medical research, researchers often deal with data on the time to the occurrence of a well-defined event—such as death of a patient. Such data are called **survival data**. Of course, the event of interest does not have to be death. In the present example, the event is smoking relapse; in other studies, it could be the onset of illness, recovery from illness, or relief from symptoms.

Typically in survival data we find a subject who is not observed to experience the event of interest during the

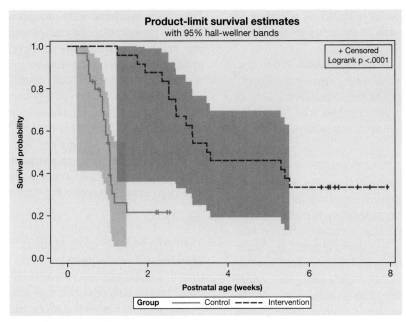

FIGURE 19-2. Kaplan–Meier curve.

study period. In our example, the subject may still be not smoking at 8 weeks. Or the subject was last observed to be nonsmoking at 6 weeks and was subsequently lost to follow up. The time-to-event for these subjects is known to exceed some number; their survival time is said to be **censored**. Partial information can be derived from the censored observations to estimate survival probability up to the last follow-up visit. Ignoring this information can seriously bias the results and is thus a mistake that researchers want to avoid.

Because of the presence of censoring, neither the t-test nor the chi-square test is useful in analyzing survival data. The statistical methods to analyze survival data belong to the domain of survival analysis. Such methods include the **Kaplan–Meier** estimate of the survival function, the **log-rank test for** comparing the survival distributions of two or more groups and the **Cox proportional hazards regression model** to assess the simultaneous effect of multiple independent variables (say, treatment group, age, sex, and race) on survival time.

Figure 19-2 shows a hypothetical Kaplan–Meier survival curve that can possibly arise from the study. Suppose that these are indeed the survival curves drawn using data obtained by the researchers. At what time did 50% of the mothers in the intervention group resume smoking?

A. Between week 2 and week 3
B. Between week 3 and week 4
C. Between week 4 and week 5
D. Between week 6 and week 7
E. None of the above

Discussion

The correct answer is **B**. Kaplan–Meier survival curves are stepwise, not smooth. Any jumping point represents a time when a mother resumed smoking. One way to compare survival curves is by looking at what is called **median survival**, the length of time when 50% of a group is smoke free. Half of the mothers in the control group resumed smoking in week 1. Half of the mothers in the intervention group resumed smoking between weeks 3 and 4.

To formally compare the survival curves, researchers often report the p-value for the log-rank test, which is shown in Figure 19-2 to be less than 0.0001. What does this p-value suggest?

A. The survival curves of the intervention and control groups are significantly different
B. The survival curves of the intervention and control groups are not significantly different
C. It is unclear whether the survival curves of the intervention and control groups are significantly different

Discussion

The correct answer is **A**. The null hypothesis is that there is no difference between the two survival curves. When the p-value for the log-rank test is very small, the null hypothesis is rejected. In this case, the researchers conclude that the intervention worked. The graphs actually support the small p-value. Starting from week 1, the proportion of smoke-free mothers is always higher in the intervention group than in the control group, and the gap between the groups does not decrease over time.

CASE 4

The effect of asthma medications taken by expectant mothers during early pregnancy on birth outcomes is largely unknown. An ongoing, multicenter, population-based, epidemiological study was conducted to examine genetic and environmental risk factors for birth defects.[4] Active surveillance of clinical and vital records was used to identify all infants in a given catchment area with a major birth defect. To form a comparison group, a random sample of infants without apparent birth defect was selected from vital records. In each case, families were subsequently approached and invited to participate in the study interview and consent to medical record review. The interview surveyed the participants regarding various exposures, including medication use before and during pregnancy. Data from this study were used to examine the association between maternal periconceptional asthma medication and occurrence of individual major birth defects in their offspring.

What type of epidemiological study design was used in this case?
A. Nested case-control
B. Case-control
C. Case-only
D. Case–case

Discussion

The correct answer is **B**. The study utilizes is an observational **case-control** design where mothers in the study were enrolled on the basis of presence or absence of the outcome (i.e., a major birth defect in their offspring). The relation between an exposure and the outcome is examined by measuring how frequently the exposure occurs in the case and control groups. Case-control studies differ from cohort studies primarily in that for case-control studies, participants are selected and categorized on the basis of their outcome after it has happened, whereas in cohort studies groups are defined based on their exposure as measured before the outcome occurred. Birth defects, both major and minor, are relatively rare occurrences, affecting a total of 3% of all births in the United States. A case-control study aids in evaluating associations for rare outcomes by allocating greater relative study resources to the diseased, with only a representative sample of the "nondiseased" comparison group. It is worth noting that the use of the word "control" in "case-control" is misleading, as there has been no random assignment of exposure or control status. A better name would be "case-comparison" study. The advantages of case-control studies are that they are time saving and cost effective. Disadvantages are the increased risk for biases including information bias resulting from differential recall of exposure among individuals with disease as compared to nondiseased individuals. (For description of other types of studies including nested case-control, case-only, case–case, please refer to glossary.)

Case mothers were enrolled in the study if they had a baby born with one or more of 40 selected birth defects between October, 1997 and December, 2005. Live births, still births, and elective terminations were all eligible to be in the case group. All birth defects were identified from the surveillance systems in each participating state that contributed to the study. Birth defects were further confirmed by clinical geneticist using standard criteria. Control infants included nonmalformed live born infants.

To have a valid comparison group, controls in the study will be most eligible if
A. They were born during the same time interval as cases (October 1997–December 2007)
B. Randomly selected from the source population which gave rise to the cases
C. Did not have any malformations (major or minor)
D. All of the above

Discussion

The correct answer is **D**. An important aspect of a case-control study is selection of controls. Controls should be similar to cases in their characteristics, but not have the disease or outcome of interest. Controls should be representative of the population from which the cases are drawn. There are several sources for identifying and recruiting potential controls in a case-control design, including community or hospitals (with a different disease or diagnosis than that being studied in cases). To increase comparability, controls can be matched to cases by age, race, sex, socioeconomic status, geographic location of residence or work, etc. Matching can be done on a group level or at individual level. However, it is important to not overmatch as it may lead to difficulties in recruitment and analysis. Once the controls are matched to cases on selected characteristics, one cannot examine the role of those characteristics on disease risk, because the prevalence of these factors has already been manipulated by the investigator. Also, a study can use various ratios of case and control groups, for example, two controls for each case, or three controls for each case, which provides greater statistical efficiency than a 1:1 case-control ratio. Finally, multiple sources can be used simultaneously to identify controls, such as hospital based, community based, etc. and associations can be analyzed separately.

Associations between maternal characteristics and each birth defect were evaluated using statistical tests. Confounders were selected on the basis of statistical significance tests, where a variable is significantly associated with both maternal periconceptional asthma medication use (exposure) and having an offspring with birth defect (outcome). As an additional means, prior literature was searched to identify other potential confounders. Using multivariable regression models, adjusted odds ratios were estimated to evaluate the association between selected exposure and outcome for each birth defect.

What measure of association was used to estimate the risk in the study?
A. Odds ratio
B. Relative risk
C. Risk difference
D. None of the above

Discussion

The correct answer is **A**. An **odds ratio** is the only measure of association available from a case-control study, in contrast to longitudinal cohorts and randomized clinical trials where odds ratios, risk ratios, and risk differences are all possible. The odds ratio is defined as the ratio of the odds that the exposure occurred in cases to the odds that the exposure occurred in controls. As with the risk ratio (relative risk), the exposure is not related to a disease if the odds ratio is equal to 1. Disease is more common among the exposure (positive association) if the odds ratio is greater than 1. Disease is less common in the exposed (negative association) if the odds ratio is less than 1. Although the odds ratio is the only measure directly estimable from a case-control study, under certain conditions the odds ratio is a good approximation of risk ratio, which is a more valid measure of association obtained in cohort studies when the cases and controls are representative of the population from which they are selected, and the disease being studied is rare.

What are the advantages of case-control studies?
A. Inexpensive and quick
B. Useful to study associations in rare outcomes by enrolling fewer subjects
C. More than one exposure can be identified at the same time in the same study
D. All of the above

Discussion

The correct answer is **D**. There are several advantages to case-control studies. Case-control studies are relatively inexpensive and can be conducted with fewer subjects than larger cohort and prospective studies. Case-control studies are design of choice to study drug exposures and adverse reactions among those exposed compared to unexposed subjects. However, there are several limitations and biases in case-control studies to be mindful of. Case-control studies are often retrospective and may lack needed information as it is either unavailable or not recorded specifically for the study purpose. There may be recall errors leading to bias. Cases may recall events and exposures differently compared to controls. Reporting errors are common in severe diseases where patients yield to societal norms, and report exposures inaccurately (e.g., maternal smoking during pregnancy). Control selection is an important aspect of a case-control study and can lead to bias if not representative or based on the source from which the controls are drawn (hospital-based vs. population-based).

CASE 5

Preterm infants are at elevated risk of NEC and nosocomial sepsis. More than a dozen randomized trials of varying sizes and quality have been conducted to determine whether prophylactic enteral administration of probiotics reduce risk for NEC, sepsis, and mortality. However the results of these trials have been mixed with some showing a protective effect of prophylactic probiotic administration to infants at risk for NEC and sepsis, and others showing no effect at all.

A qualitative review of all or a well-defined subset of studies on a given exposure-outcome association is called a
A. Meta-analysis
B. Systematic review
C. Consensus guideline
D. Standard-of-care

A study which quantitatively combines the effect estimates from a set of similar trials in order to produce a summary exposure-outcome measure of association is called a
A. Meta-analysis
B. Systematic review
C. Consensus guideline
D. Standard-of-care

Discussion

The correct answer for question number 1 is **B**, systematic review, and the correct answer for question number 2 is **A**, meta-analysis. It is a rare test of hypothesis that is fully accepted with a single study, and as such replicability and reproducibility of findings is a hallmark of the scientific method. However it is not uncommon for multiple studies to produce different results, casting doubt on the clinical implications. These differences could arise simply due to random error or due to systematic differences or biases which differ across studies. Novel hypotheses are rarely tested with large expensive trials, and thus the smaller sample sizes of early trials raise the possibility that a given randomized controlled trial either incorrectly identified an association between therapy and outcome when in fact none existed, or alternatively failed to find an effect when in fact it existed. It is also possible that differences in conduct of a trial such as participant selection, blinding, dose, duration of treatment, participant compliance with assigned protocol, or adequate measurement of outcome result in a biased estimate of effect.

With the rapid growth in the volume of the biomedical literature, the importance of systematic qualitative and quantitative reviews of the literature has become increasingly important. A systematic review refers to a well-defined approach to identifying all relevant literature on a given topic. Conduct of a good systematic review requires concise definition of the study exposure and outcome, a priori listing of inclusion and exclusion criteria for studies, a systematic approach to finding studies using search databases such as PubMed or a clinical trials registry (e.g., http://www.clinical.trials.gov). A meta-analysis is a quantitative extension which seeks to summarize the statistical measure of effect from several studies into a single summary measure (e.g., odds ratio, risk ratio, hazard ratio) which pools information across all included studies.

In order to synthesize the current literature on prophylactic probiotic administration in neonates at risk for NEC and sepsis, the Cochrane Review conducted a systematic review and meta-analysis of 16 randomized controlled trials of the association.[5] For each of the 16 studies, the

Cochrane Review provides a summary of the inclusion criteria, the type and duration of probiotic administered, the measured outcomes, and assessment of adequacy of randomization, study arm allocation concealment, and measured outcomes.

What is the easiest source of error in the original studies for meta-analysis to overcome?
A. Selection bias
B. Confounding bias
C. Information bias
D. Random error

Discussion

The correct answer is **D**. In general a statistical meta-analysis improves the precision of a measure of effect (e.g., an odds ratio or risk ratio) by pooling the study populations across multiple studies and effectively increasing the sample size. While it is occasionally possible for investigators to variably weight studies based on a subjective assessment of their quality with regards to systematic bias, it is not at all easy to fully correct for systematic sources of bias in calculating a summary measure of effect. As such systematic meta-analyses can provide very useful information, but are ultimately limited by the net quality of the constituent studies.

The Cochrane Review found that the summary association of probiotic administration as compared with placebo for severe stage II–III NEC among preterm low–birth-weight infants in the NICU was a risk ratio of 0.35 (95% CI 0.24–0.52). The risk difference was –0.04% (95% CI –0.06 to –0.02) with a number-needed-to-treat (NNT) of 24.

For sepsis, the summary risk ratio was 0.90 (95% CI 0.76–1.07).

For mortality the summary risk ratio was 0.40 (95% CI 0.27–0.60) and the risk difference was –0.04% (95% CI –0.06 to –0.01) and a NNT of 25.

Looking at the risk ratios and CIs what is the most accurate summary of the results above?
A. There is no significant association between probiotic administration and severe NEC, sepsis, or mortality
B. Probiotic administration significantly increases the risk of severe NEC and mortality, but not sepsis, as compared with placebo
C. Probiotic administration significantly decreases the risk of severe NEC and mortality, but not sepsis, as compared with placebo
D. There is a significant protective effect of probiotic administration on severe NEC, sepsis, and mortality

Discussion

The correct answer is **C**. The risk ratios for all three outcomes are below 1.0 (the null value for a ratio) suggesting that the treatment is associated with lower risk than the placebo. However the 95% CIs exclude the null value of 1.0 for only two of the outcomes: severe NEC and mortality. For sepsis, the CI spans the null value of 1.0. At an α of 0.05, this would be interpreted as a nonsignificant association.

What is the interpretation of the number-needed-to-treat (NNT) of 24 for severe NEC?

A. No effect of enteral prophylactic probiotics can be observed until at least 24 infants with severe NEC have been treated

B. Only the most severe 24th percentile of infants needs to be treated with enteral prophylactic probiotics to prevent NEC

C. One case of severe NEC can be prevented for every 24 preterm low–birth-weight infants treated with enteral prophylactic probiotics

D. None of the above

Discussion

The correct answer is **C**. **NNT** is a tool for interpreting population study findings in a more clinical context. The NNT is calculated as the inverse of the absolute risk difference. The pooled risk of severe NEC among all infants receiving probiotics was 32/1, 371 or 2.3%. The pooled risk of severe NEC among all infants receiving placebo was 90/1,376 or 6.5%. The risk difference is thus 4.2%, the inverse of which is 1/0.042 = 24. This suggests that on average 24 infants must be treated in order for one case of NEC to be prevented.

CASE 6

The standard method for diagnosing congenital cytomegalovirus (CMV) infection is traditional virus isolation from saliva or urine specimens in tissue culture. This process, however, is labor and resource intensive and requires tissue culture facilities. A study was conducted to determine whether dried blood spot (DBS) polymerase chain reaction (PCR) assays are useful in screening newborns for congenital CMV infection.[6] Of the 11,407 infants, 60 were confirmed to have congenital CMV infection. Each of the 11,407 infants was screened for congenital CMV infection using the single-primer DBS PCR assay. The single-primer DBS PCR assay identified only 17 of the 60 confirmed to have congenital CMV infection. Moreover, four were wrongly identified by the DBS PCR assay as having congenital CMV infection.

Calculate and interpret the sensitivity of the single-primer DBS PCR assay in identifying infants with confirmed congenital CMV infection

A. 0.1%

B. 0.5%

C. 28.3%

D. 3.5%

E. 80.9%

Discussion

The correct answer is **C**. **Sensitivity** is the ratio of positive DBS PCR results to all true positives. Sixty were confirmed with a gold standard to have the disease. Of the 60, 17 were identified by DBS PCR assay as having the disease. Hence, sensitivity is estimated to be 17/60 = 28.3%. This suggests that about 28.3% of those who have congenital CMV infection will be correctly identified by DBS PCR.

A similar concept is **specificity**, which is the ratio of negative DBS PCR results to all true negatives. There were 11,347 (=11,407 – 60) who did not have congenital CMV infection. Of the 11,347, four were misidentified as having the infection (i.e., false positives). Hence, 11,343 (=11,347 – 4) were correctly identified as not having the infection. Hence, specificity is estimated to be 11,343/11,347 = 99.9%. It is almost certain that infants who have been confirmed to have no congenital CMV infection will test negative using the DBS PCR assay.

Sensitivity and specificity are estimated using sample data. Ninety-five percent CIs usually accompany such estimates.

Calculate and interpret the positive predictive value

A. 19.0%

B. 80.9%

C. 99.6%

D. 28.3%

E. 0.3%

Discussion

The correct answer is **B**. The **positive predictive value (PPV)** is the ratio of true positives to all positive DBS PCR results. There were 21 who tested positive; of the 21, 17 had confirmed congenital CMV infection. Hence, PPV is estimated to be 17/21 = 80.9%. This suggests that about 80.9% of those who test positive actually have the disease.

A similar concept is **negative predictive value (NPV)**, which is the ratio of true negatives to all negative DBS

PCR results. There were 11,386 (=11,407 − 21) infants who had negative DBS PCR results. Of these 11,386, 11,343 did not have the infection. Hence, NPV is estimated to be 11,343/11,386 = 99.6%. This suggests that virtually everybody who test negative do not have the disease.

PPV and NPV are estimated using sample data. Ninety-five percent CIs usually accompany such estimates.

Likelihood ratios (LRs) are often calculated to summarize the diagnostic accuracy of the DBS PCR assay. Calculate and interpret the positive LR

A. 28.3%
B. 3.5
C. 80.9%
D. 0.7
E. 803.7%

Discussion

The correct answer is **E**. Combining sensitivity and specificity into one measure, the **positive LR** is the ratio of sensitivity and (1 − specificity). It is the ratio between the probability of observing a positive result among patients with the disease and the probability of observing a positive result among patients without the disease. In our example, positive LR is estimated to be 0.2833/(1 − 0.9996) = 803.7. In other words, an infant with the disease is 803.7 times as likely as an infant without the disease to have a positive result. Generally, if the positive LR is greater than 1, a positive test is more likely to be observed in people with the disease than in people without the disease.

A similar concept is **negative LR**, which is the ratio of (1 − sensitivity) and specificity. It is the ratio between the probability of observing a negative result among patients with the disease and the probability of observing a negative result among patients without the disease. In our example, negative LR is estimated to be (1 − 0.2833)/0.9996 = 0.7. In other words, the probability that an infant with the disease has a negative result is 0.7 times that of an infant without the disease. Sometimes taking the reciprocal of the negative LR can facilitate interpretation. Knowing that 1/0.7 = 1.4, we say that an infant without the disease is 1.4 times as likely as an infant with the disease to have a negative result. Generally, if the negative LR is less than 1, a negative test is more likely to be observed in people with the disease than in people without the disease.

The patient's chance of having the disease prior to the diagnostic test is called pretest probability; the patient's chance of having the disease after the diagnostic test is administered is called posttest probability. The LR aids in calculating the patient's posttest probability.

Positive and negative LRs are estimated using sample data. Ninety-five percent CIs usually accompany such estimates.

This question is taken from a puzzle aired on June 7, 2004 in the radio show Car Talk. A dreaded new disease is sweeping across the countryside. It is called "The Bucolic Plague." If a person is afflicted with it, he begins wandering around the woods aimlessly, until he finally collapses and dies. The remedy is to lock oneself in the bathroom for two or three days, until the urge passes. A test has been developed that can detect the disease. The test is 99% accurate. That is, if the person has the disease, there is a 99% chance that the test will detect it. If the person does not have the disease, the test will be 99% accurate in saying a negative result. In the general population, 0.1% of the people have the disease. A randomly selected person tests positive. The person wants to know if he should lock himself in the bathroom and ask for a constant supply of magazines.

What is the probability that the person actually has the Bucolic Plague?

A. 99%
B. 68%
C. 50%
D. 25%
E. 9%

Discussion

The correct answer is **E**. The sensitivity of the test is 99%, which is the probability of testing positive among those who have the disease. But this is not the same as the probability of having the disease among those who test positive. What is thus being asked is not sensitivity but the positive predictive value. Say there are 1,000,000 people in the population. With prevalence = 0.001, there are 1,000 people in the population with the disease and 999,000 without the disease. Because sensitivity is 99%, of the 1,000 people who have the disease, 990 of them will test positive. Because specificity is 99%, of the 999,000 people who do not have the disease, 989,010 will test negative. We thus have Table 19-3.

To calculate PPV, we divide 990 by 10,980, which is 9%.

TABLE 19-3. **Predictive Value**

		DISEASE		
		YES	NO	
Test	+	990	9,990	10,980
	−	10	989,010	989,020
		1,000	999,000	1,000,000

GLOSSARY

Descriptive Statistics

Incidence: Incidence is the new occurrence of disease or other event in a previously unaffected individual. Incident occurrence of disease is necessary for calculation of incidence rates or risks.

Prevalence: Prevalence is a count of the number of individuals in a population with a disease at a given point in time or over a given period of time. Prevalence is often estimated as a proportion of the number of affected individuals in the population divided by total number of individuals at risk. Point prevalence is measured at one point in time and does not have units. Alternately, period prevalence is measured over a period of time, and is defined as total number of affected individuals and new cases in the population over a period of time divided by total number of individuals at risk during the same period.

Rate: A rate is a ratio of the number of incident events to the amount of person-time (e.g. person-days or person-years) at risk for the event in a defined population during a specified period of time. Rate allows for comparison of frequency of events between populations at varying times, geographical areas, or with different attributes.

Risk: Risk is a proportion, and is defined as the probability or likelihood that a particular event (e.g., illness) will occur during a period of time.

Odds: The odds of an event are related to the probability of the event. Odds are expressed as the chance of the event occurring as compared to the chance of it not occurring (e.g. odds = $P/(1-P)$, where P = probability of event). If there is a 75% probability of an event occurring, the odds are 3:1 in favor of the event occurring. Odds enter into biomedical studies primarily as a component of the odds ratio, which is a common measure of association between an exposure or treatment and an outcome or disease.

Validity

Face Validity: A measure of how representative a questionnaire or a study appears to measure what is supposed to be measured. Face validity is generally established by a superficial or face value using common-sense criterion. It is considered as a weak measure compared to other types of validity.

Construct Validity: A construct is an attribute based on established theories. Construct validity is a measure of how well a questionnaire or a study is able to assess the construct both conceptually or theoretically.

Content Validity: A measure of how well a questionnaire or a study is able to represent the domain of the study. Content validity is usually established by experts in the field of study.

Criterion-related Validity: A measure of correlation of results between a new a questionnaire and an external existing criterion that is well-accepted.

Predictive Validity: A measure of correlation of results between two questionnaires, where the response on one test predicts the outcome on the other test.

Reliability

Inter-observer reliability:

Kappa: Kappa is a measure of the degree of agreement that occurs non-randomly, between two or more observers. It can also be applied to agreement between two or more measurements of the same categorical variable. Kappa is a value between -1 and 1. If the agreement is concordant, the value of kappa is positive, if the agreement no more or less than chance concordance then the value is 0, and if the agreement is discordant more than expected by chance, kappa is negative.

Chronbach's alpha reliability coefficient: Measure of internal consistency in reliability assessment of items measured on a scale. The Chronbach's alpha takes the value between 0 and 1. The closer the coefficient is to 1, higher the internal consistency of items on the scale. A value of 0.8 or higher is recommended for favorable reliability of a scale.

Bias

Selection Bias: Systematic differences in the characteristics of the chosen study sample compared to the population from which they are selected from. This systematic difference leads to errors in study results. Random selection strategies are recommended to reduce selection bias.

Misclassification Bias: Falsely classifying of a subject, value, exposure or an attribute to a category that it does not represent leads to misclassification. There are two types of misclassification. Non-differential misclassification occurs if the probability of misclassification is same in all the categories or groups. Differential misclassification is when the probability varies between groups.

Information Bias: An error in the measurement of exposure or outcome leading to differential ascertainment of information between the comparison groups in a study.

Case Studies

Nested case-control study: A case control study is nested in an ongoing cohort study. The baseline cohort is established at a specific point, and followed prospectively over time. During the follow-up, a small percent of the subjects may develop a disease and form the cases, while the others are disease free, and are candidates for being controls. The design is efficient when possibly expensive assays, exams, or evaluations are required of the controls; by selecting a representative sample of the cohort population, the controls successfully represent the exposure experience of the population while minimizing the cost of measurement. The risks of disease can then be analyzed as a nested case-control design. Limited recall bias exists as the exposures are assessed at the baseline, and multiple outcomes can be studied.

Case-only study: A study design that examines exposures from a case series, without a control group. Selected exposures are based on assumed or theoretical data on prior distribution before the disease occurrence. This method is widely used to study gene-environment risks for a disease.

Case-case study: A study in which cases with selected characteristics are compared to cases without these characteristics. This method allows examining associations which are specific to cases that share some similar characteristics.

REFERENCES

1. Rouse DJ, Hirtz DG, Thom E, et al. A randomized, controlled trial of magnesium sulfate for the prevention of cerebral palsy. *N Engl J Med.* 2008;359(9):895–905.
2. Terrin G, Passariello A, De Curtis M, et al. Ranitidine is associated with infections, necrotizing enterocolitis, and fatal outcome in newborns. *Pediatrics.* 2012;129(1):e40–e45.
3. Phillips RM, Merritt TA, Goldstein MR, et al. Prevention of postpartum smoking relapse in mothers of infants in the neonatal intensive care unit. *J Perinatol.* 2012;32(5):374–380.
4. Lin S, Munsie JP, Herdt-Losavio ML, et al. Maternal asthma medication use and the risk of selected birth defects. *Pediatrics.* 2012;129(2):e317–e324.
5. Alfaleh K, Anabrees J, Bassler D, et al. Probiotics for prevention of necrotizing enterocolitis in preterm infants. *Cochrane Database Syst Rev.* 2011;(3):CD005496.
6. Boppana SB, Ross SA, Novak Z, et al. Dried blood spot real-time polymerase chain reaction assays to screen newborns for congenital cytomegalovirus infection. *JAMA.* 2010;303(14):1375–1382.

INDEX

Note: Page numbers followed by f and t indicates figure and table only.